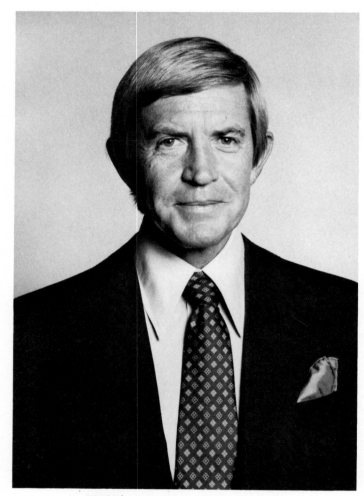

THOMAS D. REES, M.D., F.A.C.S.

VOLUME II

AESTHETIC PLASTIC SURGERY

THOMAS D. REES, M.D., F.A.C.S.

Clinical Professor of Surgery (Plastic Surgery),
 New York University School of Medicine;
Chairman, Department of Plastic Surgery,
 Manhattan Eye, Ear and Throat Hospital;
Attending Surgeon,
 New York University—Bellevue Medical Center

Illustrations by Daisy Stilwell

Assistant Editor for **Body Contouring**

SHERRELL J. ASTON, M.D., F.A.C.S.

Assistant Professor of Surgery (Plastic Surgery),
 New York University School of Medicine

W. B. SAUNDERS COMPANY
Philadelphia   London   Toronto

W. B. Saunders Company: West Washington Square
Philadelphia, PA 19105

1 St. Anne's Road
Eastbourne, East Sussex BN21 3UN, England

1 Goldthorne Avenue
Toronto, Ontario M8Z 5T9, Canada

Apartado 26370—Cedro 512
Mexico 4, D.F., Mexico

Rua Coronel Cabrita, 8
Sao Cristovao Caixa Postal 21176
Rio de Janeiro, Brazil

9 Waltham Street
Artarmon, N.S.W. 2064, Australia

Ichibancho, Central Bldg., 22-1 Ichibancho
Chiyoda-Ku, Tokyo 102, Japan

Cover: "Nude" by Mario Korbel (Fogg Art Museum, Cambridge).
Photograph by Robert G. Davis, reproduced with permission.

Aesthetic Plastic Surgery

ISBN Volume I   0-7216-7519-0
ISBN Volume II 0-7216-7521-2
ISBN Set 0-7216-7522-0

Last digit is the print number: 9   8   7   6   5   4   3

This book is dedicated to my wife, Nan, and to Tom, David, and Liz, who have with equanimity borne my detachment on weekends and holidays and plane trips for too many years while preparing this book. I hope I can make it up to them.

CONTRIBUTORS

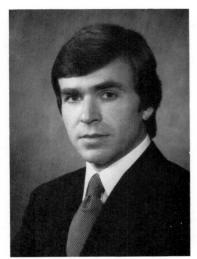

SHERRELL J. ASTON, M.D., F.A.C.S.

Assistant Professor of Surgery (Plastic Surgery), New York University School of Medicine; Attending Surgeon, Manhattan Eye, Ear and Throat Hospital; Associate Attending Surgeon, Institute of Reconstructive Plastic Surgery, New York University Medical Center, and Bellevue Hospital; Staff Member, Doctors' Hospital, New York

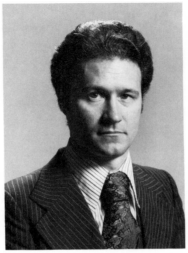

DANIEL C. BAKER, M.D.

Assistant Professor of Surgery (Plastic Surgery), New York University School of Medicine; Assistant Attending Surgeon, Institute of Reconstructive Plastic Surgery, New York University Medical Center; Associate Attending Surgeon, Manhattan Eye, Ear and Throat Hospital, New York

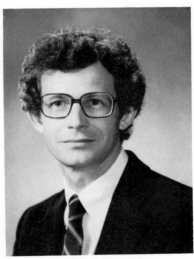

JOHN BOSTWICK, III, M.D., F.A.C.S.

Associate Professor of Surgery (Plastic and Reconstructive Surgery), Emory University School of Medicine; Attending Surgeon, Emory University Hospital, Crawford W. Long Hospital, and Grady Memorial Hospital, Atlanta, Georgia

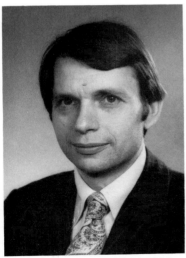

RICHARD J. COBURN, D.M.D., M.D.

Clinical Associate in Surgery, Mount Sinai School of Medicine; Attending Plastic Surgeon, Doctors' Hospital and St. Luke's Hospital, New York

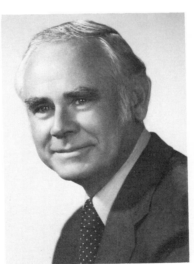

RAY A. ELLIOTT, JR., M.D., F.A.C.S.

Clinical Associate Professor of Plastic Surgery and Clinical Associate Professor of Orthopedics (Hand), Albany Medical College; Attending Plastic Surgeon, Albany Medical Center Hospital, Albany V.A. Hospital, Albany Memorial Hospital, and Child's Hospital, Albany, New York

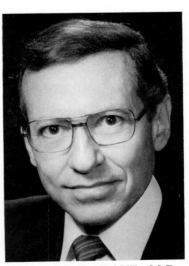

BERNARD L. KAYE, M.D., F.A.C.S.

Clinical Professor of Surgery (Plastic Surgery), University of Florida School of Medicine; Chief, Section of Plastic Surgery, Baptist Medical Center, Jacksonville, Florida

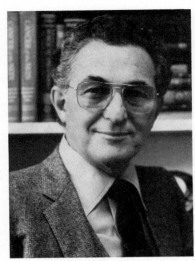

NORMAN ORENTREICH,
M.D.

Clinical Associate Professor of Dermatology, New York University School of Medicine; Attending in Department of Dermatology, University Hospital, New York University Medical Center, New York

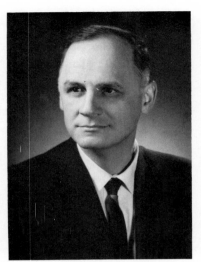

CHARLES P. VALLIS,
M.D., F.A.C.S.

Instructor in Plastic Surgery, Tufts Medical School, Boston, Massachusetts; Senior Attending Surgeon, Lynn Union Hospital, Lynn, Massachusetts

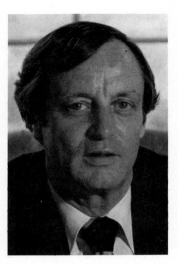

DONALD WOOD-SMITH,
M.D.

Associate Professor of Surgery (Plastic Surgery), New York University School of Medicine; Attending Surgeon, University Hospital, New York University Medical Center, Bellevue Hospital, Manhattan Veterans Administration Hospital, New York Eye and Ear Infirmary, and Doctors' Hospital; Attending Surgeon and Surgeon Director, Manhattan Eye, Ear and Throat Hospital, New York

SIDNEY HOROWITZ,
D.D.S.

Professor of Dentistry and Director of the Division of Orofacial Development, School of Dental and Oral Surgery, Columbia University, New York

SEAMUS LYNCH, M.D.

Chief of Anesthesiology, Central Suffolk Hospital, Riverhead, New York; Attending Anesthesiologist, Eastern L.I. Hospital, Greenport, New York; Consulting Anesthesiologist, Manhattan Eye, Ear and Throat Hospital, New York

FRANCES C.
MACGREGOR, M.A.

Clinical Associate Professor of Surgery (Sociology), Institute of Reconstructive Plastic Surgery, New York University Medical Center; Consultant in Social Psychology, Plastic Surgery Department, Manhattan Eye, Ear and Throat Hospital, New York

FOREWORD

This book is the experience of a life dedicated to teaching, art, and the practice of surgery. Such an endeavor could come only from someone who is constantly pushed by an intimate sense of harmony, creativeness, and duty.

In this volume, the author brings together a full description of his proven techniques and their importance to the surgeons dedicated to plastic surgery. All the steps of the operative procedures are fully illustrated with pictures and drawings of high quality. Dr. Rees highlights not only the teaching of techniques but also the discussion and management of many complications and rare and difficult problems. This volume is sure to be a success in the field of aesthetic surgery.

IVO PITANGUY, M.D.

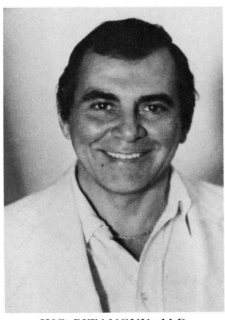

IVO PITANGUY, M.D.

PREFACE

Historically, surgery has been performed for the treatment of organic disease. It was considered to be the ultimate tool for relieving human suffering when all other forms of therapy were exhausted. The concept that surgery can also be performed on an elective basis to improve the quality of life is a relatively modern idea that has grown at an accelerated rate throughout the world during the past decade. This extraordinary increase in public demand for a medical service was not predicted by anyone—certainly not by surgeons already practicing the profession.

Several factors converging at the same time in history are responsible for this boom in aesthetic surgery. The public has been continuously bombarded by the communications media. The general medical profession has become better educated about aesthetic surgery and has accepted the fact that it is safe. There is a growing awareness that the role of modern therapy should not be limited only to the treatment of organic disease but that it should alleviate human suffering in all its forms. Survival is no longer the only principal effort; improvement of the quality of life is also important.

It is impossible to measure human suffering. A minor physical irregularity can be of no consequence to one individual and yet can be of major significance to another. Vanity is a natural phenomenon not limited to Homo sapiens. Undergoing surgery to improve one's self-image can be the ultimate form of catering to vanity, but it is only one more modality in a long list since the beginnings of man that includes the constant changing of styles of clothes, hair, self-adornment, and even self-mutilation.

A bump on the nose may be unimportant to one individual; however, in another it can produce a range of problems from emotional discomfort to mental decompensation. The latter extreme is, of course, pathologic and bears little relationship to the physical problem. No one denies the tragic consequences of major facial disfigurement. Operations devised to improve such deformities are justified without question by all. Major surgery to correct significant craniofacial deformity is commonplace today. In the final analysis, these procedures are performed for aesthetic reasons.

Demand stimulates supply; however, there has been a woefully inadequate number of surgeons trained in these techniques to meet the need. It is hoped that this deficiency will be rectified in the near future as more and more residents graduate from programs well versed in the necessary skills.

This book was written expressly for the younger surgeon with a solid background in plastic surgery, in order to serve as a reference while he accumulates the experience required to season his judgment and surgical skill. Experience is still the best teacher in aesthetic surgery. If the older and more experienced surgeon finds some pearls herein, I will be pleased.

It was not intended that this book represent an encyclopedia of technique in aesthetic surgery. The literature is suffused with myriad solutions to every surgical problem. Many are useful and valid, but unfortunately, others provide many pitfalls for the inexperienced surgeon. As in the book that served as a precursor for this one (*Cosmetic Facial Surgery*), it is my intention to provide basic, practical, and tested surgical maneuvers that have withstood the tests of time. A few techniques of significant historical impact are also included. My contribution to this book is the result of personal experience gained in over 20 years in the practice of plastic surgery in New York City. It is a personal statement of an experience earned by observation, trial and error, and building upon the knowledge of those who taught me.

As each year passes, new techniques that promise to have an ultimate bearing on aesthetic surgery are introduced into the specialty of plastic surgery. The role of microvascular surgery with all the potential of free flaps has yet to be assimilated into aesthetic surgery. The implications of these techniques are not yet understood, except in breast reconstruction. Research in wound healing will eventually have direct application in aesthetic techniques and will eliminate some of the anxiety now associated with these procedures. The aging process is under intense investigation. It is doubtful that aging will be controlled; yet there is little doubt that human life will continue to be extended. The demand on aesthetic surgery will certainly increase — not to maintain eternal youth but to stave off the ravages of advanced years. Older people desire to look good in the same way that adolescents with physical defects do.

An effort has been made throughout this book to identify problems and pitfalls at the precise point in the procedure at which they can occur, and to indicate both the prevention and the treatment thereof. This dispenses with secondary problems throughout the text, but it seems to be a more practical approach than devoting an isolated section to secondary problems.

Our job as surgeons is to meet the needs of our patients with safety and perfection. It is the aim of this book to help provide the technical knowledge to meet this goal.

THOMAS D. REES, M.D., F.A.C.S.

ACKNOWLEDGMENTS

Cosmetic Facial Surgery (1973), co-authored with Donald Wood-Smith, can be considered the forerunner of this book. *Cosmetic Facial Surgery* was written because it was apparent that no work dealing specifically with cosmetic surgery had been produced for some years. In 1973, it seemed reasonable to assume that there would not be sufficient growth in the field of aesthetic surgery to warrant another edition for many years to come, to say nothing of a total rewrite. That assumption was wrong. *Cosmetic Facial Surgery* went into three printings and was well received. Its popularity can only be attributed to intense interest in the subject by surgeons throughout the world. The field of aesthetic surgery has grown at a surprising pace. A sufficient number of technical advances have occurred to justify this new book, which has been expanded to include the body as well as the face.

Much of the material was published previously in *Cosmetic Facial Surgery*. For the sake of completeness and to avoid repetitive references, this fact is hereby acknowledged.

Many of the illustrations and case studies are new or thoroughly revised to accommodate current changes and new developments. The authors make specific contributions based on their personal experience. Dr. Norman Orentreich, for example, invented the punch graft technique of hair transplantation and is an acknowledged expert on the subject of baldness.

I was particularly delighted that Dr. John Bostwick agreed to write the chapter on breast reconstruction. Postmastectomy patients present the most trying emotional handicaps imposed by a physical (aesthetic) deformity. Recent advances in techniques for reconstructing the female breast have improved the results dramatically. Thousands of women annually are seeking breast reconstruction. The contributions to improving the results in breast reconstruction utilizing myocutaneous flaps—pioneered by Dr. Bostwick and his associates, Dr. Louis Vasquonez and their mentor Dr. Josh Jurkiewicz—have revolutionized the technique. Breast reconstruction is clearly an "aesthetic" operation and as such deserves a prominent place in the repertoire of the plastic surgeon.

I am also very grateful for the contributions made by Drs. Richard Coburn, Sidney Horowitz, Bernard Kaye, Sherrell Aston, Richard Vallis, Seamus Lynch, and Ray Elliot. I realize very well the effort and the time put into preparing their chapters. I hope they will feel personally rewarded by the book, since I cannot adequately compensate their splendid effort in any other way.

The superb artwork is again the product of the mastery of Daisy Stilwell. Probably no other artist has her experience and knowledge of plastic surgery. Miss Stilwell translates the surgeon's thoughts and plans to paper with clarity and precision. Without her ability to interpret my scribblings and instructions, this book would probably never have been completed.

The photography is mostly the work of Don Allen in New York City, one of the best medical photographers in the world. His detail is brutal; this is the best way for a surgeon to evaluate his work.

I would also like to acknowledge Dr. Frances Macgregor, who contributed a chapter reflecting her deep commitment to the special psychosocial problems of those with physical irregularities. Dr. Macgregor has committed most of her professional life to working with patients undergoing plastic surgery. She has a profound knowledge and understanding of their problems. I recommend her chapter for intense study and reflection by the young surgeon, for it is this area of aesthetic surgery that is the least understood.

I would also like to thank Dr. Ralph Millard of Miami, Florida, and Dr. Ivo Pitanguy of Brazil, two surgeons of world renown, for their forewords. These two surgeons, legends in their own lifetimes, have been close friends and colleagues of mine throughout my training and experience in plastic surgery. We have often traded ideas, dreams, and experiences, as well as shared disappointments. I am envious of both Ralph and Ivo, as they both have extraordinary energy, multifaceted personalities, incredible skill, great charm, and considerable athletic prowess.

I owe much to my teachers, colleagues, and pupils over the years, who have prodded me, guided me, and stimulated me to search constantly for better answers and ways of doing things.

I offer sincere thanks for the endless help and encouragement from my staff and associates, who helped with secretarial work, gathering the case materials, and the manuscript. Special thanks to Miss Karola Noetel, Mrs. Charles (Sharee) Sorenson, Sandi Sledz (no task could be done soon enough), Mary Dean, Carole Cannataro, and Pauline Porowski.

I am also grateful to Mr. Al Meier, Ms. Jill Goldman, and Ms. Karen McFadden of W. B. Saunders Company, who guided this book through to the end, making the whole experience not only bearable but even fun.

THOMAS D. REES, M.D., F.A.C.S.

CONTENTS

VOLUME II

AESTHETIC PLASTIC SURGERY

Part 3

BLEPHAROPLASTY

Chapter 15

History

Thomas D. Rees, M.D., F.A.C.S.

"Doing the eyelids is like slip-covering a chair; it makes the rest of the room look tired."

A Patient

BACKGROUND

The beginnings of eyelid surgery go back to the 10th century in Arabia. Even at that early date, the surgeon Avicenne (980–1036) — and somewhat later, Ibn Roshd (1126–1198) — noted the effect of excess skin folds of the upper eyelids in impairing vision and thus, according to Sichel (1844), devised ways to excise them. Reports of such skin folds did not appear in the European literature until 1792, when Beer described them in his textbook published in Vienna. The first illustration of this eyelid deformity was not published until 25 years later, in a subsequent edition of Beer's text.

In 1818, von Graefe first used the word "blepharoplasty" to describe reconstructive techniques used to repair deformities caused by excision of eyelid carcinoma. Apparently, however, he did not envision the potential of a similar procedure to correct eyelid defects caused by heredity or the ravages of age.

During the early 1800's, European surgeons began to develop many new and imaginative techniques of cosmetic and reconstructive surgery. The pages of the *Journal Universel et Hebdomadaire de Médecine et de Chirurgie Pratique et des Institutions Médicales* of the 1830's are filled with colorful descriptions of procedures devised by Serre, Morax, Roux, Goyrand, and others for the repair of eyelids and adjoining facial structures. Although many of their methods have since proved to be more fancy than fact, this was, nonetheless, the dawn of the coming era of eyelid surgery.

Reports of excess skin folds of the eyelid were also published by Mackenzie (1830), Alibert (1832), Graf (1836), and Dupuytren (1839), who noted poetically as well as accurately: "On rencontre cette singuliére maladie chez des jeunes filles d'une constitution lymphatique, ayant la peau blanche, les cheveux blonds et les formes empâtées." (One finds this curious disease in young girls of a lymphatic constitution, with a white skin, blond hair, and thick features.) Apart from Graf and Dupuytren, these authors confined their interest to the upper eyelids only. All of them advised excision of the excess skin alone.

Sichel (1844) provided one of the first accurate descriptions of herniated orbital fat:

The lid is smooth and swollen, and presents a tumor that may be elastic on palpation. Most commonly, this tumor is circumscribed between the adherent part of the lid and its transverse fold. Often it hangs in front of the inferior aspect of the lid as a bulge or a little transverse bag. Its weight, more considerable than the one of a simple skin fold, makes movements of the lid more difficult. . . . It is a rare condition. . . . It is most often found in children.

In 1899, a description of a case of "fat hernia" of the upper lid was published by Schmidt-Rimpler, but this diagnosis was discounted in 1930 by Elschnig, who remarked that it was, in all probability, merely a lipoma.

In 1880, Hotz defined the difference between ptosis atonica and the excess skin folds caused by old age. He pointed out that in ptosis atonica, the skin does not remain attached on top of the tarsus as it does in elderly people. Fuchs (1899) attributed this to the fact that the bands of fascia connecting the skin with the tendons of the levator and with the upper margin of the orbit were not sufficiently rigid. Thus, in ptosis atonica, the skin could not be properly drawn up when the lid was raised, but it hung down in the form of a flabby pouch.

Three years earlier, Fuchs had reported a case of recurrent swelling of the eyelids of four years' duration in a 20-year-old female. This had produced wrinkles and vasodilatation of the superficial veins of the skin with marked redness and atrophy, prolapse of the orbital fat, and ptosis of the skin above the tarsus and in front of the eye. He called this condition "blepharochalasis."

A certain amount of confusion still exists regarding the term "blepharochalasis." In recent years, it has been increasingly used as a diagnostic term to describe almost any degree of excess skin or fat of the eyelids, when, classically, the diagnosis should be reserved for patients — usually young and female — with advanced skin folds of the eyelids and the atrophic changes described previously, associated with recurrent bouts of swelling or edema. Panneton (1936, a, b) further limited the term to apply only to the most advanced stages of "baggy eyelids" of familial origin.

The familial nature of the disorder was emphasized by Panneton (1936, a, b) when he reported 51 cases in a family of 79 members. Based on this study, he advanced the hypothesis that baggy eyelids were the first stage of an inherited deformity, the second stage of which corresponded to a mild ptosis atonica, and the third stage to blepharochalasis.

True blepharochalasis is apparently a rare entity, for in a review of the world literature, Panneton (1936, a) mentioned only 93 reported cases and indicated that only 63 of these truly met his criteria for the disease. Not aware of the earlier reports of Graf (1836), Kreiker (1929), Elschnig (1930), and Stein (1930), Panneton described what he believed to be the first case of blepharochalasis of the lower eyelids published in the literature.

All the authors thus far mentioned advocated removal of excess skin and protruding fat only when it was markedly obvious. Cosmetic surgery of baggy eyelids did not develop until later.

The earliest attempts to correct "l'oeil poché" were designed to remove excess skin only. Contributions were made by Miller (1908, 1924), Kolle (1911), Bourguet (1921, 1929), Noël (1926), Hunt (1926), Bettman (1928), Joseph (1928), Kahn (1934), Barsky (1938), Arruga (1952), and others.

Some of the prescribed incisions were more conjecture than reality. Miller, for example, imagined 13 different incisions to correct 13 possible deformities. Some of these operative procedures were apparently maintained in secrecy by their originators. Passot (1919) complained of such secrecy, particularly among German surgeons, protesting that ". . . ceux-ci, gardant secrètes leurs méthodes, ont, par ce silence, laissé peser sur leur procédé une vague suspicion. . . ." (By keeping their methods secret, they allow a certain suspicion to exist about their procedures.) However, he did pay special tribute to the open publications of Kolle (1911), which he considered scholarly.

One of the procedures widely employed in Europe throughout this period was popularly known as the "temporal lift," a technique that has recently regained popularity in the press as the "minilift." As early as 1921, this type of surgery was condemned by Bourguet. The efficacy of the technique, which provides for the excision of temporal and preauricular skin to corret small wrinkles of the skin lateral to the eyelids ("crow's-feet"), is still disputed by most surgeons.

Bourguet (1929) was apparently the first to advocate fat removal in eyelid surgery, doing so in the same paper in which he identified the two different fat compartments of the upper eyelids. He was also first as far as we know to report the transconjunctional approach to the periorbital fat accumulation in the lower lid. The transconjunctional approach was later championed by Claoué (1931), Passot (1931), Fomon (1939), and others. Closure of the defect in the orbital septum with fascia lata strips was advised by Sakler (1937).

In a rather detailed paper, Madame Noël (1928) described her technique for correcting the different morphologic deformities of baggy eyelids; that is, the eyelid with fat, the eyelid with excess or wrinkled skin, and the flaccid (bypotonic) lid. The early history (before 1930) of blepharoplasty was summarized well by Kathryn Stephenson (1977).

From the 1940's on, most publications, including textbooks by May (1947), Padgett and Stephenson (1948), and Spaeth (1948), described fat excision as an integral part of the operative procedure. But it was not until 1951 that a full description of the fat compartments of the eyelids was provided by Castanares. Such compartmentalization of the fat was subsequently challenged, however, on the basis of dye injection studies in cadavers (Hugo and Stone, 1974). In 1951, the term "supraorbital adipocele" was proposed by Holden, and in 1952, Fox suggested "dermachalasis" as a descriptive addition to the diagnostic terminology.

TERMINOLOGY

Despite the various terms proposed over the years to describe the condition of baggy eyelids — e.g., ptosis atonica, ptosis lipomatosis, blepharochalasis, dermachalasis, herniated orbital fat, and so forth — there is still no general agreement as to what the various degrees of this condition should be properly called. From the foregoing, it is clear that some of the terms proposed describe only one component of a more complex defect.

True ptosis exists only rarely in patients with

baggy eyelids. As early as 1844, Sichel demonstrated that if one supports the skin fold with a forceps, the movement of the lids usually becomes normal again. Loose eyelid skin is due, most often, to age alone. Although it rarely interferes with sight, it may encroach on the superior portion of the visual field in its extreme degrees. Nevertheless, many patients claim a sense of improved vision after surgery.

The term "fat hernia" appears to be a misnomer. Although the periorbital fat may be excessive in amount and may bulge against the orbital septum and orbicularis oculi muscle, it is more likely to be a pseudohernia than an actual one. The septum and muscle are frequently attenuated, but herniation of the fat into the subcutaneous tissue rarely occurs.

The word "blepharochalasis" ($\beta\lambda\epsilon\phi\alpha\rho o\sigma$ = eyelid, $\chi\alpha\lambda\alpha\sigma\iota\sigma$ = relaxation) means, in itself, no more than the sum total of its parts: relaxation of the eyelids. Likewise, "dermachalasis" signifies only relaxation of the skin. True blepharochalasis and ptosis atonica are found only rarely. The deformity of "baggy" eyelids is, however, much more common and causes the same symptoms of heaviness and fullness of the eyelids.

TECHNIQUES

Modern variations in the evolution of the technique of blepharoplasty were provided by Holden (1951), Bames (1951, 1958), Fox (1952), Dufourmentel and Mouly (1958), Reidy (1960), Erich (1961), Ginestet et al. (1967), González-Ulloa and Stevens (1961, 1967), Smith and Fasano (1962), Converse (1964), Castanares (1951, 1964a, 1967), Johnson and Hadley (1964), Beare (1967), Rees and Ristow (1968), Rees and Dupuis (1969), Rees (1969, a, b), Lewis (1969), Silver (1969), Loeb (1971, 1977), Cronin (1972), Sheen (1974), Flowers (1976), Furnas (1978), and others. These techniques differ only in their interpretation of anatomic detail and fine points of surgical approach.

The techniques of González-Ulloa (1961) and Lewis (1969) differ significantly in the design of the skin incision and, therefore, they bear comment. The "racquet" incision of González-Ulloa, which joins the incision of the upper with the lower eyelids on the temporal side of the lateral canthus, seems to produce satisfactory results in his hands. Some surgeons have criticized this design because hypertrophy of the lateral limb can occur, edema of the skin "trapped" by the scar is conceivable, and secondary operations are more difficult to plan and execute.

The z-plasty technique of Lewis also differs significantly from other techniques. He utilizes the z-plasty principle as an interpolation flap at the lateral commissure to elevate the corner of the eye and to eliminate overhang of the upper incision. Further experience by other surgeons is necessary before this procedure can be adequately evaluated.

The operational procedure published by Silver (1969) is sensible and would seem well adapted to certain cases in the older age group.

The role of the orbicularis oculi muscle in the morphology of baggy eyelids along with redundant fat and skin in the lower lids was recently emphasized by Loeb (1977) and Furnas (1978). Both authors recommend excision of offending redundant muscle after careful study of the problem. Orbicularis excision in the lower lid is unquestionably helpful in certain morphologic problems, but it is a step to be taken with extreme caution. Furnas goes further and recommends plication or fixation of the orbicularis to the periosteum of the orbital rim. Sheen (1978) recommends fixation of the orbicularis to the lower lid tarsus to recreate a natural muscle fold there.

Refinements of upper lid blepharoplasty have been suggested by Sheen (1974, 1977), Flowers (1976), and Baker, Gordon, and Mosienko (1977). These refinements are based primarily on developments in surgery of the Oriental eyelid to create a permanent supratarsal fold and on the early recurrence of the upper lid deformity encountered in some patients. Sheen (1974) suggested fixation of the levator expansion to the tarsus in select problems. Later (1977), he changed his technique and abandoned tarsus fixation, recommending instead fixation of the levator to the lower cut edge of the orbicularis in patients whose skin fold is lower than 10 mm from the ciliary border, a distance he arbitrarily considered to be the norm. When the supratarsal fold occurs at a level higher than 10 mm above the ciliary border, Sheen did not consider the patient a candidate for this procedure. He reported improved long-term results with levator fixation in patients with folds located less than 10 mm from the ciliary border (in the midpupillary line).

Flowers, who has done considerable work in non-Caucasian surgery, developed the "anchor blepharoplasty," which is an adaptation of non-Caucasian surgery to Caucasians. He, too, fixes the levator. Both Sheen and Flowers excised a strip of excess orbicularis oculi from the upper lids during their procedures. Baker et al. (1977) believed that this excision of muscle is responsible for the improved results reported in levator fixation by Sheen and Flowers. They showed convincing photographic evidence to support their view.

After extensive experience in blepharoplasty, the author believes that levator fixation is occasionally but rarely indicated in patients whose supratarsal fold is attenuated or nonexistent (Caucasian or non-Caucasian). Also, in agreement with Sheen, when such a fold exists in a low position (below 10 mm in most cases), excision of a strip of muscle along with redundant skin and fat suffices to produce an excellent result in most cases, as described by Baker, Gordon, and Mosienko.

(For references, see pages 577 to 580.)

Chapter 16
Baggy Eyelids
THOMAS D. REES, M.D., F.A.C.S.

ETIOLOGY

Blepharoplasty is performed to correct deformities of inheritance, disease, or increasing age. It is perhaps the most exacting and demanding operation in the field of cosmetic plastic surgery. Probably in no other procedure are even minor errors in surgical judgment or technique more apparent. The surgeon must constantly strive for perfection yet maintain a conservative attitude in his operative approach.

The eyes form the very basis of individual recognition and account for a large part of the expressiveness of the human face. It is the eyes that first establish contact when people meet. The eyes project sorrow, happiness, elation — the gamut of human emotions. It is interesting to consider what actually provides expression to the eyes. Certainly the globes themselves are entirely expressionless structures, unless one considers constriction and dilatation of the pupil as a form of expression. It is, in fact, the contour of the skin, the subcutaneous tissue, muscle, and fat, the hair, and the lashes around the eyes that convey expression

We think of lines of expression about the eyes as being "earned" with age. The eyes of a child or baby are relatively free of wrinkles or bulges and are therefore thought to have a much "clearer" expression than those of an adult. With the passage of time, wrinkles and deep lines of expression, as well as the gradual formation of puffs or bags of the lids due to relaxing skin, and muscle or underlying pseudohernias of fat, begin to develop.

Some of these signs of advancing age are thought to be attractive in certain individuals, but they are generally the cause of constant worry and anguish, notably in women. For example, "laugh lines" radiating laterally from the outer canthus of the eye convey much of the expression of the eyes of the adult and are not generally regarded as unattractive. However, the situation assumes quite a different dimension when these lines are accompanied by deep furrows, creases of the skin of the upper and lower eyelids, overhanging skin and muscle folds, and bulging fat pockets.

Baggy eyelids can actually occur at any age from a wide variety of causes. In young children, they may be the result of edema that accumulates during sleep, or they may be caused by such widely diverse conditions as local allergy or thyroid or chronic renal disease. In older children, adolescents, or young adults, they are usually the result of an overabundance or pseudoherniation of orbital fat and are generally hereditary. Recurrent swelling in this age group can also be caused by allergy, hormonal influence (the menstrual cycle), overindulgence in alcohol, too little or too much sleep, and edema of thyroid, cardiac, or renal etiology. During the middle years and beyond, characteristic changes of aging occur in the eyelid and brow region. Extra skin folds, wrinkles, ptosis of the brows, and degenerative changes of the skin and orbicularis oculi muscle may herald the onset of baggy eyelids or may compound the fat bags of youth. Again, chronic or intermittent edema from a wide variety of causes will accentuate these changes. Because these changes of age were considered, until recently, to be part of the normal course of events, it is understandable why most older people accepted their occurrence with little overt complaint and did little to remedy the situation.

Today, however, blepharoplasty has become a commonplace operation that is sought by the public and sanctioned by the general physician. A number of operative techniques for the procedure have been described. No one technique is suitable for all patients. Each operation must be highly individualized to meet the needs of the patient at hand. Appropriate teaching of these techniques and their variations is a necessary part of the training program for all plastic surgeons.

MORPHOLOGIC CONSIDERATIONS

Perhaps in no other form of corrective surgery, with the possible exception of nasal plasty, is careful preoperative evaluation of each and every detail of the morphologic defect more important. Such objective and meticulous study is essential in planning a personalized operative procedure. It is inexcusable for any surgeon to use only one blepharoplasty technique for all patients. He must be reasonably imaginative and inventive, even in minor details, to achieve the naturalness of expression that differentiates a good from a mediocre result.

The morphologic and histologic changes attending the aging process of the skin and subcutaneous tissue are varied. Microscopic findings are reflected in the obvious, visible changes that become increasingly apparent with age. These changes are frequently first manifested in the eyelid area and are often more severe and progressive there than they are in other parts of the face. Many of these changes are thought to be the result of a progressive dehydration of the skin that occurs with age. Thinning of the skin is attendent with other described degenerative changes such as loss of elasticity, acanthosis, hyperkeratosis, diminution of dermal collagen, and so forth.

In addition to senile changes in the skin of the eyelids, there frequently is bulging of the periorbital fat, often erroneously referred to as "herniated fat." The orbital septum as well as the orbicularis oculi may be attenuated.

In a classic paper, Castanares (1951) classified the collection of periorbital fat in both upper and lower lids into compartments. He also distinguished three types of eyelid deformity, which he subsequently expanded into a more complete classification (1977) that included six types: (1) blepharochalasis — axony and relaxation of the lid skin (Figure 16–2), (2) dermochalasis (ptosis adiposa of Sichel) — hypertrophy of the upper lid skin, which hangs "like a curtain" (Figure 16–3), (3) hypertrophy of the orbicularis muscle — horizontal bulging of the muscle immediately below the lower lid margin, (4) protrusion of intraorbital fat — pseudoherniation, (5) combination of any of the above, and (6) hooding of upper lids due to ptosis of the brows. Such a classification may be useful to

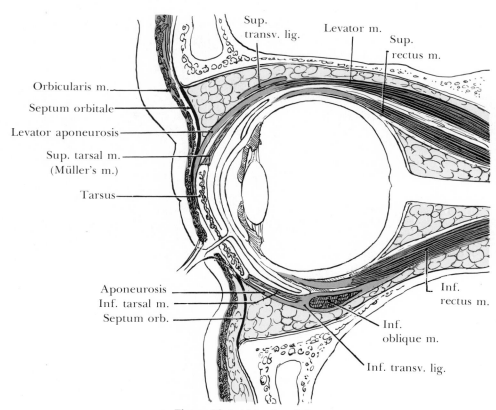

Figure 16–1. Muscles of the eye.

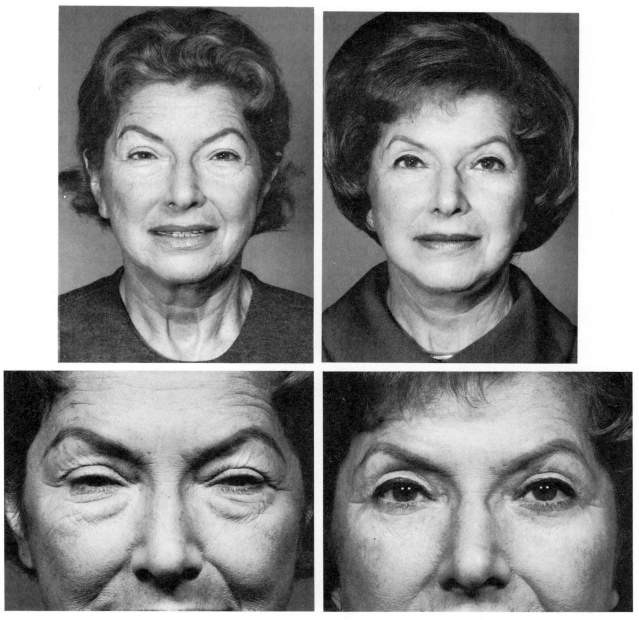

Figure 16–2

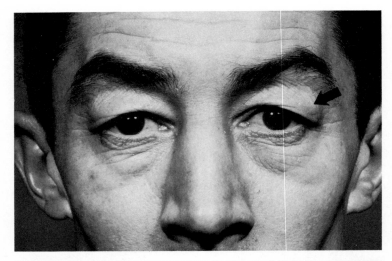

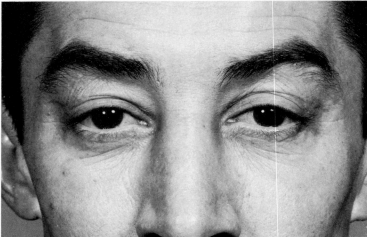

Figure 16–3. The arrow in the preoperative photograph points to an unusual bulge at the lateral margin of the orbit in the upper eyelid. Ballottement and palpation revealed a rounded, smooth tumor beneath the skin, which protruded farther with pressure on the eye. These masses, one on each side, were ptotic lacrimal glands, which should be suspected and looked for in patients with marked fullness in this region. At operation the glands can be delivered through a small incision placed laterally through the orbicularis muscle and the septum. A major portion of a lacrimal gland can be resected without untoward effects, provided lacrimation is normal. About one half of the gland was resected in this patient.

the surgeon in helping to identify the morphology in each case and to plan his surgical approach accordingly.

The compartmentalization of the periorbital fat is generally accepted as a useful clinical concept. However, it was challenged by Hugo and Stone (1974) after injecting 54 orbits in 27 cadavers with Evans blue dye followed by dissection. They found generalized diffusion of the dye throughout the orbit, leading them to believe that there is no true compartmentalization of the fat.

From a practical clinical standpoint, there seem to be two distinct types of fat in the upper lid that appear to be separated from each other if only by an exceedingly thin capsule. There is a horizontal, sausage-shaped, butter-yellow fat accumulation lying between the orbital septum and the levator, and a more medially located, fibrous whitish fat pocket. Both of these require extensive removal in most patients.

Lower lid excision of fat must be more carefully assessed clinically. There seem to be at least two

(and maybe more) distinct accumulations of fat separated by the inferior oblique muscle. The medial collection is pale yellow to white in color and appears to have many fibrous strands. The middle compartment is (like the upper lid) butter-yellow in color and seems separated from the other by a thin capsular membrane. The lateral collection of fat resembles the medial one. It is pale yellow to white and has connective tissue strands. It may well be contiguous with the medial collection.

All periorbital fat in the lower lid is found deep to the orbicularis oculi and the orbital septum. If the fat accumulation is marked, the force of the bulge can with time exert pressure on and attenuate both the septum and the muscle, so that a pseudohernia of fat is apparent. Often, such marked fat accumulations are associated with engorged veins that lend a bluish cast to the lower lid. Likewise, large fat bags cast a shadow with tangential light that intensifies the dark rings. Hyperpigmentation of the skin is also a factor in heightening the dark ring effect, and it is important to distin-

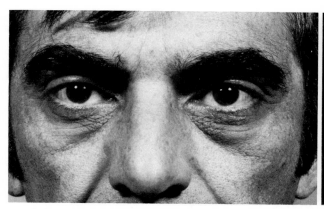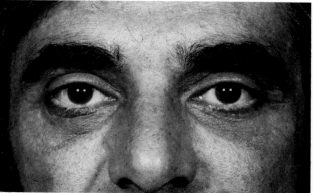

Figure 16–4. This patient has the typical appearance of a person with Horton's venous lake syndrome—a syndrome characterized by dark circles and bags under the eyes with a history of intermittent edema of the lids and associated with severe migraine-type headaches.

guish between all three elements before prognosticating the possible results of blepharoplasty in patients whose chief complaint is "dark circles" under the eyes, since hyperpigmentation of the skin is the one factor of the three that will not be improved by surgery (Figure 16–4).

In some younger patients and most older patients, excessive fat is accompanied by redundant skin and muscle of varying degrees. As noted previously, the role of hypertrophied or excess muscle and its position has been recognized only recently by Castanares, Loeb, Furnas, Sheen, and others who have devised operative procedures to deal with the muscle. Furnas (1978) aptly described redundant muscle as "festoons of sagging orbicularis." Clearly, caution and judgment must be exercised in resecting or plicating the orbicularis muscle, as a postoperative shortage cannot be replaced by free grafts as can a shortage of skin. Care must also be taken to study the configuration of the bony infraorbital margin preoperatively and its relationship to the soft tissue configuration caused by the skin, muscle, and fat. Overresection of fat can, under such circumstances, result in permanent enophthalmos, which cannot be corrected (see section on complications).

The amount, distribution, and type of excess skin should be carefully noted. The thin skin usually found in the older patient tears easily and will have to be handled with great care. Thickened skin contracts more following surgery and is also more likely to retain edema for a longer period.

The position of the eyebrows should be observed in order to determine if it will be necessary to elevate these structures during the procedure.

It is important to inform the patient beforehand of the limitations of the procedure. For example, bulges, depressions, or bags of cheek skin below the eyelid itself cannot be eliminated. Marked skin bags of the eyelids themselves may require a two-stage procedure with an interval of several months between operations to permit accurate determination of the exact amount of excess skin remaining. Wrinkled skin, whether caused by actinic exposure or age, may be improved, but it will not be completely smoothed out. Wrinkles that occur in animation likewise will not be eradicated. Subsequent chemical abrasion may be necessary to improve the result further. Hyperpigmentation of the skin and prominent bony rims should also be noted and explained.

SYSTEMIC AND OPHTHALMOLOGIC CONSIDERATIONS

The surgeon must not allow all his interest to be focused solely on the eyelids when considering blepharoplasty for a patient with palpebral bags. A number of systemic conditions can directly affect the eyes and the eyelids and should be kept in mind. A thorough history and physical examination are needed to rule out any systemic contribution to the baggy lids. If the plastic surgeon is not inclined toward such a time-consuming examination, he should request a complete workup from an internist or the family doctor.

PREVENTION OF COMPLICATIONS

Prevention of complications is an important aspect of aesthetic blepharoplasty. It begins long before the surgery, starting with the first consultation. An adequate general and ophthalmologic history followed by an ophthalmologic examination is considered basic procedure. This includes examination of the adnexal structures, the bony orbit, and the extraocular muscles; a visual acuity test; and ophthalmoscopic examination for lenticular opacities or obvious retinal pathology. A slit lamp examination should be done when indicated — for instance, if there is a history of recurrent corneal abrasions or "dry eye syndrome." The systems review should probe for a history of thyroid disease, allergy, diabetes, and cardiovascular disease, since these conditions in particular may effect the eyes and adnexae. The ophthalmologic review should include specific questions about irritative symptoms, corneal abrasions, epiphora, glaucoma, detached retina, cataract, or surgical operations as well as visual disturbances. It is astonishing how frail the memory is. In their desire to have aesthetic surgery, patients may forget or not recognize the significance of such symptoms. In fact, some even suppress a positive history for fear that the surgeon will refuse to perform the operation.

Examination of the eyes, orbits, and related structures requires only a few minutes. A portable Snellen chart is convenient for testing acuity, and it can be used by a nurse or an assistant. Each eye should be tested separately. Examination of the extraocular muscles is important to determine if a paresis or paralysis exists that could lead to troublesome or serious postoperative consequences. Paralysis of the superior rectus, for example, with an absent Bell's phenomenon, could promote dessication leading to ulceration of the cornea, since temporary lagophthalmos after blepharoplasty is not uncommon. Spasm of Müller's muscle is normal in some individuals; on the other hand, it can herald early thyrotoxicosis or expanding intraorbital lesions long before other symptoms occur.

A sign of levator spasm is a staring look caused by scleral "show" above the limbus of the cornea. Spasm may or may not be associated with exophthalmos. Such eye signs can precede the symptomatology of hyperthyroidism and even the changes in protein-bound iodine fractions by many months. A slight bulging of the globes, so-called normal exophthalmos or proptosis, occurs in some individuals without thyroid disease or ocular pathology. It can be a trait that is genetically inherited. Asymmetry is also common. Unilateral exophthalmos may suggest occult orbital lesions. Investigations of the orbit by tomography may be indicated if suspicion of a space-filling lesion or bony deformity exists.

Familial exophthalmos is normally identified by taking the patient's history. The exophthalmos is usually bilateral, and the patient acknowledges the presence of the protruding eye syndrome in the family.

Thyroid disease can produce localized signs in the eye and orbital regions in addition to exophthalmos, including excessive edema, which can occur in both the hypothyroid and hyperthyroid states. Chronic recurrent edema with interstitial fibrosis and pronounced palpebral bags suggests hypothyroidism. Eyelid surgery in myxedematous patients is disappointing; therefore, if the symptoms and signs are suggestive of thyroid disease, a thorough thyroid workup is in order.

Intermittent eyelid edema in women is often related to cyclical hormone influence (Figure 16–5). Many females are prone to collect periorbital edema in the immediate premenstrual days of their cycle. Fluid retention is common with interruptions of the normal hormonal balances at menopause. Periorbital edema related to hormonal influence can often be identified by the medical history. The patient should be informed that swelling of the eyelids will continue, even after a successful blepharoplasty with removal of redundant fat and skin.

Allergy may be manifested not only as allergic dermatitis of the eyelid skin but also as recurrent episodes of intensive periorbital edema. An unusual but typical localized edema can occur over the malar eminences, just below the bony infraorbital rims and not involving the eyelid skin itself. This small sac-like area of edema is usually intermittent and may eventually result in subcutaneous fibrosis. It is typical, and once recognized, it is never forgotten. It can be the source of misunderstanding between patient and surgeon unless it is identified preoperatively, since it is unlikely to be abated by blepharoplasty. The patient should be so advised. It is helpful to point out this localized area of edema formation on the preoperative photographs. Extensive undermining of the skin, which may be repeated in several months, and postoperative intralesional injections of minute doses of steroid may be helpful, if not curative. Significant periorbital edema can result following a local antigenic challenge to a body part remote from the eyelids, such as a bee sting of the leg.

Certain localized conditions can also result in hypertrophy of the lids and therefore also have to be considered in the differential diagnosis. These include lymphangiomas, hemangiomas, mixed lymphohemangiomas, neurofibromatoses, lipomatoses, foreign body reactions (from paraffin or silicone injections), and low-grade inflammatory processes. Careful and detailed local examination will often shed light on such pathologic entities. Measurement of tension can be postponed until the patient is anesthetized at surgery, unless there is a history of glaucoma or symptoms of the disease. It should be noted here that chronic glaucoma is not necessarily a contraindication to blepharoplasty.

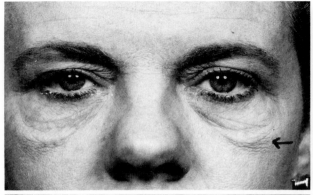

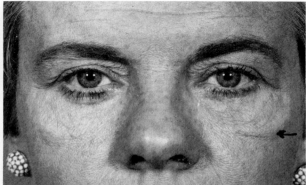

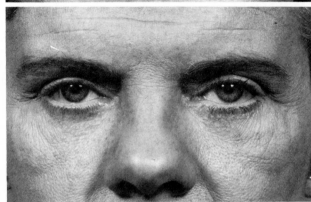

Figure 16–5. The surgeon must be wary of secondary bags over the malar eminence. Often there is a history of recurrent swelling (edema) related to the menstrual period. Such pockets of edema are not uncommon in women, and they can be the only external manifestation of edema of a systemic origin. Edema of the periorbital area can also be familial in etiology or a symptom of allergic reaction.

It is important to identify these malar pouches preoperatively (*A*), since they are often still present after primary blepharoplasty (*B*) and prove to be a disappointment to patient and surgeon. Sometimes a secondary procedure with wide undermining and minimal, repeated minute doses of intralesional steroids will do the trick (*C*).

If slit lamp examination or corroborative funduscopic testing seems indicated, or if disease is suspected, consultation with an ophthalmologist, preferably one who is surgically oriented, should be sought. Any question of muscular imbalance is of particular importance and should be clarified. If the patient's history is suggestive of the "dry eye syndrome," a Schirmer's test or a lysozyme analysis of the tears is in order.

As in other surgical procedures, it is incumbent upon the surgeon to inform the patient preoperatively of the likelihood of complications. Just how detailed it need be varies with each patient. Legal precedents exist, but they are controversial. Certainly, a discussion of the more common problems such as edema, hematoma, lid lag, or pull down (scleral show) is in order. If the patient is more persistent, rare complications such as extraocular muscle paresis or even blindness should be identified.

The author has found a printed letter of information such as the one shown in Figure 1–1, to be helpful. It should be read by the patient prior to consultation. I require all patients to sign a simple written statement that they have read and understood this document.

Suffice it to say that in elective surgery of any sort, especially that of a cosmetic nature, the consultation of a specialist colleague should be sought whenever there is any doubt. This is true not only because it helps to insure the safety of the patient but because, in the case of blepharoplasty, so many factors can have a direct bearing on the results of surgery.

(For references, see pages 577 to 580.)

Chapter 17

Surgical Procedures

Thomas D. Rees, M.D., F.A.C.S.

ANESTHETIC TECHNIQUE

Anesthetic techniques vary according to the personal preferences of each surgeon. Blepharoplasty can be done under general or local anesthesia. Either technique, however, is facilitated by the injection of a local anesthetic such as 0.5 percent procaine (Novocain) or lidocaine (Xylocaine) containing epinephrine 1:200,000 to help delineate tissue planes and promote hemostasis.

Since adequate removal of intraorbital fat does require considerable traction on deep structures, which causes pain difficult to block with local anesthesia alone, I prefer a basal narcosis supplemented by local infiltration. The surgeon can use various tricks to help him judge the safe amount of skin to remove with either local or general anesthetic. These will be discussed later in the chapter.

This combination of sedation and analgesia is administered under the direction of a competent anesthesiologist. The details of anesthesia for facial surgery are described in Chapter 3.

OPERATIVE TECHNIQUE

The design of incisions to correct palpebral defects must take into account all the different and distinct morphologic factors that constitute the composite deformity. It is the *total* defect that camouflages the natural beauty and shape of the eye, which are so important to individual expression. The most important factors to consider are (1) the degree of ptosis of the brow, (2) the amount and degree of wrinkling of the excess skin of both upper and lower lids, (3) the amount and location of protruding orbital fat in both lids with particular attention to the medial fat of the upper lid and the lateral fat of the lower lid, (4) the amount and configuration of redundant orbicularis muscle in both upper and lower lids, and (5) associated factors such as the pigmentation and senile degenera-

tive changes in the skin, the conformation of the bony orbit, the degreee of ptosis of the lacrimal gland, and the presence of irritative signs of the conjunctiva. Each person has various combinations of these defects in varying degrees of severity. It is important to analyze this combination and to define the role of each factor in order to vary the operative approach appropriately (Figures 17–1 through 17–4).

UPPER EYELIDS

The upper lids should be repaired first. In many patients, a simple elliptical excision of the excess skin or skin and muscle will suffice (Figures 17–5 and 17–6), although in those with marked ptosis of the brows due to senility or paralysis of the frontal branch of the facial nerve, this may be insufficient. In the latter group of patients, excision of the excess skin folds of the upper eyelids by standardized techniques should be augmented by excision of an ellipse of skin superior and adjacent to the brow. The net result of this is not only removal of excess skin but elevation of the brow (see Figure 24–1). It is important that the skin excision above the brow be wider in the lateral two thirds than in the medial third. The final suture line is planned to lie just within the upper hair follicle line of the brow.

The placement of the suture line of the standard upper lid excision is also of paramount importance. The lowermost line of the ellipse, which becomes the final suture line, should lie between 7 and 12 mm above the ciliary margin in the midpupillary plane, depending on the morphology of the individual patient (Figure 17–8). The final scar should fall naturally into the supratarsal fold (Figure 17–9).

The lateral extension should lie in a "crow's foot." Because the final suture line tends to ride upward, it should be drawn at a level lower than its intended destination (Figures 17–10 and 17–11). A

Text continued on page 483.

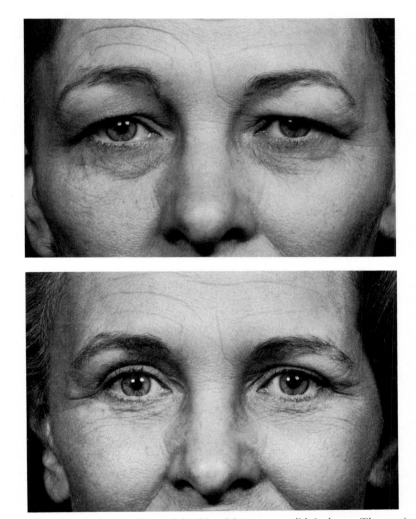

Figure 17–1.   An example of marked redundancy of the skin of the upper eyelids is shown. The surgical result was satisfactory, but only part of the patient's problem has been corrected. There is, in addition, a degree of ptosis of the eyebrows which gives the effect of a slight downward slant to the eyes. The forehead has few horizontal wrinkles (which usually appear later in life); this makes elevation of the brows difficult because the scar resulting from such a procedure would very likely be noticeable.

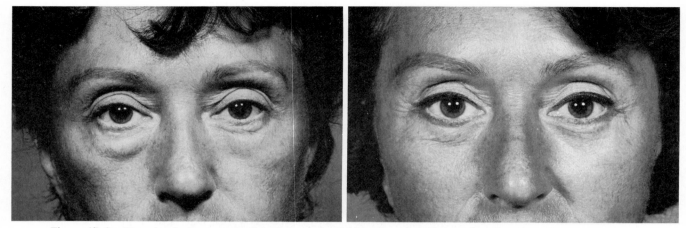

Figure 17–2.   Note that in the preoperative photograph of this patient there is a marked discrepancy between the size of the bulges caused by the orbital fat pockets of the lower lids. The right lower lid contains considerably more fat than the left. Expert professional photographs such as this (by Don Allen) are particularly important to guide the surgeon during blepharoplasty. Each detail, including asymmetrical problems such as this one, becomes apparent in the photograph, yet may not be obvious during physical examination of the patient.

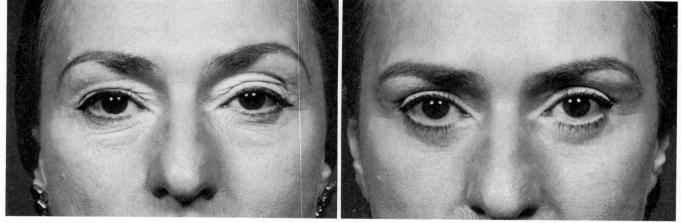

As middle age advances, certain changes occur in the eyelid skin as well as the pseudoherniations of fat, which tend to increase. The skin changes may be accentuated by exposure to the wind and sun, by diminution of the effects of female hormones, by recurrent edema and by other factors. The skin becomes thinner and therefore more wrinkled. The sebaceous glands may increase in number, and sometimes many small adenomas appear. Xanthelasma patches develop in some patients. These pictures show a typical set of changes in a patient in her fourth decade of life, and the improvement obtained by blepharoplasty. (From Rees, T. D., and Guy, C. L.: Surg. Clin. North Am. *51*:353, 1971.)

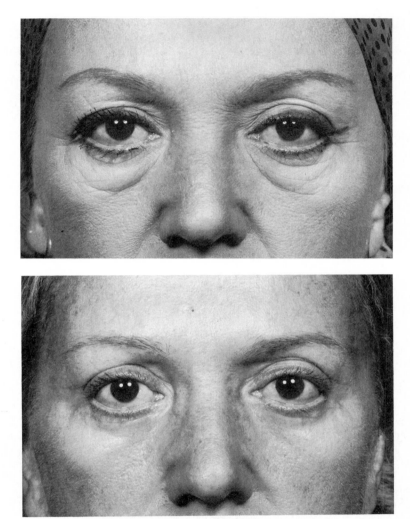

Figure 17-3. The preoperative photograph of this patient shows two unusual features that the surgeon needs to observe and discuss with a prospective patient; the moderate degree of scleral "show" and the slight exophthalmos. The scleral show cannot be improved by surgery, but it also should not be increased unless too much skin is excised. Often, however, a slight exophthalmos can be ameliorated by removal of orbital fat.

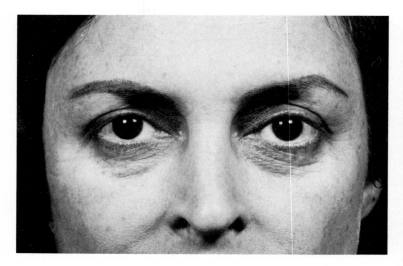

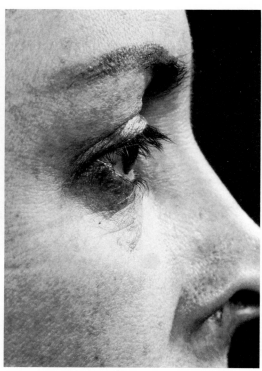

Figure 17–4. The essential problem in this woman, who is approaching middle age, is excess skin of the lower eyelids as well as increased pigmentation of the skin. Such pigmentation is common in some families and in some peoples, particularly those of Mediterranean origin. The dark coloration cannot be changed by blepharoplasty, but often it will seem to be lightened by the operation because many wrinkles are removed or smoothed out. If the fat pockets are prominent, tangential lighting will cast a shadow, further accentuating the dark circles. Patients without such dark pigmentation may occasionally show discoloration below the eyes for many months if ecchymosis following surgery was unusually severe. This results from hematoma and the accumulation of breakdown products of blood, particularly pigments; there is no known method of hastening its removal. Increased pigmentation can be improved by deep chemabrasion after blepharoplasty.

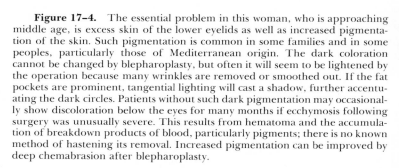

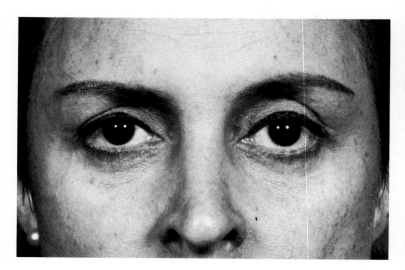

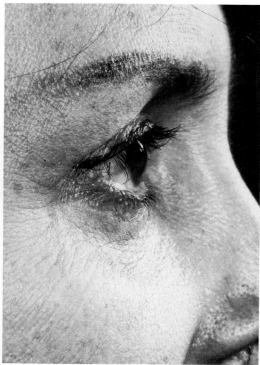

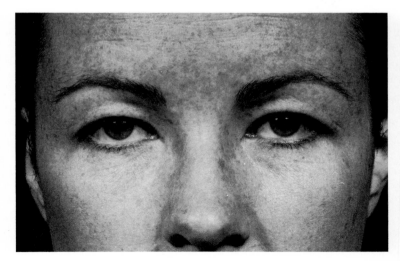

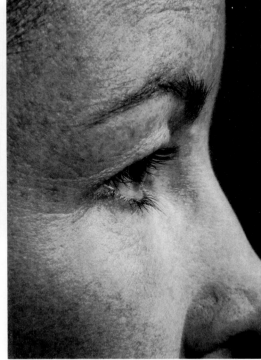

Figure 17–5.   This illustration shows a skin fold of the upper eyelids in a 22-year-old girl. Such a fold is easily removed by the technique shown in Figure 17–6. In the young patient, care should be exercised in measuring the skin with the marking forceps so that not too much skin is excised. The young eyelid is less forgiving than the senile lid, and lagophthalmos can result more easily. Very early reports in the literature described excess upper lid skin folds that were probably similar to this example. The fold may resemble the so-called mongoloid fold seen in Asians, in spite of a lack of Asian heritage.

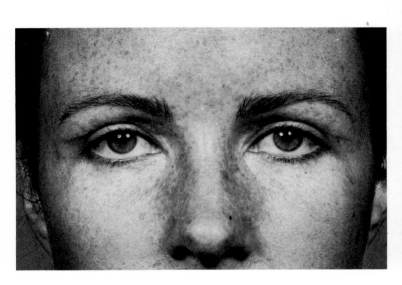

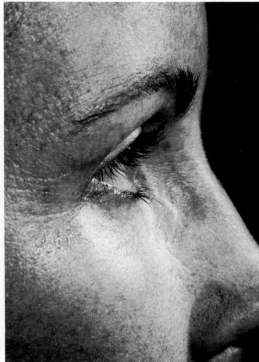

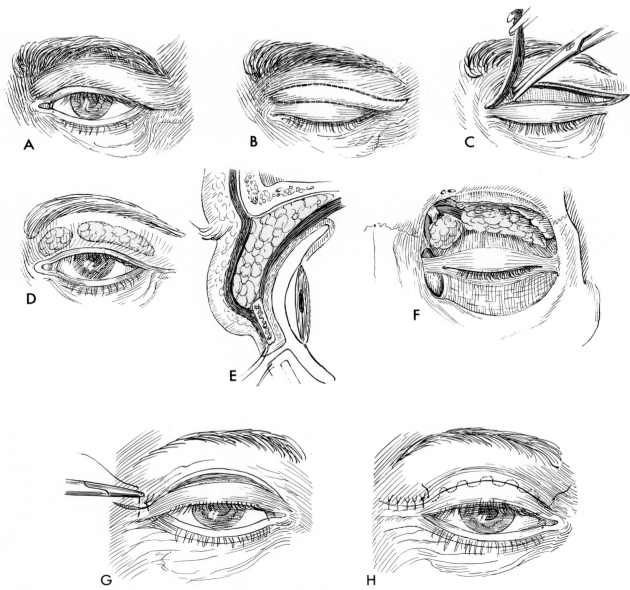

Figure 17–6. *A* and *B*, Excess skin folds of the upper eyelids are removed by designing an ellipse with a dart that extends as far laterally as necessary and is best slanted slightly upward at the lateral canthus. The lower limb of the incision is located according to the level of insertion of the levator aponeurosis and the configuration of the bony orbit. The location varies from 6 to approximately 12 cm above the ciliary margin. It constitutes the new level of the supratarsal fold. The final suture line is drawn superiorly with healing, and the final scar should be planned so as to end up in the supratarsal fold. The lateral dart, slanted upward, is to avoid a "dog-ear" at this location. It is the most visible part of the scar and is disturbing to some patients; therefore, the patient should be notified of its location and nature prior to surgery.

C, In most cases, a strip of orbicularis muscle is excised with the skin. This step has improved the results considerably in recent years and has reduced the number of secondary trims required; however, it must be done with judgment and caution since muscle cannot be replaced. Routine insertion of the levator into the skin or muscle as advocated by some is not considered necessary by the author. Excision of a muscle strip accomplishes the same effect.

D, *E*, and *F*, The location of the two major fat compartments in the upper lid behind the orbital septum. Note the location of the superior oblique muscle (*F*). It is deep, but can be damaged by deep dissection. The fat can be removed by widely opening the orbital septum or by stab wounds.

G and *H*, The upper lid is sutured with subcuticular and fine interrupted sutures.

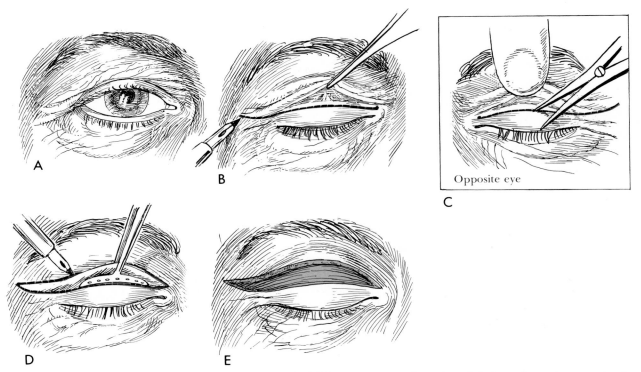

Figure 17-7.   *A*, As the lid becomes more senile, the skin fold increases proportionately and the brow descends, narrowing the space between the brow and upper lid.

B, Forceps facilitate locating the supratarsal fold. The lateral dart must be drawn further laterally.

C, Calipers are helpful to achieve symmetry in the opposite eye.

D, Green forceps are very helpful in grasping the skin fold of the "blepharochalasis" while designing the incision.

E, After excision of the skin, the surgeon can decide whether or not to excise a muscle strip as well, and if so, how much.

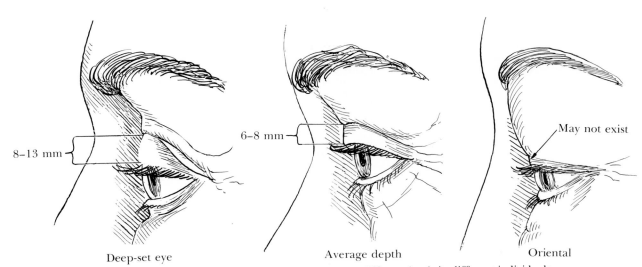

Figure 17-8.   The "normal" supratarsal fold occurs at different levels in different individuals.

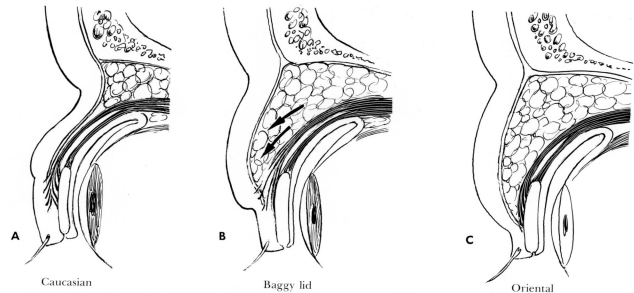

Caucasian   Baggy lid   Oriental

Figure 17–9.   The supratarsal fold is present because of the insertion of fibrous aponeurotic slips from the levator expansion into the dermis of the skin. (*A*) In the Caucasian the fold is pronounced. (*B*) In the baggy eyelid, the bulging fat and/or redundant skin can camouflage the natural fold. (*C*) In many Orientals the fold does not exist because of the absence of these fibrous slips. Recreation of the attachment of the levator into the skin or muscle forms the basis of the operations for the Oriental eyelid, and has been adapted in certain cases to the Caucasian eyelid by Sheen and Flowers.

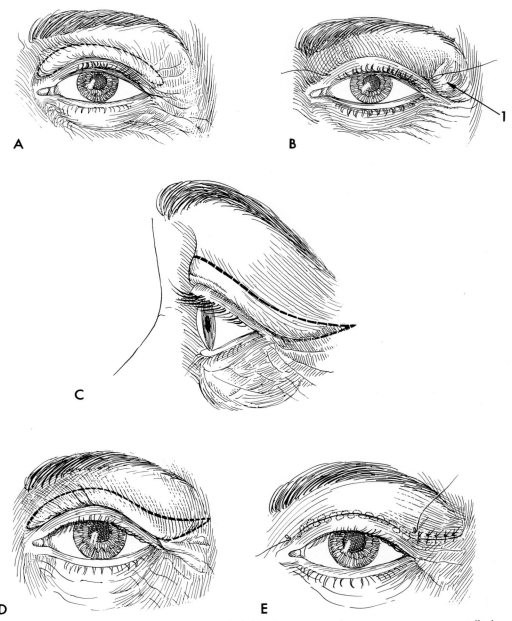

Figure 17–10.   In the senile patient or in those with marked skin changes secondary to exposure, accurate tailoring of the upper lid excision is most important. Ending the lateral extent of the incision at the lateral canthus *(A)*, as can be done in the young patient, results in a "dog-ear" or pucker of the skin laterally *(B* 1*)*. In such patients it is best to extend the lateral incision quite far laterally in natural skin creases and slanted slightly superiorly *(C and D)*. This eliminates the skin fold and tailors the incision to prevent a dog-ear while at the same time tightening the skin lateral to the canthus, which aids in the lower eyelid surgery *(E)*.

One disadvantage is that the eyebrow may end closer to the lid margin after such trimming. It may be necessary to elevate the brow simultaneously, or to advise the patient to pluck the eyebrows of the lateral two thirds of the brow and create a new line with makeup pencil. (Rees, T. D.: Technical Considerations in Blepharoplasty and Rhytidectomy. Transactions of the Fifth International Congress of Plastic and Reconstructive Surgery, Australia, 1971. Sidney, Butterworth & Co. (Australia), Ltd., 1971, p. 1067.)

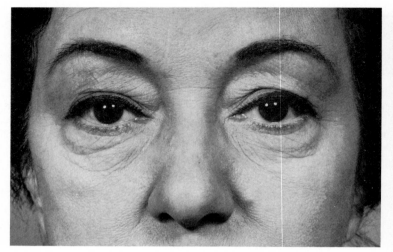

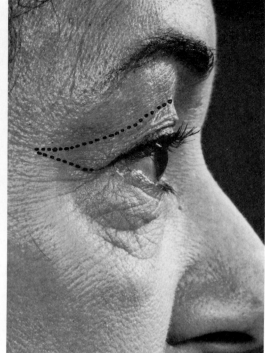

Figure 17–11.   An attractive woman of middle age had marked palpebral bags of the upper and lower eyelids caused by a combination of overabundant periorbital fat and progressive degenerative changes in the skin. Correction of such a condition requires generous excision of both skin and fat. The elliptical excision of the upper eyelid skin must be carried well laterally, to or beyond the lateral corner of the eyebrow (Fig. 17–10); otherwise, a small dog-ear can appear at this angle of the wound. These extreme lateral extensions of the incision, which are carried at a slight upward angle, are quite worrisome to most patients until the scars have settled in. Their presence should be explained to the patient before the operation. The lateral dog-ear, if left, can result in a pleat or overhang as shown in Figure 17–10. The lower lids of this patient were dealt with as shown in Figure 17–10.

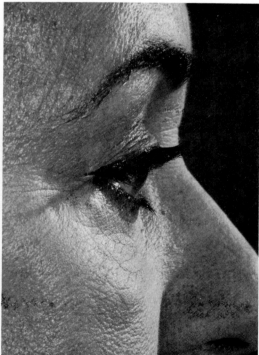

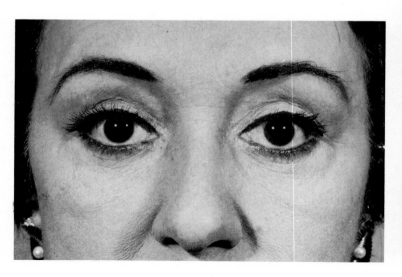

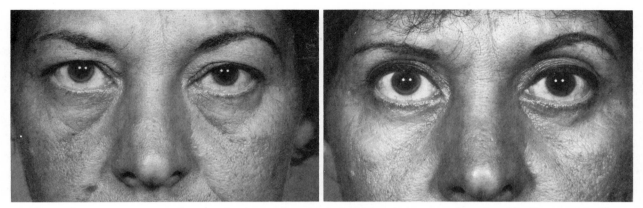

Figure 17–12. An example of levator fixation to the orbicularis. This technique was championed by Sheen and by Flowers. The same results can likely be achieved with excision of a strip of orbicularis muscle.

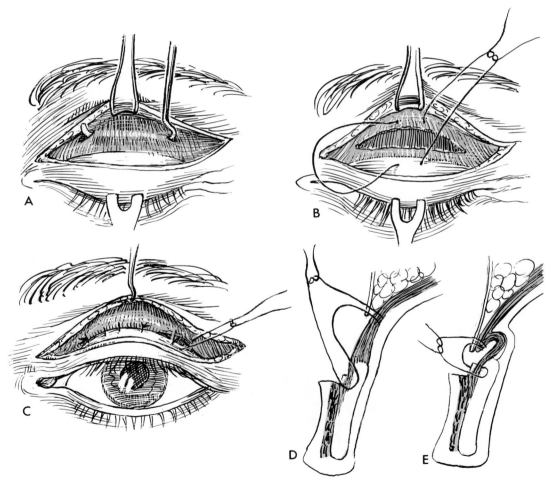

Figure 17–13. Method of levator fixation to form a supratarsal fold.

A, The levator expansion is identified. The thin aponeurosis is transected.

B, Sutures are placed to fix the incised edge of the levator to the tarsal plate and/or the dermis of the inferior wound edge.

C, A row of such sutures is placed with the knots buried. Extremely fine nonabsorbable suture material is used, such as 6-0 or 7-0 nylon.

D and *E,* The placement of these sutures is shown in cross-section. Note that if pseudoptosis is present, the levator can be reefed at the same time. Ordinarily, only the superficial layer of the levator is used in the fixation. Müller's muscle is not interfered with.

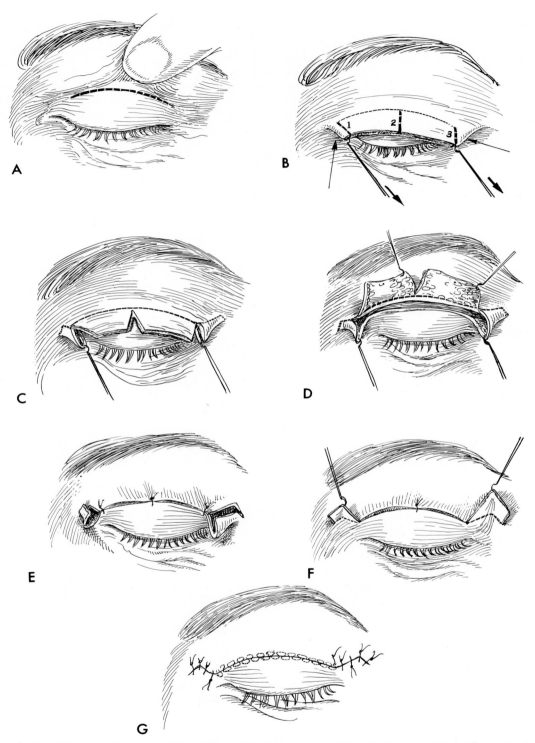

Figure 17–14.   Silver's technique for excision of skin folds of the upper eyelid. Instead of marking an ellipse of redundant skin, Silver first makes his incision in the supratarsal fold *(A)*. He then undermines the skin superiorly (toward the brow), creating an apron of skin that is allowed to hang over the lid margin *(B)*. This skin flap is split in three places *(C)* and pulled laterally *(D)*, which helps to avoid the bunching effect that so often occurs medially.

The flap is trimmed along a complex line (dotted in *C*), paying special attention to the trimming of the excess skin at the medial aspect *(E)*. Laterally, too, Silver undermines the skin to connect with his lower eyelid incisions and to help to iron out the crow's feet *(F* and *G)*.

careful and thorough removal of the medial fat pockets through a stab wound in the orbital septum is important in order to prevent a secondary postoperative bulging of the fat in this region.

The upper eyelid wound is best sutured with a subcuticular suture of fine nylon, which can be left in place four or five days. This type of suture is most helpful in preventing troublesome epithelial tunnels or inclusion cysts, which easily form around interrupted sutures after 48 hours.

When a subcuticular suture is used, it is important either to cut the medial end where it emerges from the skin so that the cut end can retract beneath the skin, or to remove this suture by the fourth postoperative day. Otherwise, for unknown reasons, a pustule forms at the site of the skin entrance, which results in an unsightly nodule of scar tissue requiring many months to absorb. The suture line in the upper lid can be further reinforced by several fine interrupted sutures, which are removed at 24 to 48 hours at the latest.

A useful technique to aid in definition of the supratarsal fold in those patients with low insertion of the levator expansion (below 10 mm) or in patients with unusual redundancy of skin and muscle, "deep set eyes," or a relative low brow position was described by Sheen (1974, 1977) and Flowers (1976) (Figures 17–12 and 17–13). These surgeons prefer to achieve a fixation of the levator to the tarsus in certain instances, or to the cut inferior margin of the orbicularis, to insure a clear-cut delineation of the fold. Baker et al. (1977) refute the necessity of levator fixation and claim equally good results with simple excision of a strip of muscle.

The reader is strongly advised to study these key publications for a better understanding of the fine points of upper eyelid blepharoplasty. However, such modifications are most useful in certain patients only. The novice surgeon is admonished to proceed cautiously with these more complicated techniques. Muscle excision should always be conservative.

Advanced degrees of blepharochalasis can interfere with the peripheral fields of vision (upward gaze). Such patients have ligitimate functional indication for surgery. Their problem should be documented by good photographs and by a visual field examination. If any question exists, consultation from a qualified ophthalmologist should be obtained.

Silver devised a novel and practical approach to the excision of skin folds of the upper eyelids that deals with the redundancy or "dog ear" that is frequently encountered at the medial angle of the wound, where the incision must be terminated be-

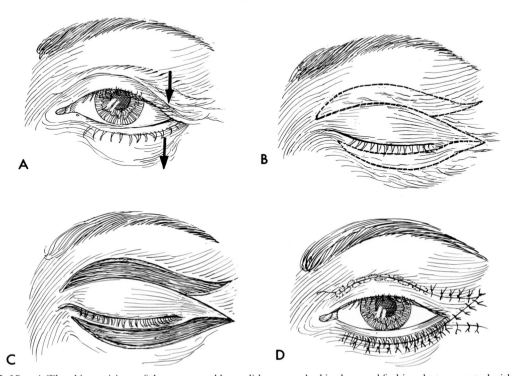

Figure 17–15. *A,* The skin excisions of the upper and lower lids are marked in the usual fashion, but connected with an oblique limb from the upper to the lower lid to convert the design to a z-plasty *(B).* The skin excision is demonstrated in the shaded areas *(C).* The flaps are then switched (interpolated) and sutured *(D),* elevating the skin strip extending laterally from the lateral canthus (Lewis. 1969).

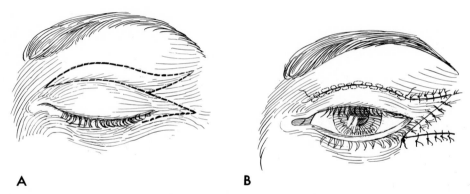

Figure 17–16. An alternate procedure recommended by Lewis to elevate the lateral canthus when there is no redundancy of lower eyelid skin, but excision of upper lid skin is required. A small interpolation flap is designed from the upper lid in the form of a z-plasty *(A)*. The flap is let into the lower lid and sutured *(B)*.

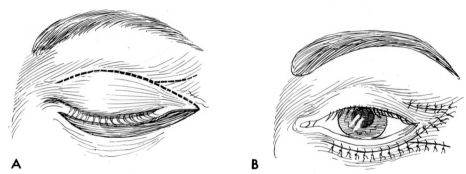

Lewis's variation for a complete lower blepharoplasty and z-blepharoplasty in the external canthal area and lateral portions of the upper lids only *(A* and *B)*. In this case the interpolation flap is from the upper to the lower lid, which helps to elevate the lateral canthus. It is useful only when little or no redundancy of the upper lid skin is present.

fore the side wall of the nose is encountered (Figure 17–14). This technique also helps to solve the problem of excess skin at the inner or medial angle of the wound and seems to help in tailoring the outer angle as well. It is most applicable in the older patient with very marked skin excess.

Lewis (1969) devised an operative variation based on the z-plasty or interpolated flap principle in order to elevate the lateral canthal region in those patients with senile ptosis and marked skin excess (Figure 17–15). The author has not used this technique but finds it intriguing. It should be remembered that the fewer incisions the better, as one should always plan for future secondary operations, which may be made more complicated by the presence of connecting incisions. When there is no redundancy of lower lid skin but excision of the upper lid is required, a small inter-

polation flap can be designed from the upper lid in the form of a z-plasty (Figure 17–16).

LOWER EYELIDS

Correction of the lower eyelid is the most challenging part of cosmetic blepharoplasty. Here, operative technique varies most considerably, and an analysis of anatomic problems is most necessary to achieve the desired correction without such postoperative problems as epiphora, ectropion, and secondary fat herniation. Absolute hemostasis with fine needle-tipped forceps and cautery is mandatory throughout the procedure to prevent hematoma, which may prolong convalescence and contribute to other complications.

In patients with only moderate protrusion of the periorbital fat and minimal skin or muscle excess, the lower eyelid is opened by an incision placed approximately 2 mm below the ciliary margin or in the first natural skin crease (Figure 17–17). This incision is carried through the skin and orbicularis muscle, thereby creating a skin-muscle flap as described by McIndoe and subsequently by Beare (1967) and Rees and Dupuis (1969) (Figures 17–17 and 17–18). The orbital septum can then be incised and excess fat can be removed from the appropriate compartments (Figure 17–17). The amount of fat removal is determined by the degree of protrusion of fat when pressure is gently applied to the globe. If necessary, a small strip of muscle and skin may be trimmed, although this must be done with caution, as these are generally young patients with tight structures and little tissue to spare (Figure 17–18). The flap is then replaced and sutured with interrupted sutures of fine black silk. Figure 17–19 shows a patient who underwent the skin-muscle flap operation.

If a moderate amount of excess skin and/or orbicularis muscle exists in addition to excess fat, conservative skin excision is done after fat removal. Excess fat is removed by making an incision splitting the orbicularis muscle or by making multiple stab wounds through the muscle and orbital septum (Figure 17–20). (See also Figures 17–21 to 17–24.) In most operations on the lower lids, the majority of excess fat is found in the medial fat compartment. Fat removal from the lateral pocket should always be conservative to prevent an unsightly postoperative contour depression.

Redundant orbicularis oculi muscle may be identified as a horizontal bulge just over the tarsus in such moderate deformities. Such a "muscle roll" is pleasing in the young lid, but when it is exaggerated, particularly upon animation, it becomes unattractive. The muscle can be trimmed or plicated, although correction should be understated and conservative (Figure 17–25). Other solutions are to excise the offending muscle cautiously or to imbricate the area with fine sutures (Figure 17–26). Obviously, either of these maneuvers must be undertaken with extreme care, because a pull on the lid will result in scleral show or ectropion. Differentials in the level and amount of excision of skin and muscle can be useful in producing more natural results. If a slight muscle bulge is desirable, more skin and less muscle is excised. The redundant muscle contracts and forms a small ridge along the tarsus (Figure 17–27).

The amount of skin to be removed can be marked prior to the incision (as recommended by Converse) or subsequent to undermining. It is usually necessary to extend the markings for the lower eyelid incision laterally into a so-called crow's foot. According to the Converse technique, the excess skin is then held with forceps in a manner similar to the method used for the upper lids, and the skin pattern is excised along the lines drawn (Figure 17–28).

According to Converse (1964), when only a moderate amount of excess skin is the problem, little or no undermining of the skin is necessary, except to make minute final adjustments to allow the skin flap to fit naturally without tension to the upper margin of the wound. Such preoperative determination is, however, hazardous in inexperienced hands and can easily result in lid pull with "scleral show." The author believes a safer technique is to remove excess skin (and muscle) after the dissection and fat removal.

Accurate determination of the exact amount of skin to be trimmed is imperative in surgery of the lower lid in order to avoid an ectropion resulting from an overambitious resection. If the operation is being performed under local anesthesia and the patient can cooperate, two maneuvers can help to avoid the removal of too much skin. The patient is asked to rotate the eyes upward to elevate the lid margin to a "safe" position. The undermined skin can then be draped over the wound edge and the excess can be removed. Safety is further facilitated by having the patient open the mouth widely to duplicate the forces of an extrinsic ectropion of the type often seen in burns of the face.

If the patient is under general anesthesia or is unable to cooperate, gentle downward pressure applied to the globe results in an upward elevation of the lower lid so the skin may be safely draped over it and excised while the lid is in an elevated position.

Patients with considerable excess of skin and/or muscle of the lower eyelids sometimes have folds extending to the cheeks. This requires wide undermining, which may extend to the infraorbital margin itself. As noted previously, true cheek pads cannot be corrected by blepharoplasty.

When wide undermining is indicated, it should be done prior to excision of fat. After fat removal, the skin flap is draped over the upper margin of the wound and drawn laterally and superiorly. A slight sling effect is the result of this rotation. The excess skin is then trimmed, mostly from the lateral triangle.

In some patients, a marked redundancy of orbicularis oculi muscle contributes significantly to the palpebral bag deformity. These ridges of muscle have been referred to as "festoons" by Furnas (1978) (Figure 17–29). This excess muscle can be trimmed as a separate muscle flap. It can

Text continued on page 503.

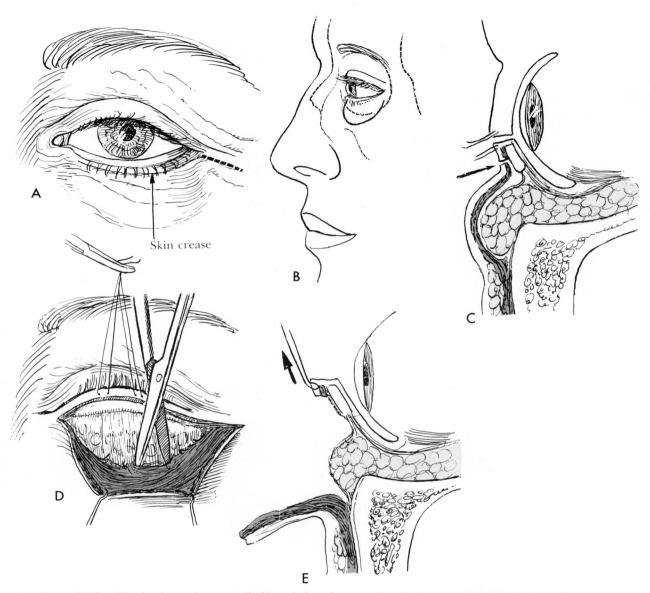

Skin crease

Figure 17–17.   The simplest and most applicable technique for correcting the lower eyelid deformity is the skin-muscle flap. It can be used in most age groups and for most baggy lower lids except for those deformities that have marked excess of skin. It is particularly useful in the young patient with familial fat bags and minimal or no excess skin to be removed. Contrary to wide skin undermining, this technique causes minimal disturbance of tissue and avoids an extensive dead space beneath a skin flap which is subject to hematoma formation, fibrosis, and contracture. The origin of the skin-muscle flap is obscure, but it was championed by Sir Archibald McIndoe, who did not claim to be its originator.

A, The incision is placed in the first natural crease below the ciliary margin, usually 2 or 3 mm. It extends laterally in a natural "crow's foot."

B, The eyelid bag superimposed on the framework of the face.

C, The incision is carried down to the tarsal plate, and the dissection then proceeds on the anterior surface of the plate and orbital septum in a caudal direction.

D, With blunt or sharp dissection, the skin-muscle flap is peeled from the underlying orbital septum caudally to the bony rim.

E, The dissection viewed laterally. The fat now bulges forward.

Illustration continued on the opposite page.

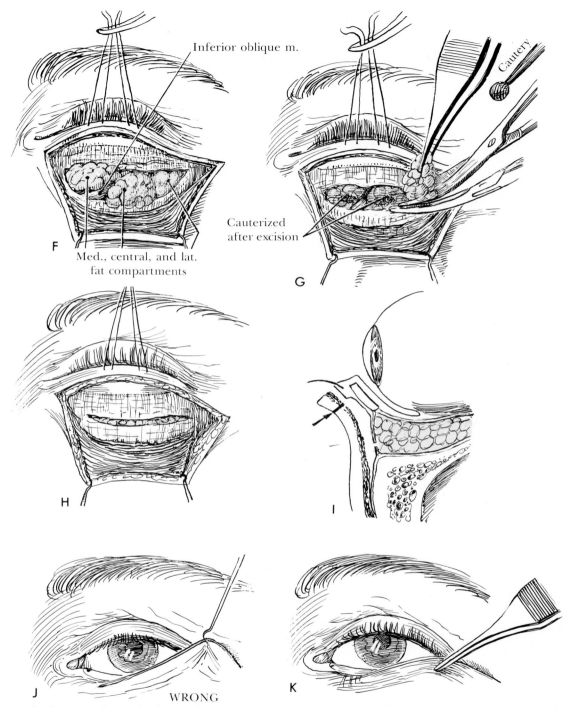

Figure 17–17 *Continued.* *F,* The three major fat compartments are readily identified as they bulge forward against the orbital septum.

G and *H,* The excess fat can be removed either by opening the orbital septum widely or by teasing open the attenuated capsule over the fat bulge. The base of the fat is best clamped with a hemostat and cauterized to avoid deep bleeding.

I, The skin-muscle flap is replaced and the excess strip is excised.

J and *K,* The skin-muscle flap must be handled carefully and correctly to avoid excessive resection and therefore pull or ectropion of the lower lid. Undue pull in a cephalic direction with a hook or forceps is dangerous and is apt to result in excessive resection. The flap should be gently draped over the wound edge, with the lid margin in a neutral position. In this way, there is little danger of over-excision. If the patient is awake, it is helpful to ask the patient to open the mouth widely. This maneuver puts tension on the lid flap. Depression of the eyeball also elevates the lid margin and helps greatly in the assessment of the amount of skin and muscle to remove.

Illustration continued on the following page.

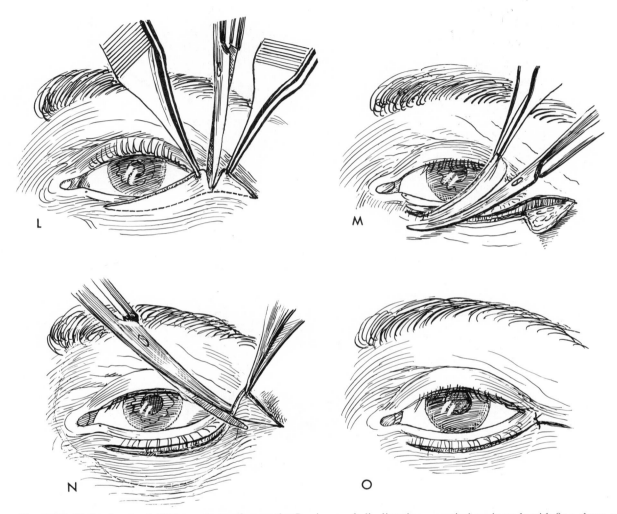

Figure 17–17 *Continued. L,* With gentle traction on the flap in a cephalic direction, a vertical cut is made with fine, sharp scissors at the level of the outer canthus. This cut provides the guideline for excision.

M, Without exerting further traction on the flap, sharp, curved scissors are used to excise the excess strip in a horizontal direction along the wound. Remember that it is always preferable to be conservative and remove too little skin rather than too much. More can always be removed.

N, The lateral "dog-ear" is trimmed.

O, The key suture is placed at the lateral canthus.

Illustration continued on the opposite page.

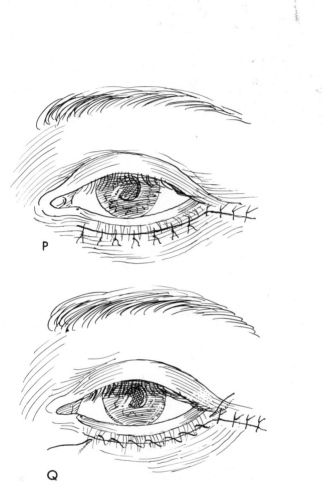

Figure 17–17 *Continued.*   *P* and *Q*, The incision can be sutured according to the surgeon's choice with interrupted, running, or subcuticular sutures.

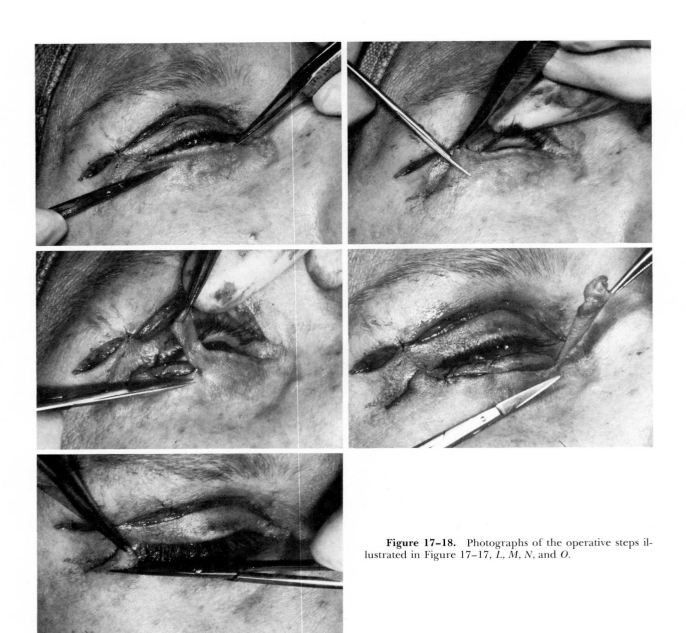

Figure 17–18. Photographs of the operative steps illustrated in Figure 17–17, *L, M, N,* and *O.*

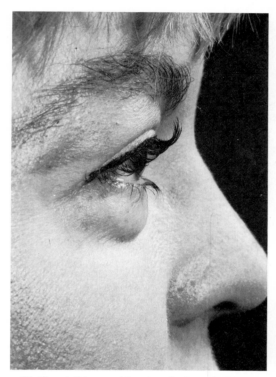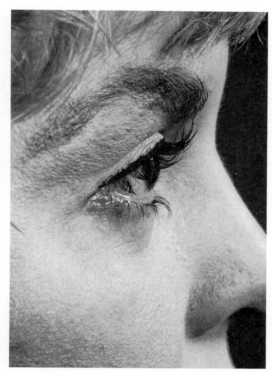

Figure 17–19. A 24-year-old patient had marked bulging of the lower eyelids caused by pseudoherniation of fat. The condition was present in her mother and grandmother as well. Correction was obtained by the skin-muscle flap technique, but it was also necessary to remove a 3 mm strip of muscle from the upper margin of the orbicularis because a localized ridge of muscle was present. Many patients have such a ridge lying horizontally just at the level of the tarsal plate, which becomes activated on facial animation. These ridges can be trimmed, but this should be done with great care to prevent a drag on the lower lid.

Figure 17–20.   Technique for limited undermining and excision of excess skin of the lower lids in a patient who requires moderate skin excision is shown. In this more advanced degree of degenerative lid change, the upper eyelids almost always require correction also. It is preferable to correct both upper and lower lids at the same operation, the upper ones first because the lateral extension of the upper eyelid design alters the skin tension lateral to the eye (in the region of the "laugh lines") and thus affects the lower lids.

The lower eyelid incision is usually located about 2 mm below the ciliary margin, as in the skin-muscle flap operation (*A* and *B*). Usually there is a natural skin crease at about that point, which can be used as a guide. The lower eyelid skin is undermined as far as necessary to reach below the redundancy. It should be separated from the orbicularis muscle and, thus, constitutes almost a full-thickness skin graft.

Absolute hemostasis is necessary (*B*). Each small vessel is coagulated with pinpoint jewelers' forceps.

Excess periorbital fat is removed from the offending compartments of the lower lid through stab wounds in the muscle and orbital septum (*C* and *D*). The medial and middle fat pockets are most commonly entered.

The authors' method of judging how much skin is to be excised from the lower eyelid is shown in *E*. After the skin is undermined and the fat is removed, the redundant skin is draped over the lid margin with traction lightly applied in a superior and lateral direction. The eyeball is depressed by finger pressure from above. This displacement of the globe elevates the lower lid margin, which must be freely mobile. The maneuver is similar to having the patient look upward during local anesthesia. Excess skin is carefully excised, being sure that too much traction is not exerted on the skin so that overcorrection will result. Pressure on the eyeball must be applied with the upper lid open. This technique has the advantage of allowing safe skin removal under general anesthesia or in the heavily sedated patient. It is generally a safer method for the inexperienced surgeon.

The wound is sutured with interrupted 6–0 black silk sutures (*F*). (From Rees, T. D.: Plast. Reconstr. Surg., *41*:497, 1968.)

See illustration on the opposite page.

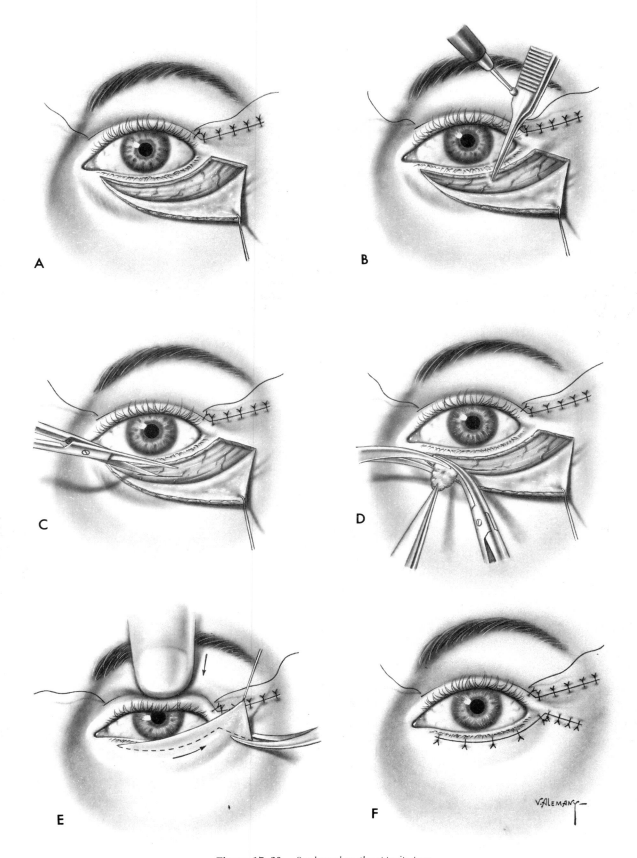

Figure 17–20. *See legend on the opposite page.*

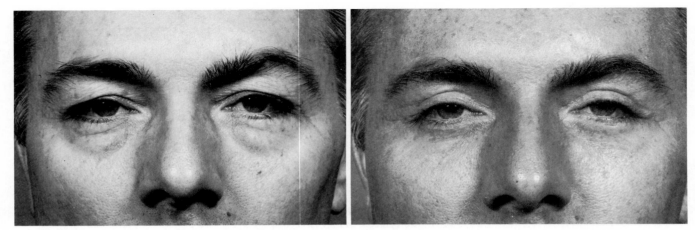

Figure 17–21. This is a 38-year-old man with moderately advanced blepharochalasis, or excess skin folds of the upper lids, and palpebral bags of the lower lids, consisting mainly of pseudohernias of periorbital fat. Correction was achieved by the technique shown in Figure 17–20.

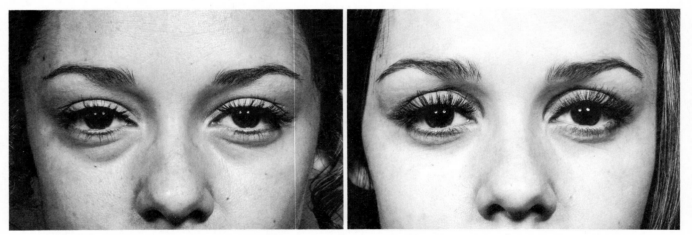

This young woman had palpebral bags of fat and skin. In such a patient skin and fat are equally at fault, and the deformity cannot be corrected with a skin-muscle flap. The skin must be undermined and redraped; the procedure for limited undermining as required in this case is shown in Figure 17–20.

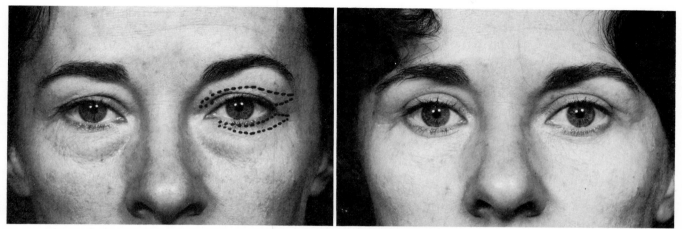

Figure 17-22.   Upper and lower palpebral bags were corrected by the technique described and illustrated in Figure 17-17. Dotted lines indicate the approximate skin incisions required; note the small amount of skin to be removed from the lower lids in spite of the relatively large visible swellings. Lid bulges in this area are primarily due to fat, and the actual skin excess is minimal to moderate.

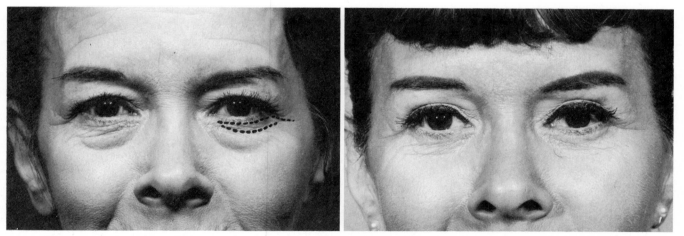

These are preoperative and postoperative views of a smiling patient. The approximate skin excision of the lower lids is marked in the preoperative photograph. Note that the fine rhytides that appear when the facial muscles are animated are still present after surgery. Patients such as this, with particularly deep wrinkles, complain that the wrinkles are even more noticeable after blepharoplasty. The reason is that the underlying fat formerly present smoothed the skin and ironed out some of the wrinkles. If wrinkling is marked after primary surgery, deep chemical peel should be considered to improve the wrinkles and possibly even to obliterate them.

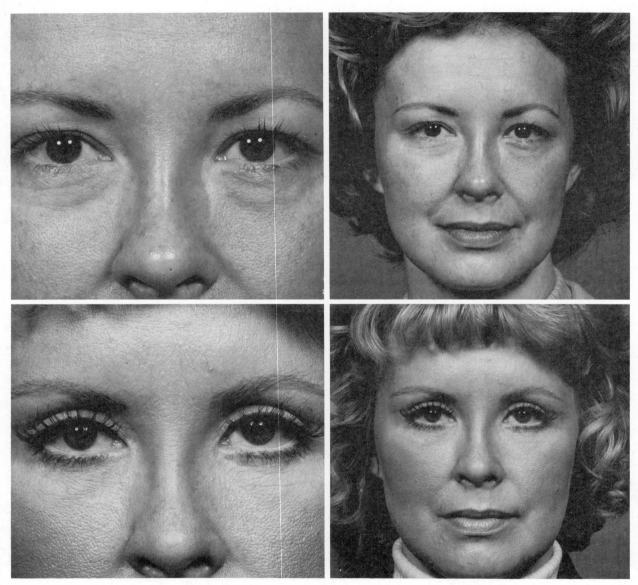

Figure 17–23. An example of results achieved by the skin-muscle flap technique.

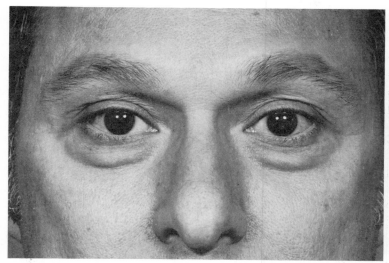

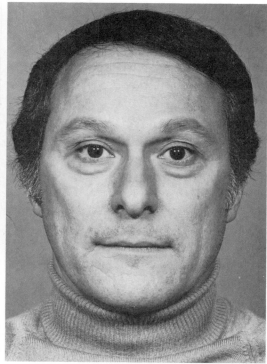

Figure 17–24. Excess fat with some redundancy of skin in a man is shown. This problem requires excision of skin as well as fat, although the skin excision is minimal. Limited skin undermining is needed, as shown in Figure 17–20. The skin-muscle flap can still be used; however, the fat can also be removed through stab wounds in the orbital septum. Note that the amount of sclera visible is only slightly increased after the operation, provided the amount of skin excised is conservative. The operation results in a brighter and clearer expression that is particularly noticeable in the full-face photographs. The facies also appears more rested.

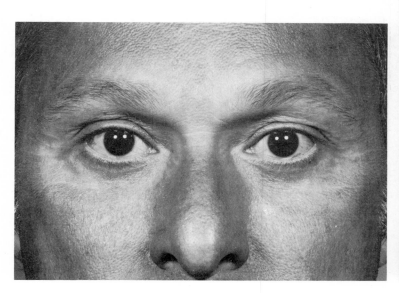

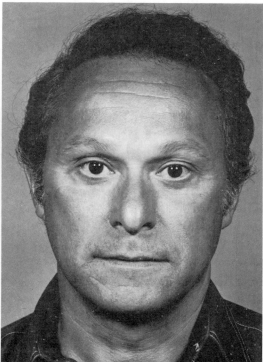

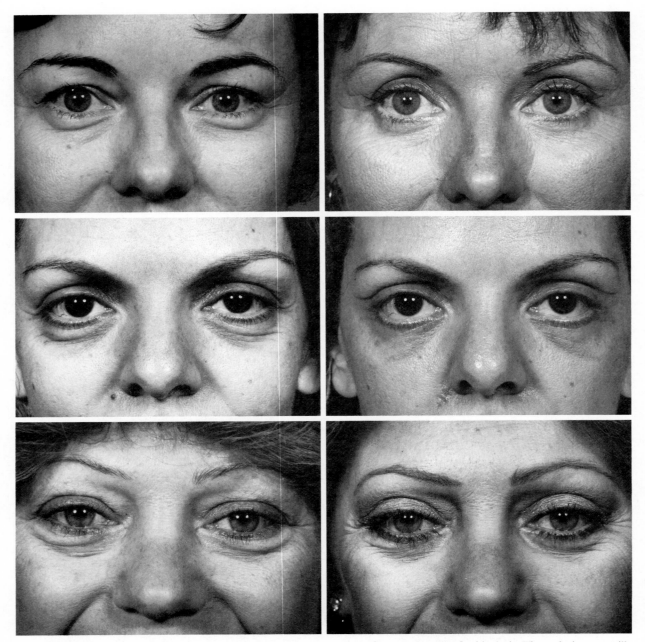

Figure 17–25.   These patients are examples of operative correction of a "muscle roll" of orbicularis. The techniques are illustrated in Figure 17–26. A small muscle roll is normal and quite attractive particularly in the young lid, but when it is exaggerated, particularly on animation, the result is not pleasing to the patient. Correction should be understated and conservative.

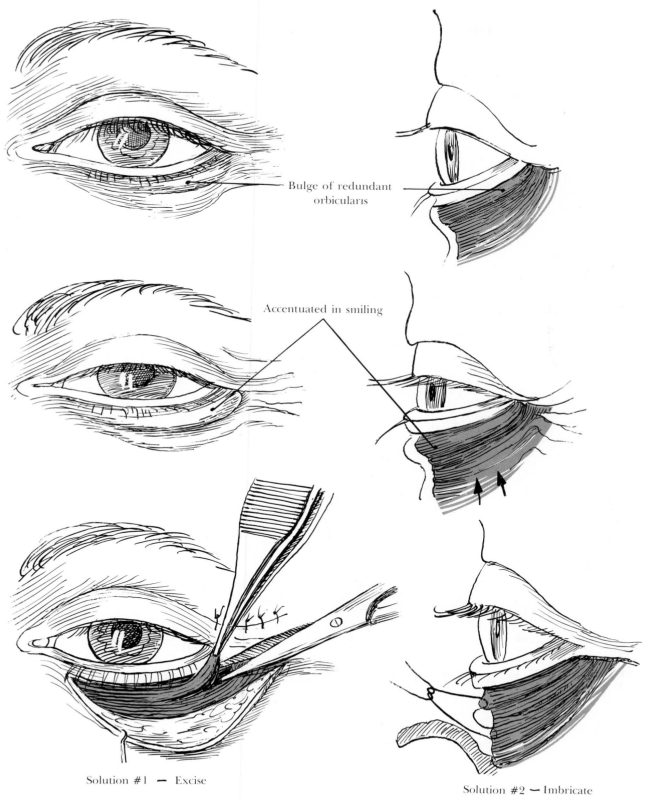

Bulge of redundant orbicularis

Accentuated in smiling

Solution #1 — Excise

Solution #2 — Imbricate

Figure 17–26

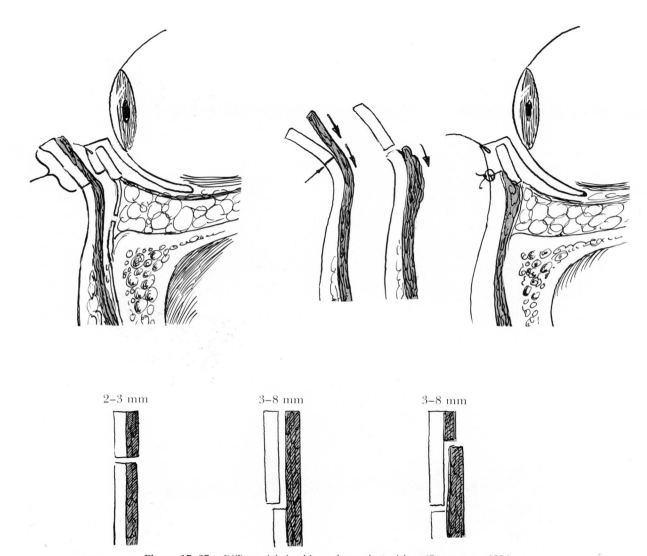

2–3 mm   3–8 mm   3–8 mm

Figure 17–27. Differentials in skin and muscle excision. (See text, p. 485.)

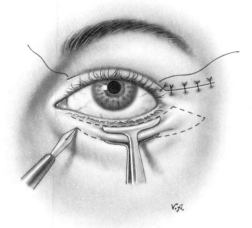

Figure 17–28. This drawing illustrates Converse's method of preoperative estimation of the amount of skin to be excised from the lower eyelids with marking forceps. The patient should be in a sitting or semisitting position for marking. Care is taken not to drag the lid margin downward. This technique requires expert judgment and considerable experience, and it should not be attempted by the beginner except as a rough means of estimating the amount of skin to be excised. Just as in the undermining technique, the majority of the skin is excised laterally as a triangle. This Converse technique of preoperative skin marking is best used in those patients with marked skin excess and minimal fat bags. These are, in general, the characteristics of the senile lid.

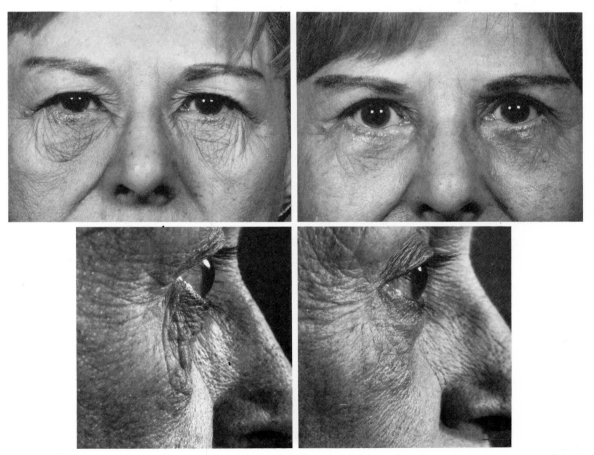

Figure 17–29. This patient had what appears to be a marked excess of skin on first glance. However, more careful examination indicates that there is also considerable excess or "festoons" of muscle. Improvement was obtained according to the technique illustrated in Figure 17–30. The redundant muscle was excised and tightened laterally.

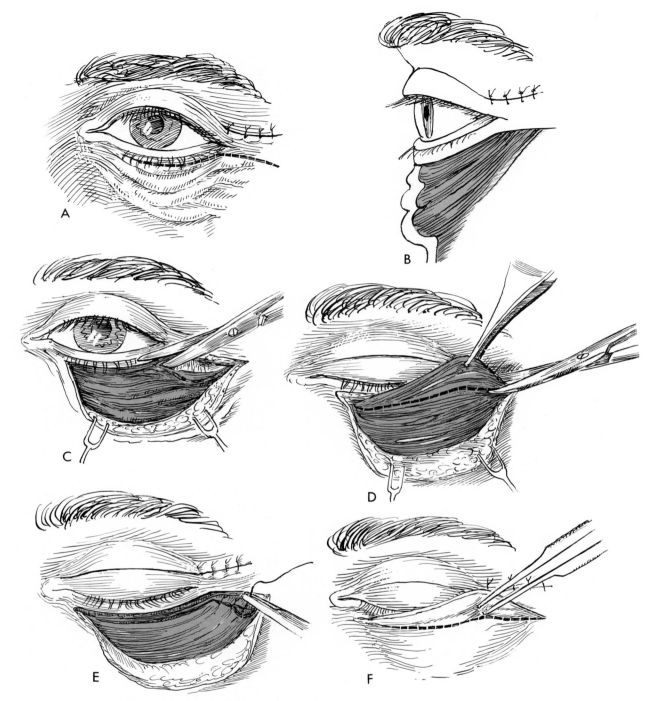

Figure 17–30.   The surgical correction of muscle excess is shown (Furnas).

A, The deformity and usual location of the incision.

B, A lateral view of the deformity.

C, The skin has been extensively undermined. The muscle is incised separately.

D, The muscle is pulled gently in a cephalic and slightly lateral direction to take up the slack. The excess is excised.

E, The muscle is then sutured laterally to soft tissue or, according to preference, to periosteum. The muscle acts as a hammock support.

F, The redundant skin is then excised in the manner described previously (Furnas, 1978).

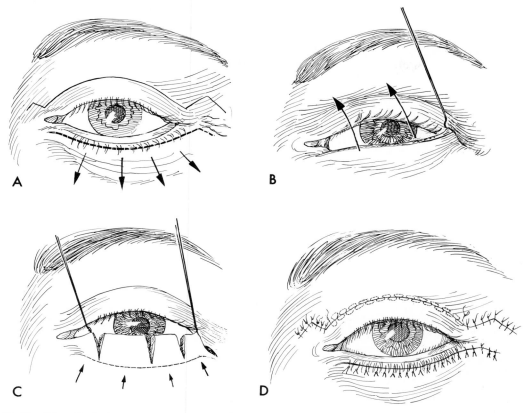

Figure 17–31.   Silver Technique.

The incision is made along the dotted line in *A*. The lower flap is undermined as far as necessary and the excess skin is draped over the lid margin (*B*). As in all techniques, it is important that the lid margin be free and lie in a natural position before skin is excised. Depression of the globe to raise the lid margin (Figure 17–20,*E*) might be helpful at this juncture. Multiple cuts are then made in the skin flap (*C*) and the excess is excised. The vertical incisions have the advantage of preventing too much skin from being removed in one cutting. Another considerable advantage of the technique is that by suturing from lateral to medial (*D*), a dog-ear at the lateral edge of the wound is avoided.

also be plicated in certain patients or fixed to the periosteum of the lateral orbit by a suture (Furnas, 1978), although this maneuver requires considerable experience (Figure 17–30).

Care must be taken to avoid undue tension on the skin flap because horizontal or vertical foreshortening of the lower lid margin can result in buckling of the tarsus, with epiphora or ectropion.

To avoid tenting of the skin flap, care must be taken to see that the entire skin flap is in approximation with all crevices and contours of the wound bed. Wound edges are then stitched with interrupted sutures of fine silk or a running suture. A temporary tarsorrhaphy suture is placed in each eye when a compression dressing is used.

The technique of Silver (1969) (Figure 17–31) is also most useful in correction of marked skin excess in the presenile and senile eyelid. Silver's method has great merit for removing redundant skin, but it must be used with utmost care, and it is of doubtful value in the young patient with only a small amount of excess skin.

It is only fair to comment at this juncture that the efficacy and safety of the skin-muscle flap as compared with wide skin undermining is not entirely established. Many surgeons employ the skin-muscle flap in all cases; other surgeons prefer skin undermining in all but the young patient with tight skin. Both groups claim equally good results. Spira (1977) attempted a clinical study to clarify the situation. In a group of 26 patients ranging in age from 35 to 68 years, he performed a skin-muscle flap on one lower lid and a skin undermine operation on the contralateral lower lid. His postoperative results were assessed from color transparencies by several plastic surgeons, residents, and students. The photographs were made from 3 to 12 months following surgery. Except for one or two minor disparities, the observers felt that there were no significant variations between the two eye-lids. Despite the lack of demonstrable difference in the results, Spira nevertheless indicated his contin-ued preference to vary the technique according to the age and degree of deformity presenting. He, like the author, seems unconvinced that one surgi-cal technique is suitable for all. The jury is still out!

In a similar bilateral clinical study in which one orbital septum was sutured and the other was not, Tipton (1972) was unable to ascertain a differ-ence in the postoperative result. Most surgeons prefer not to suture the septum, since the sutured septum might logically act as a tether on the lower lid, increasing the likelihood of pull down.

Finally, a word of caution regarding the senile lid. With age, the skin becomes more thinned and wrinkled, the lower lids lose tone, the tarsus be-comes unsupported, the muscles become weak, and all tissues become more redundant. Skin (and sometimes fat) bags of the lower eyelids form and can extend to and below infraorbital rims. The fat compartments of the lower lid become more prom-inent and sometimes seem to herniate through the overlying muscle. The orbital septum becomes in-creasingly attenuated. The brows become more

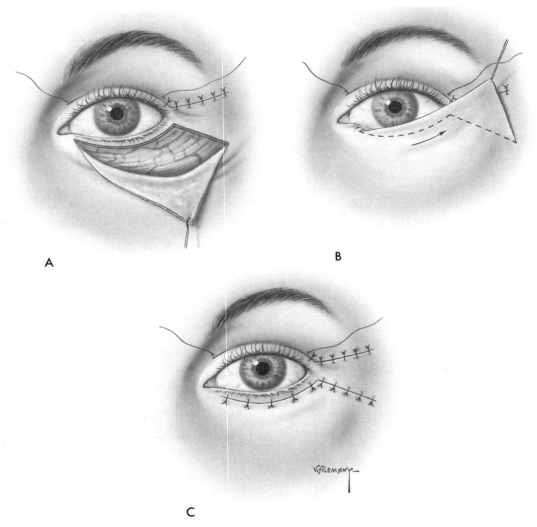

Figure 17–32.   Undermining of the skin of the lower eyelids must be quite extensive in the older patient and almost always must extend beyond the lowermost redundant skin fold *(A)*. It may be necessary to open the muscle and orbital septum widely to retrieve the fat, as stab wounds may not suffice.

Extreme caution must be exercised in removing excessive skin in these patients because of the natural tendency toward ectropion with advancing years *(B)*. As in the more moderate operation, the majority of the skin excess is best excised as a lateral triangle. He-mostasis is most important, as well as delicate handling of tissue. Senile skin can be very thin and friable and is, therefore, easily torn with skin hooks or forceps.

The authors prefer a temporary tarsorrhaphy suture for a few hours after surgery until the lower skin flap adheres to the muscle *(C)*. This is another preventive measure against ectropion.

ptotic as the years and the pull of gravity take effect.

Under these circumstances standard blepharoplasty techniques can exert unusual traction on the weakened tarsus, which can evert or buckle, thereby precipitating a senile ectropion with eversion of the lower lid margin. Loss of tone in the lower lid in the aging patient can be identified quite easily by the pinch test. The vertical length of the lower lid is grasped between the examiner's thumb and index finger to test tone and redundancy. Sagging

of the lateral third of the lower eyelid is also a useful sign of incipient senile ectropion.

Should considerable redundancy exist, it is advisable to perform a wedge resection of full-thickness lower lid (including tarsus) during primary bleopharoplasty. Experience will soon dictate the amount of excision required. The repair should be located lateral to the limbus (see the section on correction of ectropion).

Such an added step will insure a tight foreshortened lower lid and greatly reduce the

Text continued on page 518.

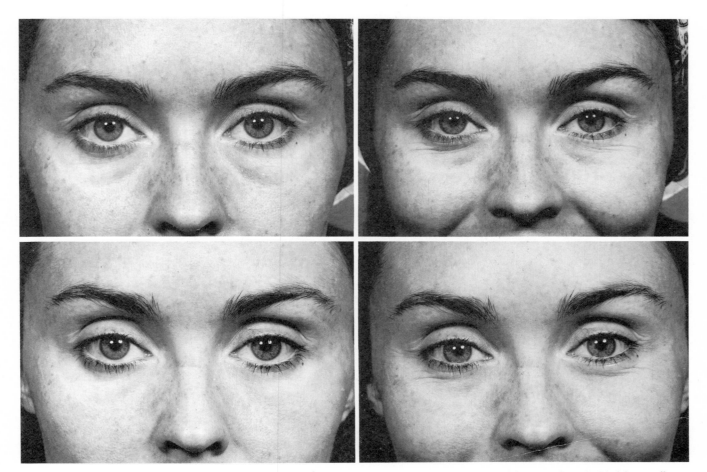

Figure 17–33.   The familial type of bulging of the lower eyelids caused by excessive (or pseudoherniated) periorbital fat usually occurs in the second or third decade of life. It is easily corrected by the skin-muscle flap technique of McIndoe and Beare (Figure 17–17), which produces minimal trauma and rarely requires any excision of skin in these young patients.

The incision is placed 2 to 3 mm below the ciliary margin. The offending fat compartments are usually found to be the medial and middle ones, as described by Castanares (1951). Fat is removed through stab wounds in the orbicularis muscle and the orbital septum. Four to six sutures suffice to close the wound. On occasion, a small strip of skin and muscle can be trimmed if these tissues are redundant. Sutures are removed in 48 hours.

Preoperative views are at the top; postoperative views are below. In the two photographs on the right, the patient is smiling. Comparison with the left-hand views will demonstrate that, on animation of the facial muscles, even in such a young adult, fine lines or rhytides remain after surgery, though they are usually improved by the procedure. Patients should be advised that these "laugh lines" will not be eradicated by the operation. (From Rees, T. D., and Dupuis, C. C.: Plast. Reconstr. Surg., *43*:381, 1969.)

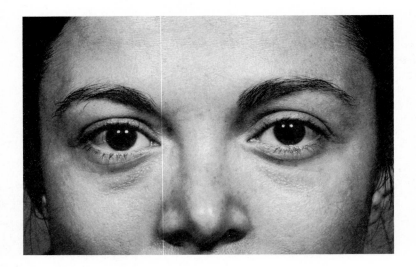

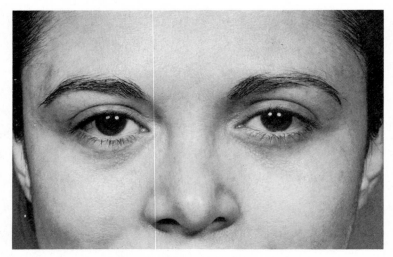

Figure 17–34. A similar problem of familial palpebral bags is shown in a young patient in whom the condition is slightly more advanced. Familial fat bulges are progressive and should be removed early in their development. The upper eyelids may or may not be involved in a similar manner.

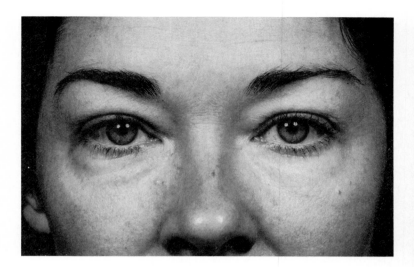

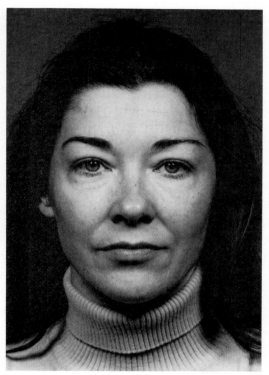

Figure 17–35. This attractive young woman represents an ideal patient for blepharoplasty. She had been aware of her "puffy" eyes since childhood, for the condition was transmitted through the maternal side of her family. With age, the patient began to notice a definite sense of heaviness in her eyes and complained that her eyes fatigued easily. A standard skin-muscle flap blepharoplasty was done, with removal of a small strip of skin and of medial fat from the upper eyelids. Note the dramatic effect of this surgery on the patient's facial expression: the "dissipated" look has vanished.

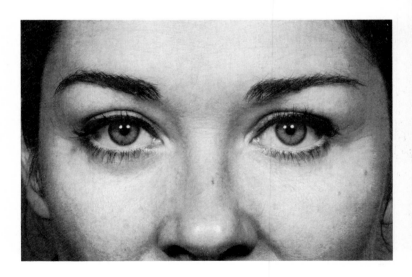

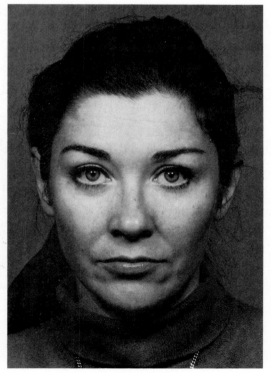

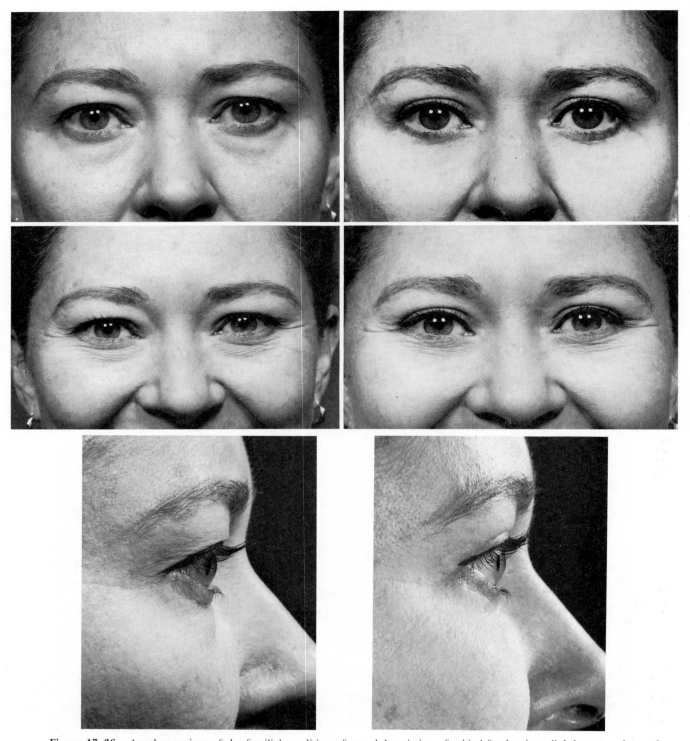

Figure 17–36.   Another variant of the familial condition of pseudoherniation of orbital fat, but in a slightly more advanced state, is demonstrated by this patient, whose upper lids are involved as well as the lower lids. The fat pockets of the upper lid in such patients consist of a medial collection of whitish "fibro-fat" as well as a sausage-shaped horizontal fat pad that is butter-yellow in color and lies between the orbicularis oculi muscle and the levator expansion.

The operative procedure is slightly more complicated. It is necessary to remove an ellipse of excess skin from the upper lids and take out the offending fat from the upper lid compartments. The lower eyelids will also require removal of a small strip of skin, but the skin-muscle flap operation can be used, after which a small amount of undermining is done to provide a skin cuff for excision.

Again, note that the fine wrinkles of facial expression are *not* eliminated by the surgery. The lateral views show how the appearance of the eye is "cleared" by this technique.

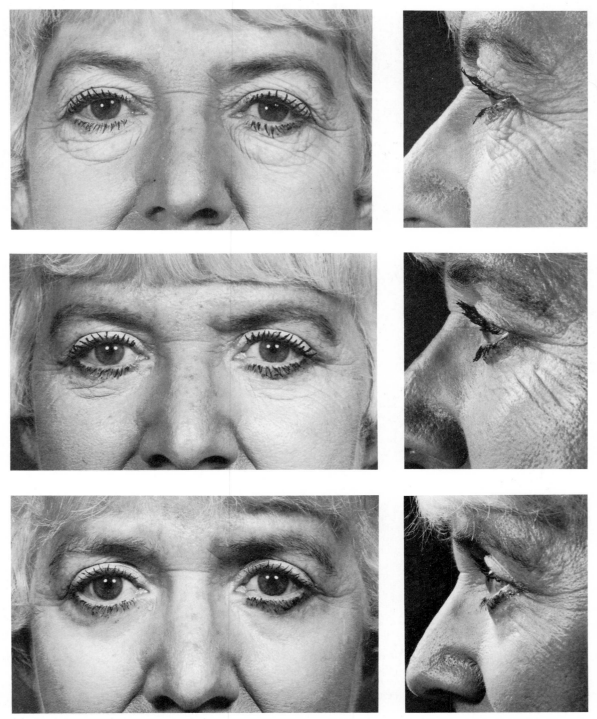

Figure 17–37. This patient shows marked rhytidosis of the face and eyelids. Improvement in such a patient can be obtained only by blepharoplasty with wide undermining, followed in several weeks by a deep skin peel that can be done selectively to the eyelids and not necessarily to the entire face. This patient's peel followed her blepharoplasty by six weeks.

The preoperative condition is shown in the upper views, the postoperative in the center, and the final result after chemical peel at the bottom. Note the smoothness in skin texture obtained from peeling.

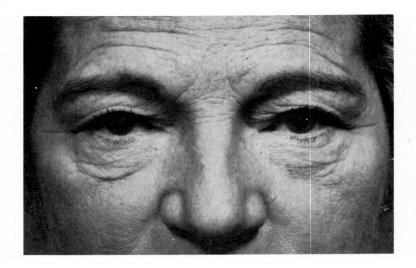

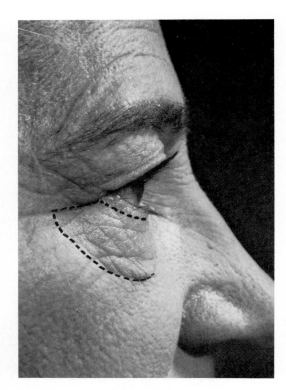

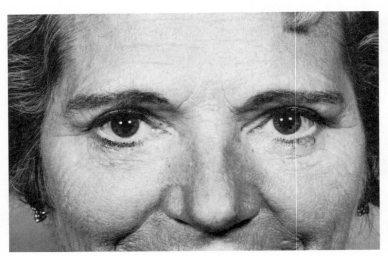

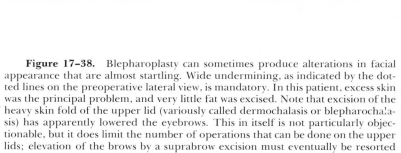

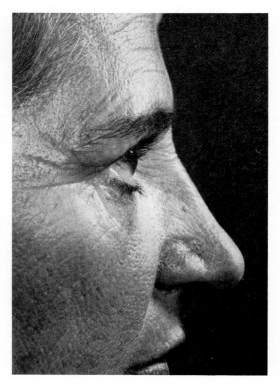

Figure 17–38. Blepharoplasty can sometimes produce alterations in facial appearance that are almost startling. Wide undermining, as indicated by the dotted lines on the preoperative lateral view, is mandatory. In this patient, excess skin was the principal problem, and very little fat was excised. Note that excision of the heavy skin fold of the upper lid (variously called dermochalasis or blepharochalasis) has apparently lowered the eyebrows. This in itself is not particularly objectionable, but it does limit the number of operations that can be done on the upper lids; elevation of the brows by a suprabrow excision must eventually be resorted to.

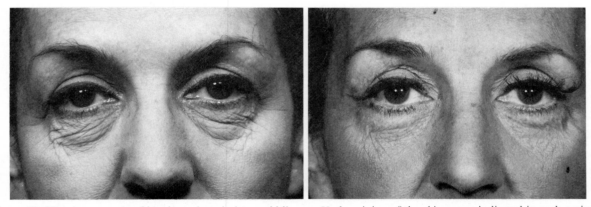

Figure 17–39. An example of blepharoplasty in later middle age. Undermining of the skin seems indicated in such patients.

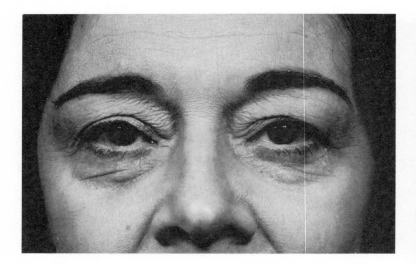

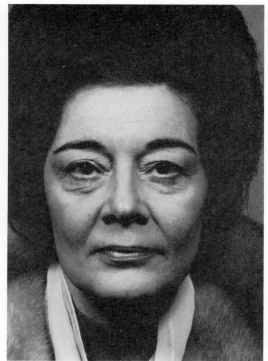

Figure 17–40.   A thorough and quite extensive blepharoplasty with generous skin excision can often result in a remarkable improvement in the entire facial appearance, particularly when the rest of the face is much younger looking than the eyelids. In this respect blepharoplasty can have a much more profound effect on the facial appearance than a face lift, because the eyes are the real focal point of facial expression. It is the eyes, too, that are first noticed when one meets a stranger.

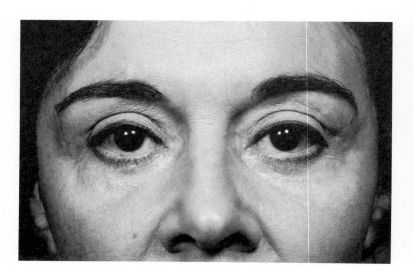

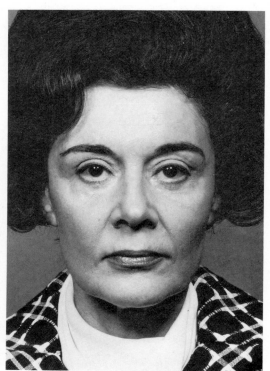

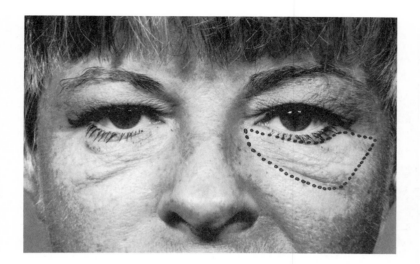
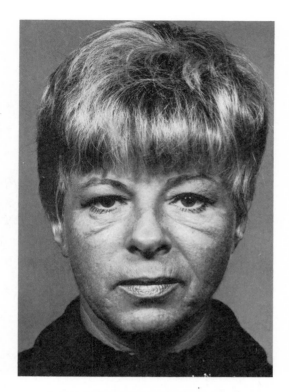
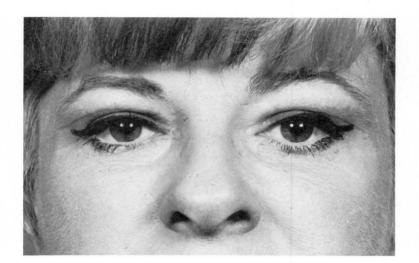
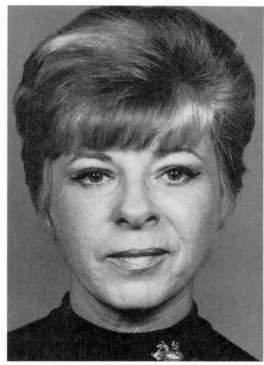
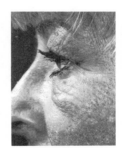
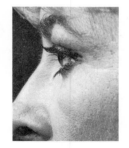

Figure 17–41.   This woman, aged 40, shows marked premature aging of the skin of the eyelids in the preoperative photographs. The skin is wrinkled and thickened, and the "bags" extend well down into the cheeks. This condition is partly the result of a hereditary predisposition, but it has been hastened considerably in this patient by excessive exposure to actinic rays. The dotted line in the preoperative close-up indicates the area that must be undermined in order to achieve correction of the loose skin. Note that the undermining extends down to the cheek. Skin like this is quite leathery and thick. There is considerable inherent support, so that ectropion is unlikely; nevertheless, great care must be exercised as usual in the resection. The technique shown in Figure 17–32 is particularly useful in this type of patient. The marked change in the patient's entire facial appearance from blepharoplasty alone is most noticeable. (From Rees, T. D.: Technical Considerations in Blepharoplasty. Transactions of the Fourth International Congress of Plastic and Reconstructive Surgery. Excerpta Medica Foundation, Amsterdam, 1969, p. 1084.)

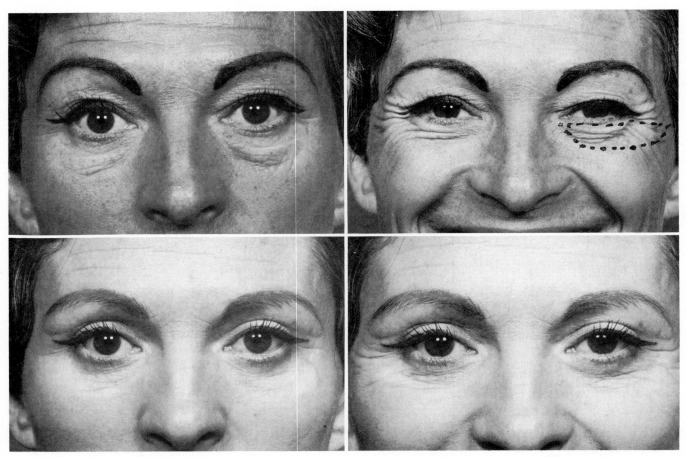

Figure 17–42. This patient has had excessive exposure to the sun for many years, which has caused severe degenerative changes in the skin. There are many deep lines and wrinkles, which are markedly aggravated by any kind of facial animation. Definite but somewhat limited correction can be achieved by wide undermining of the affected skin. Fat removal, on the other hand, was conservative in this patient. Undermining must extend far enough laterally to include the "laugh lines," as has been pointed out by Gurdin (dotted lines in the preoperative "animated" photo). Wide wedges of skin are also removed from the lateral extensions of the incisions. The postoperative view showing the patient smiling demonstrates the amount of correction possible with this technique. Before surgery it should be made clear to patients with weatherbeaten skin and rhytidosis that blepharoplasty will not eliminate the deeper lines.

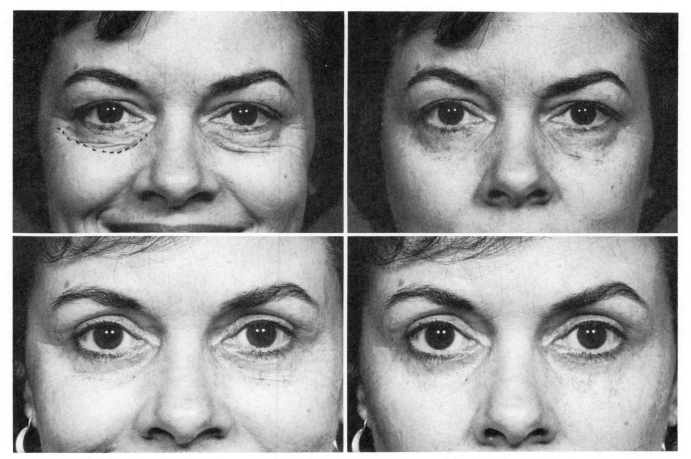

Figure 17–43.   Sometimes in patients approaching or in middle age the excess of skin of the lower lids is more apparent in animation than when the face is in repose. The excess becomes apparent on animation because of the interaction of the underlying orbicularis oculi muscle fibers and the flaccid skin on top. This is often the chief complaint of a patient in this age group and may be associated with little or no excess fat.

Blepharoplasty in such patients does not eliminate these expression wrinkles, but with very wide undermining, as indicated by the dotted line in the preoperative animated (smiling) photo, the postoperative result can be quite an improvement. This degree of change cannot be expected in all patients, a fact that is best pointed out to the patient before surgery.

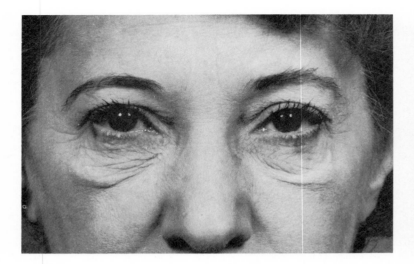

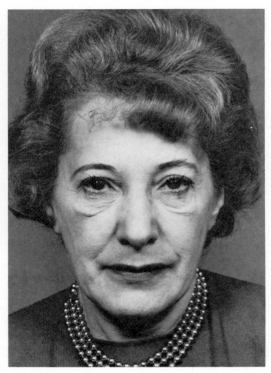

Figure 17–44.   A patient had marked skin bags but little periorbital fat. Skin folds that extend to the cheeks or even lower can be very difficult to eradicate. Improvement will be obtained only by extensive undermining. Small bags or depressions of the cheeks themselves cannot be greatly improved by operation, even with wide undermining. These cheek bags, or "malar bags," should be spotted by the surgeon preoperatively and pointed out to the patient. (From Rees, T. D., and Guy, C. L.: Surg. Clin. North Am. *51*:353, 1971.)

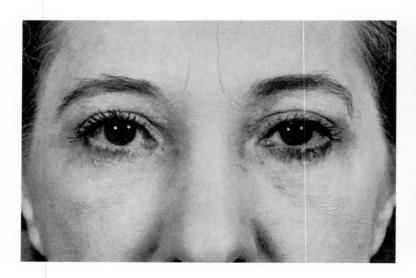

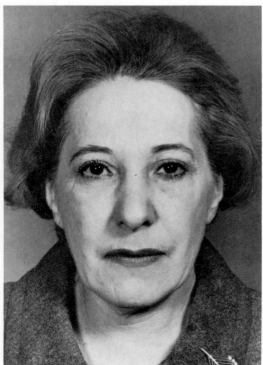

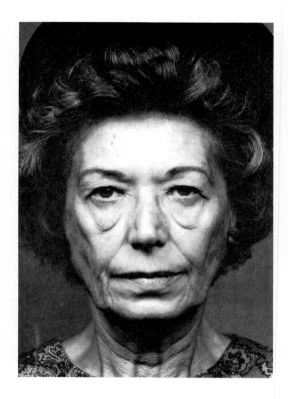

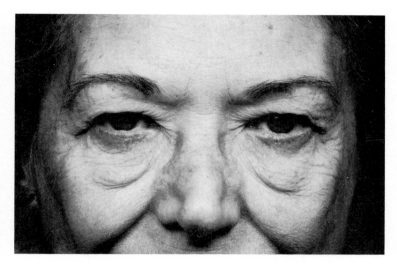

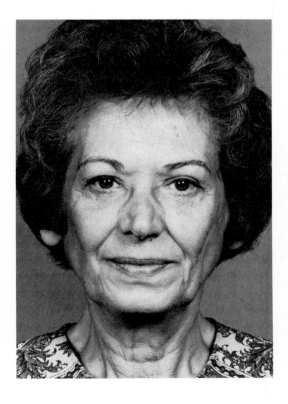

Figure 17–45. Blepharoplasty may be performed for advanced senile-type eyelids. Undermining must be extensive but tempered by conservative skin excision; the danger of inducing ectropion is great in the older patient. Lid structures are apt to be attenuated and weakened, particularly the orbicularis oculi muscle. The aim of surgery is to "clean up" the facial expression, not to change it, and certainly not to produce an illusion of youth. Certain limitations of a morphological nature exist in older people, and they must be accepted as part of the postoperative appearance too. Skin wrinkles will still be present, and in spite of extensive removal of upper eyelid skin folds, these cannot be completely obliterated. Ptosis of the brows is almost always a strong factor in the older patient, who also usually has considerable horizontal wrinkling of the forehead skin. These wrinkles facilitate elevation of the brows, inasmuch as the resulting scar is more easily camouflaged. When a face lift is done in conjunction with blepharoplasty, a strong temporal lift also helps to raise the brow, but the final result of direct brow elevation and temporal lift is still less than optimal.

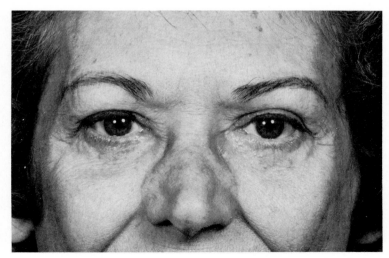

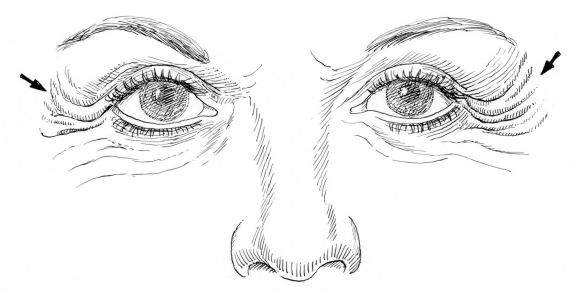

Figure 17–46

changes of ectropion. Of course, an exact and accurate repair of all structures is required, most especially of the lid margin and the tarsal plate.

The following photographs illustrate some of the special problems encountered in blepharoplasty patients (Figures 17–32 through 17–45).

THE ORBICULARIS OCULI FLAP

Elimination of the lateral orbital wrinkles ("crow's feet") is one of the most difficult feats in facial cosmetic surgery. Rhytides lateral to the orbit are the result of intricate interaction between the orbicularis oculi muscle and the skin (Figure 17–46). Only in total paralysis of the facial nerve do these wrinkles disappear. Total paralysis is not practical in the patient. During facial animation, the muscle exhibits an accordion-like effect on the overlying skin, accentuating the folds and wrinkles as the muscle shortens and the skin is thrown into furrows and depressions. Such skin folds and wrinkles do not respond to standard blepharoplasty and facial plasty techniques.

Skoog (1974) advocated a direct surgical approach to the orbicularis to correct this problem. To correct wrinkling at the lateral canthus, he split the muscle partially so that it could be "splayed out." The muscle was sutured in this splayed posture. He advised that the muscle be incised in a horizontal direction from its lateral border and the cut ends would be separated and sutured without significantly disturbing eyelid function. The technique has not gained wide usage because of the inherent danger to the orbicularis branch of the temporal branch of the facial nerve; however, the results are rewarding in patients with such a problem. Aston (1980) adapted the Skoog technique and reported his experience with several patients.

TECHNIQUE

The lateral orbital border of the orbicularis oculi muscle is exposed through the temporal and standard face lift incision (Figure 17–47). The skin flap is elevated by sharp dissection. As the skin flap approaches the lateral border of the orbicularis,

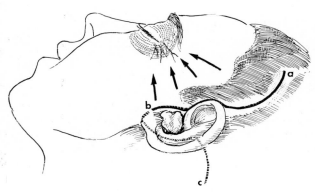

Figure 17–47

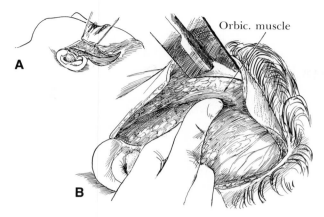

Figure 17–48

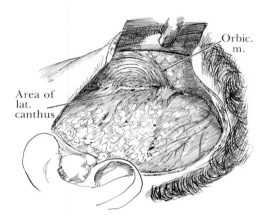

Figure 17–49

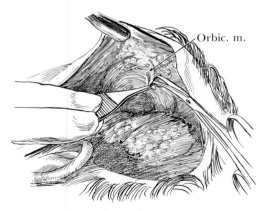

Figure 17–50

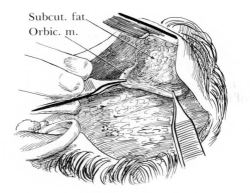

Subcut. fat.
Orbic. m.

Figure 17–51

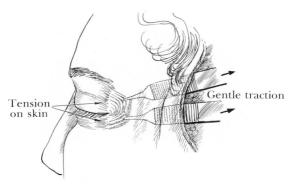

Tension
on skin

Gentle traction

Figure 17–52

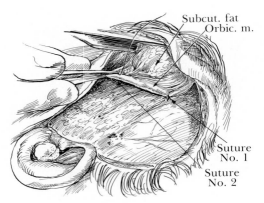

Subcut. fat
Orbic. m.

Suture
No. 1

Suture
No. 2

Figure 17–53

blunt finger dissection is employed to lessen the likelihood of damage to the temporal branch of the facial nerve. Blunt dissection elevates the flap from the underlying fascia (Figure 17–48). Blunt dissection readily identifies the lateral border of the orbicularis with less danger of incising the muscle until the precise point of muscle incision is identified. The border of the muscle is ordinarily found 3 to 5 cm lateral to the orbital rim, where it is closely adherent to the under surface of the skin flap (Figure 17–49). (There is considerable difference in the thickness of the muscle among patients.) After the border of the muscle is identified, blunt dissection is continued deep to the muscle between the muscle and the deep fascia, leaving the muscle attached to the skin flap. Dissection is continued in a medial direction towards the orbital rim.

After the lateral border of the muscle is developed by blunt dissection, it is grasped with tissue forceps. Small blunt scissors are used to separate the muscle from the thin layer of subcutaneous fat between the muscle and the overlying skin (Figure 17–50). The muscle is carefully dissected and separated from the subcutaneous fat and skin medial to the lateral canthus, then splayed out and held by two pairs of forceps. Traction is exerted in a cephalic, caudal, and lateral direction (Figure 17–51). The pull on the muscle is transmitted to the skin of the lateral canthal region. Desired tension is determined by trial and error (Figure 17–52). The muscle is then sutured in its "splayed out" configuration to the temporal fascia (Figure 17–53). The gap between the two key sutures is sutured with a running catgut (Figures 17–54 and 17–55).

In some instances in which the muscle is extraordinarily thick or the skin folds are very prominent, the muscle is split along a horizontal line

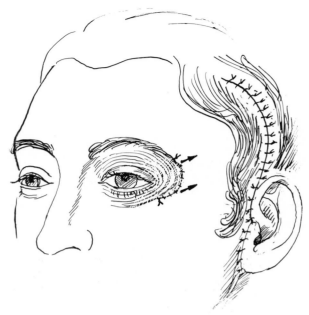

Figure 17–55

extending to a point just lateral to the lateral canthus (Figure 17–56). The divided edges of the muscle can then be separated and sutured under tension. Excessive tension on the divided muscle can result in too much pull at the lateral canthus, which may persist for several months. After suture fixation of the muscle flap, the overlying skin flap is redraped, the excess skin is excised, and the skin wound is sutured.

The effects of such a direct surgical approach to the orbicularis muscle unquestionably enhances the result of facial rhytides that are enforced by animation. The only hazard of the procedure is division of one or more fine branches of the se-

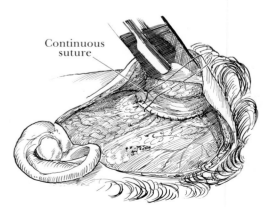

Continuous suture

Figure 17–54

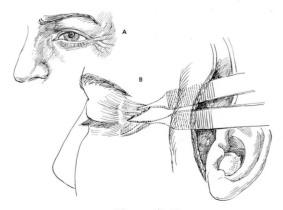

Figure 17–56

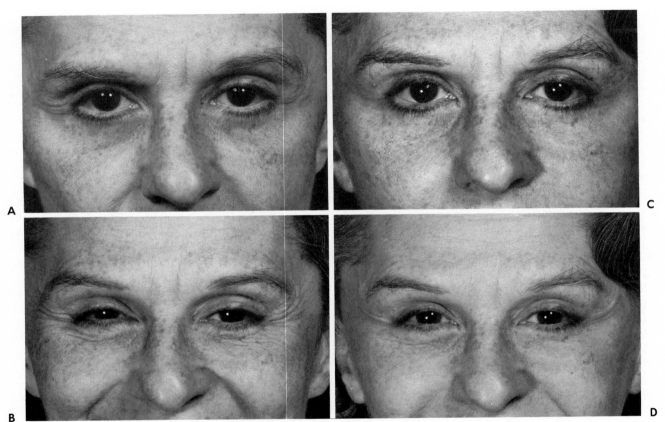

Figure 17–57.   *A,* A 59-year-old female with skin folds and wrinkles in the lateral canthal area. Upper- and lower-lid blepharo-plasty had been performed one year earlier.

B, Smiling increases folds and wrinkles.

C and *D,* Postoperative photographs show folds and wrinkles in lateral canthal area reduced and lateral brow lifed after facial plasty and splaying out the orbicularis oculi muscle bilaterally. (Courtesy of Dr. S. J. Aston.)

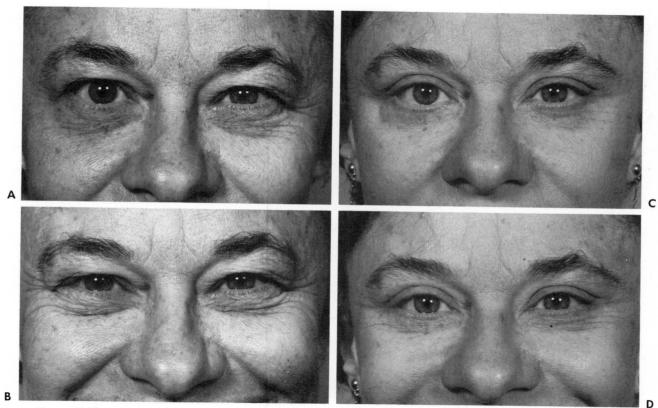

Figure 17–58. *A* and *B*, Preoperative status showing excess skin folds, and lateral brow ptosis.

C and *D*, Following facial plasty, upper- and lower-lid blepharoplasty, and division of the orbicularis oculi muscle ring at the lateral canthi. (Courtesy of Dr. S. J. Aston.)

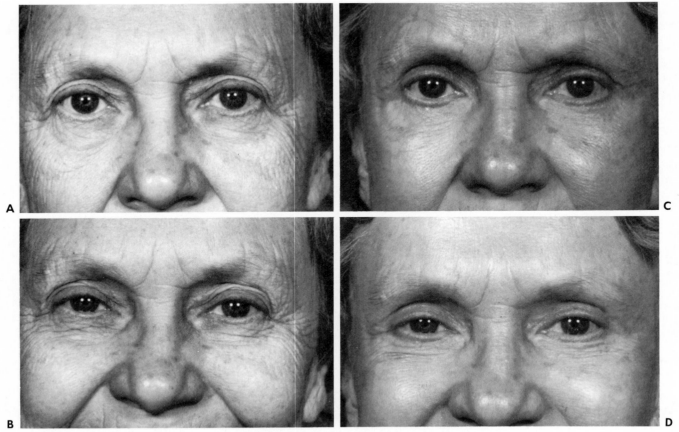

Figure 17–59.   Preoperative status in repose *(A)* and smiling *(B)*.

C, Following facial plasty and upper- and lower-lid blepharoplasty, orbicularis oculi muscle flaps splaying out the muscle on the right side, and muscle ring division on the left side.

D, During smiling, orbicularis oculi muscle activity at the lateral canthus is greater on the undivided side (right) as compared with the divided side (left), which shows no folds and wrinkles. (Courtesy of Dr. S. J. Aston.)

venth nerve to the orbicularis muscle. Since the muscle has many nerve filaments, considerable overlap exists. The damage inflicted by severing one or more branches may well account for at least part of the result. Improvement in the "crow's foot" effect is further enhanced by the redistribution of the muscle and the skin flap. The author is indebted to Dr. Aston for revitalizing Skoog's technique and for the illustrations and patient photographs (Figures 17–57 through 17–59).

(For references, see pages 577 to 580.)

Chapter 18

Postoperative Considerations and Complications

THOMAS D. REES, M.D., F.A.C.S.

EYE DRESSINGS

Bandaging of the eyes following operation is not essential. The author has vacillated about bandaging during the past several years. Theoretically, at least, a moderate pressure dressing for the first few hours following surgery would seem beneficial to help to control oozing, edema, and hematoma.

Certainly, if bandages are not used, it is important to make sure that the cornea is covered and that the eyes are well lubricated during recovery from anesthesia. For this purpose, liberal instillation of a bland ophthalmic ointment is recommended. Application of iced sterile compresses as soon as possible, preferably commencing in the recovery room, is important for the same reasons that pressure bandages are used.

If bandages are used, only moderate pressure is necessary. It is highly important to assure that the lids that were operated on are in proper position under such dressings. This is especially true for the lower lids, which must be maintained in the "normal" position and not depressed in a caudal direction by the upper lid or by the bandage. Such depression of the lower lid can result in adherence of the skin flap to the wound in the orbital septum or to a lower than normal level on the muscle bed. Either can result in ectropion and eversion and must be treated by immediate reoperation and adjustment of the skin flap. Proper positioning of the skin flaps and lids can be provided by the temporary tarsorrhaphy suture, which is placed through the gray line of the lid, and by the careful application of a wrap-around dressing over two eye pads placed on each eye (Figure 18–1).

If dressings are applied, they are removed the following morning along with the tarsorrhaphy sutures. Application of ice compresses is then commenced and continued for the next two days.

Eye dressings may cause some patients to experience severe claustrophobia. When this is the case, sedatives or tranquilizers may be helpful in alleviating the patient's anxiety. The dressings are removed at once, however, if the patient cannot be controlled by these medications.

Perhaps the main purpose of dressings is to provide an added insurance against reactive bleeding during the immediate recovery phase. Every surgeon has experienced, to his consternation, the development of a hematoma or active bleeding from the wound edges in patients in the recovery room who vomited or retched following general anesthesia, despite the excellence of the anesthetic technique, and sometimes even following local anesthesia.

Most interrupted sutures, including the subcuticular suture, are removed on the fourth postoperative day. Sutures left longer than this often result in the formation of epithelial tunnels or sinuses, which can be most troublesome. Wound agglutination can be insured even when sutures are removed at this early time by the application of small sterile strips of paper adhesive across the tension lines of the incision. Paper adhesive has proved to be virtually nonreactive in most patients and is extremely effective in maintaining apposition of the wound edges during the period of maximal weakness.

All crusts and scabs are gently cleansed away from the wound at the end of the first week. A bland eyewash is sometimes beneficial if the patient

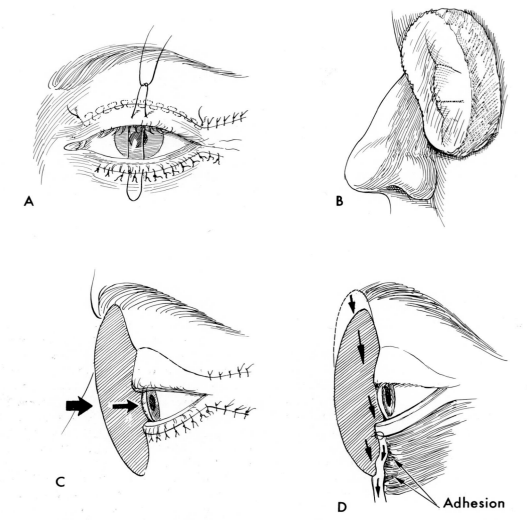

Figure 18–1. When compression dressings are to be used, a tarsorrhaphy suture is important to prevent possible abrasion of the cornea (*A*). Even more important, such a temporary suture keeps the dressing (*B*) from pushing the lower lid downward by shearing force so that it adheres to the muscle at a lower level, resulting in ectropion (*C* and *D*).

complains of irritation, scratchiness, or marked itching. Some patients find the intermittent application of ice compresses to be soothing even several days after the operation, and they are encouraged to continue them if they feel they are helpful.

Exercising of the orbicularis muscles by "squeezing" the eyelids closed at intermittent time intervals is helpful in reducing edema and regaining mobility after the first week. The use of oral or parenteral enzymes has not generally been proved effective in the control of postoperative wound edema.

Women may apply eye makeup on about the tenth postoperative day, but it is advisable to remove it thoroughly and carefully after each use.

Oiled eye pads are recommended for this purpose.

Management of minor complications such as inclusion cysts, hematomas, and scar thickening are described in the following section.

COMPLICATIONS OF BLEPHAROPLASTY

Complications of cosmetic blepharoplasty may be divided into two groups: those that are relatively temporary and those that are persistent or even permanent. The latter problems often require subsequent surgical intervention to attempt correction. Temporary complications are usually self-limiting and generally appear almost immediately after surgery.

DRY EYE SYNDROME

Minor or subclinical forms of the dry eye syndrome are more prevalent than commonly believed. When fully developed, the syndrome is known as keratoconjunctivitis sicca or Sjögren's disease, and it can result in blindness from corneal opacities. Diminution in tear production occurs normally with advancing age. It also may be hereditary or a consequence of certain systemic diseases such as thyrotoxicosis. A history of recurrent bouts of irritation of the eyes with burning and itching often combined with a slight protrusion of the globe (exophthalmous) is suggestive. A preoperative Schirmer's test is then advisable to determine the amount of tear production. A small strip of absorbent paper is inserted into the anesthetized inferior fornix. Tear production is measured in millimeters over a given period. A Schirmer's test seems unnecessary in every potential blepharoplasty patient, but it can suggest the diagnosis when positive. The diagnosis is further confirmed by a lysozyme test. The absence of lysozyme in the tears is diagnostic.

Slit lamp examination of the cornea and conjunctiva reveals minute filamentous ulcerations in more advanced cases. Staining with rose bengal or fluorescein will identify the lesions.

The dry eye syndrome can be complicated and exacerbated by lid surgery because of the normal forces of wound contracture with the slight lagophthalmous and ectropion that frequently occur during the healing period. Patients with slight exophthalmous, a dropped lower lid, and "scleral show" before surgery, are particicularly prone to these mechanical forces of wound healing that can

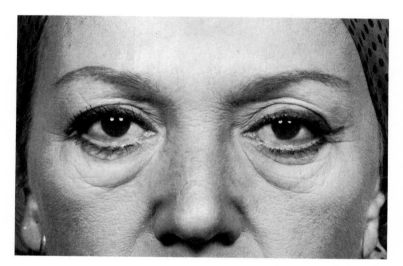

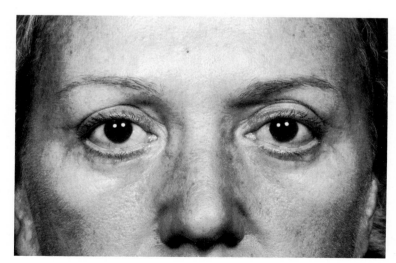

Figure 18–2. The preoperative photograph of this patient shows two unusual features that the surgeon needs to observe and discuss with a prospective patient: the moderate degree of scleral "show" and the slight exophthalmos. The scleral show cannot be improved by surgery, but it also should not be increased unless too much skin is excised. Often, however, a slight exophthalmos can be ameliorated by removal of orbital fat. Such a configuration of minimal scleral show and exophthalmos are frequently associated with the dry eye syndrome.

aggravate the symptoms (Figure 18–2). Patients with such contours should be carefully questioned about irritative eye symptomatology.

Full blown keratoconjunctivitis sicca is a serious and debilitating disease that can lead to xerophthalmia with multiple small filamentous ulcers of the cornea. Cicatricial replacement of the cornea with blindness can eventually result if the disease is untreated.

Cosmetic blepharoplasty is not necessarily precluded because of diminished tear production, but extreme caution in the surgical approach should be exercised. Skin and fat excision must be conservative. If the surgeon and patient elect to proceed with the surgery, a two stage procedure seems advisable: operation of the upper lids first followed a few weeks later by operation of the lower lids. Levator fixation to the upper lids is probably unwise in such patients. Should the dry eye syndrome develop after aesthetic blepharoplasty, protracted conservative treatment must be anticipated. Protection and lubrication of the cornea is the only treatment, and it is important at night when lagophthalmous and corneal drying from exposure is likely to result from loss of the normal air seal of the lids. Bland protective agents such as Lacrilube or Duralube and a complete air seal of the lids may be required at night for weeks or months until the lids seal naturally again during sleep. An artificial lid seal eye dressing is available commercially, or it can be fashioned by applying thin plastic sheeting such as saran wrap over the eye and sealing it to the skin with Vaseline. During the day, frequent application of "artificial tears" may be required to maintain corneal lubrication. Several such compounds are available. Valium (diazepam) may be helpful, since the combination of sleep loss and constant irritation of the eyes can extract a heavy emotional toll.

Many months may pass before significant improvement occurs. Ophthalmologic consultation should be obtained when the problem is first recognized.

EPIPHORA

Epiphora is not uncommon after blepharoplasty and is likely to persist for the first few days of the postoperative period. A temporary derangement in the mechanical outflow system of the tears, the result of normal wound edema and reaction, is often the cause. The lower eyelids serve as a gutter that drains the tears medially by gravity. Tears are drained through the inferior and superior canaliculi into the lacrimal sac and hence through the nasal-lacrimal duct into the nose. A high percentage of normal tear volume is dissipated by evaportion. Of the remainder, 85 per cent is drained via the inferior canaliculis. Blockages or mechanical derangements of the outflow tract of the lacrimal system can result in little or no overt tearing, except with stress. Epiphora in the immediate postoperative period is usually dissipated shortly. However, with persistent epiphora, a possible mechanical interference with the gravitational system of tear collection and drainage or a source of chronic irritation should be investigated. A caudal "drag" on the lateral third of the lower eyelid is a common cause of persistent epiphora. It can result from temporary scar pull or excessive skin excision of the lid.

Blockage of the canaliculi or duct system is not uncommon in unoperated patients. The canaliculi, ductile system, or lacrimal sac can become obstructed by concretions or mucous plugs requiring mechanical irrigation or dilatation to restore drainage. Persistent epiphora suggests distortion or deflection of the canaliculi, the inferior canaliculus being far more important in the drainage system than the superior canaliculus, since it drains most of the tears. Probing of the lacrimal system should be performed by experienced hands, since injury to the thin walls of the ducts or sacs that could further aggravate the condition by stenosis can occur.

Disturbance of the orbicularis muscle in and around the medial lower lid can aggravate epiphora. The orbicularis muscle is believed to serve as an assist pump by its squeezing action; severance of the canaliculi could conceivably occur during surgery, thus requiring reconstruction.

CORNEAL INJURY

Injury to the cornea is very difficult to treat, and prevention should be of the utmost importance. Gauze sponges should be replaced with atraumatic nonabsorbable synthetic sponges because gauze is abrasive to the delicate cornea. A protective corneal shield is favored by many surgeons during the operation; however, a corneal lens shield can itself cause an abrasion if inserted improperly. It is important to prevent desiccation of the cornea during surgery, as drying can result in abrasion, which can progress to ulceration because of the avascularity of the cornea. Frequent irrigations with sterile saline during the operation is therefore a good practice, particularly during the final suturing, when the lids are apt to be open and the cornea is exposed. At the conclusion of the procedure, a bland lubricating ointment should be applied liberally to the incisions and the conjunctival sac to protect the cornea during the first few hours following surgery until muscular closure is reestablished.

Thorough irrigation of the conjunctival sac at the end of the procedure helps to remove foreign matter such as bits and pieces of suture. Foreign material can cause corneal abrasion, a most uncomfortable and even painful condition.

Pain in the eye after surgery is a warning signal that requires investigation. Corneal injury such as abrasion must be ruled out. The cornea and conjunctival sac can be stained with fluorescein or rose bengal dye. Minute abrasions are sometimes only detected with a slit lamp. One is available in most hospitals. If a corneal abrasion is found, the eye should be treated with appropriate topical medication and put at rest with an occlusive dressing until healing has occurred.

DERMATOLOGIC COMPLICATIONS

Small, preexisting telangiectasias of the eyelid skin are likely to be intensified in size and numbers after surgery, particularly along the margins of the upper eyelids below the incision. Patients with such lesions may be advised of this possibility. Application of camouflaging cosmetics is the best treatment, since telangiectasias are not likely to improve.

Hypertrophic scarring of eyelid wounds is unusual but can occur, particularly in fair-skinned individuals. True keloids in the eyelid skin have not been reported and probably do not occur. Scar hypertrophy is most common along the medial portion of the incision near the epicanthus and treatment consists of watchful waiting. The surgeon should not be in a hurry to perform Z-plasties, V-Y plasties, or other maneuvers, since these may only complicate and prolong the scar resolution. Intralesional injections of minute doses of steroids may accelerate resolution of the hypertrophy;

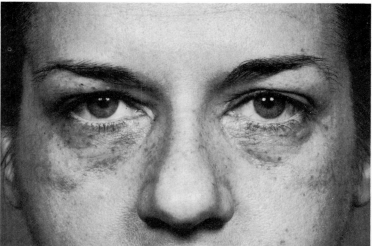
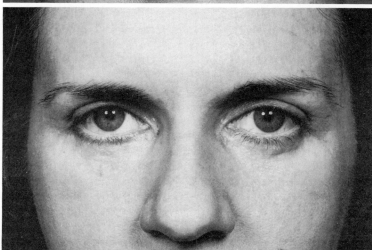

Figure 18–3. In certain types of pigmentation, the pigment is quite superficial and responds to chemabrasion. The irregular and unsightly pattern of pigmentation seen in this patient had been present since her childhood. Blepharoplasty followed in six weeks by deep chemical peel achieved the result shown in the postoperative view, which has persisted for two years.

however, improvement almost always occurs with the passage of time.

Increased pigmentation of the skin should be noted prior to surgery because it is unlikely that the operation will improve the problem and may in fact aggravate it. Sometimes, reducing the convex lid contour caused by bulging periorbital fat and redundant eyelid skin apparently improves dark pigmentation by flattening the highlights. Prolonged postoperative ecchymosis can result in dark discoloration of the eyelids sometimes for many months following surgery. This problem is, fortunately, uncommon and usually self-curing. Observation is the proper method of treatment. Discoloration disappears even after 12 to 18 months, except in exceedingly rare individuals in whom it can apparently persist for life.

Superficial melanotic pigmentation of the eyelid skin can often be improved or eliminated by a deep chemical peel (Figure 18–3). Chemical peel can be done six to eight weeks after blepharoplasty. It can enhance the result of blepharoplasty not only by reducing superficial pigmentation but also by removing many of the remaining fine rhytides that cannot be removed safely at operation.

The eyelid skin is very thin and rich in epithelial cells. Postoperative milia inclusion cysts are common after surgery, as epithelial debris may become trapped in the wound. Milia are easily evacuated through a stab wound made with a small hypodermic needle or a #11 blade. Larger inclusion cysts require excision. Epithelial tunnels will result if sutures are left in the eyelid skin for longer than four or five days (Figure 18–4). The epithelium grows rapidly along the suture tract and lines it to form a tunnel. It is therefore important to remove all interrupted sutures in the eyelid skin within 48 hours after surgery, leaving only subcuticular sutures and those in the lateral skin of the orbital region for another two or three days where epithelial tunnels are not likely to occur. If tunnels form, they are treated by exteriorization. A fine scissor blade is inserted into the tunnel and the covering epithelium is snipped away.

HEMATOMA

Hematomas can occur anywhere in the blepharoplasty wound. Localized subcutaneous or submuscular hematomas following surgery often are not recognized until after much of the immediate swelling and ecchymosis have subsided. Such localized hematomas become liquified in approximately seven to nine days after the surgery. They should be thoroughly evacuated. It is rare that aspiration of hematomas is completely effective; therefore it is best to reopen the blepharoplasty

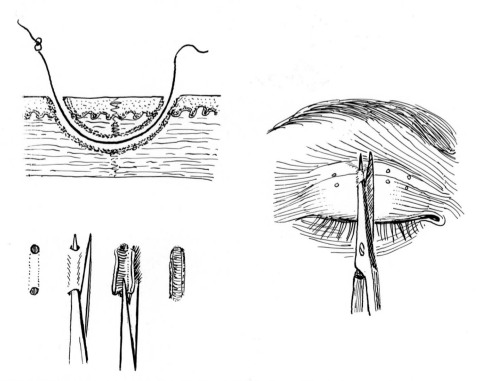

Figure 18–4. Epithelial tunnels that result from leaving sutures in the eyelid skin for more than four or five days are treated by unroofing them (marsupialization). The technique is simple and efficient. (After Converse.)

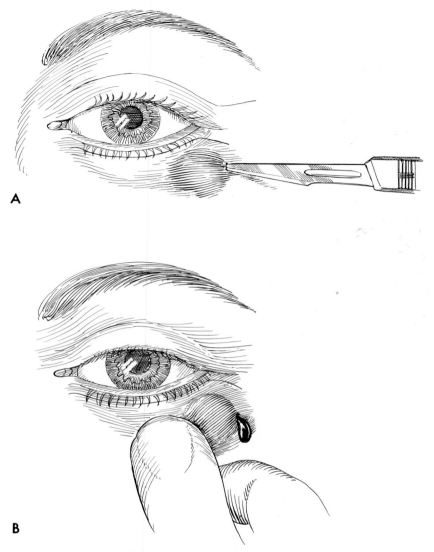

Figure 18–5.   If a small, localized hematoma of the eyelid develops postoperatively (*A*), it should be removed at about eight days by making a stab wound with a #11 blade and pressing out the contents with the thumb (*B*).

incision adjacent to the hematoma or make a separate stab wound over it with a #11 blade (Figure 18–5). The clot should be painstakingly and thoroughly evacuated. Every effort should be made to evacuate the hematoma completely during its liquid stage (Figure 18–6). Any residual clot will contribute to the formation of a firm organizing scar, which may persist for many months and be a source of annoyance to the patient. Such persistent scar nodules are best treated with injections of very dilute, small doses of intralesional steroids, such as triamcinolone acetate. Caution is advised in the use of steroids because there is considerable individual variation in response to these injections. Significant subcutaneous atrophy can occur in some patients. Rarely more than 2 mg of triamcinolone or related compounds are required at

any one injection. It is wise to space the injections at least two to three weeks apart so that the effect can be measured and a cumulative effect can be avoided.

An acute hematoma discovered immediately following surgery is better left undisturbed until liquification occurs. Early clots are poorly defined, adherent to surrounding muscle, and difficult to evacuate.

Retrobulbar hematoma

Retrobulbar hematoma is a feared and spectacular complication of blepharoplasty. Blood collects in the deep tissues throughout the soft tissues of the orbit behind the orbital septum. Puncture of a small vessel during deep injection of the fat pock-

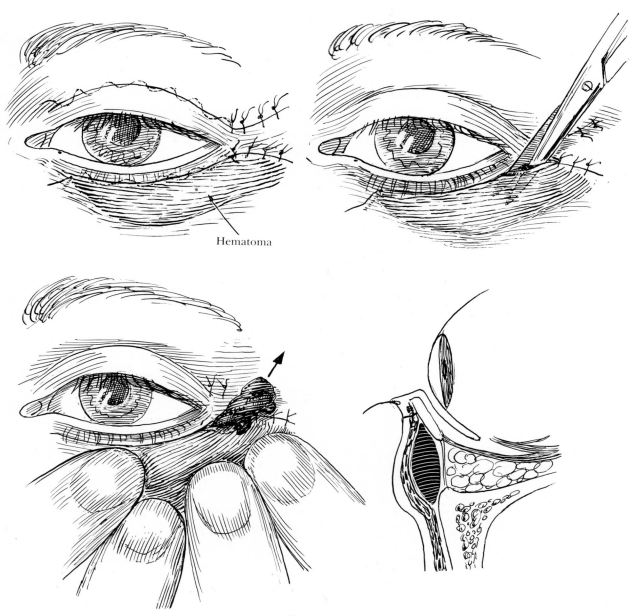

Hematoma

Figure 18–6

ets is the usual cause. It is therefore best to delay deep injections of local anesthetic into the fat pockets until immediately before making an incision into the orbital septum. Bleeding from open vessels of the fat pedicle stumps can also cause retrobulbar hematoma, but much less frequently than do punctured vessels. The offending bleeder in a fat pedicle can often be identified and coagulated, whereas in the retrobulbar hematoma caused by deep needle injection, the exact point of bleeding is rarely distinguishable.

Signs of retrobulbar hematoma are unmistakable: the eye becomes stony hard and proptotic and the lids are forced back from the globe, causing the eye to protrude further and further. Treatment during operation consists of opening the orbital septum extensively and exploring the deeper orbit insofar as is safe and practical. As stated, it is rare that the offending bleeding point is found. The blood is not locally collected as it is in localized hematoma but is infiltrated throughout the fat and soft tissues, making effective drainage difficult or impossible. It is probably just as wise to continue the operation as it is to stop it. It seems reasonable to assume that decompression of the orbital contents by opening the orbital septum

widely would help. Likewise, the remote possibility of identifying the bleeding point is enhanced.

When retrobulbar hematoma is apparent, the intraocular pressure should be measured with a tonometer. A moderate elevation of pressure is not unusual and may persist for several hours. A temporary tarsorrhaphy suture through the eyelids may be helpful as a postoperative measure to protect the cornea if the proptosis is not too severe. Pressure dressings are not required in the author's opinion, since further pressure on the globe and central retinal vessels seems inadvisable.

Postoperative treatment of retrobulbar hematoma consists primarily of observation, application of cold compresses, use of diuretics to reduce the extracellular fluid volume, and medical reduction of the blood pressure when elevated. The consultation and advice of a qualified ophthalmologist should be sought. Paracentesis of the anterior chamber of the eye in order to decompress the elevated intraocular pressure has been suggested. Such treatment is controversial. Until the rationale is established by further investigation, the technique must be considered inadvisable in most cases unless strongly suggested by a qualified ophthalmologist who is familiar with the problem. In the

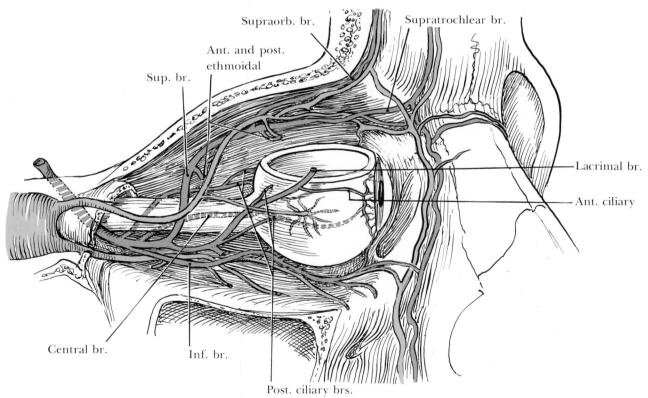

Figure 18–7.   Retrobulbar hematomas on rare occasions may produce pressure on the central retinal vasculature and cause temporary or permanent loss of vision. This complication is extraordinarily rare, considering the vast numbers of blepharoplasties done each year. Permanent blindness has not been satisfactorily reproduced in experimental animals.

author's experience with five instances of retrobulbar hematoma, paracentesis was performed in none and a prompt recovery was experienced in all. A recent clinical report by Huang et al. (1977) of ten cases of retrobulbar hematoma from trauma or elective surgery showed no permanent visual disturbances. In their series, temporary elevation of the intraocular pressure readings were common. Anterior chamber paracentesis was not performed, despite elevated pressures.

Retrobulbar hematoma, so frightening at onset, most often subsides dramatically within 12 to 24 hours following surgery. Blindness has been attributed to retrobulbar hematoma; however, a direct cause and effect relationship has not been established. The mechanism is thought to be pressure on the central retinal vessels (Figure 18–7). Fry (1969) injected large volumes of blood into the posterior orbit in monkeys. Although he produced temporary interference with vision, permanent blindness did not occur with this technique in any animal. Similar experiments in rabbits by DeMere et al. (1974) and Huang et al. (1977) failed to produce permanent blindness in these animals. Retrobulbar hematoma is well known to eye surgeons who administer large numbers of local anesthetics by deep orbital injection. The general consensus is that it is more frightening than threatening. However, the patient should be carefully followed until complete resolution has occurred.

BLINDNESS

Blindness is the most feared complication of eye surgery, yet knowledge of its relationship to the blepharoplasty operation is scant. Existing documentation seems too flimsy to invite definite conclusions — the patients were dissimilar and related disease processes such as hypertension and diabetes were present in many. It seems probable that progressive and unrelieved pressure from retrobulbar hematomas could result in blindness by choking the ophthalmic vessels, but such an end result must be exceedingly rare. Retrobulbar hematoma from all causes occurs with insufficient frequency to identify a causal relationship to blindness. Blindness associated with blepharoplasty or retrobulbar hematoma is exceedingly rare.

Idiopathic optic atrophy has been reported as a cause of blindness following blepharoplasty but could well have been incidental to the surgery. It seems reasonable to assume that many cases of blindness following blepharoplasty have not been reported, although it is important that such patients be documented. Preoperative binocular ophthalmologic evaluation of the patient is obviously essential from a legal point of view, in the event such a serious problem as blindness should be discovered in the postoperative period.

A review of seven cases of blindness following blepharoplasty was reported by Moser et al. (1973). The data was obtained through a comprehensive international survey of plastic surgeons. They were able to uncover only seven instances of unilateral blindness occurring simultaneously with blepharoplasty or in the immediate postoperative period. The authors concluded that the coincidence was "extremely rare, as the surgeons surveyed had doubtless done tens of thousands of blepharoplasties." In the group, they found three cases reportedly due to retrobulbar optic neuritis and one to an optic nerve injury that was unproven. They speculated that such changes were probably the results of fascicular changes of an unrecognized central nervous system disease such as multiple sclerosis or toxic amblyopia. Thrombosis of the retinal artery and vein was reported as the cause of two cases of blindness. The final conclusion of these investigators was that no causal relationship could be established.

Hueston and Heinze (1972) told of a 37-year-old patient who, following an uneventful blepharoplasty, developed severe orbital ecchymosis and swelling and a rise in the intraocular tension that led to blindness. This patient apparently had a retrobulbar hematoma and was noted to have a general interstitial extravasation of blood. They could not determine a discrete orbital hematoma, which is not unusual since retrobulbar hematomas are not usually so circumscribed. A cessation of blood circulation in the retina and optic disc was noted. Paracentesis of the anterior chamber was performed, and the patient made a complete recovery. This experience led to the authors' primary recommendation, which was careful observation of patients following surgery and prompt anterior chamber paracentesis at the onset of increased intraocular pressure (Hueston, 1977).

ENOPHTHALMOS

Enophthalmos following blepharoplasty can often be anticipated and therefore avoided by careful preoperative examination. Patients with "deep set" eyes or prominent infraorbital bony margins present an ideal anatomic predisposition for developing enophthalmos following removal of redundant periorbital fat (Figures 18–8 and 18–9). Great care should be exercised in such patients to remove a minimal amount of fat (Figure 18–10). If

Text continued on page 540.

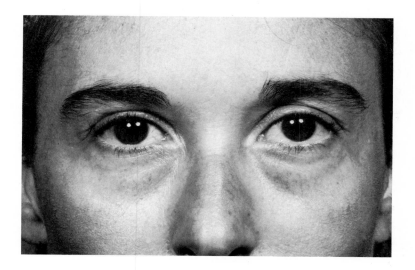

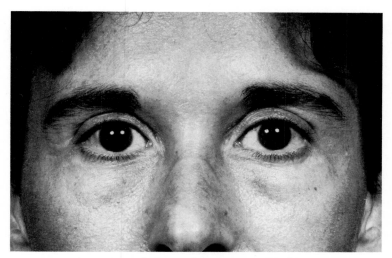

Figure 18–8.   This young woman demonstrates bulging of the lower eyelids from what was thought to be protruding fat. However, as can be seen in the postoperative view, blepharoplasty with removal of the fat pockets did not entirely correct the appearance of swelling in the lower lids. On careful postoperative examination, it was determined that these remaining ridges were caused by prominence of the bony infraorbital rim. It behooves the surgeon to examine each patient carefully before the operation to avoid disappointment with the operative result.

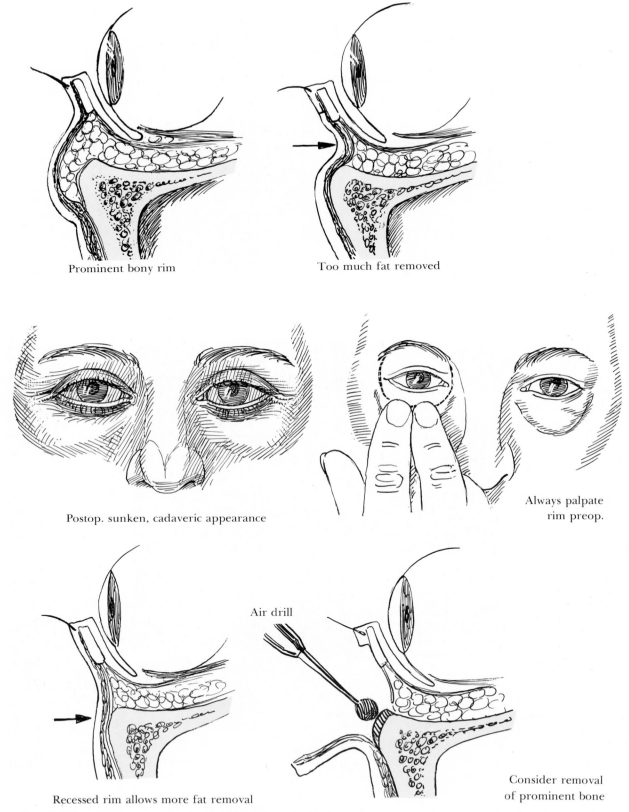

Prominent bony rim

Too much fat removed

Postop. sunken, cadaveric appearance

Always palpate
rim preop.

Air drill

Recessed rim allows more fat removal

Consider removal
of prominent bone

Figure 18–9.   The amount of bulging fat and the anatomic characteristics of the bony rims are important in order to anticipate the results of fat removal. In the presence of strong, forward-projecting bony infraorbital rims, excessive fat removal can result in enophthalmos. The treatment of enophthalmos still is quite unsatisfactory. A possible solution is to bur down the bony rim carefully.

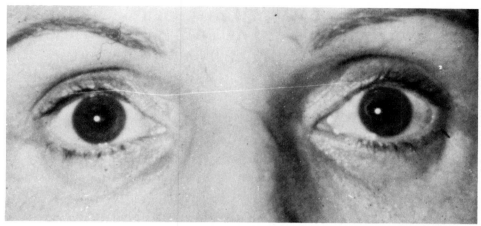

Figure 18–10. Marked enophthalmos with a cadaveric sunken appearance resulted in this patient following blepharoplasty. Too much fat was removed in the face of strong bony rims. Free fat grafts from the submental area have been used by Loeb (1979) to correct this problem.

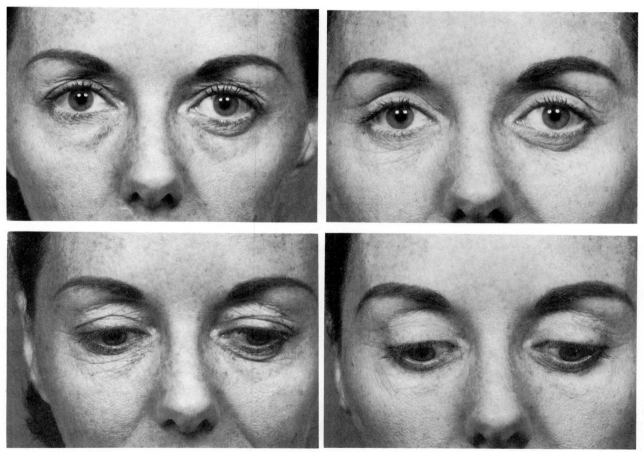

Figure 18–11. Postoperative problems and dissatisfied patients can often be avoided more easily if the surgeon exercises all his powers of perception in studying each patient preoperatively. Professional photographs such as these are sometimes more revealing than personal examination. This patient underwent a standard blepharoplasty but was not happy with the result; friends said that she looked "peculiar" and that her eyes were different. Because she was a photographer's model, her problem was acute. Examination of the photographs in retrospect clearly showed that the two eyes were indeed quite different, the left appearing much larger than the right — an asymmetry camouflaged preoperatively by excess skin and small fat bags.

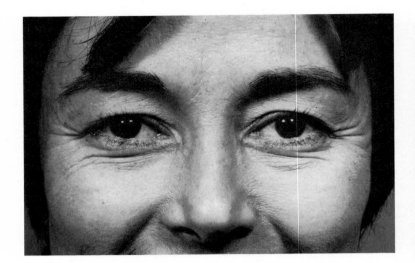

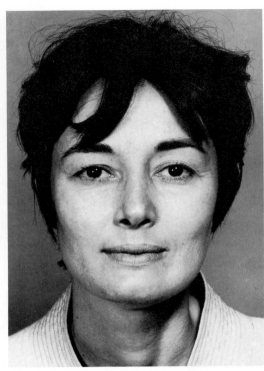

Figure 18–12.   This patient was in her early thirties and had a typical familial skin fold of the upper lid, the type that was described in the early literature on the subject and that has been termed "blepharochalasis." Note the natural asymmetry of her eyes. The left eye is larger than the right.

Illustration continued on the opposite page.

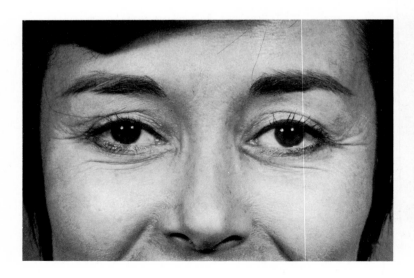

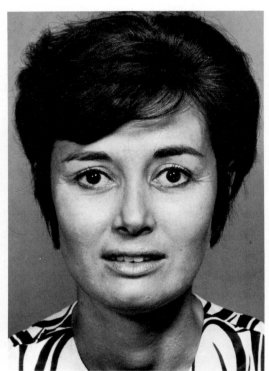

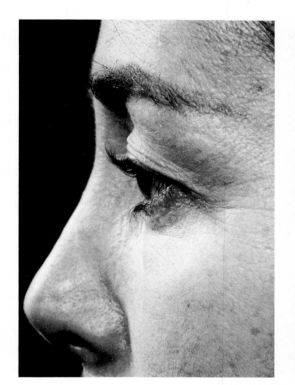 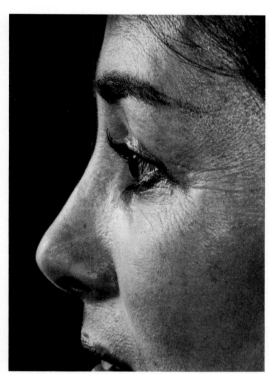

Figure 8–12   *Continued.*

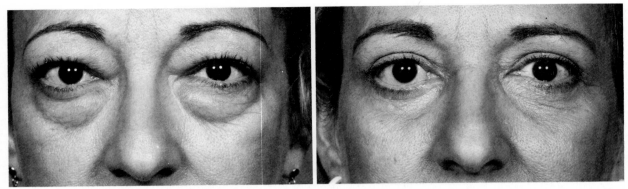

Figure 18–13. Most people have asymmetry of the face and therefore of the eyes to some degree. Some have significant asymmetry that they are often unaware of. The eyes can be markedly different in both size and shape. When the redundant skin and fat of the lids is considerable, as in the preoperative photograph of this patient, asymmetry can be camouflaged, only to become quite evident after surgery. Asymmetry should be noted in the preoperative examination and called to the attention of the patient to avoid postoperative surprises. Notice how much larger the right eye is than the left in this patient. This problem was difficult to see in the preoperative photograph. In fact, this patient had a measurable exophthalmos in the right eye without a history of thyroid disease.

the surgeon suspects that he has removed too much fat during surgery, an appropriate amount can be reinserted through the rent in the orbital septum in order to fill out the defect. When fat is replaced, the orbital septum should be sutured to retain the graft. The author has replaced small fat grafts in such a manner on a number of occasions with apparent success. It is unknown whether the fat survives as a free fat graft or simply fills in the contour from fibrous organization of the transplant.

Once established, it is exceedingly difficult to correct the cadaverous appearance of enophthalmos. Dermis-fat grafts performed subsequently were not successful; however, Loeb (1979) has recently reported successful correction of the problem in several patients with free fat grafts from the submental fat pad placed deep into the orbital septum. The use of prosthetic substances in the periorbital tissues in the absence of blindness is considered unwise under most circumstances.

Careful reduction of the prominent bony orbital margins with an air-driven polishing bur might well be effective in some cases.

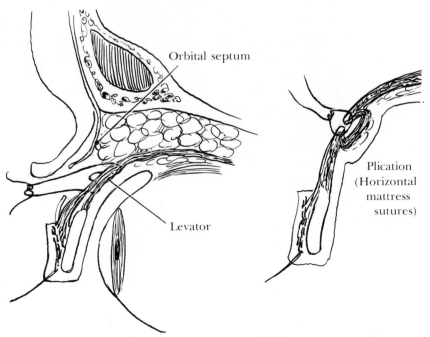

Orbital septum

Levator

Plication
(Horizontal
mattress
sutures)

Figure 18–14. Levator plication.

ASYMMETRY

Almost everyone has some degree of asymmetry of the eyes, adnexae, and orbits. When camouflaged with redundant skin and/or periorbital fat, asymmetry may not be obvious to the patient until after aesthetic blepharoplasty. Although asymmetry is significant in many patients, it is astonishing how few people are aware of it. It is good practice to point out such differences preoperatively (Figures 18–11 through 18–13).

Asymmetry may be related to unilateral ptosis. Plication of the levator expansion or fixation to the tarsal plate on one or both sides can correct or improve the asymmetry in such patients (Figure 18–14). Often, asymmetry can be improved if not completely corrected by varying the soft tissue resection from side to side during surgery.

The levator expansion inserts into the superior border of the tarsus with fibrous attachments to the dermis that form the supratarsal fold. The smooth muscle component that lies behind the aponeurosis is known as Müller's smooth muscle (Figure 18–15). It is spasm of this muscle in Grave's disease that elevates the lid and produces the characteristic stare (Figure 18–16).

Figure 18–17 shows the improvement in a patient with marked spasm of Müller's muscle in both eyes. The thyrotoxicosis was under control for several years. Müller's muscle was sectioned subtotally under local anesthesia. Exophthalmos with spasm of Müller's muscle can be the only sign of Grave's disease and can precede protein changes in the blood or systemic signs and symptoms by many months and sometimes years. These eye signs can be hidden by blepharochalasis and palpebral bags. If not discovered during the preoperative examination, a surprise is in store for both patient and surgeon. Careful examination before surgery will usually reveal both exophthalmos and levator

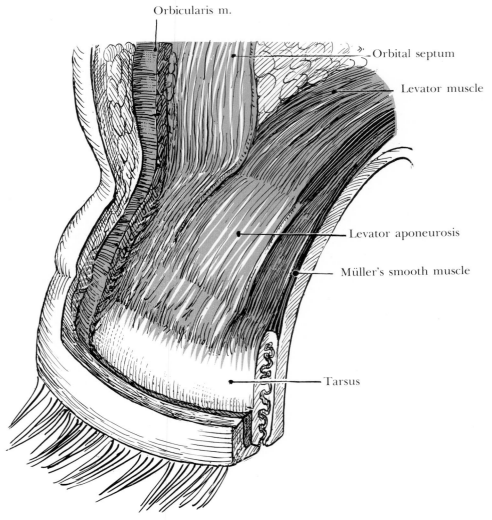

Orbicularis m.

Orbital septum

Levator muscle

Levator aponeurosis

Müller's smooth muscle

Tarsus

Figure 18–15

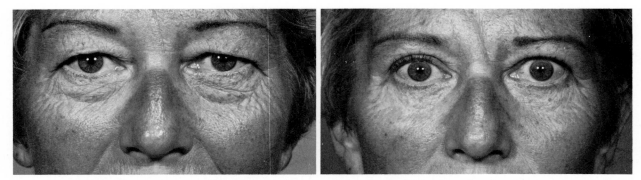

Figure 18–16.   The typical "stare" of thyroid disease caused by spasm of Müller's muscle became evident in this patient after correction of her blepharochalasis. Careful preoperative examination will disclose this problem before surgery.

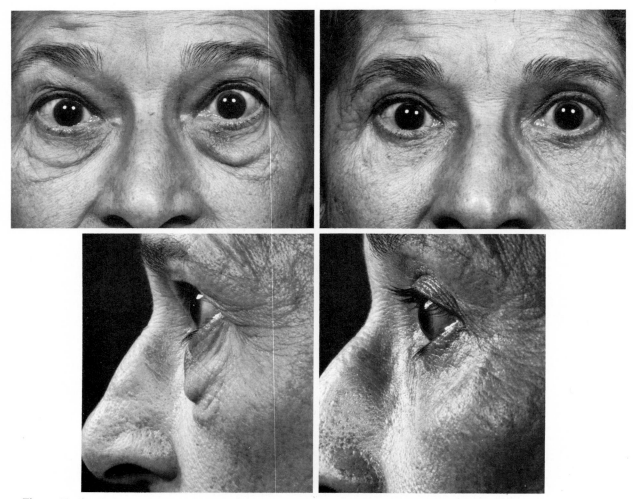

Figure 18–17.   Subtotal resection of Müller's muscle produced some correction of the muscle spasm and lid retraction in this elderly patient with long-standing disease.

spasm. Levator spasm in the patient with quiescent Grave's disease can be improved by partial sectioning of Müller's smooth muscle.

PTOSIS

Ptosis can be inherited or acquired. Marked excessive skin, soft tissues, and fat of the upper eyelids (blepharochalasis) can cause relative ptosis. Excision of redundant tissue in such cases can correct the condition. Loss of power of the levator muscle results from a variety of local, neurologic, or systemic causes (Figure 18–18). A simple reefing of the levator expansion may improve the situation in minor paresis (Figures 18–14 and 18–19). On the other hand, sudden onset of ptosis may be associated with neuromuscular disorders. Investigation should rule out such factors; for example, ptosis can be the first symptom of myasthenia gravis. Mustardé (1975, 1976) recently provided an excellent review of ptosis and corrective techniques.

Disparate resection of soft tissue or imbalance in the level of levator fixation can also result in "relative" ptosis. Unquestionably, levator fixation into the dermis or tarsus as advocated by Sheen (1974), Flowers (1976), and others is a useful procedure in selected patients; however, great care should be exercised to suture the levator at exactly the same level on either side to prevent asymmetrical ptosis, although such disparity usually corrects itself with time.

POSTOPERATIVE WRINKLING

It is not uncommon for patients to complain of the appearance of small wrinkles of the eyelid skin after cosmetic blepharoplasty, particularly when the main problem to begin with was redundant fat (Figure 18–20). This is often a real observation rather than imagined, and it may be the result of reducing the ballooning effect on the skin caused by the bulging redundant periorbital fat and the interaction of the animated orbicularis oculi muscle with the skin. When the maximal

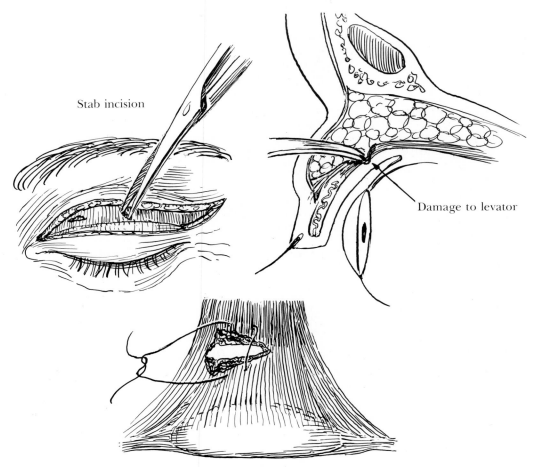

Stab incision

Damage to levator

Figure 18–18.   The aponeurosis of the levator can be damaged when the orbital septum is incised to remove fat. Such rents in the muscle expansion should be repaired primarily if recognized. Secondary repair is instituted if ptosis should result.

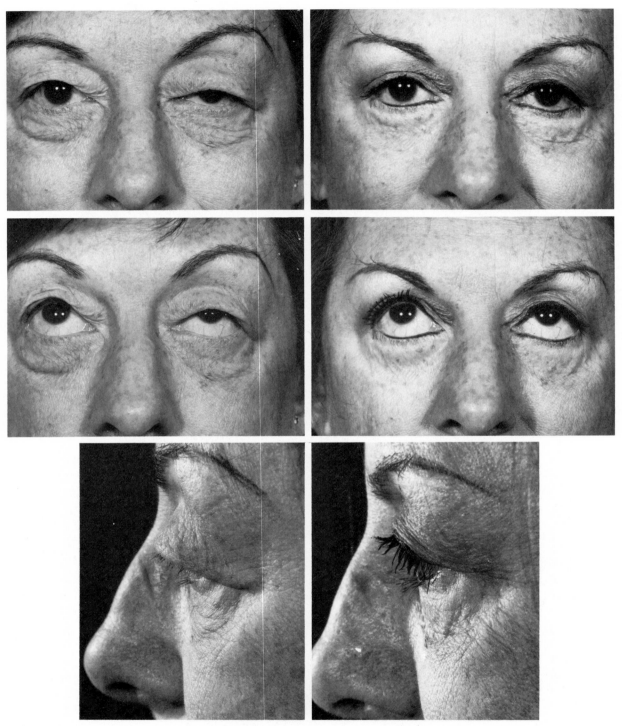

Figure 18–19. Severe, long-standing blepharochalasis in association with a slack levator expansion results in a form of pseudoptosis that can be improved and sometimes completely corrected by appropriate trimming of the skin fold, judicious resection of excess orbicularis muscle, and plication of the levator expansion. (See Figure 18–14.)

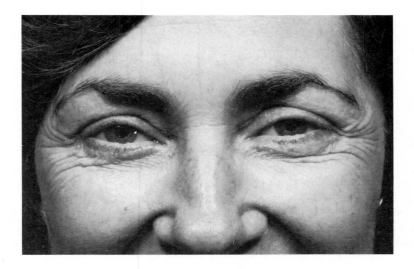

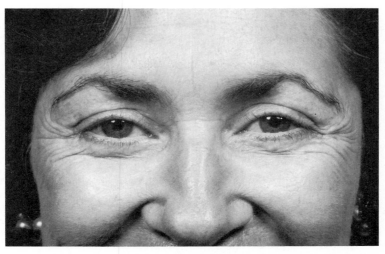

Figure 18–20.   As in primary blepharoplasty, note that the wrinkling present on animation in the secondary case can be improved but by no means eliminated. In the preoperative photograph, wrinkling is accentuated by the scars, which act as contracting bands. Smooth redistribution of the skin at the second operation helps to improve the situation.

amount of skin as well as fat has been resected in such an individual, a chemical abrasion may substantially improve such wrinkles. This has been effective in a number of our patients. Such a technique is also helpful in certain types of superficial increased pigmentation.

ECTROPION

"Scleral show" can occur in some patients no matter how conservatively the blepharoplasty was carried out (Figure 18–21). In some patients, such mild ectropion may be temporary, lasting several months, but in others, it is permanent. It sometimes can be anticipated before surgery if one takes note of unusual bulging of the globe, a relative shortness of soft tissue, or excessive pseudoherniation of orbital fat.

Minimal postoperative ectropion or "scleral show" is often caused by the removal of fat in patients who have excessive periorbital fat with a marked convex curve of the lids (Figure 18–22). In such patients, it is extremely important to recontour the skin flap so that it fills all contours of the dissected muscle beneath (Figure 18–23).

The immediate problem of ectropion is usually the result of chemosis and generalized wound edema and reaction. Such ectropion is not the result of excessive tissue resection and it is usually resolved within a few days. Severe chemosis can be rapidly resolved by the local application of topical steroids, often within a few hours. (See Figure 18–24.)

Text continued on page 550.

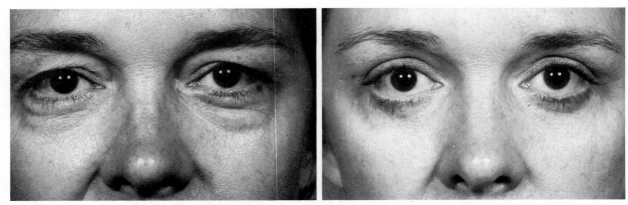

Figure 18–21.   In the author's opinion scleral show sometimes occurs following blepharoplasty despite every possible precaution to prevent it. It can occur both after skin-flap dissection and after the skin-muscle flap technique, and even when little or no skin is excised. The forces of wound contraction are probably responsible. It is unwise to promise any patient that scleral show after surgery will not exist. On the other hand, its occurrence in careful surgery is unusual enough that it need not be part of a routine "informed consent." In this patient, scleral show was present after a skin-muscle flap technique in which *no* skin or muscle was excised, only fat.

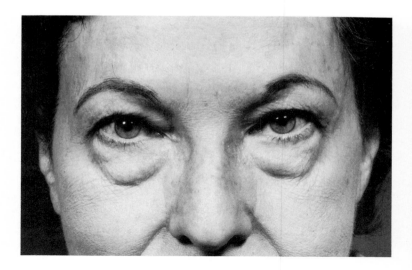

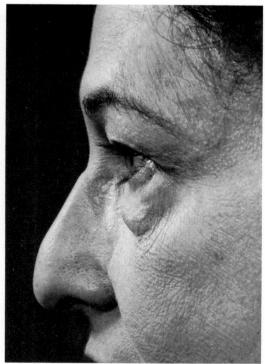

Figure 18–22. The author has been impressed by several patients with very large fat pockets of the lower eyelids who had some degree of scleral show or even mild ectropion after surgery, even when minimal skin was excised. Preoperative estimates of the skin excision in patients such as this are obviously valueless and even dangerous.

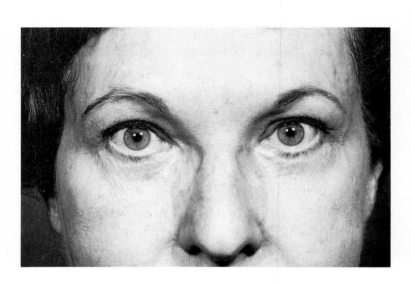

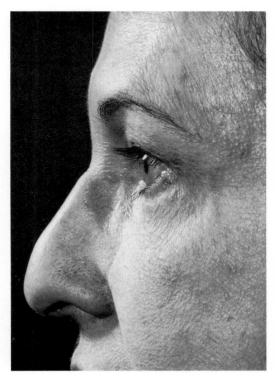

Figure 18–23.   One of the pitfalls of blepharoplasty is to be found in the patient with large fat bags of the lower lids, but with virtually no excess skin (*A*). In fact, the skin is stretched tight by the bulging fat, and removal of the fat may produce a slight concavity (*C* 2). No skin is excised in such patients. Instead, the undermined skin is looked upon as a full-thickness skin graft (*B*) and is draped over every contour of the wound exactly as a graft would be applied. Bridging over pockets or concavities can create a dead space (*D* 3), where fluid or blood can accumulate; subsequent contracture of the flap (*E* 5) can cause ectropion (*E* 4). The surgeon must always be cognizant of the fat that under anesthesia (even local anesthesia), the lower eyelid is relaxed and tends to sag. Failure to take this into account can result in too much skin being excised. Pressure on the globe elevates the lower lid skin into true position (*H*), and this maneuver can safely be exaggerated somewhat in many patients.

The skin flap (which is actually more of a full-thickness graft) must be applied exactly to the somewhat concave surface beneath (*F* and *G*). This usually leaves little excess to be resected in such patients.

See illustration on the opposite page.

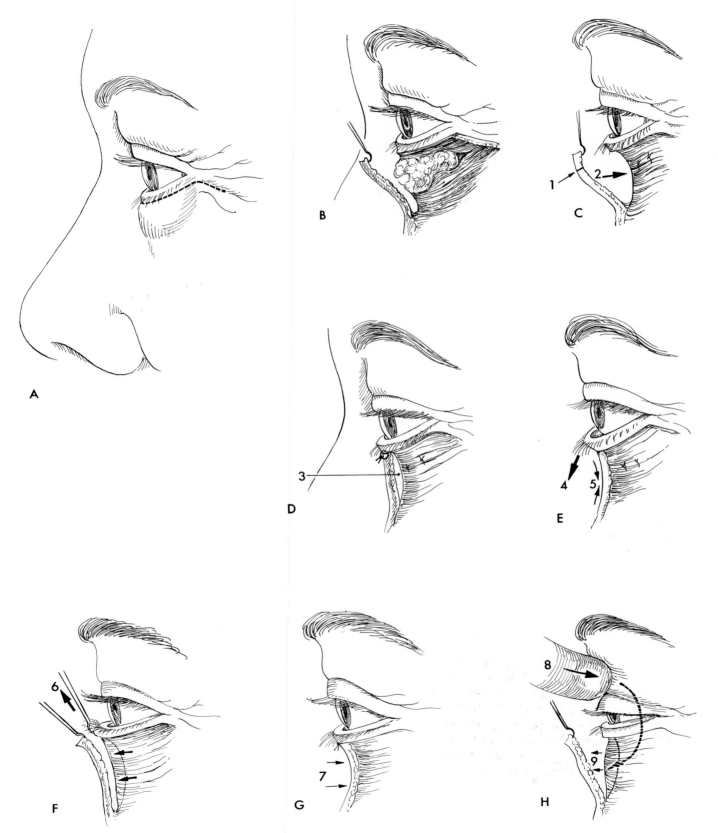

Figure 18–23. *See legend on the opposite page.*

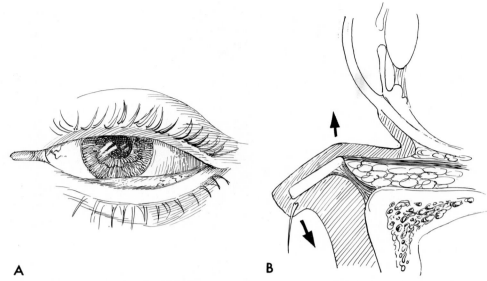

A   **B**

Figure 18–24. Temporary ectropion can result from a combination of edema and normal wound contraction; however, resolution occurs in a few days when these factors are resolved. Permanent ectropion such as this is the inevitable result of removal of too much skin and sometimes muscle. The lid is everted and held away from the eyeball because of scar contraction and outward and downward buckling of the tarsal plate (*B*). Chronic chemosis of the conjunctiva results (*A*), as well as chronic irritation of the conjunctiva and occasional secondary bacterial infection. Exposure keratitis or corneal ulceration usually does not occur unless excessive skin has also been removed from the upper lid, resulting in lagophthalmos.

If the lower lid is sufficiently pulled or everted in correction of permanent ectropion, the tear drainage mechanism is distorted, with the canaliculus pulled away from the globe. This gives rise to chronic epiphora, which is most distressing to the patient.

Another cause of temporary pulldown of the lower lid in the immediate postblepharoplasty period is a temporary paresis of the orbicularis oculi muscle, which results from surgical interference with terminal branches of the facial nerve and from wound edema and reaction within the muscle itself. Such muscle paresis is ordinarily short lived and clears up promptly following resolution of the acute wound reaction or following reinnervation of the muscle from undamaged nerve filament.

Permanent ectropion, such as that shown in Figure 18–25 is the inevitable result of the removal of too much skin and sometimes muscle. The lid is everted and held away from the eyeball because of scar contraction and outward and downward buckling of the tarsal plate (*B*). Chronic chemosis of the conjunctiva results (*A*), as well as chronic irritation of the conjunctiva and occasional secondary bacterial infection. Exposure keratitis and corneal ulceration usually do not occur, unless excessive skin has also been removed from the upper lid, resulting in lagophthalmos.

If the lower lid is sufficiently pulled or everted in an attempt to correct permanent ectropion, the tear drainage mechanism is distorted with the can-

aliculus pulled away from the globe. This leads to chronic epiphora, which is most distressing to the patient.

Cicatricial ectropion is the result of excessive removal of skin or muscle or damage to the orbital septum. If the surgeon is suspicious that he has removed too much skin at surgery, it should be replaced immediately as a free, full-thickness graft (Figures 18–26 and 18–27). Usually, such small grafts survive intact and are difficult to identify in several months. Donor sites for these grafts are shown in Figure 18–28.

The technique of skin excision of the lower eyelids is particularly important to prevent ectropion. The surgeon can use several "tricks" in excising the proper and safe amount of skin. Exerting downward pressure on the eyeball will elevate the lid (Rees, 1972); opening the mouth widely stretches the lower lid downward and is useful with local anesthesia. The lid margins should be free and the resected fat stumps should be tucked beneath the orbital septum to prevent adherence to this structure. The author's technique of skin excision has changed in recent years. I no longer routinely excise a lateral triangle but carefully drape the skin in a cephalic direction and then make one

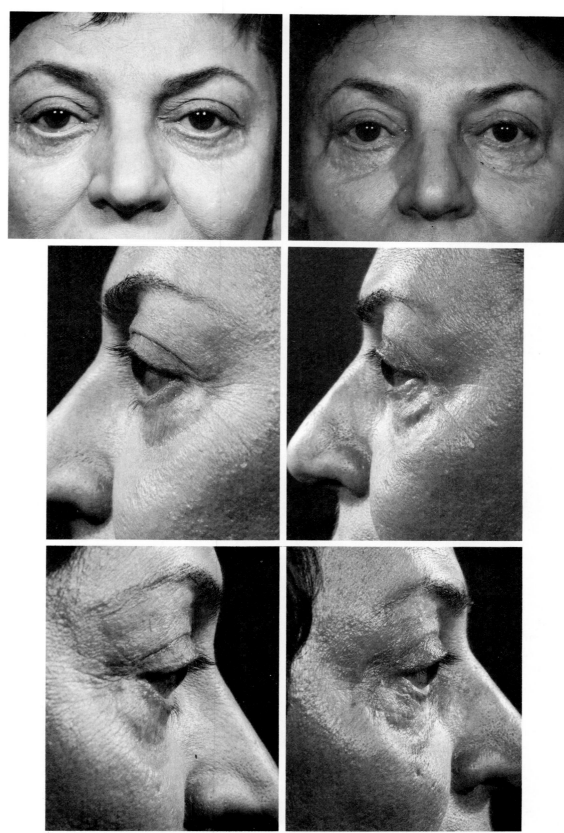

Figure 18–25. Cicatricial ectropion. An overcorrection was initially performed in each lid. Results of attempts to alleviate this problem are rarely perfect because of the considerable deep scar tissue that is usually present when the orbital septum is involved. Very large full-thickness grafts were used in each lower lid at two successive stages in addition to a full-thickness wedge resection of the lower lid, including the tarsus. The result is shown one year after the operation. Considerable improvement was achieved.

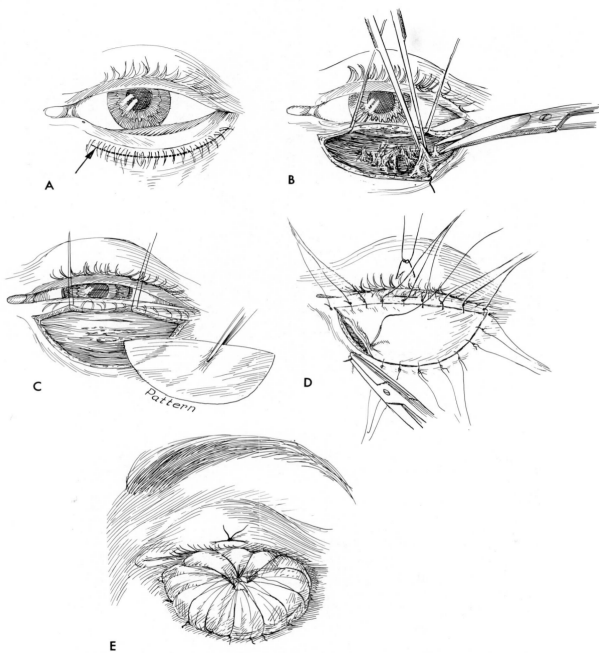

Figure 18–26.   Correction of ectropion requires replacement of the missing skin. The old wound is opened widely and all scar tissue is excised (*A, B*). The wound edges should not be undermined, because dead spaces beneath the skin can be the site of fluid accumulation or hematoma formation, which mitigates against graft survival. A pattern of the defect is then constructed with a thin sheet of plastic (*C*), and a full-thickness skin graft of the exact size is cut from the upper lid — provided a sufficient amount of skin is available. The graft is trimmed of all subcutaneous fat and sutured into place (*D*). A tie-over dressing is left in place for seven to ten days (*E*). The lids are closed during this period with a temporary tarsorrhaphy suture. A certain amount of contraction of the graft must be expected in the few weeks following surgery, but this is minimal with full-thickness grafts. If there is not enough skin on the upper lid to provide a graft of proper size, the graft should come from the retroauricular region, or, as a last resort, the supraclavicular area. The scar that results will probably be unsightly in this area, especially in a woman.

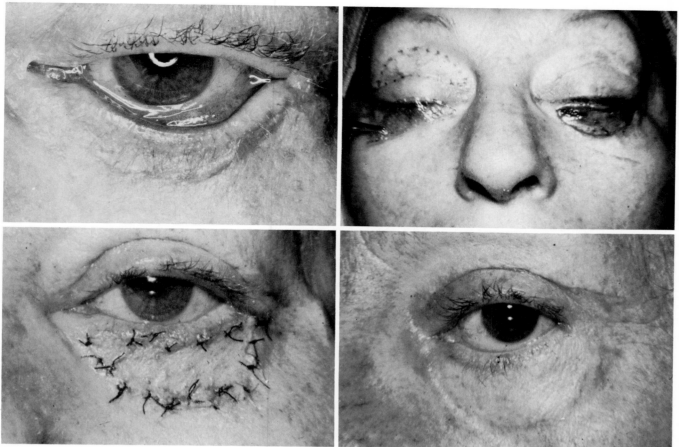

Figure 18–27. Ectropion of left lower lid treated by full-thickness skin graft according to the technique shown in Figure 18–26.

or two vertical cuts with small scissors down to the line of proposed skin excision. The redraped skin is then excised exactly along the incision line with very fine scissors. Such a maneuver has increased the safety of skin excision. Forceful lateral traction on the skin flap can actually cause ectropion in some cases (Fig. 18–29).

Observation for several months, during which time wound reaction subsides and scar tissue resolves and softens, is the best course for cicatricial ectropion. When the wound stabilizes, the defect is surgically recreated and resurfaced with full-thickness skin grafts. Occasionally, split-thickness skin grafts are required if excessive scarring is present or the defect is very large (Figures 18–30 through 18–33). The deficiency is always larger than anticipated; therefore, the graft should not be measured or cut before the wound is made. Some degree of contraction of all skin grafts must be expected, and some residual "scleral show" will probably exist after the most successful reconstruction.

Redundancy of the lower lid with its tarsal plate is common in older patients. A full-thickness wedge V-excision lateral to the corneal limbus and repair of the defect should accompany aesthetic skin corrections. Patients with a tendency to senile ectropion should have wedge-resection at the time of blepharoplasty to prevent eversion of the lid margin. The technique is simple. Repair is accomplished by an accurate approximation of the tarsal plate with fine interrupted sutures or a Mustardé pullout suture (Figures 18–34 and 18–35). Careful lineup of the lid margin is crucial to success. Marked redundancy of herniated fat or skin can easily mask early senile ectropion or loss of lid tone. A slight drooping of the lateral third of the lids, the "hound dog look," should alert the surgeon.

Diagnosis is confirmed by testing the lower lid redundancy. The lid is grasped between thumb and forefinger and stretched (Figure 18–36). Excess tissue or loss of tone is readily apparent by comparison with young lids that are tight. We do

Text continued on page 562.

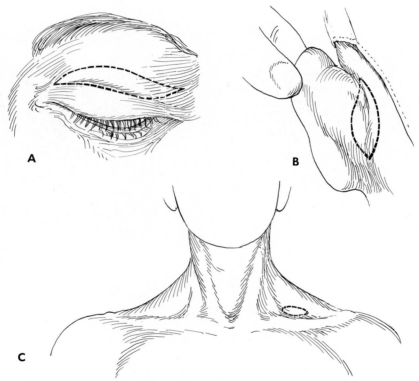

Figure 18–28. The preferred donor sites for full-thickness skin grafts in eyelid reconstruction are shown in order of their preference for color match, texture, and donor-site scarring; these are skin from the upper eyelid (*A*), retroauricular skin (*B*), and supraclavicular skin (*C*).

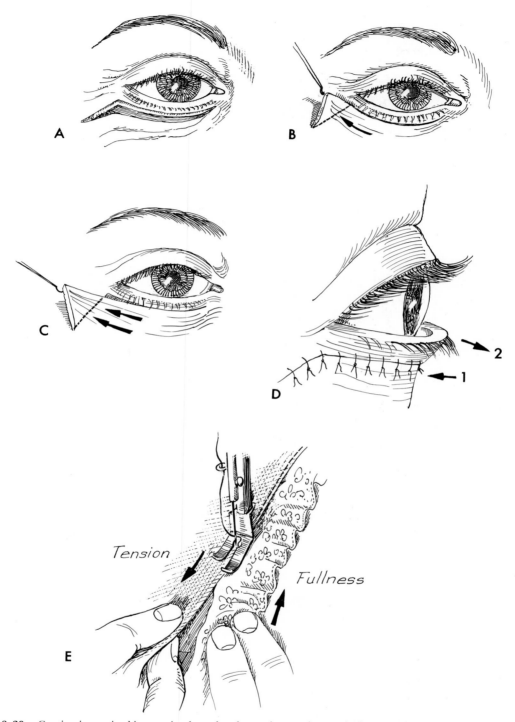

Figure 18–29. Caution is required in exerting lateral and superior traction on the lower lid skin flap preparatory to excision of the excess. If traction is excessive and the incision is located just below the tarsal plate, an outward buckling of the plate can occur because of the shortness of the skin and the tightness of the closure. The mechanism can be likened to the dressmaker's trick of making a ruffle (*E*). The lid will not be in contact with the globe, and tearing can result as well as conjunctival irritation from exposure.

The usual method of trimming excess skin of the lower lids is to exert lateral traction on the skin flap (*A* and *B*) and to remove most of the redundancy as a lateral triangle (*C*) rather than as a horizontal strip along the lower lid, which promotes the possibility of pull down. If too much is excised as a lateral triangle, the lower border of the tarsal plate can buckle forward (*D*) (From Rees, T. D.: Technical Considerations in Blepharoplasty and Rhytidectomy. Transactions of the Fifth International Congress of Plastic and Reconstructive Surgery, Australia, 1971, Sidney, Butterworth & Co. (Australia), Ltd., 1971, p. 1067.)

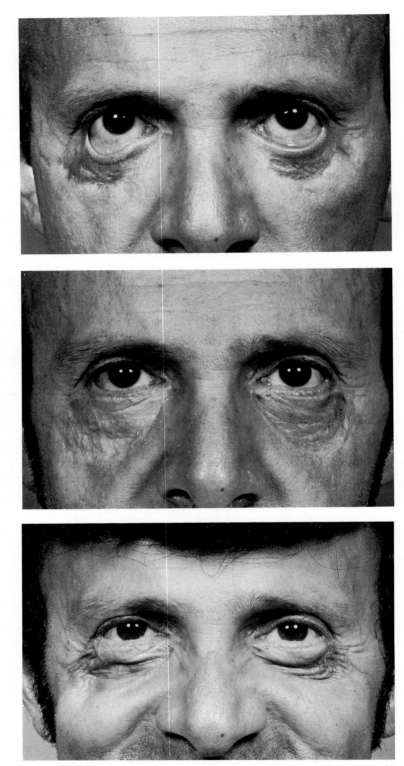

Figure 18–30.   Severe ectropion can result from excessive skin removal and poor timing of operations aimed at correcting the initial problem, as shown in this patient. Several attempts had already been made to correct bilateral ectropion that resulted from cosmetic blepharoplasty performed by another surgeon. Each of these procedures consisted of split-thickness skin grafting, and they were performed within several weeks of each other, during the period of maximum wound reaction and scar contracture. The final result consisted not only of severe ectropion but also of extensive scarring of surrounding skin and underlying muscle. The patient was not able to close his eyes.

The postoperative photographs of this patient demonstrate correction of the ectropion, but the large skin grafts are permanent cosmetic defects that cannot be eradicated.

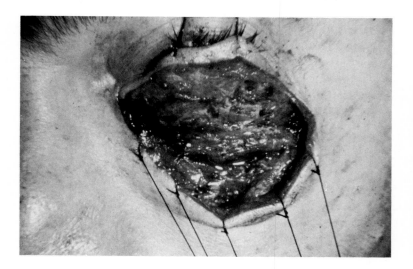

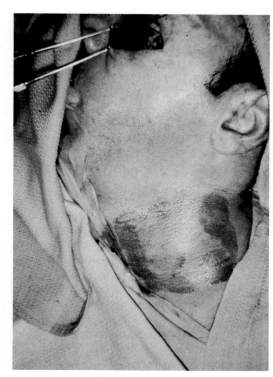

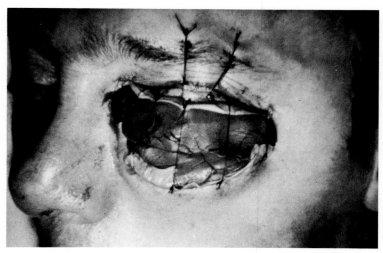

Figure 18–31.   Correction of the difficult problem shown in Figure 18–30 was undertaken by first re-creating the original defect. The remnants of the split grafts were excised, one side at a time. All scar tissue was dissected from the orbicularis muscle, and the septum orbitale was released along its entire attachment to the infraorbital rim (upper left). This was necessary in order to increase the vertical length of the lower lid, which had been firmly bound to the orbital rim by scar tissue. The skin edges of the inferior margin of the wound at the junction of the skin of the cheek were undermined to create a pocket after the method of McIndoe (Figures 18–32 and 18–33).

The neck was chosen as the donor site for a skin graft because a superior color match could be obtained (right). A thick split graft was used because of the size of the defect and because the scarring was so extensive that a full-thickness graft would have less of a chance of obtaining an adequate blood supply for survival. It is possible to obtain a rather large graft from the neck with a dermatome. The technique is facilitated by extending the skin by means of subcutaneous injections of large volumes of saline solution. Thus "blown up," the skin presents a sufficiently large and flat surface for the dermatome to be operated.

The graft is carefully draped into the pocket-like defect so that it is in contact with all raw surfaces and has a cuff of excess skin (lower left). Dental wax is then used to make an exact impression of the defect, taking care to fill all of its ramifications. The skin graft is applied to this stent with the raw surface up, and the stent is held in place by tie-over sutures. Note that the lower lid margin is elevated in a cephalad direction and maintained in an exaggerated position by sutures fixed to the forehead skin. This technique of overcorrection allows for subsequent contraction of the split-thickness graft.

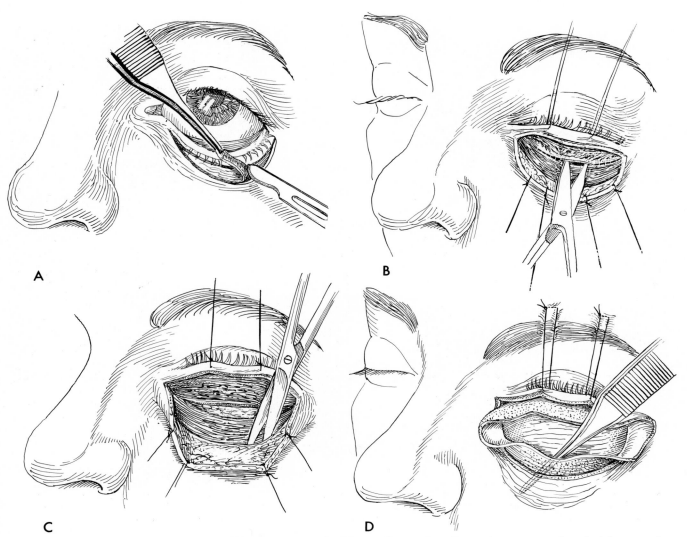

A

B

C

D

Figure 18–32.   Severe cicatricial ectropion of the lower lids with extensive scarring of normal structures and marked shortage of skin may simulate the deformity seen following burn injury. Such deformities may not be correctable with full-thickness skin grafts when circulation is in question because of thick scar tissue. Repair demands excision of all scar tissue (*A*) and dissection of a large pocket (*B* and *C*) into which a split-thickness skin graft molded around dental compound or similar material can be fitted (*D*).

One eye should be treated at a time. The stent is left in place for about 10 days. The immediate postoperative result is somewhat unpleasant, even with the ectropion corrected. The deep groove or pocket that is created is unsightly, but with the passage of several weeks, during which the graft contracts, the pocket will be greatly reduced in size. After contraction is complete and the scar tissue is sufficiently softened and matured, a secondary trim and correction of the junction between graft and skin can be undertaken.

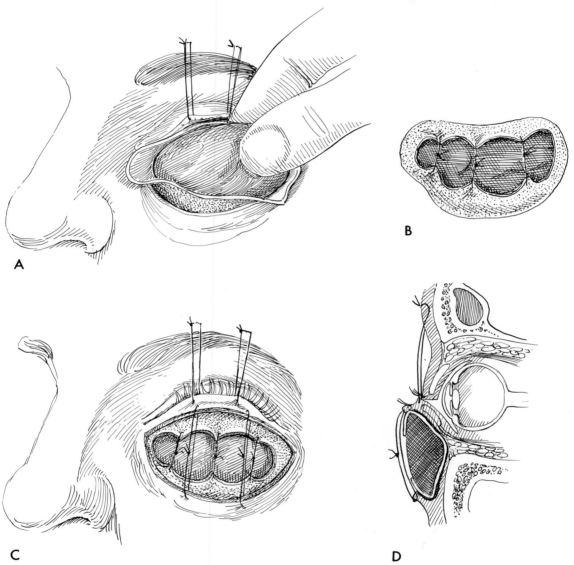

Figure 18–33. Split-thickness skin grafts for correction of ectropion are sometimes favored over full-thickness grafts in the repair of very large defects of the lids (Figure 18–30) when thick scar tissue precludes early vascularization of full-thickness grafts. Such split grafts can be taken from the neck skin if donor-site scarring is of secondary importance; otherwise, they are taken from the buttocks or thighs. The graft is applied to the stent mold of dental compound with the raw surface out (*A*). Dermatome glue can be applied to the mold for fixation, or sutures may be used to bridge across the mold (*B* and *C*). The lower lid is sutured to the brow for several days (*C* and *D*). Subsequent trimming of the raised edges of the recipient pocket may be necessary after contraction has occurred.

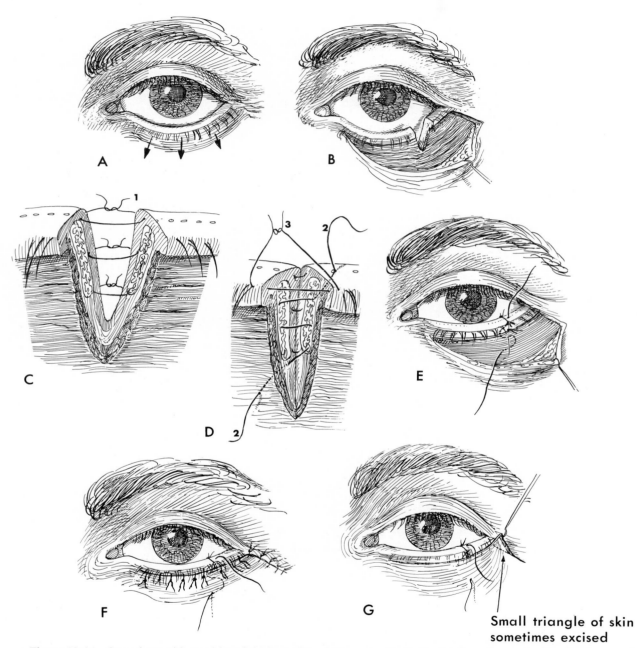

Small triangle of skin
sometimes excised

Figure 18–34.   In patients with atonicity of the lower lid, which can be familial in origin or the result of senile changes, the tendency toward ectropion can be aggravated by blepharoplasty. This is particularly true in males for some unknown reason. If ectropion develops after cosmetic blepharoplasty, and atonicity seems the primary cause (*A*), correction can be achieved by incising along the old blepharoplasty incision, undermining the skin flap, excising a suitably sized full-thickness wedge lateral to the limbus (*B*), and repairing the defect according to Mustardé's technique, with layer closure and a pull-out as shown in *C, D, E, F,* and *G.*

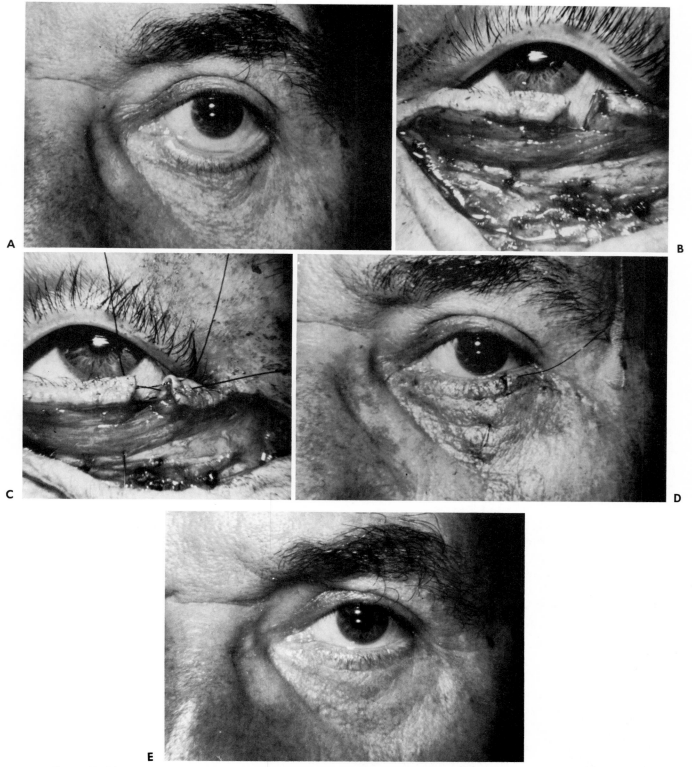

Figure 18–35.   Postoperative ectropion related to atonicity and not to excessive tissue removal is shown in *A*. The defect was recreated and a wedge was excised (*B*). A Mustardé repair was then accomplished (*C*). The immediate postoperative correction is shown in *D*; the final result is shown in *E*.

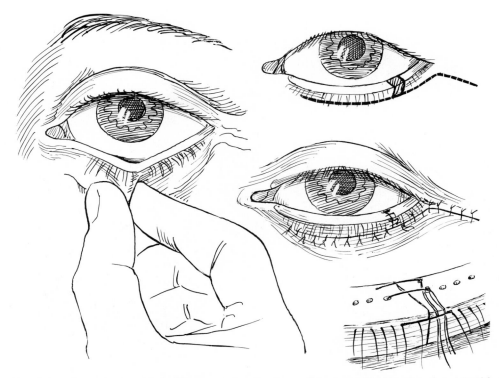

Figure 18–36. A useful test for loss of elasticity or tarsal redundancy of the lower lid is the "pinch test." With experience, the surgeon will be able to make an educated guess as to whether or not he should proceed with a wedge resection of full-thickness lid at the time of blepharoplasty in the older patient.

not hesitate to perform a V-excision routinely in older patients in whom a redundancy of lower eyelid is present.

SKIN SLOUGH

It seems remarkable that skin slough does not occur more often after complete undermining of the lower eyelid skin, since this maneuver results in what is almost a full-thickness skin graft. Skin necrosis is exceedingly rare because of the excellent blood supply in the area. The patient in Figure 18–37 appeared to have incipient slough of the skin of both lids following blepharoplasty. Typical blue-black superficial eschars developed. Treatment was expectant observation, and the result was

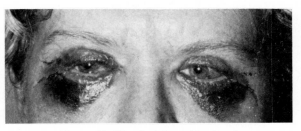

Figure 18–37. Incipient skin slough.

complete survival of both skin flaps without any loss whatsoever. Incipient or suspected slough should be treated conservatively (as is a frostbite injury), since the extent of tissue viability beneath the eschar is unknown until the eschar has separated. Complete epithelial healing usually occurs beneath the eschar. The surgeon should not be in a hurry to debride such wounds. A conservative policy is best. When healing is complete, any remaining skin deficiency can be repaired with a full-thickness skin graft.

EXTRAOCULAR MUSCLE IMBALANCE

The inferior oblique muscle occupies a position straddling the medial and middle fat compartments of the lower eyelid. Because of its relatively superficial position and its anatomic location, it can be damaged during the course of blepharoplasty when these two fat compartments are decompressed (Figure 18–38). The muscle can be injured by the cautery when the stumps of the excised fat are cauterized. It can also be traumatized by instrumental dissection in the area. Partial injuries usually heal without residual deformity shortly following the operation. Accidental complete resection of the muscle during the course of blepharo-

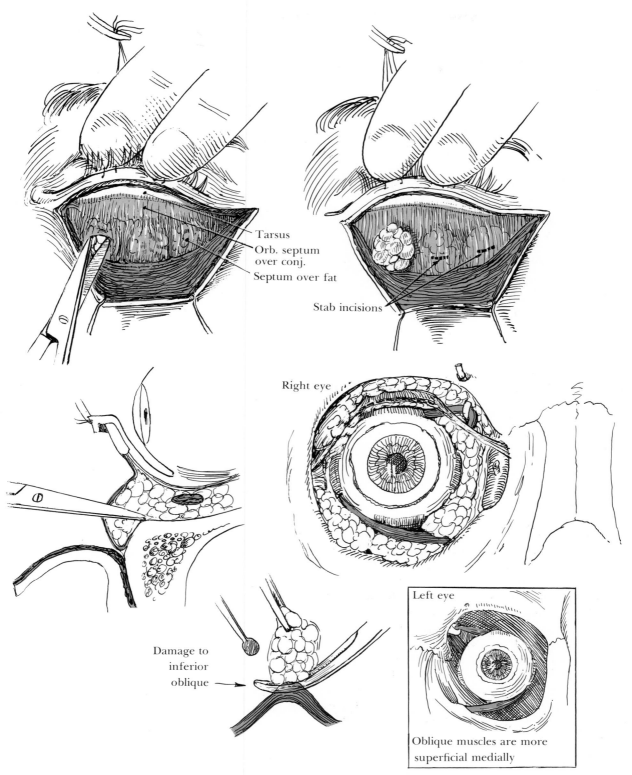

Tarsus

Orb. septum
over conj.

Septum over fat

Stab incisions

Right eye

Damage to
inferior
oblique

Left eye

Oblique muscles are more
superficial medially

Figure 18–38.   Extraocular muscle injury.

plasty is not unknown. It is recognized by persistent postoperative diplopia in which damage to the inferior rectus muscle is readily identified by ophthalmologic and visual field examination. Temporary palsy of the muscle is usually restored within six months. If damage to the muscle is proved and persists beyond this time, a resection of the inferior rectus muscle should be performed along with simple repair of the severed ends. In rare cases, if the deviation is severe enough, resection with a recession of the superior rectus muscle may be required to restore extraocular muscle balance.

Very rarely, the superior oblique muscle can be inadvertently severed at the tendon. In this situation, the superior oblique muscle should be freed from all scars in the area and a fat flap should be mobilized within the orbit and placed anterior to the tendon to prevent recurrence of adhesions to the old scar.

WOUND SEPARATION

Separation of the wound immediately after suture removal is not unheard of after blepharoplasty. It usually occurs along the lateral segment of the incision in the superior eyelids lateral to the outer canthus. Should dehiscence occur, the wound can be promptly resutured or brought together and splinted with sterile paper tape strips (steristrips).

INFECTION

Significant infection of blepharoplasty wounds is exceedingly uncommon, undoubtedly because of the rich and abundant blood supply to the area. Most surgeons do not employ prophylactic antibiotic therapy for blepharoplasty, as infection is so rare. If it occurs, however, prompt treatment with an appropriate antibiotic is indicated along with the application of warm compresses. Superficial pustules will occur around suture ends — in particular, at the medial suture exit of the subcuticular suture of the upper eyelid — if the sutures are left in place more than four or five days. The exudate should be gently expressed, and it usually causes no further problem.

LAGOPHTHALMOS

Lagophthalmos — the inability to close the eyes completely —is a common complaint during the immediate postoperative period. This can result in drying of the cornea and general desiccation and irritation of the conjunctiva and lid margins. A bland eye ointment is prescribed to use at night for patients with this problem. Methylcellulose or other protective solution eyedrops on retiring also provides protection until the condition has corrected itself. Daytime irrigation of the eyes with saline solution or any of the bland proprietary eyewashes is also helpful. Occasionally, lagophthalmos will continue for several weeks or months. The problem is rarely serious but can be a considerable nuisance.

Lagophthalmos may result from excision of too much skin from the upper eyelids. Careful preincision marking of the ellipse to be removed from the upper lids, using the Green forceps, will help to avoid this mistake. The upper lid should not remain open more than 3 mm at the end of the procedure.

If the skin shortage causing lagophthalmos is severe, a serious situation exists, for the cornea is no longer covered and protected by the upper lid. This results in desiccation, exposure keratitis, and eventual ulceration of the anterior chamber with possible perforation — a set of circumstances frequently seen following thermal burns of the eyelids. This severe degree of what is really ectropion of the upper lid requires emergency consideration, with release of the lid and immediate skin grafting. Such a problem must be exceedingly rare in cosmetic blepharoplasty; the author is aware of only one case.

CHRONIC BLEPHARITIS

Chronic blepharitis of a nonspecific nature has been seen following blepharoplasty. In my opinion, it is surprising that this problem is not more common. It is, in fact, so rare as to lead one to the conclusion that its occurrence may be coincidental. Obvious deformities of the lids such as lagophthalmos or ectropion can obviously lead to blepharitis. Treatment by a competent ophthalmologist is recommended. Recurrent chalazions or styes have also been seen following blepharoplasty, but these are usually considered coincidental since there is frequently a history of prior occurrence.

LOSS OF EYELASHES

Spontaneous loss of eyelashes has occurred twice in the author's experience. In both patients, the process proved to be reversible, however, and the lashes grew in again.

SECONDARY OPERATIONS

Secondary blepharoplasty is one of the most challenging and hazardous operations in the field of cosmetic surgery. It even ranks ahead of secondary rhinoplasty in technical difficulties and pitfalls awaiting the unwary surgeon. Such surgery should be undertaken only if, after careful assessment, the surgeon is certain that he can achieve a reasonable correction without creating further deformity. It is particularly perilous to undertake correction of minor secondary deformities in patients who have been operated on by another surgeon. Unfortunately, minor degrees of improvement are not always appreciated by the patient, even though the surgeon may feel he has accomplished a virtual miracle.

The most common deformities requiring secondary surgery after a primary eyelid repair are (1) bulging of the media fat pockets of the upper eyelids; (2) recurrence of a skin fold of the upper eyelid (Figure 18–39); (3) ptosis of the brow, often with a marked lateral skin fold (Figures 18–40 and 18–41); (4) residual herniated fat pockets of the lower eyelids, usually medial and middle and less often lateral; (5) elevated, irregular, or uneven scars, or scar contractures such as webbing near the lateral canthus (Figure 18–43); (6) varying degrees of ectropion because of excessive resection of the lower eyelids (Figure 18–44); (7) inability to close the upper lids, with corneal exposure; (8) excessive skin of the lower eyelids because of inadequate excision at the primary operation, best demonstrated on facial animation or squinting; (9) excessive pigmentation of the skin, more common after secondary blepharoplasty; and (10) the appearance of many fine wrinkles not visible before the original surgery and thought to be the result of the release of skin tension after fat removal.

Of prime importance in such surgery is the fact that there is rarely sufficient skin to spare at a secondary operation, particularly on the lower lids. This is an essential factor in planning the operation. It is *never* advisable to preestimate the amount of skin to be resected prior to a secondary procedure. Such advance planning will most often lead to the embarrassing situation of a serious skin shortage. Removal of secondary fat pseudohernias in patients in whom there is no skin to spare can also cause an acute shortage of skin, similar to that in the patient who, at the time of primary surgery, had very large fat bags and little or no excess skin.

In removing skin folds of the upper eyelids during a secondary operation, it is advisable to mark the estimated amount of skin to be removed by using a marking forceps, and then to excise *less* than this estimated amount. A further strip of skin can be excised if the first amount proves insufficient. If too much skin is excised, however, an immediate free graft may be necessary. Should the skin excision of the upper eyelids prove to have been overestimated, it is sometimes possible to narrow the defect by undermining the skin edges of the superior wound margin so that closure can be accomplished without a graft.

Even slight excess skin removal from the lower eyelids can result in a minor degree of ectropion. Lower lid ectropion is the most serious of the secondary complications requiring correction and is discussed elsewhere in this chapter.

Among the more common problems requiring a second operation are residual fat pockets in the medial corners of the upper or lower lids. Occasionally, the lateral fat compartments also require attention. If the skin excision was adequate, the surgeon need only incise the original wounds, separate the fibers of the orbicularis muscle, locate the bulging orbital septum over the offending fat pocket, and tease out the fat. It is then excised. A wide incision and exposure of the orbital septum is rarely necessary and should be avoided when possible.

In rare, selected cases, direct excision of persistent malar pouches resulting from edema, fibrosis, or unknown causes may be very helpful provided the patient will accept an external scar (Figs. 16–5 and 18–42).

BLEPHAROPLASTY OF THE ORIENTAL EYE

Since World War II, operations designed to construct a superior palpebral fold in the Oriental eyelid have become increasingly popular. According to Boo-Chai (1963), such operations have been performed for many decades by ophthalmologists in China and Japan, but have only recently been documented in the English language. In many cities of the Orient, as well as in areas containing large Oriental populations, such as Hawaii, this surgery has become commonplace. Except for Hawaii, however, these operations are infrequently performed in the United States.

In the typical mongoloid type of upper eyelid, the superior palpebral fold is absent. This condition occurs in about 50 percent of Orientals and is apparently caused by a dominant gene. Fernandez (1960) points out that some Orientals refer to the eye without a palpebral fold as the "single eye," and the eye with the fold as the "double eye." Just why many Orientals prefer to "Westernize" their eyes is not known, although it is thought to stem from the influence of motion pictures and the increasing intermarriage of Asian women and Caucasian men, particularly since the Second World War.

Text continued on page 572.

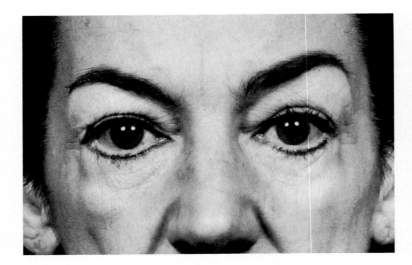

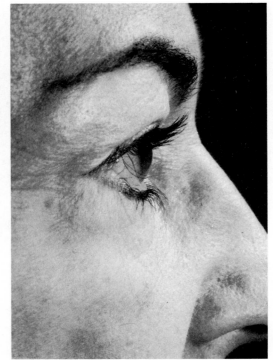

Figure 18–39. Blepharoplasty was performed in this patient several years earlier with good results. The views prior to secondary blepharoplasty show typical changes that can be expected to occur with the passage of time and that indicate the necessity for a secondary operation. Note that excess skin folds of the upper lids have reappeared, the result partly of gravity and partly of aging of the skin. Medial fat pockets are present in the upper lids, being worse on the left. These may have recurred because their removal at the original operation was too conservative. There is a very slight excess of fat in the lower lids as well.

The secondary procedure in this patient consisted of a standard removal of the upper lid skin fold, vigorous fat removal from the upper lids, and a very conservative fat removal and redraping of the skin of the lower lids after moderate undermining. No skin was excised from the lower lids since a slight shortage of skin already existed.

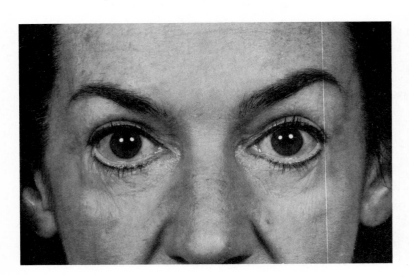

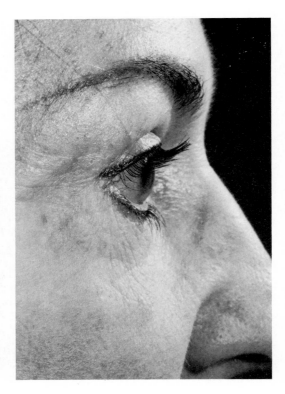

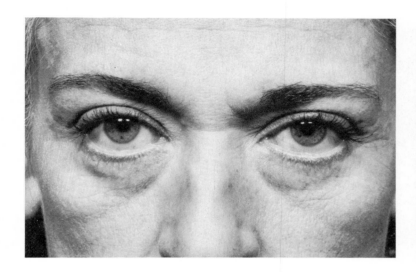

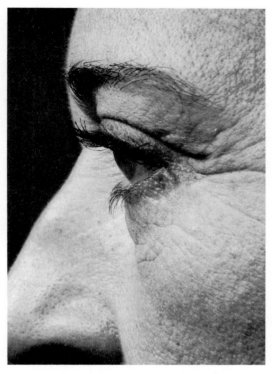

Figure 18–40. Another patient demonstrating the sort of minor defects that commonly follow blepharoplasty, in this case performed elsewhere. In the preoperative view note a recurrent skin fold of the upper lids, not necessarily because too little skin was removed, but more likely the result of ptosis of the brow. Imperfect results in the upper lids must be expected in such patients unless the brow is elevated. There is also a small residual medial fat pocket of the right lower lid and a small degree of ectropion at the lateral third of the left lower lid.

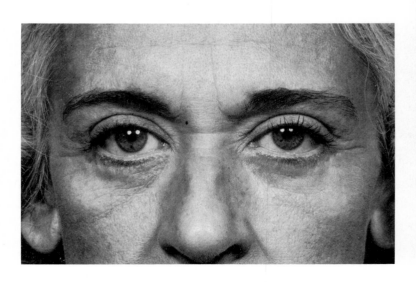

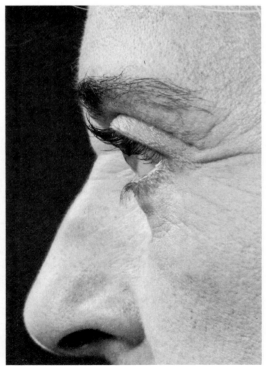

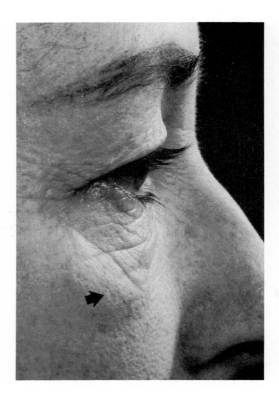

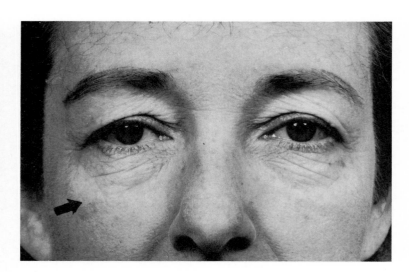

Figure 18–41. Excision of skin from the upper eyelids produced a slightly less than optimal result in this patient. One of the reasons for the limited improvement is the presence of brow ptosis; elevation of the brows was decided against.

The small cheek pouch or elevation indicated by the arrows in the preoperative photographs was of particular interest. These pouches overlying the malar eminence are often found in association with, but not necessarily related to, palpebral bags. Sometimes they are improved by very wide undermining during blepharoplasty, but the improvement is minimal. It is most important to discover these cheek deformities prior to surgery and to point them out to the patient, for they will not be removed by the operation and some patients expect that they will be.

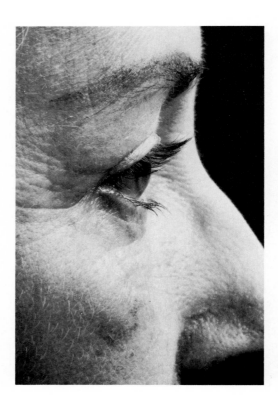

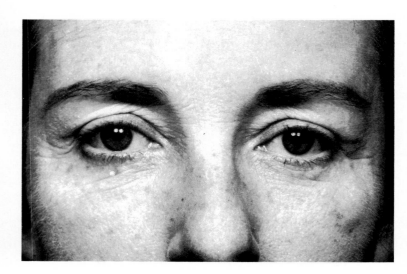

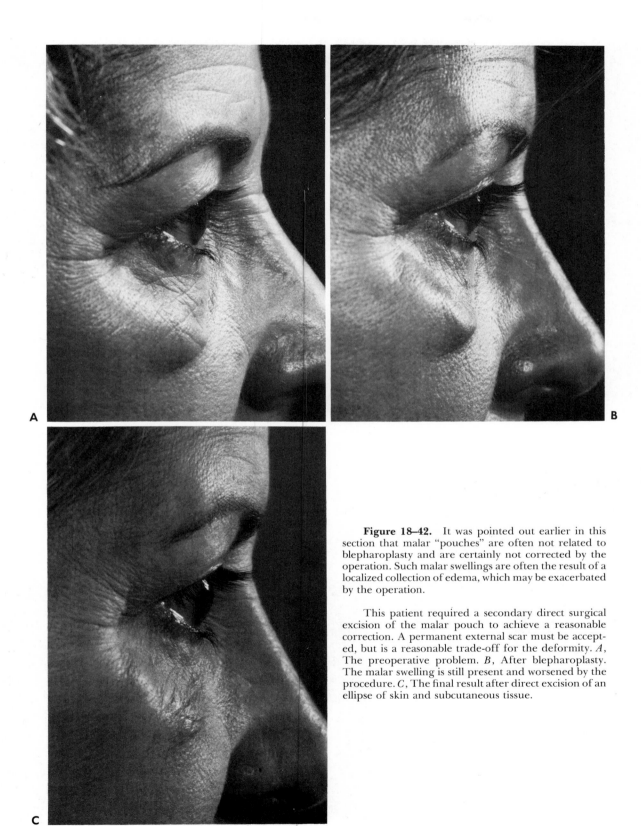

Figure 18–42.   It was pointed out earlier in this section that malar "pouches" are often not related to blepharoplasty and are certainly not corrected by the operation. Such malar swellings are often the result of a localized collection of edema, which may be exacerbated by the operation.

This patient required a secondary direct surgical excision of the malar pouch to achieve a reasonable correction. A permanent external scar must be accepted, but is a reasonable trade-off for the deformity. *A*, The preoperative problem. *B*, After blepharoplasty. The malar swelling is still present and worsened by the procedure. *C*, The final result after direct excision of an ellipse of skin and subcutaneous tissue.

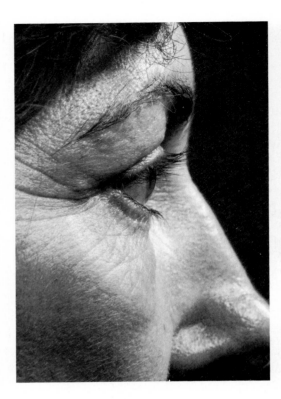

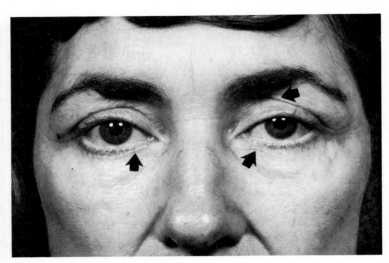

Figure 18–43.   Cosmetic blepharoplasty by another surgeon left this patient unhappy about the deep depression at the medial region of the left upper lid as well as the marked scar ridges with small suture marks still present six months after surgery in the lower lids (arrows in the preoperative photograph). Such persistent suture marks result from allowing sutures to remain in place for more than four days. The previous scars were excised, but no skin was removed, at a secondary operation. Exploration of the left upper eyelid revealed that the medial levator expansion was severed at the first operation, which may have occurred when the surgeon sought the medial fat pocket. The edges of the interrupted levator were located and united with sutures.

The postoperative result was satisfactory to the surgeon except for the small cyst seen in the lower left incision, which had to be removed later. The patient, however, was still unhappy — a not uncommon phenomenon when blepharoplasty must be repeated. There is a slight increase in scleral show in spite of the fact that only the scars of the lower lids were excised, with no removal of additional skin.

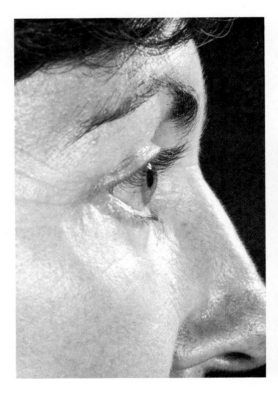

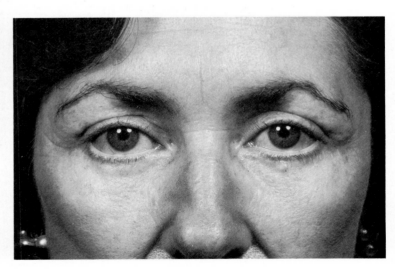

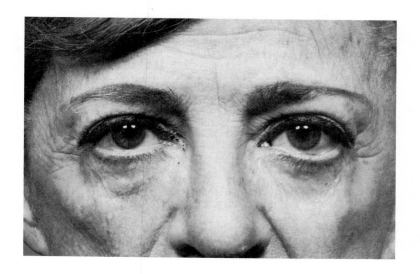

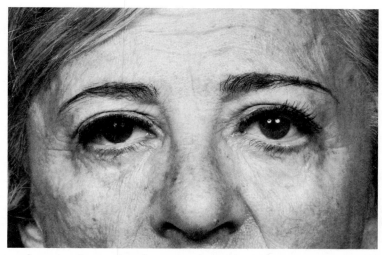

Figure 18–44.   The secondary operation consists of removing the residual fat pocket through a stab wound in the orbital septum, opening the original subciliary incision for the length of the lid, and rather wide undermining and redraping of the skin of the left lower lid to allow the lid to relax and relieve some of the skin pull responsible for the ectropion. No skin is excised.

The Oriental or "slit" eye differs from the Western eye in several important anatomic ways. There is more fat in the loose subcutaneous tissue than there is around the Caucasian eye. There is also an encapsulated, canary yellow fat pad just beneath the orbicularis muscle and above the levator expansion.

Undoubtedly the most important anatomical difference between the Oriental and Occidental eyelid is the absence of the cutaneous insertion of the levator palpebral superioris in the mongoloid lid (Figure 18–45, *A, B*). Sayoc (1954) described the double insertion of the levator into the skin and the superior border of the tarsal plate in the Caucasian eye. He pointed out that when the muscle belly of the levator contracts, the entire transverse aponeurosis is "swung backward over the glove like a visor of a helmet, pulling with it the skin of the lid, into which its terminal fibers are inserted, thus deepening and forming the superior folds." This fold formation is not caused solely by the insertion of the aponeurosis into the skin, but is aided by its main attachment along the superior border of the tarsal plate which causes the tarsus to be elevated upon contraction of the muscle.

In the Oriental, however, the absence of the cutaneous insertion is sufficient to cause the absence of the orbital palpebral sulcus and the palpebral fold. The cutaneous extension of the levator expansion ends as a ridge of thickened fascia in the Oriental. The typical mongoloid eyelid also contains a medial epicanthal fold which hides most of the caruncle.

Valuable contributions to the techniques of operating on Oriental eyelids have been made by Sayoc (1954, 1956), Millard (1955), Fernandez (1960) (Figures 18–45 through 18–47), Boo-Chai (1963a and b) (Figures 18–48 and 18–49), Uchida (1962) and others. They have devised varying ways to construct the supratarsal fold. The simplest of these procedures has been widely advertised as the "20-minute eye operation" and is done in outpatient clinics and offices throughout the Orient. Boo-Chai (1963b) advocates this simpler technique in most cases of the younger age group in whom there is a minimum of excess fat and skin (Figs. 18–48 and 18–49). He places three mattress sutures transconjunctivally, which fix the levator to the skin at a level 5 to 8 mm from the ciliary margin. These sutures are of fine nylon and are carefully placed to construct a normal shape and curve to the fold. He excises excess fat through a small stab wound in the supratarsal fold, unless there is a considerable amount of fat, in which case a larger incision is required for removal. Boo-Chai claims this simple technique is effective in most patients

and has the additional advantages of minimal scarring and distortion of lids and lashes. He further claims the method is not irreversible in that adjustments can be made if the sutures are not placed in exactly the right position.

Although Boo-Chai states that this simple technique can provide natural results of a permanent nature, other surgeons prefer a more radical approach via a long supratarsal incision with extensive reattachment of the levator expansion to the skin, as well as removal of all excess fat. In patients with more advanced deformities, i.e., more fat and skin, Boo-Chai also does the more radical procedure of the type advocated by Millard (1955), Fernandez (1960), and others.

The extensive and complete procedure described by Fernandez is preferred by the author and has proved successful in his hands (Figs. 18–45 to 18–47). In this procedure the excess skin of the upper eyelid is grasped with a marking forceps very much as in a routine blepharoplasty in a Caucasian, and the excess skin is marked and excised. The incision is planned to lie about 6 mm above the lid margin. The orbicularis muscle is then split transversely along almost the entire length of the upper eyelid. Immediately beneath the orbicularis muscle a fusiform pad of yellow fat will usually be found lying transversely from medial to lateral. This fat is removed. If separate medial fat pockets exist, a stab wound is made in the orbital septum and this fat is extruded and excised. The levator expansion is found deep to the muscle and supraorbital fat. This structure is carefully dissected and cleared. The inferior thickened edge is carefully freed across its entire width. All bleeding points are coagulated. The inferior edge of the levator expansion is then sutured to the dermis (which is very thin) at the edge of the lower incision. Fine suture material such as 6–0 white nylon, Mersilene or catgut is used. The skin incision is closed with interrupted or subcuticular sutures.

Should correction of the epicanthal fold be desired, a Z-plasty may be done at the same time or at a future date. Operations to correct the epicanthal fold can be fraught with problems and may result in unsightly scarring of the eyelids. These operations are not usually performed even in the Orient and hardly ever in the United States. If excess skin and fat also exist in the lower lids, this is corrected at the same time as upper lid repair.

Uchida (1962), Koonvisal (1969) and others advocate a similar approach with certain technical variations, including anchoring the lower skin margin to the tarsus with nonabsorbable sutures in a manner similar to the original Sayoc (1954)

Text continued on page 577.

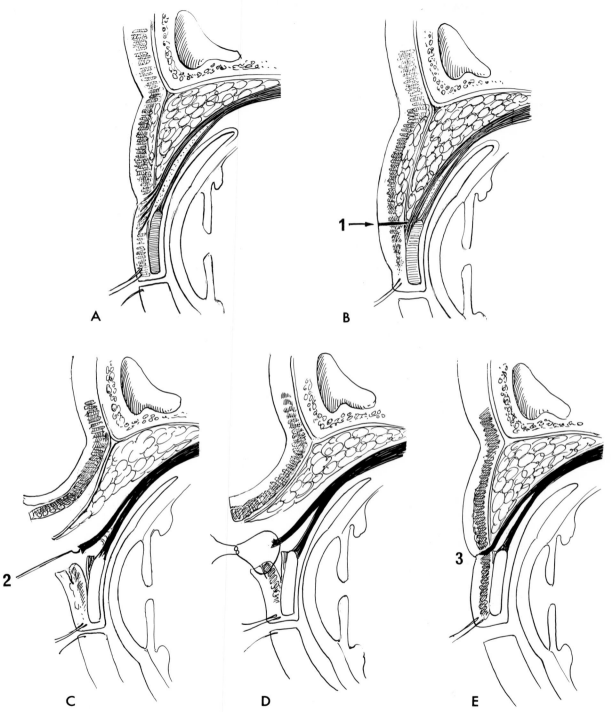

Figure 18–45.   The Caucasian eyelid (*A*) shows a dual insertion of the levator muscle into the superior border of the tarsus and a slip inserting into the dermis at the site of the supratarsal fold. The typical Oriental lid (*B*) lacks the dermal insertion of the levator aponeurosis.

The Fernandez operation in sagittal section shows the superficial layer of the levator aponeurosis dissected and held with a hook (*C*). This thin aponeurotic sheet is sutured into the dermis at the skin incision with a buried nonabsorbable suture (*D*). The desired fold is created by this insertion (*E*).

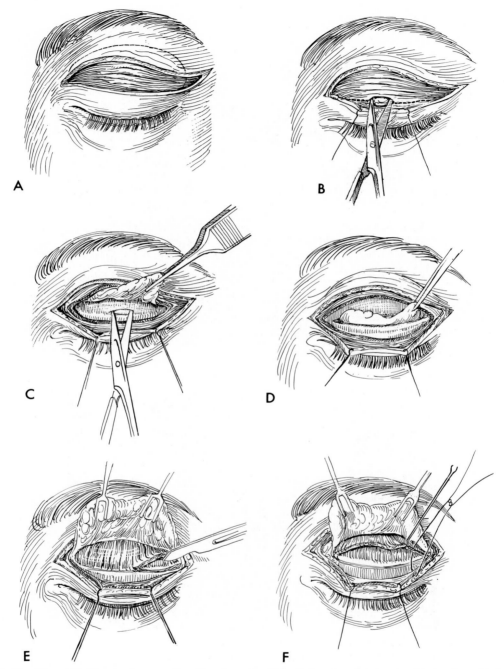

Figure 18–46. The radical Fernandez procedure for alteration of the Oriental eyelid. A strip of redundant skin is excised from the upper lid, as in cosmetic blepharoplasty; the lower limb of the incision is 7 to 8 mm from the ciliary margin (*A*). The orbicularis muscle and orbital septum are dissected along the lower edge of the incision; a small strip of muscle can be excised (*B*). The supraorbital fat is dissected free and the excess is excised (*C* and *D*). The levator aponeurosis is dissected as a thin sheet and sutured into the dermal edge of the lower wound margin, establishing a supratarsal fold (*E* and *F*). The skin margins are sutured with interrupted sutures.

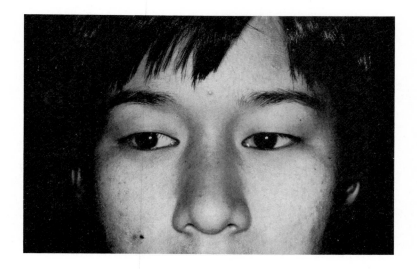

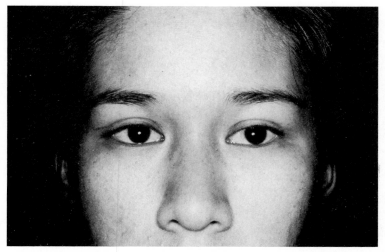

Figure 18–47.   Preoperative and postoperative photographs showing typical results from the operative procedure described by Fernandez. (Courtesy of Dr. Leabert Fernandez.)

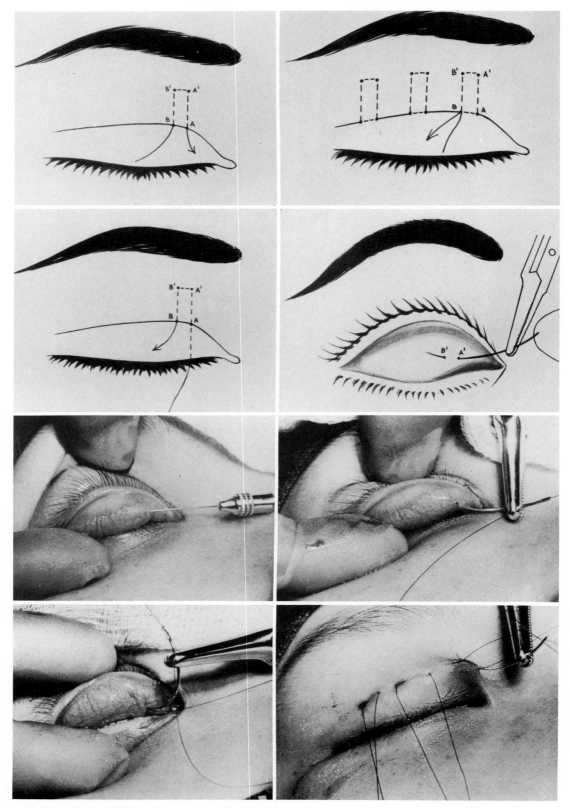

Figure 18–48.   The simplified technique of Boo-Chai for establishing a supratarsal fold in an Oriental eyelid with three mattress sutures. These sutures are passed subconjunctivally through needle puncture wounds, and they affix the levator to the skin. The knots are buried and allowed to retract through the suture holes in the skin wound. This technique is often satisfactory in younger patients who have a minimum of fat and skin. Boo-Chai advocates a more radical approach similar to that of Fernandez in more advanced deformities. (Courtesy of Dr. Khoo Boo-Chai.)

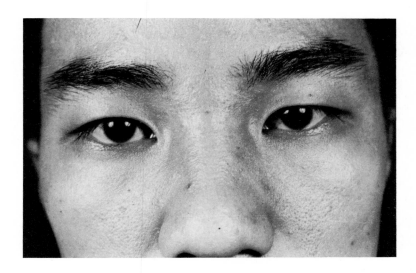

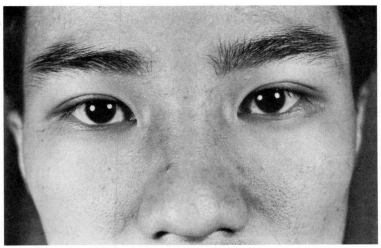

Figure 18–49. The result shown in the postoperative photograph is typical of those achieved with the Boo-Chai procedure in young patients with Oriental eyelids. (Courtesy of Dr. Khoo Boo-Chai.)

technique. This method of creating a fold by anchoring the skin to the tarsus results in a permanent fold which is present when the eye is open and when it is closed. This technique has been referred to as the "static" method.

The "dynamic" technique, championed by Fernandez (1960), produces a fold in the eye only when the eye is open. It also has the advantage of not disturbing the tarsus or the levator muscle insertion into it.

The type of fold that is acceptable in Japan and other parts of Asia is apparently somewhat different from that accepted in Hawaii or the Western Pacific. A slight crease created in the upper eyelid, which opens the eye somewhat, is considered satisfactory in Japan, whereas in Hawaii and on the mainland of the United States, the fold desired is deeper and is not rounded just above the ciliary border. In eyelids, as in so many other things, the standards of acceptability and beauty are quite different in different parts of the world.

REFERENCES

Alibert, J.-L.: Monographie des Dermatoses ou Précis Théorique et Pratique des Maladies de la Peau. Paris, Daynac, 1832, p. 795.

Arruga, H.: Ocular Surgery. New York, McGraw-Hill Book Co., 1952, p. 171.

Aston, S. J.: Orbicularis oculi muscle flaps: a technique to reduce crow's feet and lateral canthal skin folds. Plast. Reconstr. Surg. 65:206, 1980.

Baker, T. J.: Chemical face peeling and rhytidectomy. Plast. Reconstr. Surg. 29:199, 1962.

Baker, T. J., Gordon, H. L., and Mosienko, P.: Upper lid blepharoplasty. Plast. Reconstr. Surg. 60:692, 1977.

Bames, H.: (Letter to the Editor) Bags under the eyes. J.A.M.A. *146*:692, 1951.

Bames, H.: Baggy eyelids. Plast. Reconstr. Surg. *22*:264, 1958.

Barsky, A. J.: Plastic Surgery. Philadelphia, W. B. Saunders Company, 1938, p. 124.

Beare, R.: Surgical treatment of senile changes in the eyelids. The McIndoe-Beare technique. Proceedings of the 2nd International Symposium on Plastic and Reconstructive Surgery of the Eye and Adnexa, edited by Smith and Converse. St. Louis, C. V. Mosby Co., 1967, pp. 362–366.

Beer, G. J.: Lehre der Augenkrankheiten. Vienna, C. F. Wappler, 1792.

Beer, G. J.: Lehre von den Augenkrankheiten als Leitfaden Zuseinen Offentlichen Vorlesungen Entworsen. Vol. II, pp. 109–111. Vienna, Lamesina, Heubner and Volke, 1817.

Berens, C.: Aging process in eye and adnexa. Arch. Ophthalmol. *29*:171, 1943.

Bettman, A. G.: Plastic surgery about the eyes. Ann. Surg. *88*:994, 1928.

Boo-Chai, K.: Plastic construction of the superior palpebral fold. Plast. Reconstr. Surg. *31*:74, 1963a.

Boo-Chai, K.: Further experience with cosmetic surgery of the upper eyelid. Excerpta Med. Int. Cong. Series No. 66. Proceedings of the 3rd International Congress of Plastic Surgery, Washington, D.C., 1963b, pp. 518–524.

Bourguet, J.: La chirurgie esthétique de la face. Le Concours Médical, 1921, pp. 1657–1670.

Bourguet, J.: La chirurgie esthétique de l'oeil et des paupières. Monde Médical, 1929, pp. 725–731.

Callahan, A.: Surgery of the Eye: Diseases. Springfield, Ill., Charles C Thomas, 1956, p. 102.

Castanares, S.: Blepharoplasty for herniated intra-orbital fat. Anatomical basis for a new approach. Plast. Reconstr. Surg. *8*:46, 1951.

Castanares, S.: Baggy eyelids. Physiological considerations and surgical technique. Transactions of the 3rd International Congress of Plastic Surgery. Amsterdam, Excerpta Medica Foundation, 1964, pp. 499–506.

Castanares, S.: Correction of the baggy eyelids deformity produced by herniation of orbital fat. Proceedings of the 2nd International Symposium on Plastic and Reconstructive Surgery of the Eye and Adnexa, edited by Smith and Converse. St. Louis, C. V. Mosby Co., 1967, pp. 346–353.

Castanares, S.: Eyelid plasty. *In* Goldwyn, R. M. (ed.): The unfavorable result in plastic surgery: Avoidance and treatment. Boston, Little, Brown and Co., 1972, Chapter 18.

Castanares, S.: Classification of baggy eyelids deformity. Plast. Reconstr. Surg. *59*:629, 1977.

Claoué, C.: Documents de Chirurgie Plastique et Esthétique. Compte Rendu des Séances de la Société Scientifique Francaise de Chirurgie Plastique et Esthétique. Paris, Maloine, 1931, pp. 344–353.

Converse, J. M.: The Converse technique of the corrective eyelid plastic operation. *In* Converse, J. M. (ed.): Reconstructive Plastic Surgery. Philadelphia, W. B. Saunders Company, 1964, pp. 1333–1336.

Converse, J. M.: Treatment of epithelized suture tracts of eyelids by marsupialization. Plast. Reconstr. Surg. *48*:477, 1966.

Cronin, T. D.: Marginal incision for upper blepharoplasty. Plast. Reconstr. Surg. *49*:14, 1972.

DeMere, M., Wood, T., and Austin, W.: Eye complications with blepharoplasty or other eyelid surgery. Plast. Reconstr. Surg. *53*:634, 1974.

DeMere, M.: Blindness and eyelid surgery. Aesth. Plast. Surg. *2*:41, 1978.

Dufourmentel, C., and Mouly, R.: Traitement operatoire des rides et pochés palpébrales. Ann. Chir. Plast. *3*:229, 1958.

Dupuytren, G.: De l'oedéme chronique et des tumeurs enkystées des paupières. Leçons Orales de Clinique Chirur-gicale. 2nd ed. Vol. III, p. 377–378. Paris, Germer-Ballière, 1839.

Duverger, C., and Velter, E.: Thérapeutique Chirurgicale Ophthalmologique. Paris, Masson et Cie, 1926, p. 79.

Edgerton, M. T., and Hansen, F. C.: Matching facial color with split thickness skin grafts from adjacent areas. Plast. Reconstr. Surg. *21*:455, 1960.

Edgerton, M. T., Webb, W. L., Slaughter, R., and Meyer, E.: Surgical results and psychosocial changes following rhytidectomy. Plast. Reconstr. Surg. *33*:503, 1964.

Edgerton, M. T.: Causes and prevention of lower lid ectropion following blepharoplasty. Plast. Reconstr. Surg. *49*:367, 1972.

Elschnig, A.: Fetthernien, Sog. "Tränensacke" der Unterlieder Klin. Mbl. Augenheilk. *84*:763, 1930.

Erich, J. B.: Surgical elimination of wrinkles, redundant skin and pouches about the eyelids. Proc. Mayo Clin. *36*:101, 1961.

Fernandez, L. R.: The double-eyelid operation in the Oriental in Hawaii. Plast. Reconstr. Surg. *25*:257, 1960.

Flowers, R. S.: Anchor blepharoplasty. Transactions of the International Congress of Plastic Surgeons, pp. 471–472. Paris, Masson et Cie, 1976.

Fomon, S.: Surgery of Injury and Plastic Repair. Baltimore, The Williams and Wilkins Co., 1939, pp. 135–137.

Fomon, S.: Cosmetic Surgery, Principles and Practice. Philadelphia, J. B. Lippincott Company, 1960.

Fox, S. A.: Ophthalmic Plastic Surgery. New York, Grune and Stratton, 1952.

Francois, J.: Heredity in Ophthalmology. St. Louis, C. V. Mosby Co., 1961, pp. 272–275.

Fry, J. H.: Reversible visual loss after proptosis from retrobulbar hemorrhage. Plast. Reconstr. Surg. *44*:480, 1969.

Fuchs, E.: Ueber Blepharochalasis (Erschlaffung der Lidhaut). Wien. Klin. Wochenschr. *9*:109, 1896.

Fuchs, E.: Textbook of Ophthalmology. New York, Appleton, 1899, p. 553.

Furnas, D. W.: Festoons of orbicularis muscle as a cause of baggy eyelids. Plast. Reconstr. Surg. *61*:531, 1978.

Ginestet, G., Fréziéres, H., Dupuis, A., and Pons, J.: Chirurgie Plastique et Reconstructrice de la Face. Paris, Flammarion et Cie, 1967, pp. 184–187.

González-Ulloa, M., and Stevens, E. F.: The treatment of palpebral bags. Plast. Reconstr. Surg. *27*:381, 1961.

González-Ulloa, M., and Stevens, E. F.: Senile eyelid esthetic correction. Proceedings of the 2nd International Symposium on Plastic and Reconstructive Surgery of the Eye and Adnexa, edited by Smith and Converse. St. Louis, C. V. Mosby Co., 1967, pp. 354–361.

Graf, D.: Oertliche erbliche erschlaffung der Haut. Wochenschr. Ges. Heilk., 1836, pp. 225–227.

Graham, W. P., Messner, K. H., and Miller, S. H.: Keratoconjunctivitis sicca symptoms appearing after blepharoplasty. Plast. Reconstr. Surg. *47*:57, 1976.

Hadley, H. G.: Dermatolysis palpebrarum (blepharochalasis). Rocky Mt. Med. J. *37*:517, 1940.

Hartley, J. H., Lester, J. C., and Schatten, W. E.: Acute retrobulbar hemorrhage during elective blepharoplasty. Plast. Reconstr. Surg. *52*:8, 1973.

Hartman, E., Morax, P. V., and Vergez, A.: Complications visuelles graves de la chirurgie des pochés palpébrales. Ann. Oculist *195*:142, 1962.

Holden, H. M.: (Letter to the Editor) Bags under the eyes. J.A.M.A. *146*:692, 1951.

Hotz, F. C.: Ueber das Wesen und die Operation der Sogenannten Ptosis atonica. Arch. Augenheilk, *9*:95, 1880.

Hotz, F. C.: Eine neue Operation für Entropium und Trichiasis. Arch. Augenheilk. *9*:68, 1880.

Huang, T. T., Horowitz, B., and Lewis, S. T.: Retrobulbar hemorrhage. Plast. Reconstr. Surg. *59*:39, 1977.

Hueston, J. T., and Heinze, J. B.: Successful early relief of blindness occuring after blepharoplasty. Plast. Reconstr. Surg. *53*:588, 1972.

Hueston, J. T., and Heinze, J. B.: A second case of relief of blindness following blepharoplasty. Case report. Plast. Reconstr. Surg. 59:430, 1977.

Hugo, N. E., and Stone, E.: Anatomy for a blepharoplasty. Plast. Reconstr. Surg. 53:381, 1974.

Hunt, H. L.: Plastic Surgery of the Head, Face and Neck. Philadelphia, Lea and Febiger, 1926, p. 198.

Johnson, J. B., and Hadley, R. C.: The aging face. In Converse J. M. (ed.): Reconstructive Plastic Surgery. Philadelphia, W. B. Saunders Company, 1964, pp. 1306–1342.

Jones, L. T.: An anatomical approach to problems of the eyelids and lacrimal apparatus. Arch. Ophthalmol. 66:111, 1961.

Joseph, J.: Plastic operation on protruding cheek. Dtsch. Med. Wochenschr. 47:287, 1921.

Joseph, J.: Verbesserung meiner Hängemangenplastik (Melomioplastik). Dtsch. Med. Wochenschr. 54:567, 1928.

Journal Universal et Hebdomadaire de Médecine et de Chirurgie Pratiques et des Institutions Médicales, Vol. 1–13, Oct. 1830–Dec. 1833.

Kahn, K.: Plastic surgery in the removal of excessive cutaneous tissues obstructing vision. N. Y. J. Med. 34:781, 1934.

Kapp, J. F. S.: Die Technik du kosmetischen Encheiresen. Beih. Med. Klin. 3:65, 1913.

Kapp, J. F. S.: Premature Old Age in Women: A Study in the Tragedy of the Middle Aged. New York, P. L. Baruch, 1925.

Kolle, F. S.: Plastic and Cosmetic Surgery. New York, Appleton, 1911, pp. 116–117.

Koonvisal, L.: Panel on oriental eyelids. Pan-Pacific Surgical Association Congress, Oct., 1969.

Kraushar, M. F., Seelenfreund, M. H., and Frelich, D. B.: Closure of the central artery following retrobulbar injection. Trans. Am. Acad. Ophthalmol. Otolaryngol. 78:65, 1974.

Kreiker, A.: Operation der Blepharochalasis mit Hilfe der v. blaskoviesschen Lidfalten Bildenden Nähte. Klin. Mbl. Augenheilk. 83:302, 1929.

Lewis, J. B., Jr.: The Z-blepharoplasty. Plast. Reconstr. Surg. 44:331, 1969.

Loeb, R.: Aesthetic blepharoplasties based on the degree of wrinkling. Plast. Reconstr. Surg. 47:33, 1971.

Loeb, R.: Necessity for partial resection of the orbicularis oculi muscle in blepharoplasties in some young patients. Plast. Reconstr. Surg. 60:178, 1977.

Loeb, R.: Correction of enophthalmos with free fat grafts. Personal communication, 1979.

Mackenzie, W.: A Practical Treatise of the Diseases of the Eye. London, Longmans, 1830, pp. 170–171.

May, H.: Reconstructive and Reparative Surgery. Philadelphia, F. A. Davis Co., 1947, pp. 325–326.

McIndoe, A.: Personal communication. 1955.

Millard, D. R.: Oriental peregrinations. Plast. Reconstr. Surg. 16:319, 1955.

Miller, C. C.: Cosmetic Surgery. The Correction of Featural Imperfections. Chicago, Oak Printing Co., 1908, pp. 40–42.

Miller, C. C.: Cosmetic Surgery. Philadelphia, F. A. Davis Co., 1924, pp. 30–32.

Miller, C. C., and Miller, F.: Folds, bags and wrinkles of the skin about the eyes and their eradication by simple surgical methods. Med Briefs 35:540, 1907.

Moser, M. H., DiPirro, E., and McCoy, F. J.: Sudden blindness following blepharoplasty. Plast. Reconstr. Surg. 51:364, 1973.

Mustardé, J. C.: Problems and possibilities in ptosis surgery. Plast. Reconstr. Surg. 56:381, 1975.

Noël, A.: La Chirurgie Esthétique. Son Role Sociale. Paris, Masson et Cie., 1926, pp. 62–66.

Noël, A.: La Chirurgie Esthétique. Clermont (Oise), Thiron et Cie, 1928.

Padgett, E. C., and Stephenson, K. L.: Plastic and Reconstruction Surgery. Springfield, Ill., Charles C Thomas, 1948, p. 514.

Panneton, P.: Le blepharochalazis. A propos de 51 cas dans la même famille. Arch. Ophthalmol. 53:724, 1936a.

Panneton, P.: Mémoire sur le blepharochalazis. 51 cas dans la même famille. Un. Med. Canada 65:725, 1936b.

Passot, R.: La chirurgie esthétique des rides du visage. Presse Méd. 27:258, 1919.

Passot, R.: La correction chiururgicale des ride du visage. Bull. Acad. Méd. Paris 82:112, 1919.

Passot, R.: La Chirurgie Esthétique Pure (Technique et Résultats). Paris, Gaston Doin et Cie, 1931, pp. 176–180.

Personal correspondence regarding panel discussion on Oriental eyelid surgery. Pan-Pacific Surgical Association Congress, Oct. 1969.

Rees, T. D.: In panel discussion on the cosmetic eyelid plastic operation. Proceedings of the 2nd International Symposium on Plastic and Reconstructive Surgery of the Eye and Adnexa, edited by Smith and Converse. St. Louis, C. V. Mosby Co., 1967, p. 376.

Rees, T. D.: Technical aid in blepharoplasty. Plast. Reconstr. Surg. 41:497, 1968.

Rees, T. D.: Technical considerations in blepharoplasty. Transaction of the 4th International Congress of Plastic and Reconstructive Surgery. Amsterdam. Excerpta Medica Foundation, 1969a, p. 1084.

Rees, T. D.: Selection of appropriate technical variations in blepharoplasty. In Rycroft, P. V. (ed.): Corneo-Plastic Surgery. New York, Pergamon Press, 1969b, pp. 55–69.

Rees, T. D., and Dupuis, C.: Baggy eyelids in young adults. Plast. Reconstr. Surg. 43:381, 1969.

Rees, T. D., and Dupuis, C.: Cosmetic blepharoplasty in the older age group. Ophthalmic Surg. 1:30, 1970.

Rees, T. D., and Ristow, B.: Blefaroplastia consideracoes gerais sobre tecnica pos-operatorio e complicacoes. J. Brasil. Med. 15:307, 1968.

Rees, T. D.: Correction of ectropion resulting from blepharoplasty. Plast. Reconstr. Surg. 50:1, 1972.

Rees, T. D. and Wood-Smith, D.: Cosmetic facial surgery. Philadelphia, W. B. Saunders Company, 1973.

Rees, T. D.: The "dry eye" complication after blepharoplasty. Plast. Reconstr. Surg. 56:375, 1975.

Rees, T. D.: Complications following blepharoplasty. In Symposium on plastic surgery in the orbital region. St. Louis, C. V. Mosby Co., 1976.

Reidy, J. P.: Swelling of eyelids. Br. J. Plast. Surg. 13:256, 1960.

Sakler, B. R.: Plastic repair of lid hernia with fascia lata. Am. J. Ophthalmol. 20:936, 1937.

Sayoc, B. T.: Plastic construction of the superior palpebral fold. Am. J. Ophthalmol. 38:556, 1954.

Sayoc, B. T.: Absence of superior palpebral fold in slit-eyes: an anatomic and physiologic explanation. Am. J. Ophthalmol. 42:298, 1956.

Sayoc, B. T.: Blepharochalasis in upper eyelids, including its classification. Amer. J. Ophthalmol. 43:970, 1957.

Schmidt-Rimpler, H.: Fett-Hernien der oberen Augenlider. Zbl. Prak. Augenheilk. 23:297, 1899.

Sheehan, J. E.: Plastic Surgery of the Orbit. New York, The Macmillan Company, 1927.

Sheen, J. H.: Supratarsal fixation in upper blepharoplasty. Plast. Reconstr. Surg. 54:424, 1974.

Sheen, J. H.: A change in the technique of supratarsal fixation in upper blepharoplasty. Plast. Reconstr. Surg. 59:831, 1977.

Sheen, J. H.: Tarsal fixation in lower blepharoplasty. Plast. Reconstr. Surg. 62:24, 1978.

Sichel, J.: Aphorismes pratiques sur divers points d'ophtalmologie. Ann. Oculist 12:187, 1844.

Silver, H.: A new approach to the operation of blepharoplasty. Br. J. Plast. Surg. 22:253, 1969.

Skoog, T.: Plastic Surgery. Philadelphia, W. B. Saunders Company, 1974.

Smith, B., and Fasano, C. V.: The diagnosis and treatment of baggy eyelids. Bull. N.Y. Acad. Med. 38:163, 1962.

Smith, F.: Multiple excision and Z-plasties in surface reconstruction. Plast. Reconstr. Surg. 1:170, 1946.

Smith, F.: Plastic and Reconstructive Surgery. Philadelphia, W. B. Saunders Company, 1950.

Spaeth, E. B.: The Principles and Practice of Ophthalmic Surgery, 4th ed. Philadelphia, Lea and Febiger, 1948.

Spira, M.: Lower blepharoplasty — a clinical study. Plast. Reconstr. Surg. 59:35, 1977.

Steckler, M. I.: Baggy eyelids. Am. J. Ophthalmol. 37:113, 1954.

Stein, B.: Blepharochalasis des Unterlides. Klin. Mbl. Augenheilk, 84:846, 1930.

Stephenson, K. L.: The history of blepharoplasty to correct blepharochalasis. Aesth. Plast. Surg. 1:177, 1977.

Stieren, E.: Blepharochalasis. Report of 2 cases. Trans. Am. Ophthalmol. Soc. 13:713, 1914.

Swartz, R. M., Schultz, R. C., and Seaton, J. R.: "Dry eye" following blepharoplasty. Plast. Reconstr. Surg. 54:644, 1975.

Tenzel, R. R.: Cosmetic blepharoplasty. In Soll, D. B. (ed.): Management of complications in ophthalmic plastic surgery. Birmingham, Aescalapium Publishing Co., 1976, Chapter 8.

Tipton, J. B.: Should incisions in the orbital septum be sutured in blepharoplasty? Plast. Reconstr. Surg. 49:613, 1972.

Uchida, J. I.: A surgical procedure for blepharoptosis vera and for pseudo-blepharoptosis orientalis. Br. J. Plast. Surg. 15:271, 1962.

von Graefe, C. F.: De Rhinoplastice. Berlin. Dietrich Reimer, 1818, p. 13.

Weidler, W. B.: Blepharochalasis. Report of 2 cases with the microscopic examination. J.A.M.A. 61:1128, 1913.

Weinstein, A.: Ueber zwei eigenartige Formen des Herabhängens der Haut der Oberlider: Ptosis atrophica und Ptosis adiposa. Klin. Mbl. Augenheilk. 47:190, 1909.

Part 4

AESTHETIC SURGERY OF THE NECK AND FACE

Chapter 19

History

Thomas D. Rees, M.D., F.A.C.S.

"C'était pendant l'horreur d'une profonde nuit.
Ma mère Jézabel devant mois s'est montrée,
Comme au jour de sa mort pompeusement parée.
Ses malheurs n'avaient point abattu sa fierté;
Même elle avait encore cet éclat emprunté
Dont elle eut soin de peindre et d'orner sa visage,
Pour réparer des ans l'irréparable outrage."
"It was during the horror of a dark night.
My mother Jezabel appeared before me,
As on the day of her death pompously adorned.
Her misfortunes had not humbled her pride;
She still had that assumed luster
With which she carefully composed and embellished her face,
So as to repair the years' irreparable outrage."

JEAN RACINE
Athalie, Act II, Scene V (1960)

It is not known exactly who attempted the first face lift, but there is little doubt that the operation was being done in the early 1900's by many surgeons in Europe and by a few in America. Most of these early efforts were mainly in the nature of a "minilift," that is, excision of strips of skin in front of and behind the ears. Extensive undermining of the facial and cervical skin flaps was probably not done until the 1920's.

Stephenson (1970) credits von Hollanden with publishing the first paper on the correction of the sagging face in "Handbuch von Kosmetick" by Max Joseph in 1912. At about this time, there was considerable interest in facial surgery by such eminent surgeons as Lexer (1910) and Joseph (1921, 1928a and b) in Germany and Passot (1919a and b, 1931), Morestin (1915), DeMartel, Bourguet (1921), and Lagarde (1928) in France. Madame Noël (1926 and 1928), a Parisian physician and student of DeMartel, devoted most of her professional life to such cosmetic surgery.

In early 20th century Europe, the performance of such operations was often shrouded in secrecy. Individual techniques were jealously guarded by many of their originators, causing Passot to complain in the literature about such tactics, especially among the "German surgeons."

Unquestionably, this secretive attitude is the reason that not more is known about the early history and development of face lifting. Much more is known about the development of blepharoplasty, probably because the early cases were reported as being performed to correct true pathologic entities that could in some way affect vision and that were frequently familial in nature, as reported by Panneton (1936a and b). This made operations designed to correct eyelids somehow more "respectable" than face lifting, which could only be construed by most people at the turn of the century as catering to excessive vanity, and vanity was generally frowned upon in post-Victorian Europe.

Secrecy surrounded face lifting for several reasons. As just noted, public disdain for surgery catering to vanity undoubtedly forced both surgeons and patients to seek anonymity by "going underground." Much of this surgery, therefore, was done as an office procedure or in small private nursing homes. This in this own way discouraged extensive procedures (such as wide undermining) and prolonged the age of the minilift. Madame Noël was especially noted for her minor office surgery and, by description, her surgery was minimal indeed. Certainly the facial operation pub-

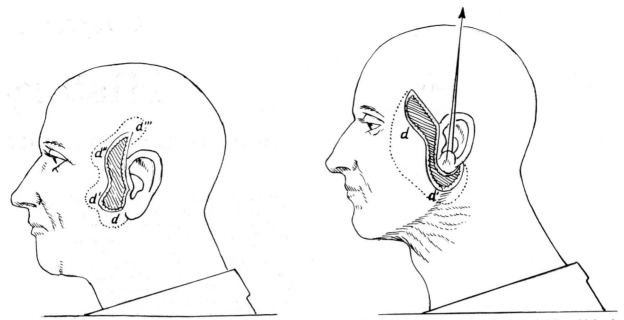

Figure 19–1.   Perhaps the first description of the "minilift" was provided by Passot; this drawing has been copied from his book on the subject, published in 1917. Preauricular skin excision accompanied by little or no skin undermining was abandoned by most surgeons because the results were short-lived. The procedure has recently regained a certain vogue, but it should be relegated to history.

lished by Passot (1931) in his "Chirurgie Esthétique du Visage" was extremely limited in the extent of undermining (Figure 19–1).

Another reason for secrecy was the low esteem in which such operations were held by many of the leading surgeons of the day. Their attitude was that no surgery, except that which was necessary to save life or to alleviate severe suffering or crippling deformity, was indicated. Many considered cosmetic surgery trivial, unnecessarily risky, and downright against the laws of nature. This attitude undoubtedly kept many talented and eminent surgeons from developing the techniques further.

Unfortunately, this unfavorable attitude by the medical profession toward facial cosmetic surgery — and face lifting in particular — persisted, although lessening in intensity, until recently. Advances in anesthesia have done much to minimize risk as well as to encourage more extensive undermining, which yields more dramatic improvements. The current widespread social demand for such surgery, as well as the improvements in results and safety of the procedure, has done much to dispel older, misguided attitudes. The face lift is finally gaining wide acceptance. Indeed, many of the patients are even members of doctor's families. Nevertheless, the condemnation or implied unacceptability of face lifting by men in powerful positions in hospitals, universities, and other institutions had a strong inhibiting effect on face lift

surgery. Many prominent plastic surgeons were forced to "hide" their face lift patients in small private hospitals or to misname the procedure purposely on the operating schedule of major hospitals. Such shenanigans still sadly persist in some medical centers.

Paradoxically, many of the most prominent plastic surgery pioneers of this century have perpetrated the secrecy and implied taint associated with cosmetic surgery. These are men who have pushed ahead the frontiers of reconstruction yet have publicly shunned "cosmetic" surgery while practicing it at the same time, often extensively. Fortunately, the young generation of plastic surgeons, as well as doctors in other disciplines, are recognizing the increasing role of cosmetic facial surgery as an integral part of modern life. Teaching in this field is now emphasized, and the livelihood of many young surgeons depends on their cosmetic surgical skill.

Still another reason for secrecy was greed, man's constant companion. The early cosmetic surgeons were well aware of the potential growth of cosmetic surgery and its financial implications. They were not eager to share their knowledge, and perhaps their profits, with others. New techniques were closely guarded by their developers and imparted only grudgingly to younger colleagues. This attitude persisted among many surgeons until very recently. In fact, it has been only in the past decade or so that many of the "tricks" or "secrets" of cosmetic surgical technique have been freely exchanged.

Even less is known about the early development of cosmetic face lifting in America or the British Isles — the Anglo-Saxon world. Very little on the subject was published, most likely because of a reticence on the part of most surgeons to be identified with "vanity surgery" by their colleagues. At the turn of the century, the Anglo-Saxon world was still very much under the influence of the post-Victorian era, more so even than continental Europe, and vanity was considered almost sinful. Miller, of Chicago, was perhaps the earliest American surgeon to publish extensively on the subject, starting in 1907 and continuing until his textbook on cosmetic surgery was published in 1924. Hunt (1926) of Scotland also openly practiced face lifting and published on the subject in his book *Plastic Surgery of the Head, Face and Neck.*

Many of the giants of plastic surgery who emerged after World Wars I and II practiced face lifting to some degree. Some of these surgeons did a great deal of "cosmetic" surgery, yet curiously they wrote very little on the subject, although they were most prolific on other topics. Gillies, Blair, Davis, Pierce, McIndoe, Mowlem, Conway, and many others performed face lifts, yet they were hesitant to publish on the subject. Many of the greatest reconstructive plastic surgeons relied on face lifting and other cosmetic operations for their livelihood, enabling them to pursue their interest in reconstruction. This same financial state of affairs still exists in many of our major cities, where reconstructive surgery alone simply cannot pay the bills.

As anesthesia became safer and techniques improved, the extent of the face lift operation became more radical. That is, the amount of skin undermining became more extensive, reaching well down into the neck and toward the corners of the mouth. The early operations, as noted, were essentially minilifts in which a strip of redundant skin in front of the ear was removed and the wound edges were undermined just enough to achieve closure, usually only 1 to 2 cm. The mastoid skin was also sometimes undermined for a short distance and a small segment was removed. The temporal lift consisted of excision of a strip of skin behind the hair at the temples. Many unique and imaginative designs, particularly in regard to the incisions in the scalp, were put forth. These very conservative techniques were as ineffective then as they are today, making it difficult to understand the current resurgence of the minilift vogue. The very ineffectiveness of such operations

and their limited period of benefit were what caused surgeons to undertake more extensive undermining in the first place in order to achieve the more lasting results now available.

The success of craniofacial surgery with its routine use of extensive scalp flaps and the coronal incision has stimulated many surgeons to reexamine and refine techniques of brow and forehead lifting. More such extensive surgery is being performed today and with better results. Similarly, some dissatisfaction with the results of face lifting by the classical skin undermine technique, particularly in the neck, has led to more extensive efforts at eliminating cervical bands (caused by the platysma muscle), fullness of the jawline, and imperfect results in the submental area. Extensive in continuity, lipectomy of the jawline and submental area along with various designs of undermining and shortening the platysma-fascial system of the neck and face, as well as actual resection of the platysma across its breadth and the formation of platysma flaps, has been championed in recent years by many surgeons including Skoog (1974), Millard et al. (1968 and 1972), Rees (1973), Guerrero-Santos (1974), Connell (1978), Peterson (1976), and others. These more extensive techniques are unquestionably improving the results. Such success is increasing the public demand for facial surgery.

Miller's (1924) textbook shows many interesting designs for excision of facial skin. It is to his credit that the basic operation performed by most surgeons today is essentially similar. As pointed out by Stephenson (1970), a review of the early literature on face lifting, limited as it is, shows that surprisingly little has been thought of since the early part of the century. Her quotation of Miller in this regard is cogent:

Operations a century old are refaced as original contributions with the slightest modifications and put forward with emphatic seriousness. Even our best surgeons, when they write upon subjects in which their experience is extensive and their understanding great, are often given to the hasty practice of crediting originality to those writers who in the previous few years have written upon similar subjects. Masterpieces of description in older literature are thus lost, and men who have made inessential changes in detail of technique are frequently credited with being originators of operations which they have really had nothing to do with developing.

These words by Miller are as true today as when he wrote them.

Although the face lift operation has been practiced for at least the past 70 years, there is no question that the demand for this type of surgery has risen very sharply over the past decade. This is not only because newer techniques yield consistently satisfactory results but also because the operation is rapidly losing the social stigma attached to it. People in all walks of life — in big cities and small and of all economic strata — are increasingly aware of the benefits of this surgery and are seeking it in ever increasing numbers. In some communities, having a face lift has almost become a status symbol.

It is interesting to note that more and more requests for face lift surgery are coming from men. Although they make up a very small segment of the overall number of rhytidectomy patients, some plastic surgeons state that up to 15 to 20 percent of their requests for facial cosmetic surgery are now coming from males. The typical man who seeks facial plasty is no longer a stage or screen star but rather a successful executive who feels a more youthful appearance will help his career, or a widower or divorcé in his 40's or 50's who is dating a younger woman. Having observed the emphasis on youth all around him — and perhaps the excellent results of face lifting on women acquaintances — the male of the species is adding to the unprecedented growth in cosmetic facial repair. In fact, the progressive rise in demand is so great that there is a considerable shortage of trained surgeons, thus making it imperative to increase the availability of training in the techniques of cosmetic facial surgery.

(For references, see pages 724 to 727.)

Chapter 20

Physical Considerations

Thomas D. Rees, M.D., F.A.C.S.

SELECTION OF PATIENTS

In selecting patients for rhytidectomy, the face lift operation, both physical and psychologic criteria must be kept in mind.

The ideal face lift candidate is usually a woman in her middle forties who is slightly on the thin side and who has prominent or strong malar eminences and mandibular angles (Figures 20–1 and 20–2). The chin, without being prominent, should be strong, and the natural cervicomental angle should approach 90 degrees when the head is held erect. Further, the skin should not be markedly degenerated from excessive actinic exposure or aging, as multiple rhytidoses, or "prune wrinkles," are not helped by the basic face lift procedure.

It is also helpful for the patient to have a full head of hair, styled in a manner that covers the ears, so that incisions can be better camouflaged. It is sometimes necessary for the patient whose hairstyle exposes the ears to change the hairdo following rhytidectomy for several weeks until the scars have faded.

Unfortunately, this type of "ideal" physical candidate is not always the one who arrives at the surgeon's office in search of a face lift. Therefore, it is important to recognize what variations of these criteria may or may not lead to good surgical results.

SPECIAL FACTORS

A strong bony framework of the face is particularly important in obtaining a good result from a face lift. This is not necessarily a racial characteristic, although it is more frequently encountered in Slavs, Scandinavians, and Asians, than, for example, in people of Mediterranean origin. High cheekbones that characterize the faces of many motion picture personalities typify this skeletal criterion. Well developed mandibular angles, often associated with prominent cheekbones, are also most helpful in providing a bony framework over which undermined skin can be drawn and redistributed. A well formed mandibular body is particularly important in eliminating loose folds of skin or "jowls." If there is retrusion of the mentum or flattening along the body of the mandible on either side, it becomes difficult to eradicate jowls despite the extent of skin undermining (Figure 20–3).

In patients with mandibular retrusion, microgenia, or retrognathia, it is sometimes desirable to insert a chin implant at the same time as rhytidectomy (Figure 20–4). Such a subtle alteration in the standard face lift technique can make a remarkable difference in the final result, particularly in the profile line. If these conditions exist, it behooves the surgeon to point them out to the patient preoperatively and to indicate tactfully that a chin implant may spell the difference between an indifferent and a superior result in surgery.

If the line of the neck and chin is more or less straight extending from the tip of the mentum to below the hyoid bone, complete redistribution of the skin — even with total undermining across the midline of the neck — may not be sufficient to restore an aesthetically pleasing cervicomental angle. There are a number of anatomic factors or combinations thereof that cause loss of the cervicomental angle. These include (1) an excess accumulation of either subcutaneous or submuscular fat, which can either be evenly distributed throughout the submental and submandibular area or can form a local lipoma; (2) excessive or redundant skin; (3) fullness of the anterior margins of the platysma muscle; or (4) low anatomic position of the hyoid bone in respect to the inferior border of the chin and the fifth cervical vertebral

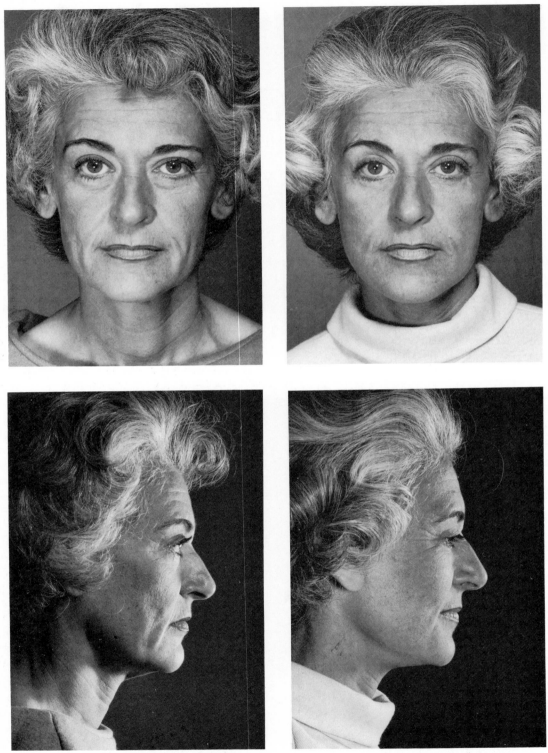

Figure 20–1.   Some patients will demonstrate slight redundancy of skin along the jaw line and on the neck as their only sign of aging. The other tissues of the face are quite healthy and relatively youthful in appearance, which is aided by a characteristic rounding of the facial outline. Even though the excess skin is not overly loose, a good result from a cervicofacial rhytidectomy requires wide undermining and redraping of the skin. It is tempting to do limited undermining in such a patient, but the result will last only for weeks or a few months at the most. This patient was an ideal candidate for the operation.

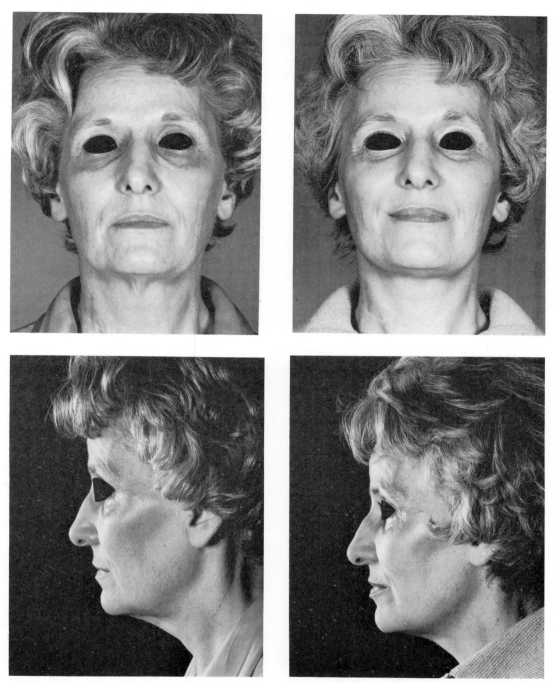

Figure 20–2.   This patient demonstrated the degree of skin laxity and ptosis of the lower face that are present in an "ideal candidate" for primary rhytidectomy (face lift) in the opinion of the author. The skin is slightly loose, there is early jowl formation, and there is minimal loose skin in the upper neck and submental region, with little subcutaneous fat. Deep nasolabial grooves are absent, and malar bone formation is strong. The texture of the skin is soft and its elasticity of good tension. There are few fine rhytides, a further promise of a good result as opposed to what can be expected in the "sunbaked" patient with dry, leathery, and wrinkled skin.

Age is less important than the factors described in obtaining an excellent result. There is no need to wait for the further passage of time and corresponding increases in laxity and ptosis before advising surgery. A second operation can always be done if it becomes necessary. Early changes such as those shown here characteristically occur in patients between 40 and 50 years of age, but there is wide variation. Heredity plays a major role in the aging process of the skin, accounting for some of the variability.

Plication of the superficial fascia is rarely necessary at this stage, as the operation will consist primarily of a readjustment of the skin envelope and removal of the excess.

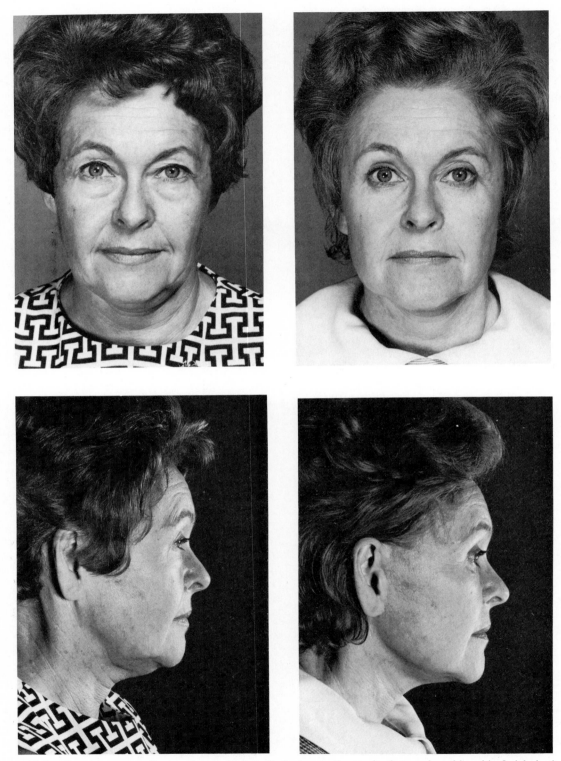

Figure 20–3.   Certain anatomic features impose built-in limitations to the results that can be achieved in facial plastic surgery. This patient, for example, has a wide or squared lower jaw and fullness of the submental tissues which is not the result of excess fat. Jowl formation takes place relatively early in such patients. Surgery must include undermining that extends to the medial edge of the jowl or beyond. The postoperative result is acceptable, as seen here; however, a slight fullness along the line of the jaw must be accepted and mars the result to a slight degree, even though it is a natural contour in this patient.

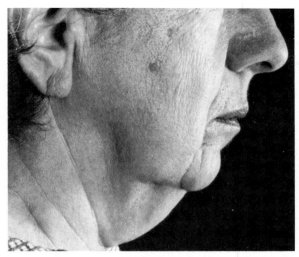

Figure 20–4. This patient epitomizes the most difficult kind of problem that can confront the surgeon in rhytidectomy. She has microgenia, a narrow mandible with depression at the angles, complete loss of a normal cervicomental angle, and submental as well as subplatysmal fat accumulations. A thorough face lift and chin implant and extensive direct surgical approach to the SMAS (platysma, superficial aponeurosis, and fibrous tissue of the face) can offer such a patient better results than ever before. It behooves the surgeon to evaluate such patients in great detail. They are poor candidates for facial surgery from an anatomic point of view.

body. When the hyoid is placed in this low position, the strap muscles of the neck do not form an acute cervicomental angle and extend more or less from the hyoid position directly to the mandible, thus obliterating the normal, more acute angle in between.

A combination of operative procedures may be required to improve the line of the jaw and the cervicomental angle. Obviously, if simple excessive skin is the cause, undermining, redistribution, and excision of the excess skin usually suffices. In practically all instances in which there is a problem beneath the mandible, a small submental incision is required. Such incisions should be made in an appropriate location, which usually is in a natural submental crease or line but not necessarily so. These incisions will be discussed more thoroughly in this chapter. If the problem is related to an accumulation of fat, either throughout the jaw and neck or as a localized lipoma on top of or beneath the strap muscles, such fat can be trimmed from side to side and under the mandible from beneath the skin flaps developed during rhytidectomy and in continuity with a submental incision. Such extensive trimming has been popularized by Millard (1972). It must be done exceedingly carefully in the submandibular area to avoid injury to the underlying ramus mandibularis (VII) nerve. It should also be done completely in continuity, almost sculpting the subcutaneous fat over the jaw

and into the submental region to achieve a more pleasing contour. It is important to maintain a small layer of subcutaneous fat on the skin flaps to prevent adherence of the skin to the underlying strap muscles, which can be most unsightly in the postoperative period. Removal of all fat may result in adhesions with fixation of the skin to muscle, causing unsightly contour irregularities that are emphasized during motion of the neck musculature (e.g., swallowing). Of course, excision of fat is no substitute at all for preoperative proper nutrition and dietary loss of fat; however, there are some individuals who have an unnatural accumulation of subcutaneous fat in this region that remains despite extensive weight loss and obesity control of their trunk and extremities.

When a submental incision is used to sculpt the fat or to gain access to the platysma, it facilitates the insertion of chin implants for augmentation when indicated. Robertson (1965) and Pitanguy (1970) suggest augmenting the chin by using the submental fat pad as a turnover flap — a most useful concept. Wilkinson has likewise suggested utilizing the redundant skin as a buried dermal flap.

Several anatomic disturbances of the area of the submental and neck region can be caused by variations in the anatomy of the platysma muscle. This subject will be discussed more extensively later in this chapter. The platysma contributes significantly to the fullness of the submental region, where it may or may not merge anatomically across the midline. Frequently, the "turkey gobbler" deformity is the result not only of redundant skin but of the redundant medial borders of the platysma muscle that fail to meet on each side. These anterior neck bands commonly occur with increasing age; however, a very strong and full platysma muscle can obliterate the normal cervicomental angle at an early age. It is possible that the low hyoid position described by Marino et al. (1963) and generally accepted as one of the major causes of a loss of the normal cervicomental angle may, in fact, be of lesser significance than the anatomic positioning of the medial margins of the platysma muscle. Only time and accumulated clinical experience will determine this issue.

Recently, considerable attention has been given to the platysma and its varying deformities, as well as to the role of these structures in face lift surgery. Various techniques have been devised to correct anatomic aberrations. Contributions have been made by Skoog (1974), Millard (1968, 1972), Rees (1973), Guerrero-Santos (1974, 1978), Connell (1978), Peterson (1976), and others. Extensive clinical experience promises to define the role of these technical procedures designed to correct the platysma and its associated fascia in face lift surgery. Unquestionably, results have been generally improved because of this attention to detail.

Marino and his group (1963) studied several patients with "double chins." Their radiographic studies indicated that when the condition is due to a low placement of the hyoid bone, the deformity cannot be corrected by conventional operations. They believe that when the hyoid bone is located higher than the inferior border of the chin, the cervicomental angle is sufficiently acute to be amenable to surgical correction by removal of subcutaneous fat and/or excess skin or platysma. If, on the other hand, the hyoid bone lies lower than the chin, the angle becomes obliterated by the geniohyoid strap muscles and is therefore not surgically correctable. Such patients should be informed of this anatomic limitation prior to operation and told that in all probability the result will be modified. Perhaps the recent concentration on the platysma of this region will further clarify the matter.

Pangman and Wallace (1961) suggested removal of excess submental fat using scissors or curettage. Maliniac (1932) and Davis (1955) stressed the need for local excisions of excessive chin and neck skin, along with the removal of submental fat pads or lipomas through submental incisions. Millard, Pigott, and Hedo (1968), on the other hand, advocated dissection and removal of excessive submental fat from beneath the skin flaps through standard rhytidectomy incisions when possible.

Adamson, Horton, and Crawford (1964) studied the necks of 12 cadavers and discovered that the submental fat pad in older individuals varied between 15 and 25 gm in weight and between 15 and 27 ml in volume. They suggested a rather aggressive technique for correction of the cervicomental angle. This method required a long transverse incision made across the neck at approximately the level of the apex of the cervicomental angle, through which the excess fat could be removed and the platysma muscle could be plicated. They recommended this procedure as an adjunct to standard rhytidectomy and emphasized the importance of placing the skin incision in the transverse neck crease. The author suggests a cautious approach to this somewhat radical technique.

Skoog (1974) recommended dissection beneath the superficial fascia of the face that blends with the platysma below and foreshortening of this fascia to improve not only the jawline but the neckline. The anatomy of this superficial muscular aponeurotic system (SMAS) was recently reviewed by Mitz and Peyronie (1976). Various procedures have been devised to transect and reposition the platysma muscle as an aid in improving the results of the jawline and neckline during rhytidectomy (Guerrero-Santos, 1974; Millard, 1972; Connell, 1978; Peterson, 1974, 1976). Since these techniques are of topical concern and seem to hold considerable promise, they will be discussed subsequently in some detail.

If the skin hangs in loose folds inferior to the level of the hyoid, it becomes necessary to undermine it above the level of the platysma muscle as far inferiorly as the thyroid gland, in order to redistribute the skin and to excise the redundancy. When marked folds or depressions extend from the lateral commissures of the mouth downward to the chin or superiorly to the alae nasi (labiomental or nasolabial folds), extensive undermining may be required to achieve improvement. Such undermining — medially to the corner of the mouth — may result in some difficulty in the postoperative period, as localized hematoma formations are commonly encountered. There is also the possibility of damage to the buccal and mandibular branches of the facial nerve, since they are quite superficial this far medially.

Correction of deep nasolabial folds is one of the most disappointing aspects in current face lift technique. Although extensive undermining can result in some softening of these deep grooves (Figure 20–5), the improvement is still limited. Patients should be advised during the preoperative evaluation that correction will be minimal in this area.

Isolated deep lines or furrows of the face, such as glabellar frown lines or the aforementioned nasolabial or labiomental creases, may be helped by liquid silicone injections. Some such lines may be ablated by this experimental technique. Injections of silicone fluid are best carried out *following* rhytidectomy, except those for the ablation of glabellar frown lines. Injections in this region may be done at the same time as the operative procedure.

Extensive undermining of the skin over the malar prominences is also fraught with hazard. The buccal, ophthalmic, and zygomatic branches of the facial nerve become very superficial in this region and can easily be damaged during dissection. The amount of redistribution of skin that can be accomplished in this area is also limited. Therefore, undermining over the cheeks should be curtailed.

A critical area over the malar eminence has been identified and referred to as "MacGregor's

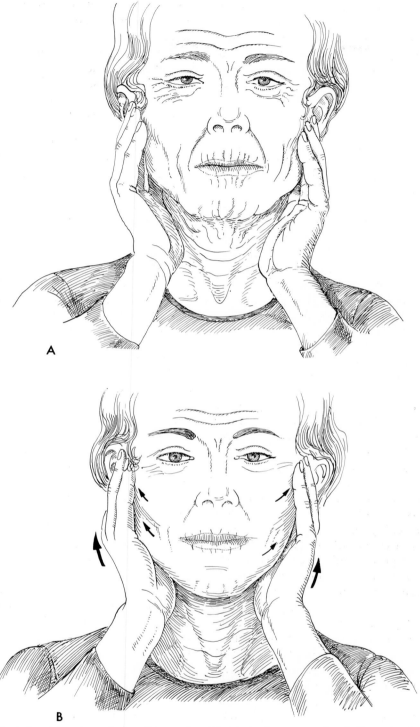

Figure 20–5. Patients inquiring about the possible results of facial plastic surgery often indicate the desired improvement by pulling the skin of the face and neck taut with their fingers (*B*). Although this maneuver gives a general idea of what may happen, it is not an accurate picture, as the correction tends to be exaggerated, particularly around the mouth and nasolabial folds. This point has to be emphasized to the patient seeking cosmetic surgery. On the other hand, the tautness of the jawline and the visible improvement of the neck will approach this simulated result. Fine rhytides in the facial skin will be improved somewhat, but not nearly to the degree that this manual tightening maneuver implies.

Immediately after surgery, particularly while postoperative edema persists, the results most often equal the patient's expectations. As time passes and edema subsides, folds and wrinkles will recur, particularly in severe cases. These shortcomings of the operative procedure must be emphasized before the operation.

patch" (1972). Not only are the facial nerve branches very superficial in this region but a significant artery penetrates the deeper structure just into the malar area that is easily severed during dissection. Division of this artery not only results in increased likelihood of hematoma but increases the possibility of avascular necrosis of the skin flaps.

Another reason for curtailing the amount of undermining over the zygoma and malar area is to lessen the danger of direct injury to the frontal branch of the facial nerve either from the dissection or from thermal injury incurred while cauterizing nearby vessels. The course of the frontal branch of the facial nerve where it emerges from the parotid gland incourses superiorly and medially to the orbicularis and frontalis muscles was described by Pitanguy and Ramos (1966). These surgeons, as well as Loeb (1970) and Correia and Zani (1973), described surgical techniques during rhytidectomy for preservation of this nerve. The nerve becomes superficial at a point midway between the anterior hairline and the lateral canthus of the eye. In fact, in this area, a bridge of soft tissue can be developed during the dissection that represents an aponeurotic neurovascular bundle in whose upper border runs the zygomatic orbital artery. Closer to the orbit, the frontal branch of the seventh nerve traverses this soft tissue bridge, which was so well described by Loeb. Extreme caution must be exercised in undermining the temporal skin in this region in order to preserve and protect these branches of the seventh nerve. If the surgeon elects to undermine the skin in the immediate subdermal plane, a nerve stimulator should be employed to identify the course of the nerve branches. Unquestionably, a safer technique of dissection is demonstrated in Figure 22–12. Because of the fusion of the temporal and superficial fascia, the dissection is extended anteriorly beneath the superficial fascia above the level of the zygoma, whereas below the zygoma, the dissection is in the immediate subcutaneous plane. In this way, the aponeurotic bridge, which carries the all important frontal branch, is maintained. Injury to this branch carries a less than 10 percent chance of return of function, even when the edges are identified and repaired.

Patients in whom the angles of the mandible are prominent and in whom the distance between the angles of the mandible is foreshortened, or those in whom the mandibular body assumes a more direct or flat course, are most apt to demonstrate a strong jowl formation from excess skin in this region. Extensive undermining and upward traction on the skin flaps is doubly important in such patients. Even then, correction of the jowls may be limited.

Patients least amenable to surgical correction by rhytidectomy are those who have demonstrable hypoplasia of the maxilla with flattening of the cheekbones and/or long narrow mandibles. This deficiency of the underlying bony architecture makes draping of the soft tissues difficult, and early recurrence of redundant skin along the jaw and neck can generally be anticipated.

As mentioned previously, patients with marked rhytidosis from extensive senile changes of the skin or from atrophy of the skin because of prolonged actinic or wind exposure can also be expected to obtain only limited improvement from a standard rhytidectomy. Such patients, however, can often benefit from a deep skin peel (chemabrasion) subsequent to operation. When ancillary procedures such as chemabrasion are thought to be necessary by the surgeon, the complete surgical program should be discussed in detail with the patient prior to the rhytidectomy.

Certain inherited or acquired conditions of the skin, while not constituting an absolute contraindication to face lift surgery, may contribute to troublesome sequelae or prolonged healing time. These conditions should be recognized prior to surgery and the patient should be advised of their potential influence on the results of the operation. For example, patients with very thin, transparent skin with hypopigmentation are prone to severe ecchymosis, which may be prolonged for many weeks or months postoperatively, particularly in the thin skin of the eyelids.

Patients with telangiectasia may experience an exacerbation of the small lesions following rhytidectomy. These may be particularly noticeable in the neck region. In some cases, these multiple telangiectases become permanent, with a resulting reddish discoloration of the neck skin and, sometimes, the cheeks. Patients with small telangiectases should be advised prior to surgery that new lesions may appear. Such disturbances in skin color can usually be camouflaged by appropriate face makeup.

A keloid diathesis does not necessarily mean that keloids will develop in the face lift scars. However, thickening or hypertrophy of the scars behind the ears is more apt to occur in such patients. They should be advised of this possibility. True keloids following face lifting are extremely rare, even in patients who exhibit true keloids of scars elsewhere on the body.

As mentioned previously, the thin patient is a

better candidate than the obese patient, not only because the immediate operative result is better but also because the obese patient has a tendency to gain and lose weight intermittently, a habit that can have disastrous effects on even the most careful rhytidectomy by causing recurrent stretching of the skin. Some obese patients can be induced to lose weight preoperatively by being made to understand that the facial plastic operation will then be more successful. The obese patient who loses significant weight and maintains the weight reduction for some time prior to surgery is often an excellent face lift candidate, for the weight loss and its maintenance indicate good motivation for the procedure. Obese patients who do not lose weight can still be helped by rhytidectomy and submental lipectomy when jowls or a double chin are the prominent factors.

Most surgeons now agree that the best time for the first facial plastic operation is whenever it is needed. In most instances, this is between the ages of 45 and 55, when the telltale signs of age usually first appear. In the author's opinion, it is unnecessary and unwise to wait for advanced signs of aging before advising surgery. When the decision to operate is postponed until the changes assume the characteristics of senility in the sixth or seventh decade, the immediate results are highly satisfying, but the improvement lasts for a shorter period than in the younger patient, and a second operation may be required sooner than if surgery was first performed in the fourth or fifth decade of life.

Uncommonly, a face lift may be required by a patient in her middle or late thirties. Early cessation of hormonal function resulting from hysterectomy or premature menopause may bring about skin changes that require surgery at an early age. Facial surgery in such patients should, however, be supplemented by hormone replacement therapy, proper skin hygiene, and related measures that will aid in maintaining the result.

(For references, see pages 724 to 727.)

Chapter 21

Preoperative Preparation

Thomas D. Rees, M.D., F.A.C.S.

The use of moulages, plaster casts, and similar three-dimensional preparations is of limited or no value in planning the face lift operation, except perhaps to impress the patient. Accurate, standardized, and realistic photographs can, however, be of immense value to the surgeon both in his preoperative planning and in the operating room. Such photographs are best taken by a professional medical photographer using standardized lighting and techniques so that every detail of the facial structure is clearly shown. However, perfectly adequate photography can be done in the surgeon's office with any one of the numerous systems available today. Care should be taken to take photographs of a high and reproducible quality. Generally an 80 to 100 mm lens takes the best "head shots" with good depth of field and minimal distortion of features. Full-face, both profiles, and three quarter views showing the face in repose and in animation can be most helpful in deciding the amount of undermining to be done and in delineating those facial configurations that can be only slightly or not at all improved by surgery.

An important view to help the surgeon assess the role of the platysma in neck deformities is the full front face taken with the chin tilted slightly upwards and the jaws clenched to contract the platysma fully (Figure 21–1). Prominent platysma borders and midmuscle bands are easily identified. It is important that all defects be pointed out to the patient on the photographs prior to surgery.

Reviewing preoperative and postoperative photographs of others with a prospective candidate for surgery seems unwise in most instances, since the patient seeks fruitlessly to identify with the photographs. Also, an "implied result" can be a medicolegal complication. Certainly if such photographs are shown, the surgeon should have written permission from the patient whose likeness is reproduced; otherwise, a serious breach of ethics

could be claimed. Perhaps a good case for showing photos can be made when the surgical candidate has an unusually difficult problem such as microgenia, an obtuse cervicomental angle, or very prominent platysmal bands. Under those circumstances, when chin augmentation or platysmal resection seems indicated, it may be helpful to use photographic documentation to illustrate possible results.

Because adequate hemostasis is so essential to a successful operative result, it is important for the surgeon to be aware of any potential bleeding problems. Patient who are on "the pill" or other forms of hormone treatment such as estrogen-replacement therapy are more apt to ooze than others. It is therefore advisable to dicontinue hormone medication in female patients 10 days to two weeks before surgery. It is also thought to be unwise to operate on patients just prior to or immediately following the onset of menses, since bleeding of the ozzing type is more apt to occur at this time.

The effect of salicylates in preventing platelet agglutination and causing distressing bleeding during and immediately after surgery seems established. All compounds that contain salicylates must be discontinued, preferably 10 days before surgery. A more complete list of these medications is provided elsewhere in this volume; however, the more commonly used ones include aspirin, Bufferin, Excedrin, and Alka-Seltzer.

Blood dyscrasias can often be discovered prior to surgery, and a history of easy bruising, and most particularly a history of prolonged bruising following minor injury, should be thoroughly investigated. Although true hemophilia does not occur in the female, certain bleeding disorders do occur. A carefully taken history should disclose if there is or ever has been any prolonged bruising, spontaneous bleeding, excessive bleeding during any previ-

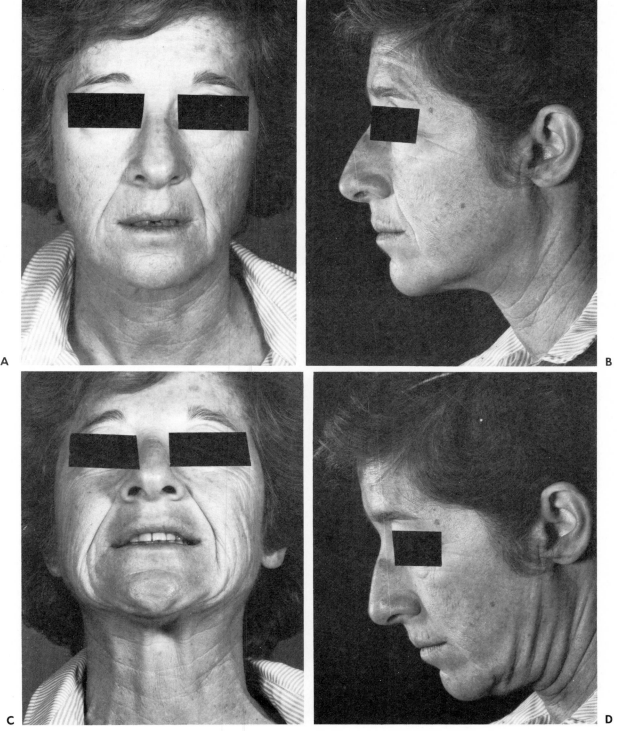

Figure 21–1. Preoperative photographs of a candidate for rhytidectomy and possible platysma surgery. Several views are advantageous in determining the technical variations in the operative procedure to be employed.

A, Frontal view, face in repose.

B, Profile view.

C, The "platysma" view, shot slightly from below with the teeth clenched. Note that the platysma is activated. The medial bands are brought into prominence by clenching the teeth.

D, The looking down, slightly flexed, "book-in-lap" view helps the surgeon to evaluate the upper neck and submental and submandibular skin, fat, and muscle.

ous operative procedures, or any bleeding problems in the family.

Preoperative antisepsis techniques are indicated in all patients to lessen the likelihood of postoperative infection, although surgical infection in rhytidectomy wounds is extremely uncommon, probably because of the rich blood supply to this region that enables the body to mobilize its natural defenses to ward off bacterial infiltration. Thorough facial washings with pHisoHex for three days preceding surgery are recommended. A 15-minute pHisoHex shampoo of the hair on the night prior to operation seems beneficial in promoting an antiseptic field in which to work. Because of the small chance of infection of the skin in this region, it is not necessary to shave the margins of the hair before rhytidectomy. Limited clipping of the hair with sharp scissors at the sites of the surgical incisions is done just prior to operation. Usually, only the areas where the excision will be accomplished are clipped, so that the eventual suture line lies mostly within the hair, particularly in the temporal scalp (Figure 21–2).

Use of various skin antiseptics immediately prior to surgery is preferred by many surgeons. Aqueous Zephiran is commonly used and not only is probably ineffective but also neutralizes much of the good achieved by the pHisoHex. Iodine releasing solutions such as Betadine are probably best; however, the skin is temporarily stained and this causes a minor distraction. In fact, pHisoHex is probably as effective alone as it is in combination with other antiseptics, and, in the author's opinion, it can be employed safely as the sole skin preparation.

Considerable controversy exists as to the value of prophylactic antibiotics. Most authorities in surgical bacteriology negate their value in elective "clean" operations such as rhytidectomy, a theory to which the author subscribes. Certainly, the antibiotics commonly employed as prophylactics by most surgeons (such as tetracycline) are ineffective against the organisms usually implicated in postoperative infections of this region. A skin concentration exceeding 10^5 is probably required as a prerequisite for infection in face lifts. Adequate skin

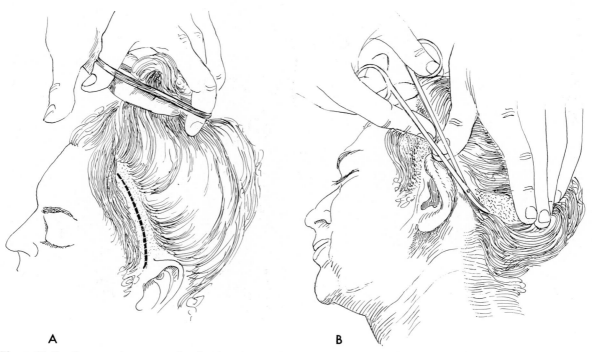

A   **B**

Figure 21–2.   Preoperative preparation for the usual face lift operation begins by combing the hair upward and fixing it with a rubber band as a top knot or "pony tail" (*A*). Sharp barber's scissors can be used to cut tracks in the temporal scalp and behind the ear to coincide with the planned incisions (*B*). These trimmed areas should be only as large as the amount of skin to be excised, so that the final suture lines lie virtually within the hair. Because preoperative preparation with pHisoHex shampoo has practically eliminated wound infections, shaving of the hair is not necessary.

preparation as described militates against such concentration. Antibiotics are no substitute for proper preparation and technique.

The patient should be placed on the table in such a way that the head can be elevated during the operative procedure. Elevation of the head is helpful in (1) control of bleeding, (2) demonstration of areas of loose or ptotic skin folds, and (3) giving the surgeon greater access to the operative field. A cerebellar head rest or similar attachment is most useful in providing access to the operative area. The access provided by the cerebellar head rest also permits suturing both sides at the same time during final closure of the wound.

The headrest should be adjusted so that the head lies in a natural position in relationship to the rest of the body. The head should be slightly flexed at the neck to permit redraping and trimming of the skin flaps at the most advantageous angle.

Chapter 22

The Classical Operation

THOMAS D. REES, M.D., F.A.C.S.

This chapter describes the classic technique of rhytidectomy that is generally accepted and practiced by plastic surgeons throughout the world. Conceptually, this procedure consists of undermining the skin and subcutaneous tissue for varying distances over the face, jawline, and neck. Skin flaps are thereby fashioned, rotated, and advanced in a posterocephalad direction and attached at their new position with key sutures. The excess skin is excised and the wounds are closed (Figures 22–1 and 22–2). The hair is not shaved; however, bare areas approximating the expected amount of soft tissue resection are cleared with sharp scissors within the hair-bearing skin so that after suturing, the incision lines lie almost entirely within the hair-bearing scalp (see Figure 21–2).

When the hairline has been rotated in a cephalic direction to the extent that there is a hairless area above the ear, it can be improved by excising a triangle along the inferior border of the temporal hair-bearing scalp to rotate the scalp flap downward as shown in Figure 22–3. Another triangle can be removed from the superior pole of the wound to avoid a dogear.

THE PROCEDURE

Planning the incisions, developing the skin flaps, and closing the skin wounds are the basic steps in all rhytidectomy procedures. The most esoteric and recent techniques involving the muscles and fascia of the face and neck are welcome additions to the basic technique, but they are not required in all patients. These techniques will be discussed subsequently. The fundamental steps of face lift surgery are illustrated in Figure 22–4.

The operation is performed with the patient under either general or local anesthetic; however, subcutaneous infiltration with dilute amounts of

epinephrine 1:200,000 is generally used to induce local hemostasis.

It is best to infiltrate the subcutaneous area prior to scrubbing. This allows at least 10 minutes for the epinephrine to achieve effect. The face is then prepared with an antiseptic solution and is suitably draped. The incisions are made and skin flaps are developed by sharp knife-scissor dissection.

The amount of undermining naturally varies from patient to patient. In the younger subject with small jowls over the body of the mandible, it is necessary to undermine only to the anterior extent of this skin fold and as much of the neck as seems necessary. Slackness of the skin over the jaw is almost inevitable in face lift patients, so that undermining is almost always required, whereas the extent of undermining on the neck depends on the configuration of the soft tissues of the neck (Figure 22–5). It may be minimal or it may cross the midline so that the skin of the neck is completely lifted. Such undermining is best kept to a superficial level to avoid damage to the seventh cranial nerve and to blood vessels, particularly the jugular vein.

The skin flap is raised with a very thin layer of fat, almost as in a full-thickness graft. When such a flap is retracted and seen from beneath, it is almost transparent. It is so thin that extreme care must be taken to preserve the blood supply and to avoid injuring the vessels. Traction is exerted only with skin hooks or traction sutures, and the flaps are not handled manually. Squeezing or excessive traction during the dissection can result in irreversible damage to the blood vessels, causing embarrassment of circulation, thrombosis, and sloughing of the skin. Minor skin sloughing is most frequently encountered over the mastoid process, where the maximum stretch is exerted, and it is also in this

600

Text continued on page 609.

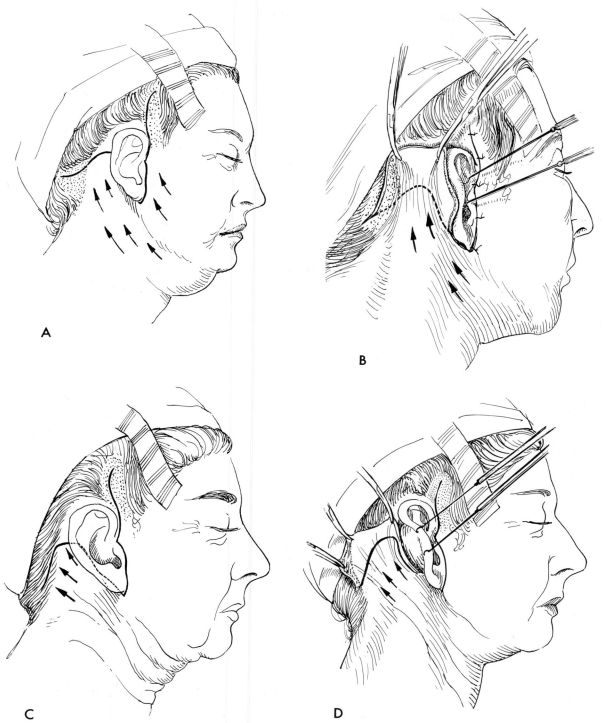

A

B

C

D

Figure 22–1. Judgment must be employed in the final draping of the skin flaps after undermining has been completed. The flaps are pulled more superiorly than posteriorly in patients whose redundant tissue is mostly in the submental area and along the jaw (*A* and *B*). If tightening of the neck is the foremost consideration, the direction of pull is more posterior than cephalad (*C* and *D*).

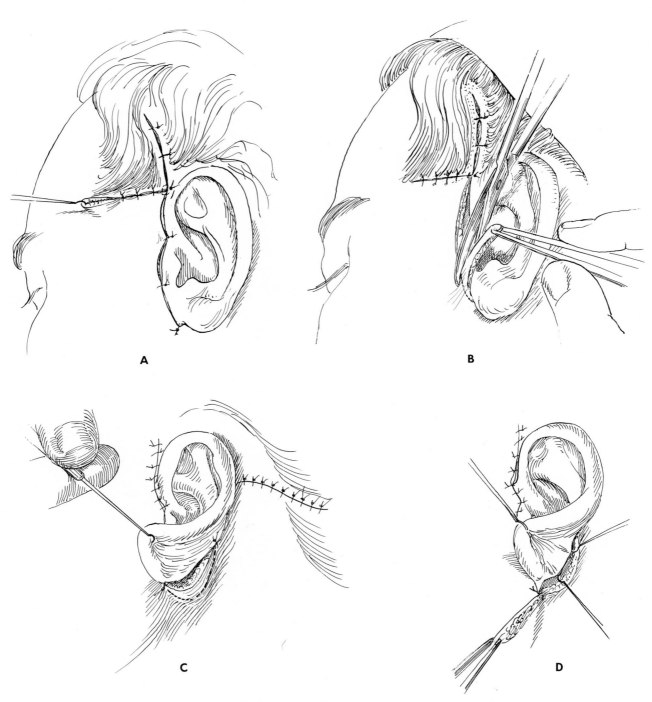

Figure 22–2. Final adjustments to excise skin are made after key sutures have been placed. A small dog-ear may present at the anterior angle of the horizontal incision (if any); it is trimmed by the conventional method of elevating it with a skin hook and removing a triangle (*A*). These small dog-ears should not be pursued farther forward than the limit of the hairline, in order to avoid visible scars. In some patients a small redundancy here may be necessary for this reason, but these usually smooth out with time.

Any excess of preauricular skin is trimmed as a final step (*B*). Trimming here should be conservative, so that there is absolutely no tension on the preauricular closure; otherwise, spreading of the final scar will result. The preauricular scar must be as inconspicuous as possible, for it is the only part of the incision that is likely to be visible.

A very small strip of skin behind the earlobe is removed to allow accurate tailoring of the wound (*C* and *D*). This is semicircular in design, conforming to the slight flange effect of the original preoperative plan.

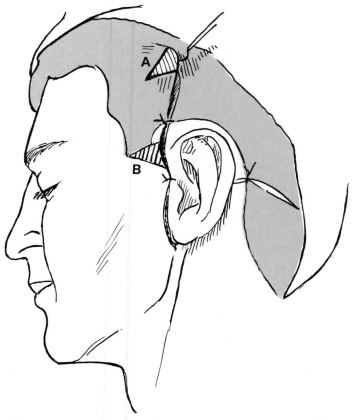

Figure 22–3.   Adjustment of temporal hairline (see text, p. 600).

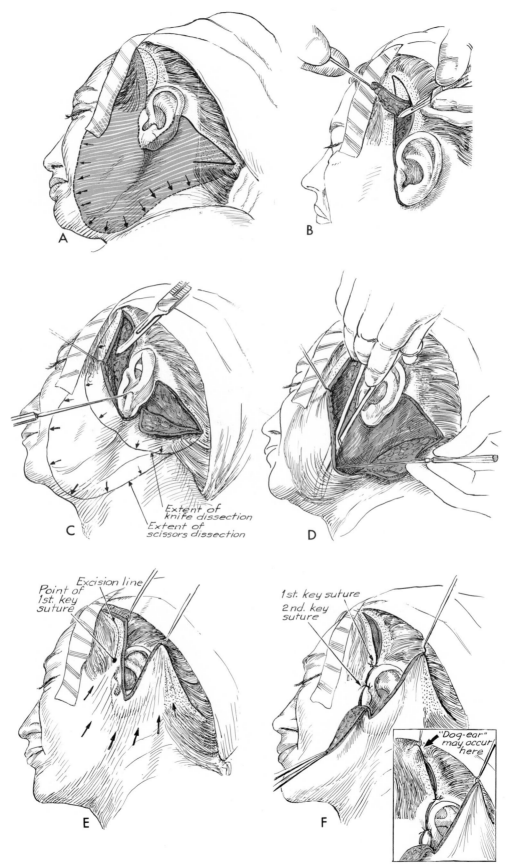

Figure 22–4. *See legend on the opposite page.*

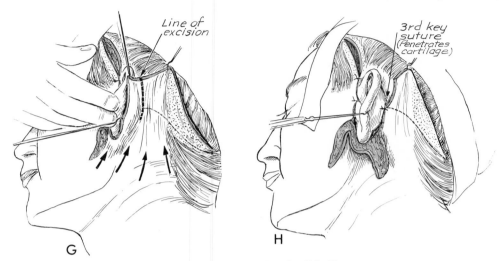

Figure 22–4.   The Classical Operation — Planning and Managing the Skin Flaps.

A, The dotted line indicates the minimum amount of undermining of skin flaps required in all patients (in the author's opinion). Undermining must extend beyond the defect. Pre-excision of the skin can be unreliable, particularly in secondary cases; however, in the temporal scalp, it is quite safe when conservatively planned. The incision into the postauricular hairline should extend into the hairline in a posterior direction, as indicated, in *most patients.* In some patients with excessive skin folds of the neck, however, the incision can follow the hairline toward the nuchal region.

B, The dissection is begun with excision of the temporal preplanned skin ellipse.

C, The undermining is best begun with a scalpel in the temporal area and over the insertion of the sternocleidomastoid muscle, where the cleavage plane is indistinct. The level of dissection in the temple is just below the superficial temporal fascia. As the dissection proceeds medially, precautions must be taken to avoid the temporal branch of the facial nerve. The extent of knife dissection usually done by the author is indicated by the first line of arrows. The absolute minimum of skin undermining is indicated by the more distal line of arrows. Scissors are used to complete the latter.

D, Double-edged scissors are utilized to extend the undermining.

At the completion of undermining of the skin flaps and whatever procedures are utilized to adjust the underlying musculature (platysma) and aponeurotic system of the face and neck, as well as excision of redundant fat, which is often done with the help of a submental incision, the skin flaps are adjusted so as to excise the redundancy and suture the wounds with appropriate support and lack of tension on the wound edges in key areas of scarring, such as the preauricular area and around the lobe.

The skin flaps are also adjusted differently in each individual, according to the problem at hand.

E, The skin flaps are generally pulled with gentle traction in a cephalic and posterior direction (arrows). The first key suture, which is a traction suture, is placed in the temporal scalp at or just above the hairline. The hairline must not be raised excessively.

F, A second suture is optional just above the tragus.

G and H, The redundant skin flap behind the ear is incised and split very cautiously to the superior angle of the postauricular incision, where a third key traction suture is placed. This suture is often anchored into the conchal cartilage.

Illustration continued on the following page.

Figure 22–4 *Continued.   I,* The excision proceeds in a piecemeal fashion, excising the redundant skin. It is important to excise the skin very accurately around the ear so that the wound edges are gently "kissing" without any tension whatsoever. Tension on the preauricular wound or around the lobule will result in forward migration of the scar and downward migration of the earlobe. Also, the possibility of hypertrophy or keloid formation is greatly increased. The temporal scalp and the wound within the posterior hairline can be sutured with some tension to relieve tension of the skin wound around the ear.

J, The posterior hairline may be difficult to adjust in some patients with a great deal of skin redundancy. Small "stairsteps" can easily be overcome with sutures. It is helpful to begin suturing the wound at the posterior angle not only to prevent stairstepping, but also to avoid dog-ears at the angle. A small irregularity in the hairline is acceptable.

K, Minute and final adjustments are made before the final wound closure.

L–O, Considerable slack in the skin flap along the jawline may require a more cephalic rotation than can be achieved with the standard incision without excessive elevation of the hairline. In such patients, a triangle can be excised at the inferior margin of the temporal hairline, not extending anterior to the hairline. This excision facilitates rotation of the cheek flap and avoids a dog-ear at the cephalic angle of the incision in the temporal scalp. The author has found this small horizontal cut almost a necessity in secondary face lifts to avoid hairline elevation. It also affords an excellent mechanical advantage in rotation of the cheek flap, as noted. As long as the anterior extent of this small incision does not violate the hairless temporal scalp, patients are unaware of it.

See illustration on the opposite page.

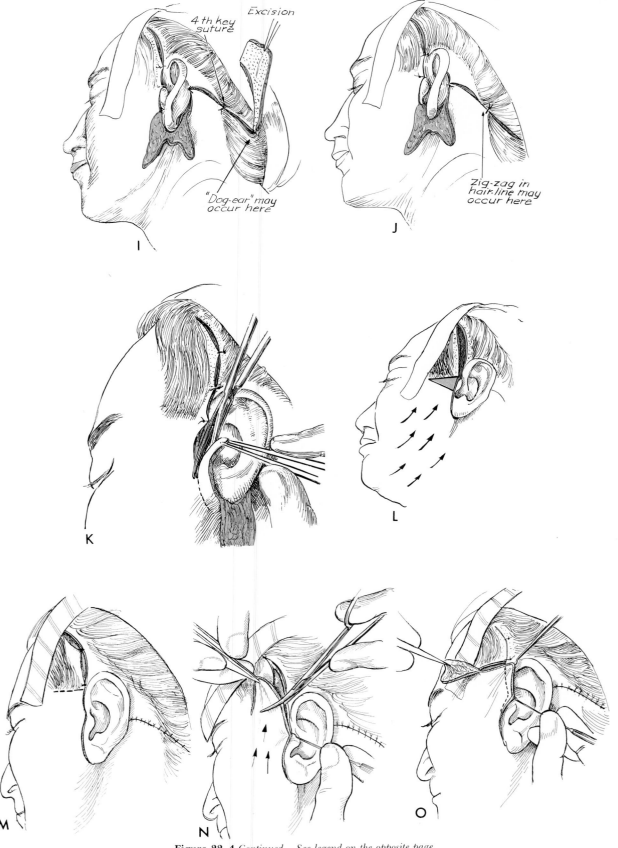

Figure 22–4 *Continued.   See legend on the opposite page.*

Illustration continued on the following page.

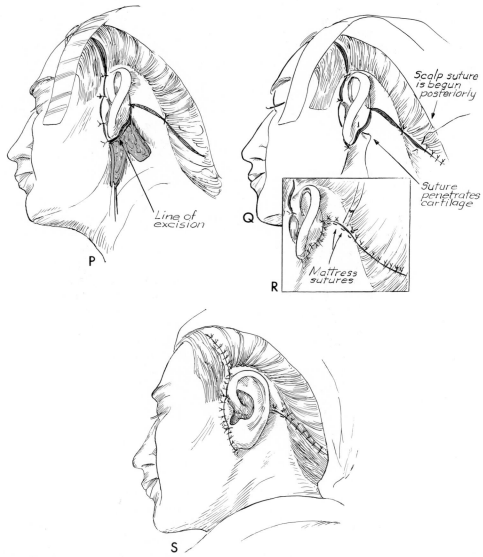

Figure 22–4 *Continued.   P,* Final trimming of the skin flaps is done behind the ear.

Q, The posterior scalp wound is sutured from the back toward the ear to avoid dog-ears and hairline stairstepping. Two or three sutures are placed through the conchal cartilage and the skin flap to relieve tension from the closure around the lobule.

R, Horizontal, half-buried mattress sutures are helpful in the bare skin of the mastoid area to avoid suture marks in this delicate skin. A better scar is produced, and it is often possible for the post–face lift patient to wear his or her hair swept backward. Fine nylon sutures are preferred for closure.

S, The final suture line.

area that skin flaps are most likely to be abused between the thumb and the forefinger during surgery.

Dissection in the loose subcutaneous and supraplatysmal tissue plane of the neck and face is best accomplished by the "spread and cut" scissor technique. Scalpel dissection serves best over the mastoid process and down the neck above the sternocleidomastoid muscle, where the skin is intimately associated with the underlying fascia. Take care to avoid injury to the postauricular nerve during these procedures. Severing this nerve produces permanent numbness of the lower part of the ear and the earlobe. If the nerve is accidentally cut and the damage is recognized during surgery, repair using 7–0 or 8–0 silk sutures in the epineurium should be carried out immediately.

Hemostasis should be meticulously carried out with fine pointed forceps and cautery. Larger vessels are ligated; if the jugular vein is cut, it is divided between clamps and tied. Pinpoint electrocoagulation of bleeding vessels is called for, without offense to the surrounding normal tissue. Excessive cauterization, especially on the underside of the skin flap, will cause focal necrosis and sometimes small perforations; scarring will mar the final result. Larger vessels, again particularly those on the flap, should be protected from the cautery when possible to avoid segmental infarction.

The facial nerve will not be endangered if the dissection can be maintained at a superficial level. Where the ramus mandibularis becomes superficial (penetrating the platysma near the external maxillary artery over the body of the mandible), particular care is required. Another dangerous area is the temporal region, and caution must be exercised to avoid injuring the temporal branch of the facial nerve. Dissection should be superficial to the temporal fascia; as it proceeds anteriorly, a nerve stimulator can be used if doubt exists as to the location of this branch.

Dissection can proceed as far anteriorly as the corner of the mouth or the nasolabial fold. However, the terminal branches of the facial nerve become extremely superficial at these places and can be easily injured, resulting in partial or complete paralysis of the muscles they innervate. It is quite true that these terminal branches may regenerate, but regeneration is not always complete, and in some instances disassociated muscle fasciculations persist indefinitely.

Dissection over the malar eminence is rarely necessary and should be undertaken with care to avoid damaging the buccal or ophthalmic branches of the facial nerve. Dissection medial to the lateral wall of the zygoma is practically never indicated.

Undermining is most effective over the lower face, jaw, and neck, where maximal improvement is achieved. Undermining extends distal to the jowl and to or across the midline of the neck. The skin flaps are then advanced and rotated, the excess skin is excised, and the wound is sutured. Maximal tension on the skin flaps occurs in the temporal and posterior scalp. There must be little or no tension where the skin flap surrounds the ear, because it produces stretched or hypertrophic scars (Figure 22–6). The preauricular scar can migrate anteriorly under stress, producing an unsightly result. The earlobe must also be fitted loosely to prevent downward traction (Figure 22–7). Hemostasis is meticulous and accomplished with cautery. Larger vessels are ligated with plain catgut.

Plication of the superficial fascia may or may not be done, according to the surgeon's preference. The lasting results of this maneuver have not been proved. The wounds are sutured with fine sutures of 4–0 and 5–0 Ethilon or Prolene. I have placed half-buried horizontal mattress sutures in the bare area of mastoid skin to minimize the scar and eliminate stitch marks in this highly visible area (Figure 22–8). Drains may or may not be used. If the wound is "moist," I prefer to use the newer suction drains. A light head dressing is applied for two days, not for its pressure effect, which is probably nonexistent, but as a protective covering for the skin flaps and to immobilize the head.

TECHNICAL DETAILS IN THE CLASSICAL SKIN OPERATION

Since the basic face lift operation involves the formation of skin flaps and the redistribution of the skin as well as excision of the excess, certain technical problems arise that are common to all flaps (Figure 22–9). Small details in the planing of rhytidectomy incisions or final adjustments of the flaps are important in the final cosmetic results in order to avoid unsightly scars or unnatural positioning of the hairline. Small dogears at the angles of the wounds within the hairline will disappear with the passage of time; however, large dogears should be avoided since they will not become completely dissipated with the forces of healing.

The problem of skin redistribution becomes more complicated with older patients whose skin is less elastic and contains many wrinkles and folds (Figure 22–10).

Text continued on page 619.

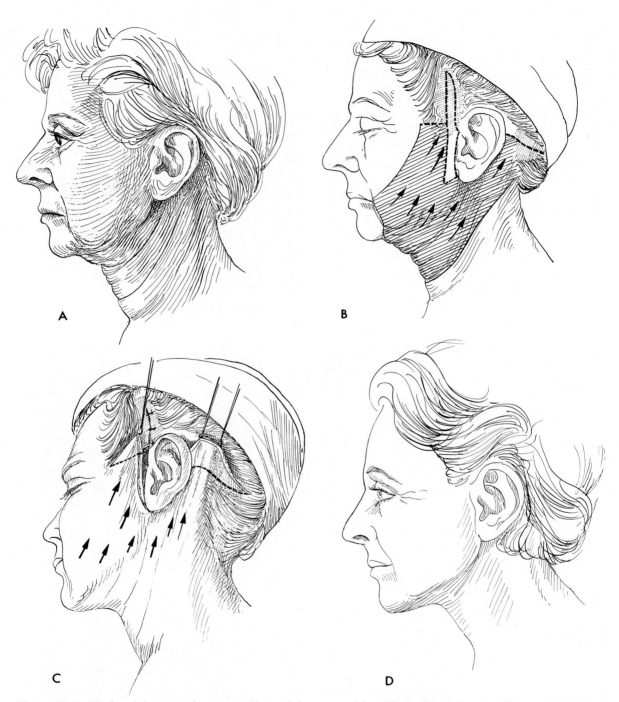

Figure 22–5. Undermining must always extend beyond the most peripheral limit of the deformity. When marked redundancy of the skin of the neck is the main problem (*A*), the undercutting must extend completely around the anterior circumference of the neck (*B*). The excess is then pulled slightly posteriorly, but mostly in a cephalad direction (*C*), where it is excised in large triangles in front of and behind the ear, leaving a pleasing result (*D*).

Illustration continued on the opposite page.

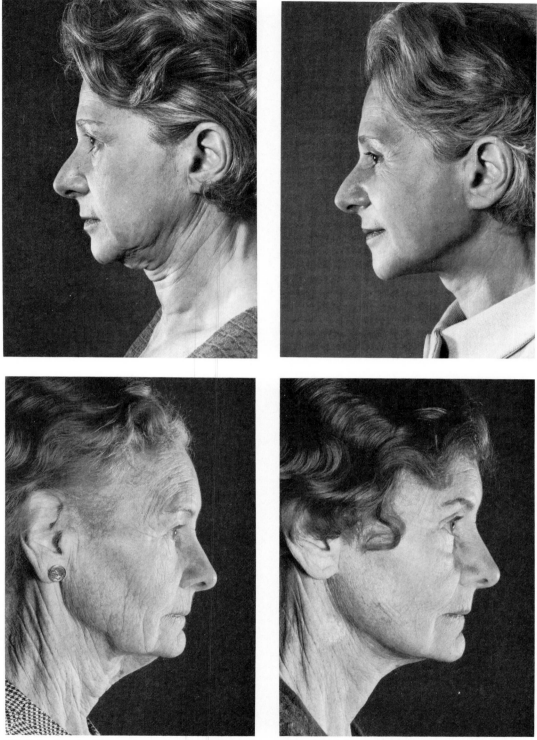

Figure 22–5 *Continued.*   Two patients with the problem illustrated in *A*, and the correction achieved using the technique shown in *B* and *C*.

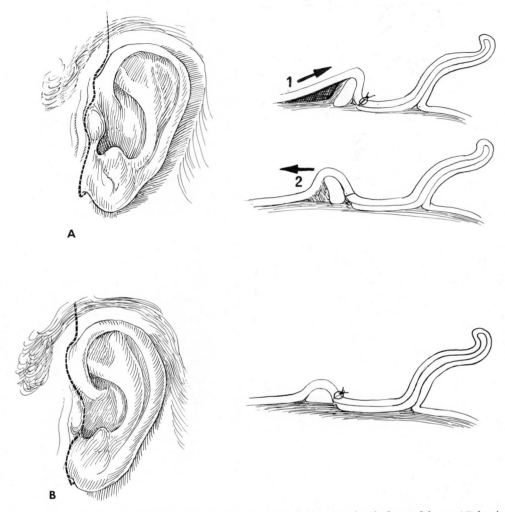

Figure 22–6.   The preauricular incision is usually placed in the normal skin crease just in front of the ear (*A*), but in some patients the incision can be carried behind the tragus so that most of the scar will be virtually invisible (*B*). This is done only in patients who have no natural line in front of the ear and who do not have a prominent or sharp tragal cartilage; otherwise, normal wound contraction may result in distortion of the tragus and an unnatural look (*A*, 1 and 2).

The usual preauricular incision heals surprisingly well and with minimal scarring, provided the sutures are removed within six days. The incision should form a slight angle at the superior edge of the tragus in order to follow the natural line of the ear.

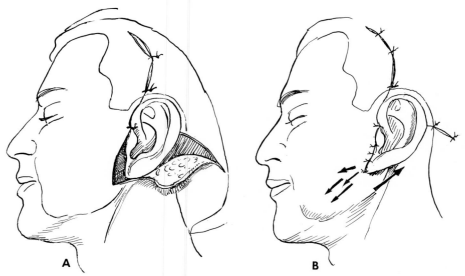

Figure 22–7. *A* and *B*, Distortion of the earlobe in the postoperative result is usually caused by untoward tension exerted on the wound by the skin flaps. One important cause of earlobe migration is excision of too much of the cheek flap in front of the ear and insufficient countertraction in a posterocephalic direction.

Illustration continued on the following page.

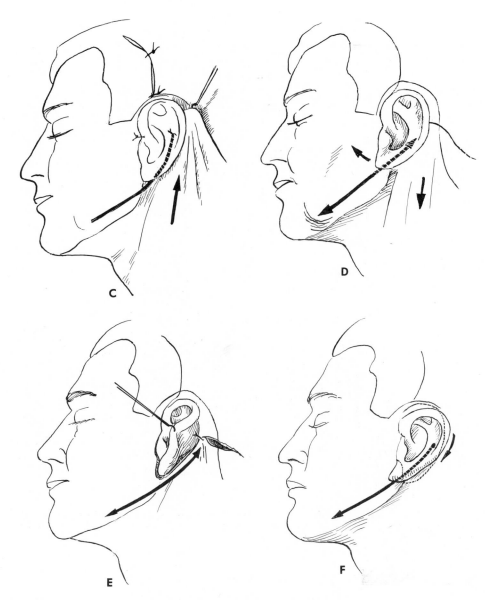

Figure 22–7 *Continued.*   *C,* Tension on the flap should be relieved by upward pull.

D, During the long-term contracture phase of healing, the flap contracts in several directions, indicated by the arrows. These forces of contraction tend to cause distortion and migration of the earlobe. This is an important reason to maintain a small cuff of redundancy around the earlobe during final adjusting and cutting of the flap.

E, The strongest line of tension on the jowl and neck flap is slightly curved and follows the line of the mandibular body in most cases.

F, The forces of healing plus gravity gradually straighten out the tension line causing forward migration of the earlobe. These forces are another good argument for leaving a redundant cuff of flap around the lobe and along the preauricular line. *There should be no tension on the preauricular incision at the end of the operation.*

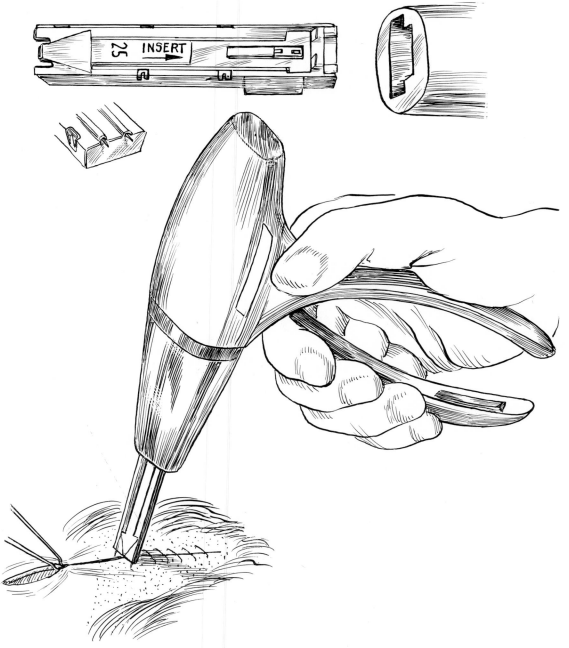

Figure 22–8. The staple gun is a useful instrument in closing the face lift wound. It is a great time-saver for the surgeon who must operate without assistants. Several models are available on the market.

The wound edges are held in direct apposition with the help of skin hooks or temporary sutures, and the staples are inserted at right angles to the skin surface.

The staples are elevated above the skin so that cross hatches of the skin wound are obviated. The author uses stainless steel staples to close incisions within the hairline and sutures to close the wounds in the visible skin areas around the ears over the mastoid.

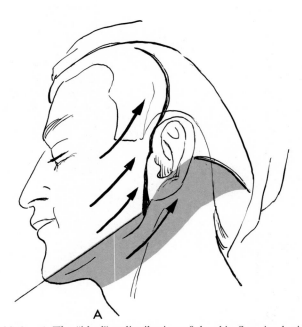

Figure 22–9.   *A,* The "ideal" redistribution of the skin flaps in rhytidectomy.

Illustration continued on the opposite page.

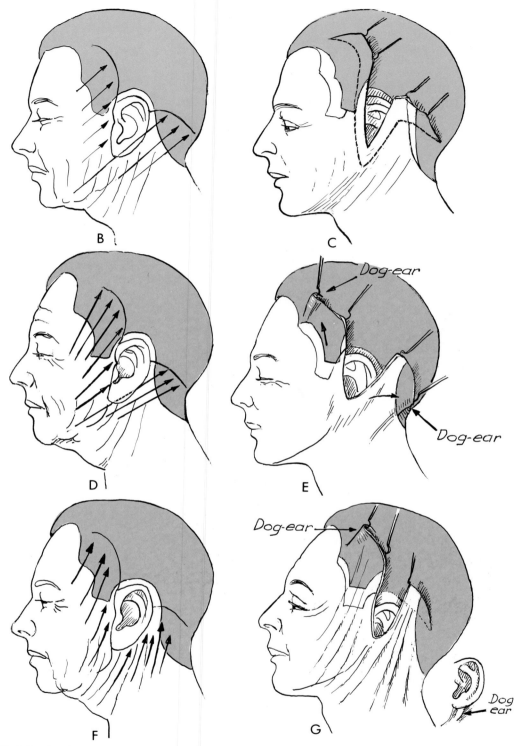

Figure 22–9 *Continued.* *B* and *C,* In patients with a moderate amount of excess skin, proper direction to pull on the skin flaps results in overlap within the hair-bearing scalp and dog-ears, which can be dealt with by even redistribution without unduly disturbing the hairline.

D and *E,* With increasingly redundant skin and more cephalic rotation of the anterior flap as well as posterior displacement of the lower flap, the size of the dog-ears increases. Stairstepping of the posterior hairline and elevation of the temporal hairline become increasingly problematic.

F and *G,* Strong cephalic tension on the flaps helps to avoid the posterior dog-ear and disturbance in the postauricular hairline indicated in *E,* however, such upward pull only raises the temporal hairline and the sideburn even higher.

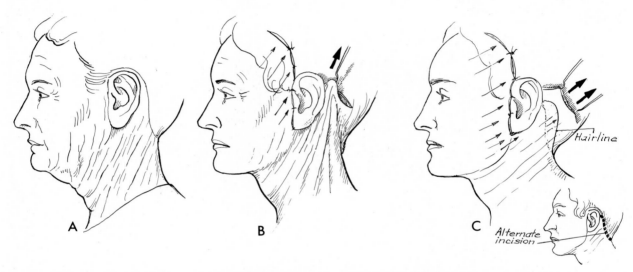

Figure 22–10. Marked redundancy and wrinkling of the neck skin is particularly difficult to solve without distorting the hairline or resorting to incisions that parallel the hairline and thereby cannot be concealed within the hair-bearing scalp.

A, The problem.

B, Strong cephalic pull draws the redundant neck skin into vertical folds.

C, Exerting tension on the neck skin in a more posterior direction improves the result but distorts the postauricular hairline considerably. The alternative incision to obviate posterior displacement of the hairline must sometimes be used; however, the scar is more obvious and difficult to camouflage.

The direction of pull of the skin flaps and the redistribution of the skin must be compromised at times to achieve a balance between the best possible end result and excessive distortion of the temporal and postauricular hairline. Such a compromise was achieved in the two patients shown in Figure 22–11, who had marked degenerative skin changes, deep wrinkling, and ptosis.

The technique must be varied from individual to individual and at times accompanied by submental dissection when correction of the submental or upper neck region is not sufficiently achieved

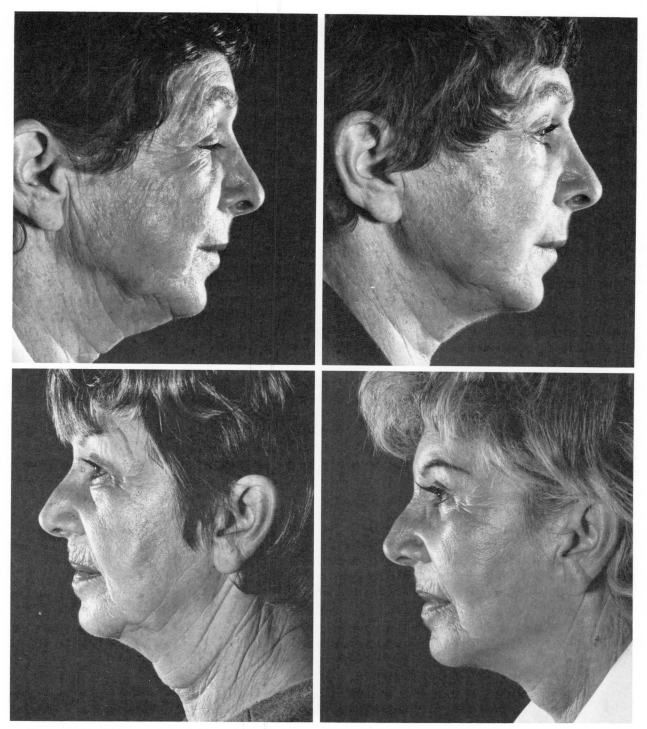

Figure 22–11.   The end result of skin redistribution must necessarily be compromised in patients with marked wrinkling and excess skin of the neck.

Figure 22–12.   To do a proper temporal lift, extensive undermining is needed (A and B). It must extend medially as far as the brow and almost to the outer canthus of the eye, and the operation is therefore anything but a "minilift." In fact, it is hazardous, because the temporal branch of the facial nerve is quite superficial in this region, coursing generally along a line drawn from the outer canthus to the external auditory canal. It is almost mandatory to use a nerve stimulator in order to avoid damage to this branch when doing a proper temporal lift.

Hemostasis can also be difficult because of the profusion of small blood vessels in the area. Excessive electrocoagulation of such vessels requires that the surgeon identify and protect the facial nerve so as not to injure its branches with the heat of the cautery. I do not subscribe to Pitanguy's advice that undermining above the theoretical transfacial course of the temporal branch can be deep to the temporal fascia while that below is superficial. On the other hand, all undermining in the temporal region should be superficial, with injury to the temporal branch of the facial nerve carefully avoided by positively identifying it.

After wide undercutting, the skin flap is rotated posteriorly with considerable posterior and cephalad traction applied (C and D). Excess skin is removed, and the wound is sutured (E). Most of the tension will be taken up in the posterior scalp, well behind the hairline; therefore, the scar in this region tends to stretch and widen with time, leaving a strip of hairless scalp.

See illustration on the opposite page.

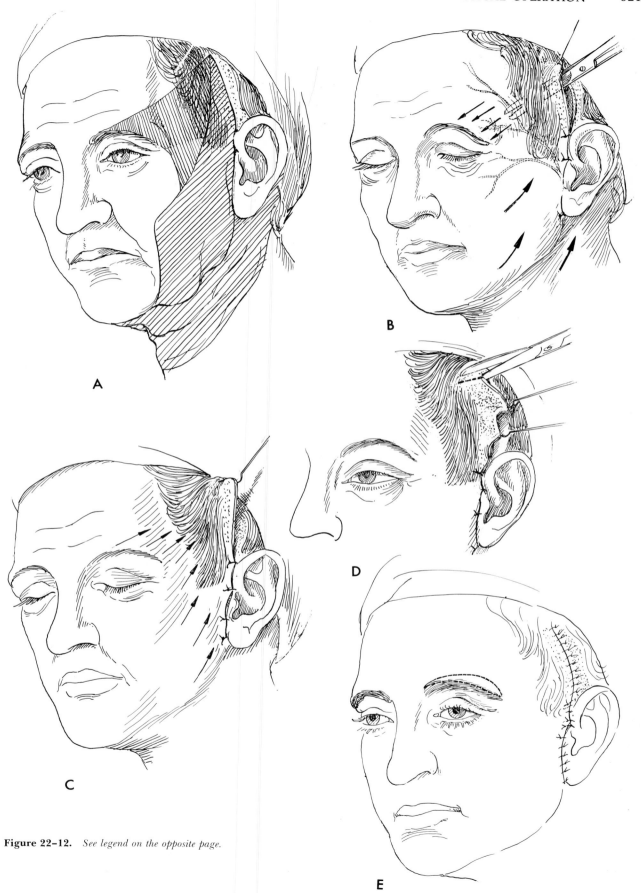

A

B

C

D

E

Figure 22–12. *See legend on the opposite page.*

by standard face lift exposure. Direct attack with defatting of the submandibular and submental areas as described by Millard (1968, 1972) has been most useful when required. Coronal incisions with reflection of a forehead flap and resection of portions of the frontalis or frown muscles to improve wrinkling of the forehead and ptosis of the brows is advocated by many surgeons. This adjunctive procedure can be done at the time of primary face lift surgery or subsequently. The author has limited experience in this ancillary technique (it is described elsewhere in this volume).

A so-called upper face lift or temporal lift may be requested by a patient with an erroneous idea of what such a procedure can accomplish. Much publicity has been given to this procedure in the popular press, where it is explained as a method of lifting the outer canthus of the eye, elevating the brow to produce an almond-eyed or slightly Oriental effect. The desired outcome will be demonstrated by the patient pulling the temporal skin upward and backward to stretch the eyelids. Some people simulate this effect by binding their temporal hair in tight twists, which tightens the temporal scalp and lifts the lids. There is no doubt that the temporal lift can raise the corner of a ptotic eyebrow or modify the advanced wrinkling of the temporal skin ("laugh lines"). But as a sole technique for a patient requesting facial plastic surgery, it is rarely justifiable. The incisions are essentially similar to the design for the temporal and preauricular area (Figure 22–12).

RESULTS

The results of this basic skin flap operation are generally salutary, and the effect is lasting. Recurrence of the initial problem inevitably occurs with the aging process and begins with placement of the final suture. It is difficult to predict the rate of occurrence, since there is so much individual variation.

Over the years, the extent of subcutaneous undermining has generally progressed in a more and more radical direction, despite sporadic attempts to limit this dissection. Unfortunately, the complication rate of the operation is directly proportional to the amount of skin undermined, and thus the surgeon and patient must accept the inherent risk of the surgical technique balanced against the results of the operation.

The main difficulty in documenting the long-term results of cervicofacial aesthetic procedures lies in our inability, as yet, to develop a valid method of evaluation. There is no acceptable laboratory model or system of controls with which to compare the results. A double-blind method of evaluation does not exist, and it seems unlikely that a truly scientific method of assessing aesthetic procedures can be devised. The long-term results of facial surgery vary considerably with individual interpretation, since the findings are subjective in nature. Indeed, few have demonstrated consistent photographic evidence in support of their chosen procedure that would withstand critical examination. Photographic documentation is notoriously subject to inaccuracies.

One of the major obstacles to developing an accurate control system is rooted in the biologic nature of the problem. People age at different rates and in different ways, depending on many factors including genetic background, environment, physiology, and emotional state. Individuals who live in temperate four-season climates age visibly at a different rate than those who live in highly actinic or dry climates. Other factors such as heavy smoking and excessive alcohol intake have also been implicated as accelerators of the aging process. The skin is our most visible yardstick for observing aging.

Aging does not appear to occur along a straight line but is cyclic in nature, progressing in short spurts followed by long periods of near quiescence, at least as far as obvious signs are concerned. It is not uncommon to see a friend who looks as though he or she has suddenly aged markedly after seeming to age very little for several years previously. Emotional problems can take a sudden and startling toll on one's appearance. Adding to the difficulties is the absence of any known accurate physiologic test to measure the aging process.

Surgeons, then, can only speculate and offer opinions as to the long-term results of their work. Careful attempts at consistent photographic documentation must be made. Third-party evaluations of results are important, since they are somewhat less prone to personal human error.

Results of aesthetic surgery should not be evaluated prior to a minimum of one year after the operation. Postoperative photographs of surgical results complete with fresh stitch marks or sutures in place and fading ecchymosis cannot be considered valid documentation of results, yet this practice is still in use.

Despite extensive undermining of the skin flaps far medially into the face, sometimes including the frontal scalp and usually extending across the midline of the neck, the one-year results in a small but significant group of patients are disappointing. The immediate result of surgery can also be disappointing in some patients in whom the skin aged with absence of elasticity, loss of turgor, and marked dehydration.

Certain results of face lift surgery have stimulated many surgeons to increase their efforts at improvement. Particularly troublesome have been the forehead, brow, anterior neck, and inframandibular, submental, and nasolabial fold regions. Recent attempts have been directed toward tightening the superficial muscular aponeurotic system (SMAS) of the face and neck. This system was recently described in excellent detail by Mitz and Peyronie (1976), who entitled it SMAS and it will be discussed in detail in a separate chapter.

A simple method of tightening the superficial musculofacial system practiced for many years was to overlap the redundancy and plicate it. Most standard publications dealing with face lift surgery contain a description of plication. Opinions vary as to the efficacy of this simple technique, yet few attempts have been made to evaluate long-term results. Tipton (1974) plicated one side and not the other. He found no difference in the results from side to side after two years. Criticism of such a study on scientific grounds is unquestionably justified; however, when dealing with the patient who is not in critical distress, acceptable methods of rational and dispassionate evaluation of results of aesthetic surgery simply do not as yet exist. Assessment of results remains one of personal opinion only. For example, the acceptance of fascial plication remains a personal choice based on experience, not on sound evidence.

Since the platysma is a superficial muscle of the cervicofacial region that apparently does not play an irreplaceable role in the human, and since it is intimately associated with the superficial aponeurotic (fascial) system of the neck and face, it became an obvious target for the attention of surgeons wishing to improve the results of face lift surgery. The anterior (medial) margins of the muscle and the configuration of the muscle in the submental region are of particular interest, since the long-term surgical results here can be disappointing. The long vertical bands of the anterior neck, which represent the medial leading borders of the platysma, often are one of the first signs of "recurrence" after face lift. Patients with marked "turkey gobbler" deformities, double chins, oblique or absent cervicomental angles (low hyoid position), and related submental and submandibular problems often share limited, even disappointing, surgical results. Intensive surgical attention to these areas was inevitable.

Anatomic repositioning, rearrangement, and selective resection of the platysma and its associated aponeurotic structures have been proposed in recent years to improve lasting results and are currently being evaluated by several surgeons. Suturing or imbricating the anterior muscle border of the platysma was reported as an adjunctive procedure in selected patients by Adamson et al. (1964) and Rees (1973). This technique has limited application but can be effective in conjunction with submental lipectomy, when convenient exposure of the upper neck is possible. Older patients in particular have platysma muscles that can easily be stretched to span the gap to the midline, where they can be imbricated or sutured together.

For several years, Skoog (1974) limited the amount of skin flap dissection in the candidate for early surgery; instead, he advocated a subplatysmal and subfascial dissection. He believed extensive dead spaces are avoided by this technique — thereby, complications associated with such dead spaces are reduced. Skoog advocated the technique particularly in the younger patient but also believed it to be effective in more advanced problems. A detailed description of this technique appeared in his superb book, to which the interested reader is referred (Skoog, 1974). Subplatysmal aponeurotic dissection is relatively bloodless and easily accomplished by blunt or sharp dissection. The branches of the facial nerve and the parotid duct must be protected. A number of surgeons have adopted this advance and have made modifications. They enthusiastically endorse this procedure.

Guerrero-Santos et al. (1974, 1978) reported improved long-term results from cervicofacial rhytidectomy by incising the platysma belly horizontally. They developed two flaps of muscle that were rotated posteriorly and to the fascia over the mastoid. They remain enthusiastic about this technique in otherwise difficult neck problems.

Resection of outstanding medial platysma borders along with varying amounts of the anterior segments of the muscle on either side of the neck was advocated by Millard et al. (1968, 1972). They improved the results of face lift surgery in the submental and inframandibular areas by contiguous and symmetric defatting of the superficial surface of the platysma. This technique obviated the unsightly depression deformity that followed localized submental lipectomy. The mandibular branch of the facial nerve must be preserved, as it penetrates the muscle during its course just inferior and parallel to the lower mandibular border where the external facial artery crosses the jaw. Except for the ramus mandibularis seventh nerve, there are few anatomic structures closely associated with the platysma that worry the surgeon.

Text continued on page 633.

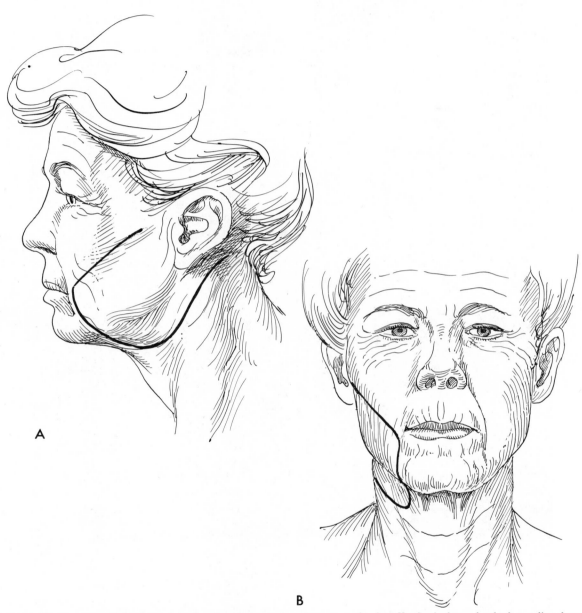

Figure 22–13. The minimal amount of undermining that can be expected to be effective is shown by the heavy line drawn over the jaw and upper neck (*A* and *B*). The earliest indications for face lifting include small jowl formation, for which the undermining must extend to the edge of the redundant skin over the jaw. Complete undermining of the neck skin is not necessary in early cases.

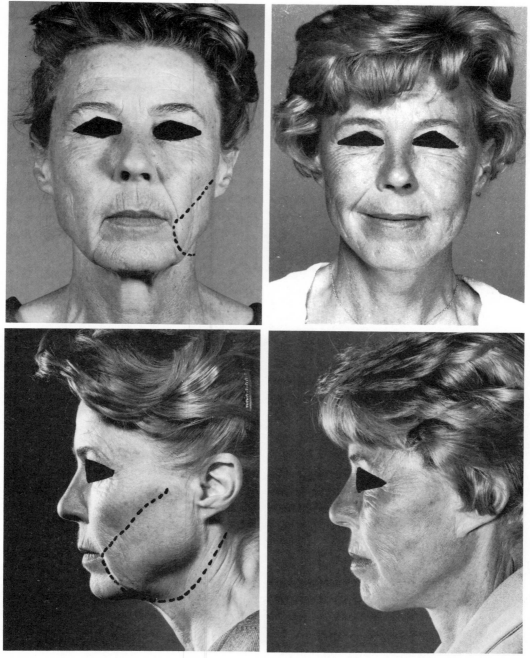

Figure 22–14.   This patient was managed as shown in Figure 22–13. Her neck skin was not particularly loose, but it was tightened as an incidental part of the face lift procedure. The neck need not be widely undermined in such a patient, but it has been our experience that we are now undermining more extensively than used to be the case in almost all patients. The rhytides of the upper lip were improved by deep chemical abrasion. Their presence, however, limits the result somewhat in comparison with the previous patient. (From Rees, T. D., and Guy, C. L.: Surg. Clin. North Am. *51*:353, 1971.)

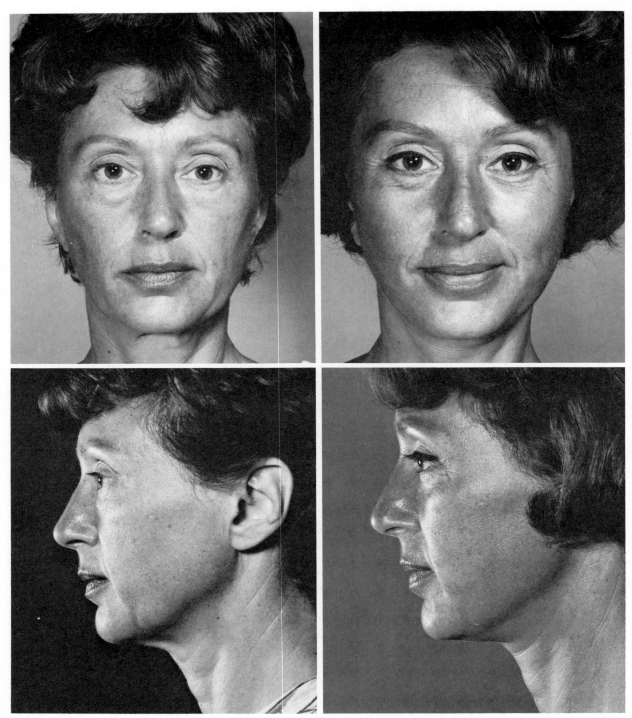

Figure 22–15. This "ideal candidate," a woman in early middle age with typical ptotic changes of the skin and musculature, underwent the classical face lift procedure with undermining of the skin only extending distal to the jowls and well into the upper neck. The SMAS was not tightened. The result is shown at two years.

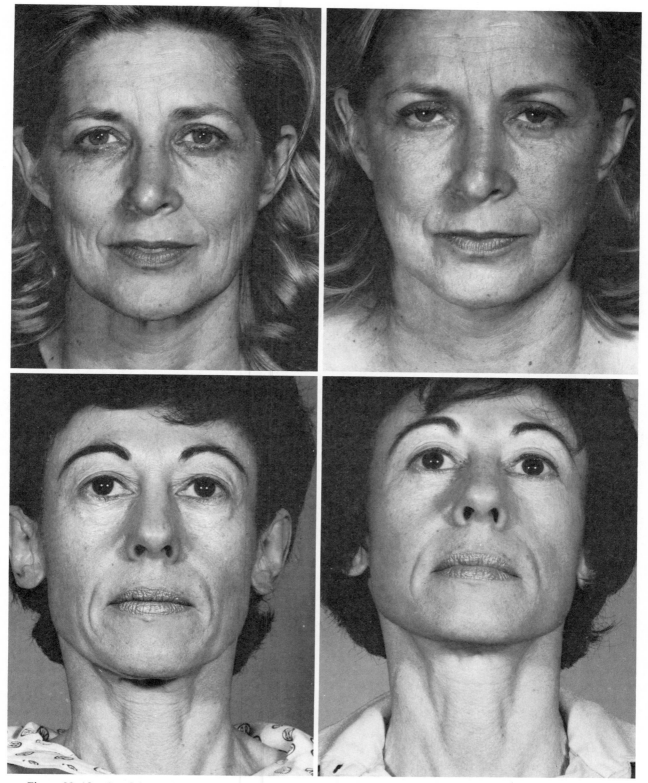

Figure 22–16.   Careful attention must be paid to specific anatomic details that require correction during face lift surgery. The amount of skin and/or SMAS dissection varies according to the problem.

These two patients demonstrate a problem of the early or young face lift candidate who is not always completely correctable: deep lines extending in rows lateral to the oral commissure. Such deep rhytides are related to the attachments of the underlying muscles of facial expression and redundant skin. Skin undermining in such patients must extend to the oral commissure to achieve improvement. Undermining and tightening of the superficial aponeurotic structures of the face and neck (Skoog) may also help the result, although that is difficult to prove (see Chapter 23).

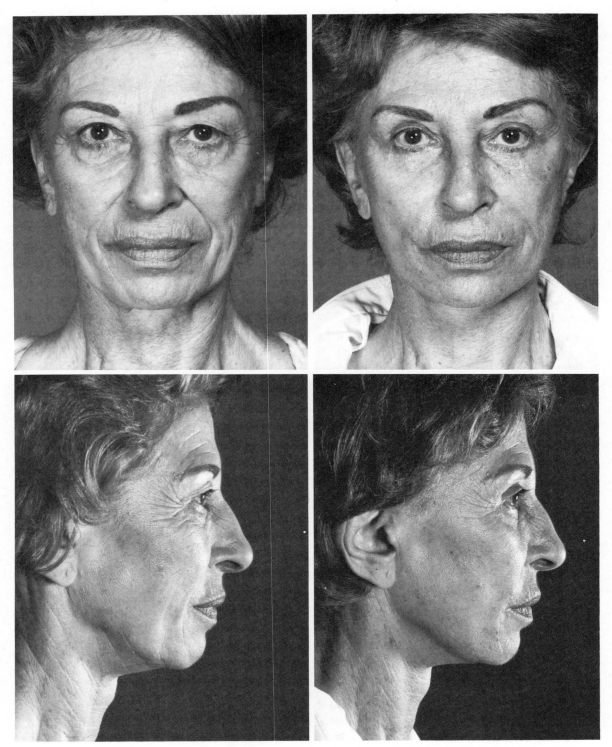

Figure 22–17. *See legend on the opposite page.*

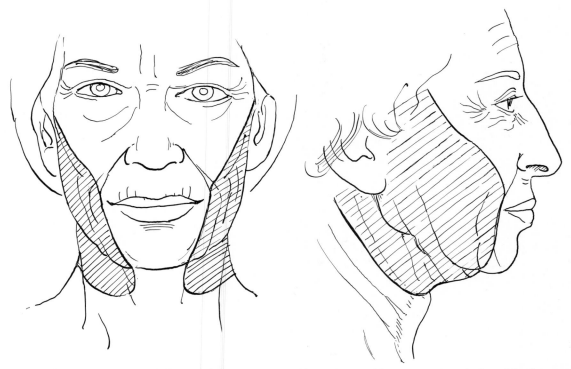

Figure 22–17.   One of the most difficult problems to correct and one that troubles many patients is that of the deep nasolabial fold. Extensive skin undermining down to and even medial to the fold can improve it to some degree; however, the final results are usually wanting. The patient with this problem should be advised that the nasolabial fold will be improved but not eliminated, as in this patient. The redundant skin folds of her lower face clearly were improved greatly by extensive skin undermining, as indicated in the drawing.

See illustration on the opposite page.

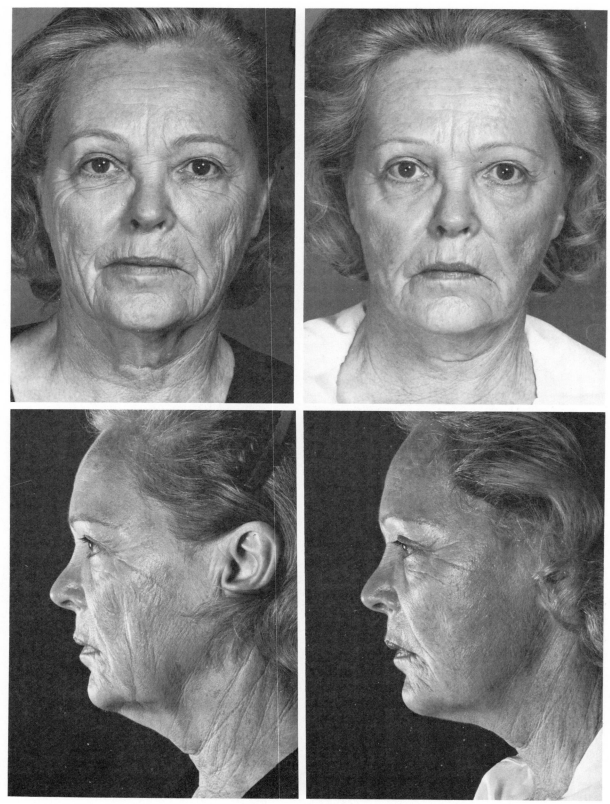

Figure 22–18. *See legend on the opposite page.*

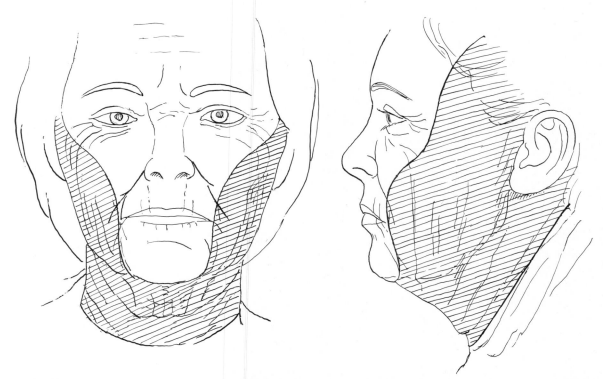

Figure 22–18. When extensive skin damage and rhytidosis are present, usually after prolonged exposure to actinic rays and the elements, with desiccation of the skin, the results of rhytidectomy are sharply limited. Skin undermining must be extensive, as indicated in the drawing. The undermining must extend completely across the midline in such patients. Fine wrinkles that remain even after such complete undercutting can only be improved further by dermabrasion or chemical peel. The author prefers the latter technique for wrinkles (see Chapter 27).

See illustration on the opposite page.

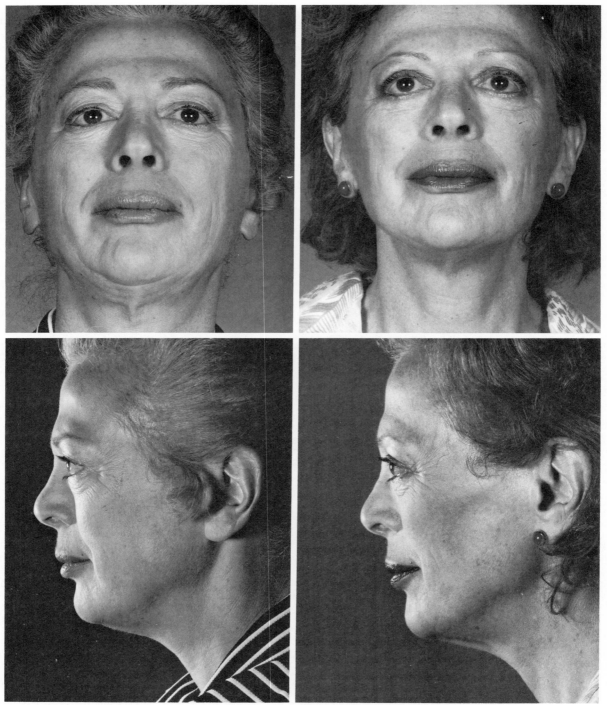

Figure 22–19.   This patient shows the results of the standard face lift procedure eight years after primary operation. The skin of the jawline and neck was undermined completely across the midline; however, no attempt was made to transect the platysma or facial aponeurosis. While the result is still excellent eight years later, it could be argued that the very small platysma band noted in the anterior neck, still present after surgery, should be transected or excised by a direct procedure. At the time of this patient's primary surgery, platysma surgery was in its infancy. In fact, eight years later, the patient underwent a second procedure. It is precisely these small imperfections in the classical (skin only) operation that have led surgeons to perform more and more surgery on the superficial fascial and muscular structures of the face and neck (SMAS). These newer procedures will be discussed in detail in a subsequent chapter.

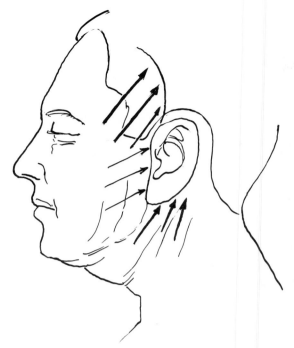

Figure 22–20. Different directions and degrees of tension (sometimes unavoidable) may be responsible for undesirable later results. Such problems are likely to occur in older patients with degenerative skin changes.

Injury to the spinal accessory nerve is conceivable during extensive surgery in the inferoposterior aspect of the neck.

Connel (1978) and Peterson (1976) advocated variations in the design of incision and resection of the platysma and musculoaponeurotic system. The enthusiasm of those surgeons who have devoted their efforts to improving the long-term results of face lifting by such techniques as musculofascial dissection is contagious. Despite a lack of "hard" evidence, these investigators seem convinced, on the basis of extensive personal experience, that the various procedures not only are efficacious but are lasting. To those surgeons who are disappointed with the results of skin flap surgery alone, such technical variations offer an attractive avenue of investigation. However, the dissection is more extensive and contains more pitfalls, such as increased danger of seventh nerve injury, than the standard skin flap technique. The experience accumulated thus far seems promising for some of these procedures; however, results are still based on the personal evaluations of a few experienced surgeons, and these procedures should not yet be accepted as a routine part of the face lift operation. These techniques are not recommended as an integral component of all face lifts, even by those who champion them; indeed, they are proposed only for difficult or unusual problems that defy perfection by standard techniques.

The limitation of skin undermining offered by the Skoog submuscular and subaponeurotic operation is attractive to all, yet the question remains —is it as lasting as the standard skin flap dissection? Supporters of the technique point out the relative simplicity of the operation and its lower morbidity from edema, ecchymosis, hematoma, skin loss, and so forth; yet, as in all other facial aesthetic procedures, there are few data to support the claims of long-term efficacy.

A principal difficulty in evaluating long-term results of subplatysmal dissection as compared with simple skin undermining lies in the realm of patient selection. The younger or "early" candidates are most likely to have good results by either wide skin undermining or submusculofascial dissection, whereas the problem cases to all surgeons are the patients with aged and redundant skin or excessive submandibular and submental fat accumulations, patients mostly in their later years and in whom the results of facial surgery are more quantitative. Long-term evaluation of these more complicated problems promises to provide us with meaningful data on the efficacy of various techniques under study. Patients in older age groups require more extensive surgery altogether; failure to dissect extensive skin flaps in such patients would seem to preclude success. It is hoped that surgery of the SMAS will prove to be a useful addition to the basic skin flap technique in many patients.

SUMMARY

The classical face lift operation has been regarded as a skin flap technique. Resection of selected portions of the platysma muscle or development of musculoaponeurotic flaps of various designs remains for the time being a promising technique in selected patients. This more complicated surgery should not be regarded as routine in all patients. Patients with prominent vertical "cords" of the anterior neck that clearly mark the protruding medial borders of the platysma muscle seem suitable candidates at this time for incision or regional excision of this portion of the muscle. After further evaluation of long-term results, the submuscular and fascial dissection with limited skin undermining may prove to be an effective substitute for extensive subcutaneous dissection in the younger face lift candidate.

Figures 22–13 through 22–20 illustrate some results of the classical standard face lift operation without dissection of the SMAS and platysma.

(For references, see pages 724 to 727.)

Chapter 23

The SMAS and the Platysma

THOMAS D. REES, M.D., F.A.C.S.

THE SMAS

Mitz and Peyronie (1976) dissected 14 hemifacial preparations on 7 cadavers and described in detail the superficial muscular and aponeurotic system (SMAS) of the face, an important concept in the recent developments of face lift surgery. Their studies indicated that this system divides the subcutaneous fat into two layers. Fat lobules lie superficial to the SMAS between the SMAS and the dermis. Fat also lies deep between the SMAS and the muscle layer.

After removing the fat lying superficial to the SMAS, Mitz and Peyronie described the fibrous longitudinal structure. This fibrous sheath is attached to the parotid sheath in the parotid-masseteric area, where it is quite thick and can readily be dissected as a layer. They considered this fibrous sheath as belonging to the cervico-cephalic fascia, continuous from the head to the neck, in continuity with the posterior part of the frontalis muscle in the upper face and with the platysma muscle in the lower face and neck. It is this structure that Skoog described in his "subplatysmal face lift." It is also this facial sheath that surgeons have been imbricating in face lift surgery for many years. More recently — since Skoog (1974) advocated his subfascial and submuscular approach — many surgeons have been performing various modified sub-SMAS dissections in the face, combined with other procedures on the platysma such as transection, plication, and flap development.

A thorough understanding of the SMAS and the related anatomy is important to the surgeon undertaking modern face lift surgery. The anatomic descriptions and illustrations that follow are taken directly from the report by Mitz and Peyronie (1976). It is important to understand that this aponeurotic structure acts as a tensor of the facial muscles from the frontalis downward to the platysma and anteriorly to the orbicularis oculi muscles. It is kept tense inferiorly by the platysma and is attached posteriorly to the fascia of the tragus and the mastoid area. It is then easy to understand how stretching the SMAS renders it an amplifier of the contractions of the facial muscles and also how direct surgical intervention of the structure such as transecting or tightening it directly affects its peripheral muscular attachments.

Ideally, extensive dissection of the SMAS in facial plasty would be ideal, since it would avoid the necessity of undermining the skin and thus inviting various complications such as slough, hematoma, and scarring. However, the branches of the facial nerve and their relationship to the SMAS impose certain limitations on the dissection and provide, in fact, the only real dangers in the technique. As seen in the accompanying illustrations (Figures 23–1 through 23–10), some anatomic areas are safe for dissection of the SMAS, such as the parotid area, and there are some areas in which the surgeon must be exceedingly cautious, such as the submusculoaponeurotic plane over the angle of the mandible, where injury to the ramus mandibularis or other branches of the lower trunk can easily occur because they emerge from the parotid gland to lie deep in the platysma and aponeurosis. Also, at the superior border of the parotid, the sub-SMAS dissection must be performed with caution anteriorly, since it is here that the frontal branch penetrates the deeper structures and becomes superficial.

THE PLATYSMA

The anatomy of the platysma varies considerably among individuals. Strong anterior or medial bands can appear at an early age and produce

Text continued on page 644.

634

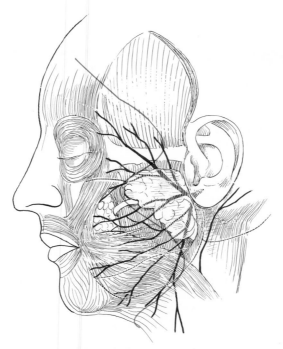

Figure 23–1.   The doubly curved red line indicates the anterior "safe" line of dissection beneath the SMAS (the submusculo-aponeurotic plane). At this line, the branches of the facial nerve become superficial from where they have coursed in the parotid gland. The danger points are easily seen over the angle of the mandible and over the zygomatic arch. The main trunk of the seventh nerve and its branches are deep in the platysma and the aponeurosis posteriorly. They penetrate the SMAS at the anterior border of the parotid.

Any dissection deeper than the subcutaneous plane anterior to the line indicated is clearly hazardous.

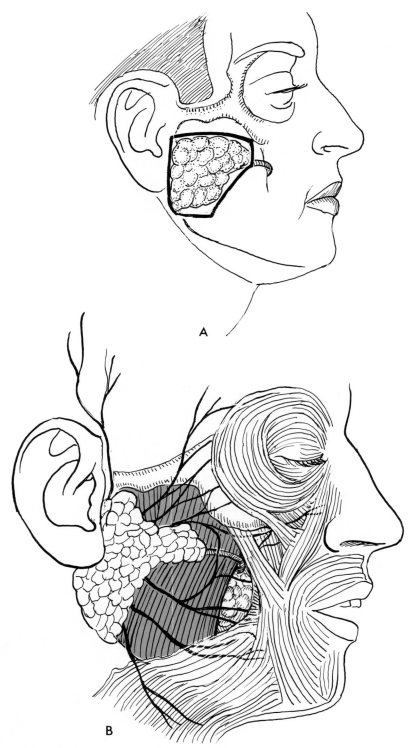

Figure 23–2. *A,* Dissection of the SMAS in the cheek area should start in front of the tragus. The dissection should extend no higher than 1 cm below the zygomatic arch, no further inferiorly than 1 cm above the inferior margin of the mandible, and no further forward than the anterior border of the parotid gland. If the dissection is maintained within these borders, there is minimal danger to the branches of the facial nerve unless aberrant branches exist. (After Mitz and Peyronie.)

B, Branches of the facial nerve can be found on the external surface of the masseter muscle, where they can easily be damaged by surgery; therefore, dissection should not proceed in this area except under unusual circumstances and with the aid of a nerve stimulator. The same is true of the fat pad of Bichat (the buccal fat pad). The buccal branch is the one most frequently injured in face lift surgery according to some reports. Return of function after injury to this branch is common, probably because of the anastomotic connections and overlay in the anterior face.

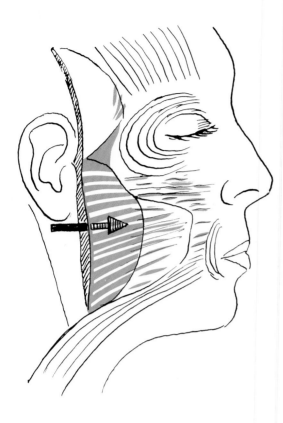

Figure 23–3. The arrow goes deep to the SMAS, indicating the depth of dissection extending from the frontalis to the platysma muscle. (SMAS layer is indicated in red.) (Redrawn from Mitz.)

Figure 23–4. *A,* In the zygomatic area, the SMAS is strongly fixed to the temporal fascia and the zygomatic arch. Emerging from beneath the parotid gland, the frontal branch of the facial nerve passes sub-SMAS over the zygomatic arch and emerges from beneath the fascia to penetrate the frontal muscles near the lateral border of the orbit (Loeb). Dissection is difficult and dangerous in this area. (Danger area is indicated in red.)

B, Safe area (blue). Over the temporalis muscle, undermining is done by digital pressure between the temporal fascia and the SMAS, until the line of fusion is reached between the SMAS and the temporal fascia.

C, Safe area (blue). Dissection is done between the SMAS and the parotid fascia. Facial nerve branches lie within the parotid gland. Integrity of the parotid fascia must be maintained.

D, Dissection in the mastoid area is difficult because the SMAS is intimately attached to the dermis and is entwined with the fibrous tissue around the insertion of the SCM muscle. Dissection is performed between the dermis and the SMAS.

E, Mandibular area. The SMAS is in close contact with the platysma. Dissection is done deep to the platysma to avoid the mandibular branch of the facial nerve.

F, In the cheek area, the SMAS is a thin covering over motor nerve branches. Sensory branches go through the SMAS to the dermis. Dissection is difficult and dangerous. Motor nerves reach superficial muscles through their deeper aspect.

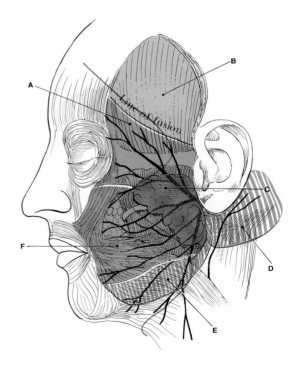

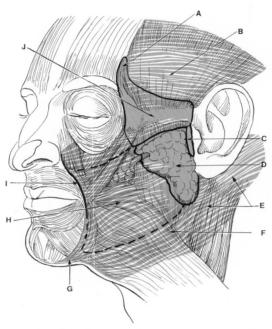

Figure 23–5. The SMAS divides the subcutaneous fat into two layers: a superficial layer and a deep layer. Superficially, small fat lobules are enclosed by fibrous septa running from the SMAS to the dermis. The deep layer of fat is not penetrated by the septa.

The SMAS invests and extends into the external part of the facial musculature, involving fibers of the frontalis, the risorius, the peripheral part of the orbicularis oculi, and the platysma. All connections of muscles to dermis are made up of SMAS fibers, which cover the facial motor nerves. The SMAS is always present in the parotid and cheek areas and has an intimate relationship with the entire superficial fascia of the head and neck. It extends from the frontalis to the platysma and is continuous with the superficial fascia over the mandible and neck and the anterior muscles of the face.

A, The SMAS is continuous with the posterior part of the frontalis.

B, The superficial fascia is loosely connected with the temporal fascia and continuous with the SMAS.

C, The SMAS is adherent in the pretragal area for 1 or 2 cm.

D, The SMAS is separate from the parotid fascia. Here, the SMAS is a dense fibrous connective tissue. Muscular fibers may be seen within the connective tissue.

E, In the mastoid area, the superficial fascia is closely attached to the fibrous layers around the ear and the insertions of the SCM muscle.

F, In the mandibular area, the SMAS is in close contact with the platysma and is directly continuous with the fascia of the neck.

G, SMAS fibers connect to the periosteum or mandible.

H, In the cheek area, the SMAS is thinner but can be followed microscopically beneath the dermis. An important layer of fat may lie between the dermis and the SMAS, separated from Bichat's fat pad by the SMAS.

I, The nasolabial fold appears to be a cutaneous fold where the SMAS ends as a distinct layer, rather than a fold caused by insertions of specific muscles.

J, The SMAS is adherent to the periosteum and fused with the temporal fascia in the temporozygomatic area (Mitz).

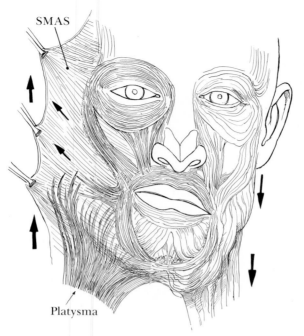

Figure 23–6.   Tension on the SMAS should tighten this structure, thereby improving the results of face lifting.

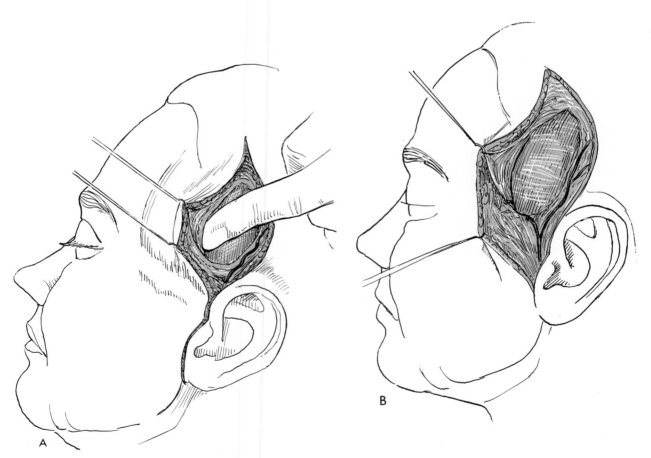

Figure 23–7.   Dissection in the temporal region is deep to the SMAS. The plane can be between the SMAS and the temporalis fascia, or it can be just beneath the temporalis fascia, provided the dissection is kept above the line of the zygoma. The superficial (SMAS) connective tissue layer actually fuses with the temporalis fascia in most instances. *A*, Superficial fascia is dissected from temporal fascia. *B*, The temporal artery has been ligated.

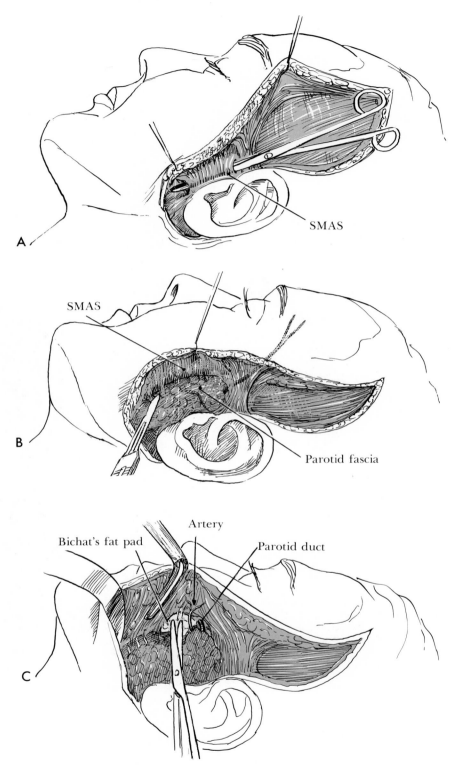

SMAS

SMAS

Parotid fascia

Bichat's fat pad

Artery

Parotid duct

Figure 23–8. *A,* Dissection of the SMAS in the cheek area can be started by inserting scissors between the SMAS and the parotid fascia, where a natural plane exists. A tunnel is easily created. The superficial layer of the tunnel is then divided.

B, The SMAS is then reflected anteriorly, and the dissection is continued by blunt or sharp dissection toward the anterior margin of the parotid gland. Note that the bridge of soft tissue over the zygoma is best left undisturbed since it contains the frontalis branch.

C, The medial or anterior border of the parotid gland marks the boundary of "safe" dissection forward. If the dissection is to proceed further, it must be done with great caution. Blunt dissection is probably best done under direct vision and with the help of a nerve stimulator. Skoog recommended ligation of a rather constant artery that is usually present in Bichat's fat pad. Branches of the seventh nerve are almost constant in the fat pad area.

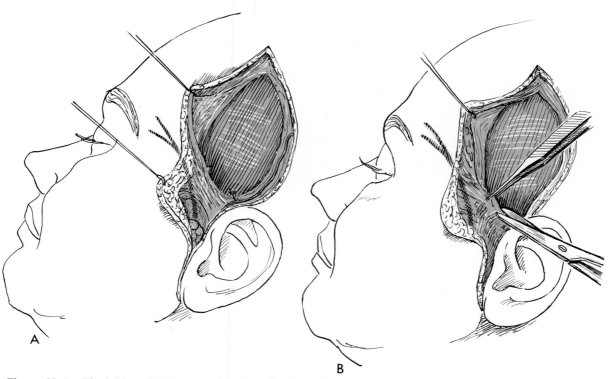

A

B

Figure 23–9. The bridge of thick connective tissue that divides the preparotid SMAS and the fusion of the SMAS with the temporal fascia can be cautiously divided as far posteriorly as possible at about the level of the zygoma. The surgeon must remember that the frontal branch penetrates this dense mass to become superficial and supply the frontalis and the related muscles of facial expression. It can be easily injured, and return of function is poor, probably less than 10 percent. *A,* The course of the temporalis nerve and the strong attachment of the SMAS to the periosteum. *B,* The SMAS can be separated 1 or 2 cm from the ear (Loeb).

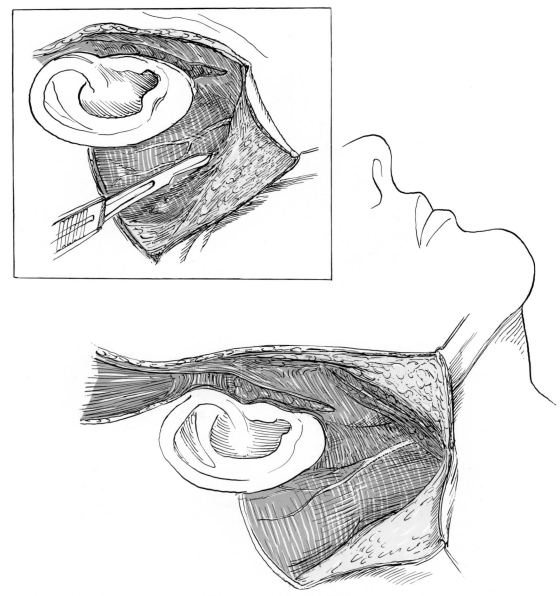

Figure 23–10. Dissection over the sternocleidomastoid muscle is difficult because of fusion of the SMAS with the muscular fascia. Virtually no plane exists. Dissection is best done with a knife, taking care to avoid injury to the underlying nerves.

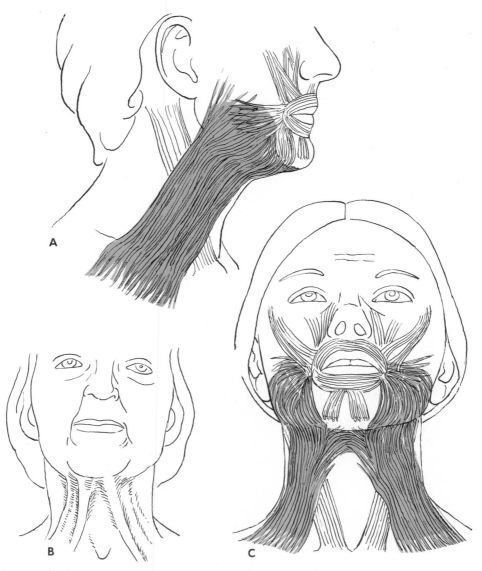

Figure 23–11. *A,* The platysma is generally a long, oblique, vertical muscle extending from the aponeurosis of the face downward to the infraclavicular area.

B, The medial bands often are pronounced and form the anterior vertical neck cords.

C, The fibers of the platysma may or may not interdigitate in the midline beneath the chin. Below the immediate inframental region, the anterior borders of the muscle separate and seep gently backward.

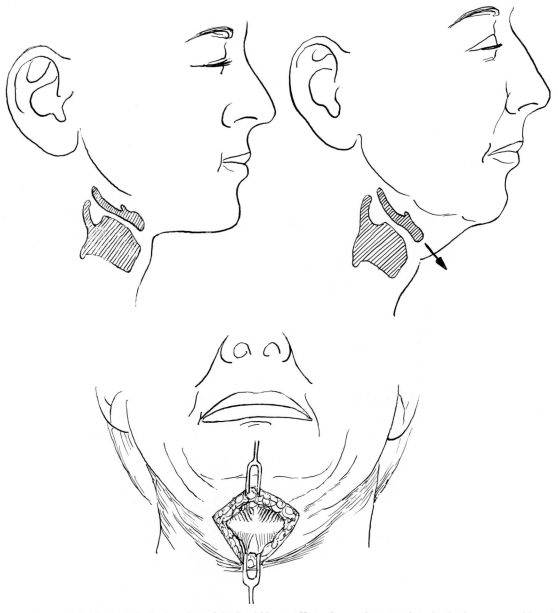

Figure 23–12.   Anterior or inferior location of the hyoid bone affects the cervicomental angle. Such an unusual location of the hyoid produces a more obtuse angle and limits somewhat the effects of sectioning the platysma.

strong cord-like structures extending vertically down the anterior neck (Figure 23–11). These medial borders of the platysma almost always occur with advancing age and become an integral part of the "turkey gobbler" deformity. Eradication of such platysma deformities has become an important part of rhytidectomy. The author believes it is important to suture the muscle together in the midline in order to reinforce the submental area. If sufficient muscle is available, it can be plicated in this region. Such reinforcement of the muscle provides a buttressing of the submental and submandibular structures.

The surgeon should be aware of the relative prominence of the thyroid cartilage (the "Adam's apple") in each patient, and what the effect of transecting the platysma above the larynx will be on this structure. Female patients in particular are not pleased to have a prominent Adam's apple as the result of platysma surgery, even though the upper neck and submental areas are vastly improved. Preoperative evaluation of the effect of sectioning the platysma or resecting the medial borders of this muscle on the prominence of the larynx should be extremely careful. A low (inferior or anterior) placement of the hyoid bone is also a factor in evaluating the results of platysma surgery (Figure 23–12).

EVALUATION OF THE PLATYSMA AND PLATYSMA SECTIONING TECHNIQUES

Although Skoog was the first to call our attention to the platysma muscle and its connecting aponeurosis of the face as important structures to adjust during face lift surgery, other surgeons have modified his work and devised varying techniques for correcting anatomic variations of the SMAS. Needless to say, the anatomic distribution of these structures varies, and no one procedure suffices to correct all neck deformities. Subaponeurotic dissection and tightening of the musculo-aponeurotic structures is sometimes all that is required in a given patient, whereas in others (most, in fact), the platysma with its prominent anterior bands and overlying fat pad must be corrected to some degree. In most younger patients who first present for a face lift operation, direct intervention of the platysma is rarely required. The exception is the patient with a loss of the natural cervicomental angle or with an unusual accumulation of fat over the muscle, both of which obscure a clean jawline and the natural curve of the neck.

The surgeon should have a thorough knowledge of the anatomy adjacent to the platysma and the superficial aponeurosis of the face in order to operate safely on these structures and to avoid untoward postoperative results (Fig. 23–13).

The Pioneer Technique of Skoog

Skoog was one of the first to operate directly on the superficial fascia and muscle system of the face and neck. He was searching for a method of face lift surgery that would avoid extensive skin undermining and yet produce a satisfactory result. The illustration in Figure 23–14 is a simplification of Skoog's technique (1974), which has been adopted by many surgeons.

Figures 23–15 and 23–16 illustrate some of the limitations of standard platysma surgery.

The Operative Approach to the Platysma Flap

The basic steps in correction with the platysma flap are shown in Figure 23–17.

VARIATIONS OF PLATYSMA SURGERY

Resection of submental and submandibular fat in continuity along with resection of the medial

Text continued on page 659.

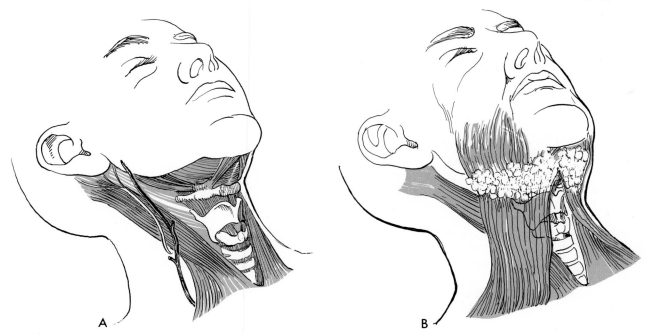

Figure 23–13. *A,* The structures of the neck immediately underlying the platysma are shown in this drawing, in which the platysma has been dissected away. Note the larynx, the hyoid bone, the position of the jugular vein, and the greater auricular nerve. Both the vein and the nerve are vulnerable during platysma surgery and should be identified during the surgery and protected.

B, There is sometimes an accumulation of fat just beneath the mandible and overlying the platysma that can be safely trimmed away (Millard) provided the sculpturing is even and the mandibular branch of the facial nerve is protected where it penetrates the muscle and becomes superficial adjacent to the anterior facial artery.

Illustration continued on the following page.

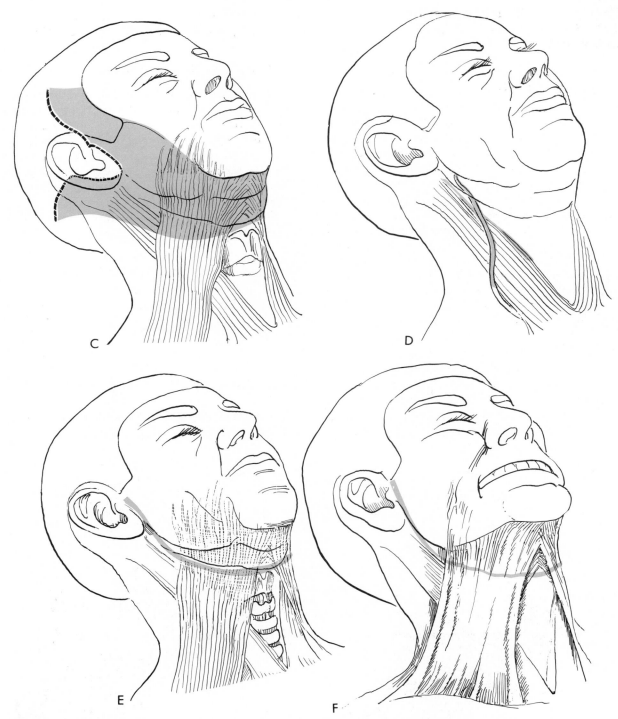

Figure 23–13 *Continued.*   *C,* The standard face lift incision and the folds of skin (and fat) are indicated (blue area).

D, The external jugular vein is shown as it courses through the neck and crosses the sternocleidomastoid muscle. This structure is easily injured during surgery; however, careful dissection and visual identification of the vessel insures its safety. Connell wisely recommends marking this structure on the skin of the neck prior to operation. If the jugular vein is injured during surgery, it is double-clamped, cleanly divided, and securely tied with a double ligature.

E, Without forced animation, the platysma is in a resting state, and the various folds and bands that are considered unsightly by many patients will not come into focus.

F, Connell emphasizes the importance of forcing the muscle into action by slightly elevating the jaw and clenching the teeth. We have found that a preoperative photograph of the patient with the teeth clenched is most helpful during surgery to identify the bands that must be divided. The anatomic variations are great and should be noted in each patient.

Illustration continued on the opposite page.

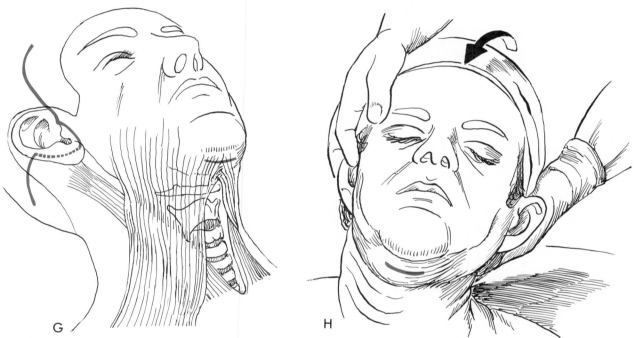

Figure 23-13 *Continued.* *G,* A small submental incision is important in most patients undergoing platysma surgery to provide visualization of and access to the submandibular and submental areas so that thorough defatting is facilitated as well as resection of the anterior platysma bands, transection of the muscle, and suturing of the muscle in the midline to buttress the submental repair and prevent lateral sagging of the divided muscle. When the muscle is divided completely and drawn laterally in the Skoog maneuver, midline suturing becomes even more important to achieve a tight and lasting sling support. The incision can be located in the natural crease beneath the mentum or 2 to 3 cm below the inferior margin of the symphysis.

H, The exact location of the submental incision is identified by flexing the head. There is no question that an added risk of keloid formation is assumed when a submental incision is used; nevertheless, the added exposure gained seems worth the risk. A fiberoptic retractor with a small blade can be used to great advantage through this very small incision. When the skin excess of the upper neck is great, the incision can be extended and redundant skin can be excised.

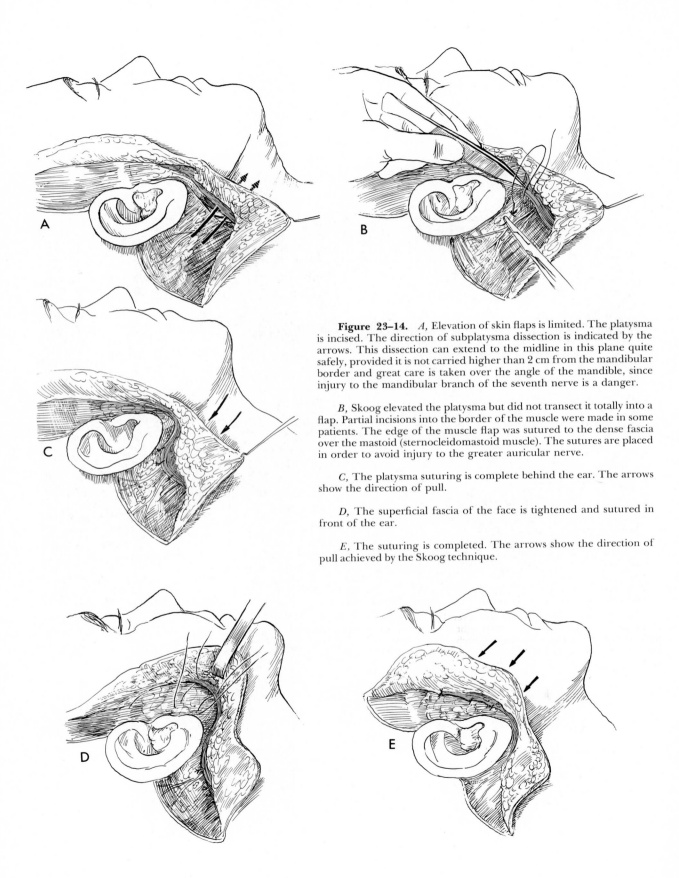

Figure 23–14. *A,* Elevation of skin flaps is limited. The platysma is incised. The direction of subplatysma dissection is indicated by the arrows. This dissection can extend to the midline in this plane quite safely, provided it is not carried higher than 2 cm from the mandibular border and great care is taken over the angle of the mandible, since injury to the mandibular branch of the seventh nerve is a danger.

B, Skoog elevated the platysma but did not transect it totally into a flap. Partial incisions into the border of the muscle were made in some patients. The edge of the muscle flap was sutured to the dense fascia over the mastoid (sternocleidomastoid muscle). The sutures are placed in order to avoid injury to the greater auricular nerve.

C, The platysma suturing is complete behind the ear. The arrows show the direction of pull.

D, The superficial fascia of the face is tightened and sutured in front of the ear.

E, The suturing is completed. The arrows show the direction of pull achieved by the Skoog technique.

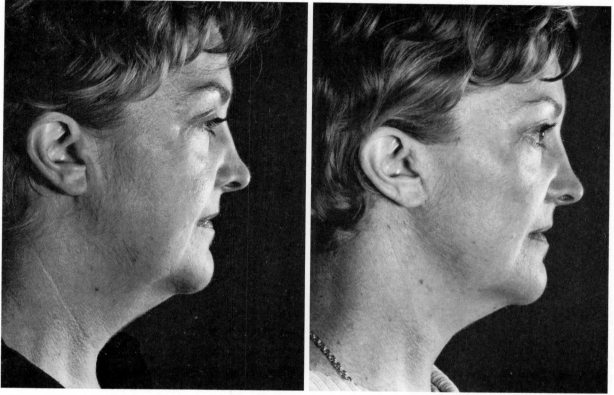

Figure 23–15.   This patient had a very difficult problem to correct when she had her rhytidectomy in 1971. Note the oblique cervicomental angle with an almost straight line from the mentum to the clavicle. This configuration is mostly muscular in this patient, with little or no fat. It was formerly thought to be a "low hyoid." The postoperative result was certainly an improvement at one year; however, more modern techniques of platysma surgery developed since 1971 would most assuredly improve this result a great deal.

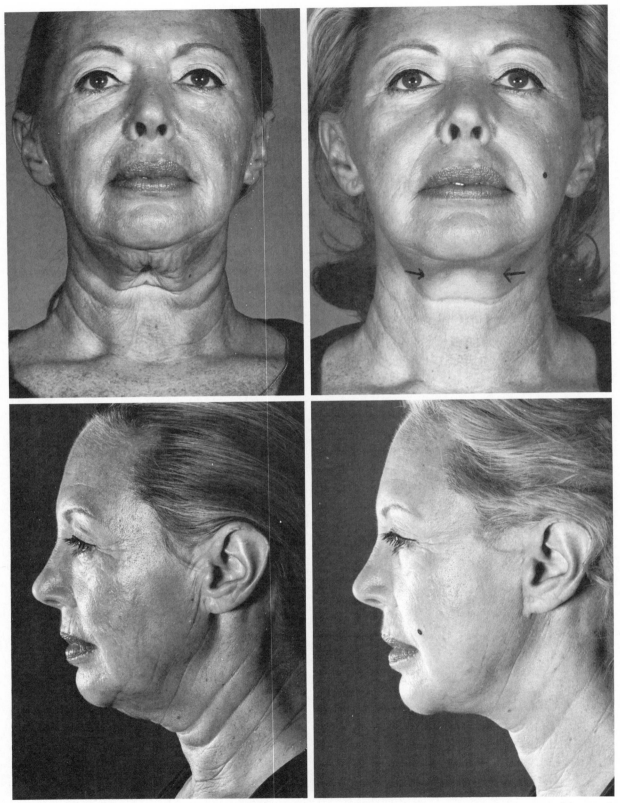

Figure 23–16. Markedly redundant skin of the neck and submental regions can be improved a great deal by standard rhytidectomy; however, the postoperative result after one or more years is often slightly disappointing to the surgeon and sometimes to the patient because of failure of the skin redraping to correct underlying platysma deformities (arrows). These shortcomings of the standard operation have stimulated surgeons to explore techniques for also correcting associated muscular irregularities.

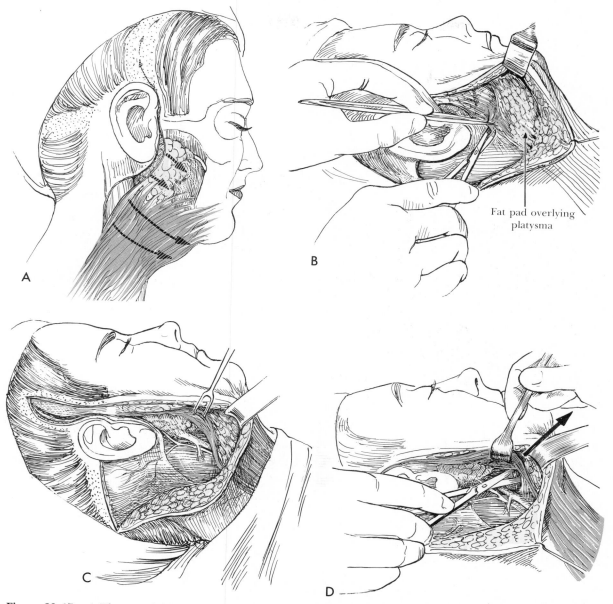

Figure 23–17. *A,* The superficial aponeurosis has been incised in the preauricular line and the platysma has also been incised where it blends with the sternocleidomastoid muscle. The upper arrows indicate the extent of dissection toward the midline to be carried out at the sub-SMAS level in the cheek and over the parotid. The lower arrows indicate the direction of dissection to the midline in the subplatysma plane.

B, The fascia of the platysma is grasped with forceps and incised with scissors. The submandibular fat is indicated. It is perfectly safe to excise this fat pad since it is superficial to the ramus mandibularis.

C, The cut edge of the platysma is retracted (double prong) and the skin flap is held with a blade retractor. Note that the superficial jugular vein and the greater auricular nerve are exposed.

D, The nerve and vein are protected, and the scissors are inserted beneath the platysma. Dissection is carried towards the midline in a slightly inferior direction. The actual line of division of the platysma that is safest for protection of the ramus mandibularis is indicated in Figure 23–22 (see subsequent plates). The nerve lies within two fingerbreadths of the mandibular border in most patients (except for the very old).

Illustration continued on the following page.

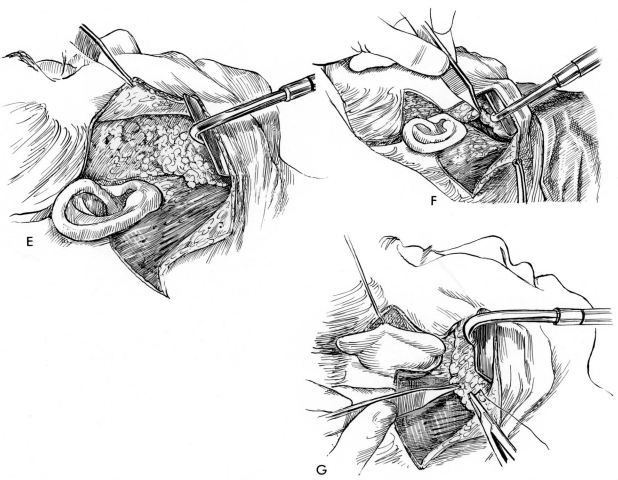

Figure 23–17 *Continued.* *E,* The fiberoptic retractor is inserted beneath the skin flap. Excellent visualization is obtained with the use of this light for excision of fat and to obtain hemostasis.

F, The free cut border of the SMAS is grasped with forceps, and traction is exerted in a posterosuperior direction.

G, A suture of strong material (Merselene, Nylon) is placed in the platysmal edge and into the fascia over the sternocleidomastoid muscle. The suture should parallel the fibers of the muscle and the course of the greater auricular nerve to avoid injury to the nerve.

Illustration continued on the opposite page.

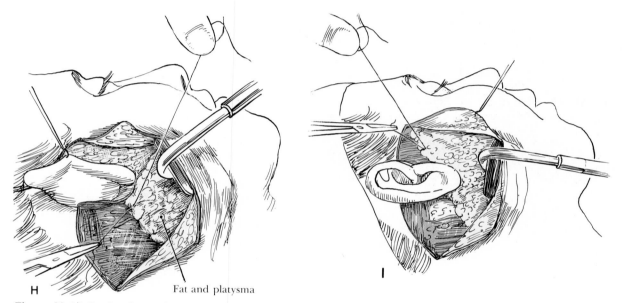

Fat and platysma

Figure 23–17 *Continued.* *H,* Several such sutures are placed to fix the platysma muscle flap to the firm fascia over the sternocleidomastoid muscle.

I, Anteriorly, the aponeurosis is sutured to the parotid fascia. The upper limits are along the zygomatic fascia.

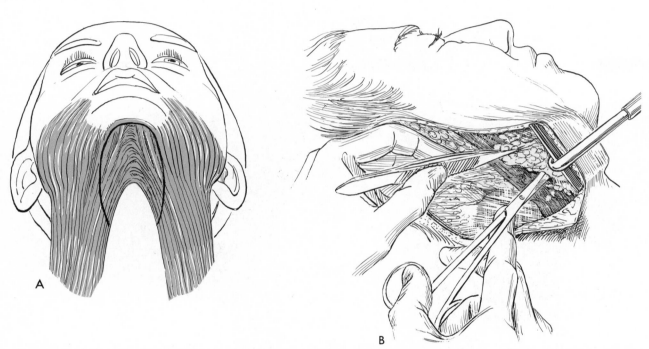

Figure 23–18. *A*, Anterior portion of the platysma can be resected. Millard does not believe that suturing of the platysma in the midline is important. The author feels that it is, except in unusual instances.

B, The fat dissection is begun laterally through the face lift incisions. The line of excision is below the mandible, and care is taken with good lighting to avoid injuring the mandibular branch where it penetrates the muscle and becomes superficial near the external maxillary artery. There is really no reason to dissect in this area, since the fat pad rarely extends to the mandibular border.

Illustration continued on the opposite page.

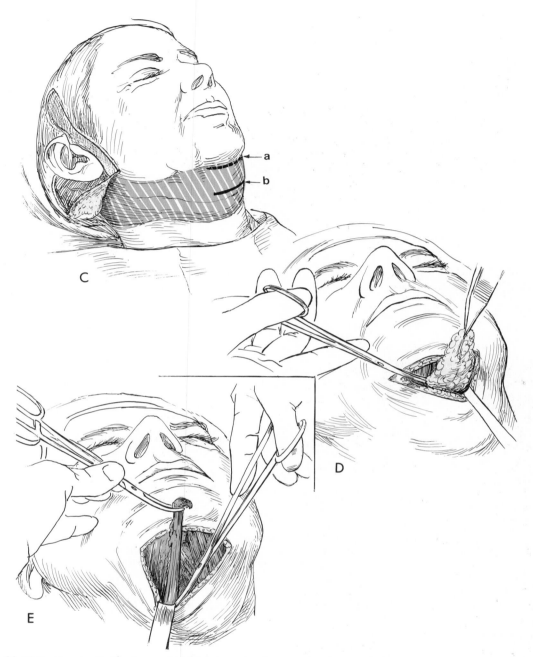

Figure 23–18 *Continued.   C,* A submental incision is made wherever the surgeon desires.

D, The fat excision is continued in continuity with the lateral submandibular excision. Care should be taken to leave a small fat layer on the skin flaps for contour purposes.

E, If the medial borders of the platysma are prominent, they can be resected.

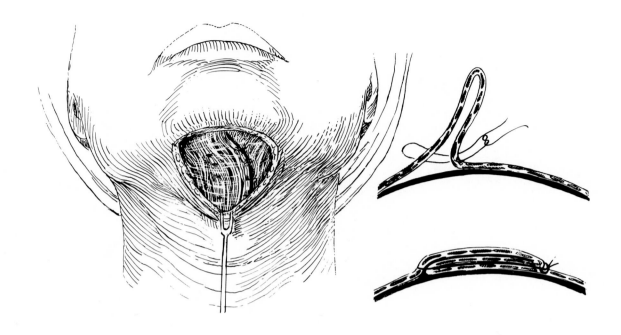

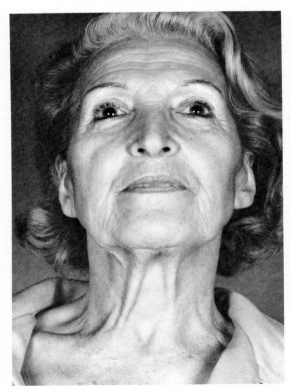
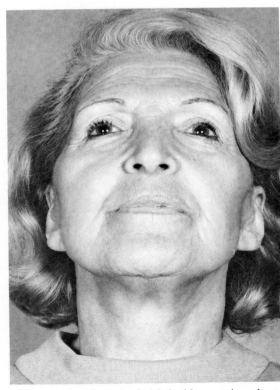

Figure 23–19.   Plication of the platysma muscle was required in this patient along with cervicofacial rhytidectomy in order to correct the vertical neck folds.

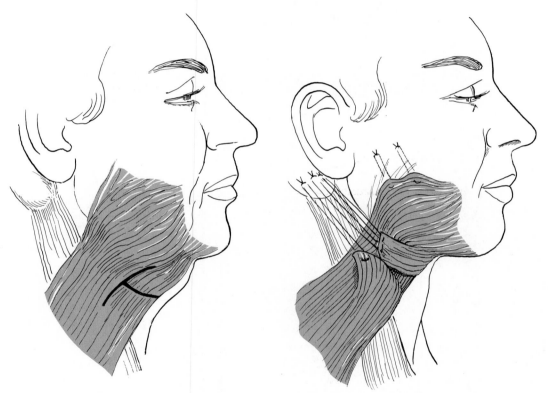

Figure 23–20.   The Guerrero-Santos platysma flap fashioned from the medial margins of the muscle.

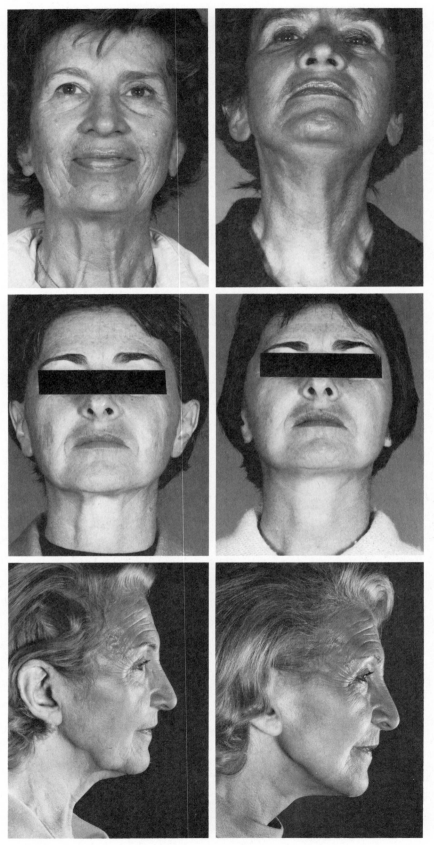

Figure 23–21. Correction of medial platysma folds by the Guerrero-Santos technique of partial transection of the muscle and the formation of small flaps.

borders of the platysma muscle according to Millard is shown in Figure 23–18. Fat resection has been a considerable step forward in improving the results of face lift surgery, particularly in patients who are unable to lose the fat in this area by dieting. In such patients, fat accumulation in the neck is often hereditary. The dissection of fat in continuity avoids the typical problem that occurs when only submental fat is excised; that is, unsightly postoperative contour bulges on either side of the excision, necessitating secondary surgery to correct the "dogears."

A simple technique for correcting or improving prominent medial borders of the platysma is to suture the muscle across the midline with or without partial transection or excision of the offending muscular band. When the medial muscular folds are lax enough, they can be plicated, as shown in Figure 23–19. Access is obtained through a small submental incision that connects the undermining across the midline. Exposure is facilitated by a small fiberoptic retractor. This technique has been in use for many years (Rees, 1973).

Guerrero-Santos was one of the first surgeons to develop flaps of platysma muscle. He advocated partial transection of the muscle from its anterior border extending midway through the muscle posteriorly (Figure 23–20). The superior flap thus formed was turned on itself and sutured to the fascia over the mastoid with bridging sutures. The

Text continued on page 683.

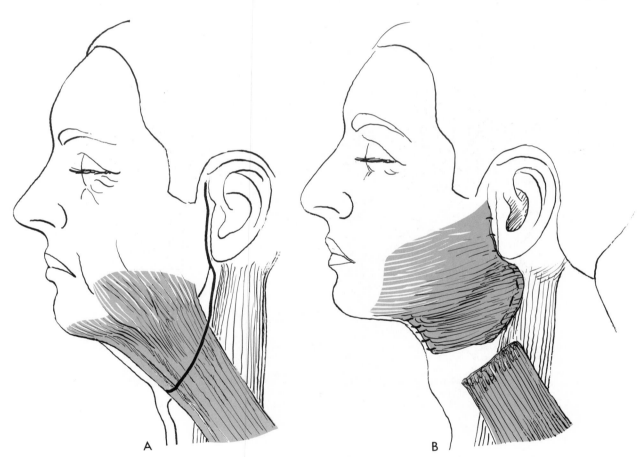

Figure 23–22. *A* and *B*, The solid line indicates the safest and most desirable level to cut across the platysma. Note the incision is quite low. In this way, injury to the ramus mandibularis of the seventh nerve is avoided, since the nerve courses beneath the platysma before it becomes superficial. The nerve is assumed to be within 2 cm of the mandibular border in most patients, although clinical experience has shown that there is considerable variation — all the more reason for keeping the incision into the muscle at a low level. In older patients with considerable tissue, ptosis of the nerve can be found in a more caudal position than one would expect. The muscle should be incised, usually in small segments at a time, with blunt scissors so that the surgeon can visualize what lies beneath. In this way, there is less likelihood of damaging the nerve or the jugular vein.

The muscle is transected to the level of the deep fascia; however, the fascia should not be violated. Care should be taken to cut all fine strands of the muscle; otherwise small bands resembling contracture bands can result in the late postoperative period. Excellent exposure is assured by good lighting with a fiberoptic retractor. Small vessels can be identified and cauterized during the transection.

After the muscle has been completely divided, it can be undermined slightly along the superior cut edge.

Illustration continued on the following page.

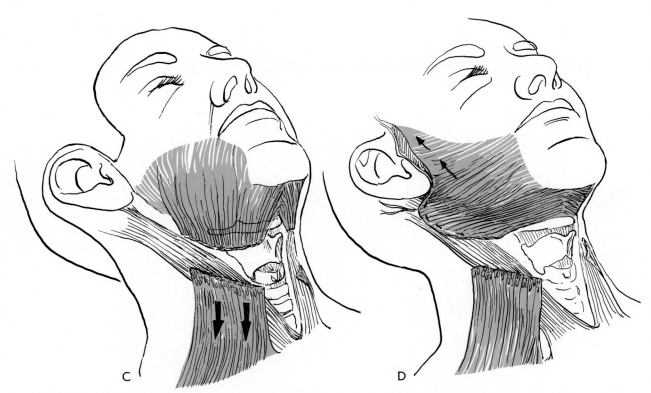

Figure 23–22 *Continued.   C,* Complete division of the platysma muscle results in a contraction of the unsatisfied ends. The lower muscle contracts resulting in a definite gap that is seen clearly after transection.

D, With or without minimal undermining of the superior cut edge, the muscle, in continuity with the facial aponeurosis (which has been undermined according to the technique shown in Figure 23–17), is rotated in a cephalic and posterior direction, where it is fixed with sutures to the fascia of the sternocleidomastoid muscle. These sutures are best placed in a vertical direction to avoid injury to the great auricular nerve.

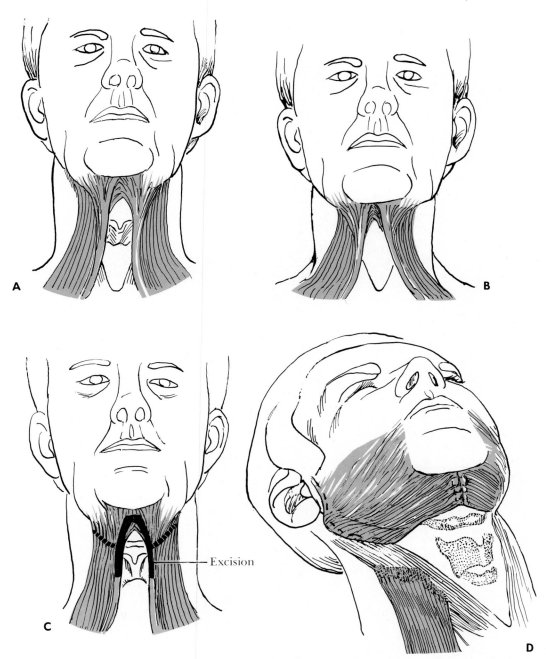

Figure 23–23. Correction of ptotic neck muscle (after Connell). *A* and *B,* A lax platysma with strong medial bands.

C, The medial bands are resected as indicated, and the muscle is transected. (In actuality, it is *important* to transect the muscle lower than is interpreted here. Muscle transection should be at least below the cricoid cartilage level to avoid "masculinizing" the neck and to preserve the ramus mandibularis.

D, The midline is buttressed with sutures, and the superior platysma flap is sutured to the muscular fascia.

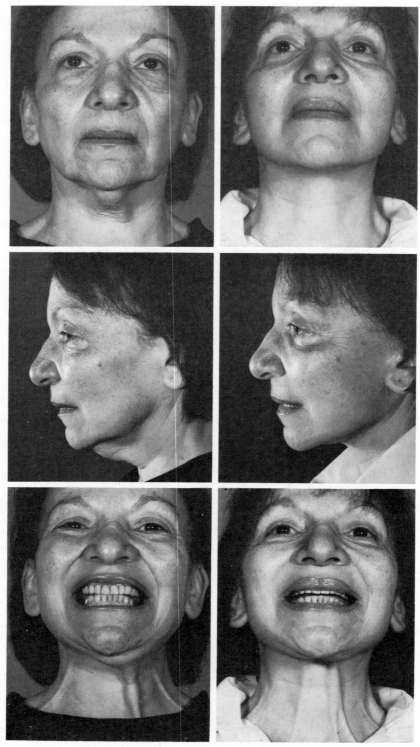

Figure 23–24. *See legend on the opposite page.*

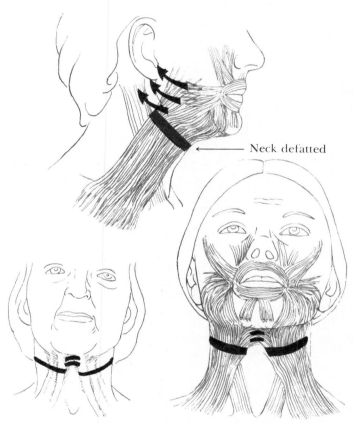

Neck defatted

Figure 23–24. Surgical problem corrected according to the platysma flap technique described in Figure 23–23. In this patient, there was also a midline "wattle" of fat (and muscle). Note the very strong platysma band on the left side in the preoperative animation photograph. The muscle was severed completely on both sides, yet several months after operation, a much attenuated band had reformed. This phenomenon has been noted by several surgeons. It may be the result of fibrous reunion of the muscle, incomplete division of the muscular band, or reinnervation of the muscle. However, the original deformity did not recur.

See illustration on the opposite page.

Figure 23–25. *A* and *B,* Marked "turkey gobbler" neck can be caused by excess submental fat or redundant medial platysma, or both.

C and *D,* Correction of such a deformity is best achieved by resection of fat and plication of the redundant muscle (Rees, 1973). The submandibular midline is strengthened by this maneuver, and the medial portion of the newly formed muscular sling is firmly fixed so that postoperative ptosis of the muscle does not occur. If the midline is not strengthened in this way, unsightly bulges along the mandibular borders on the other side can result.

See illustration on the opposite page.

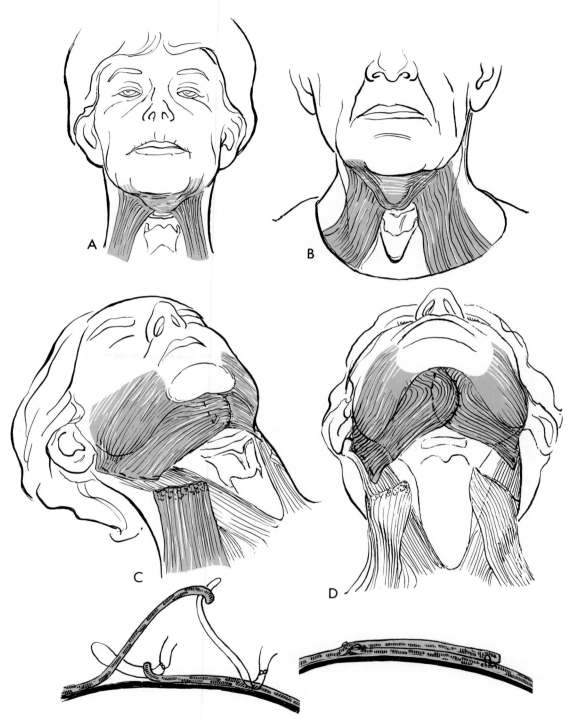

Figure 23–25.   *See legend on the opposite page.*

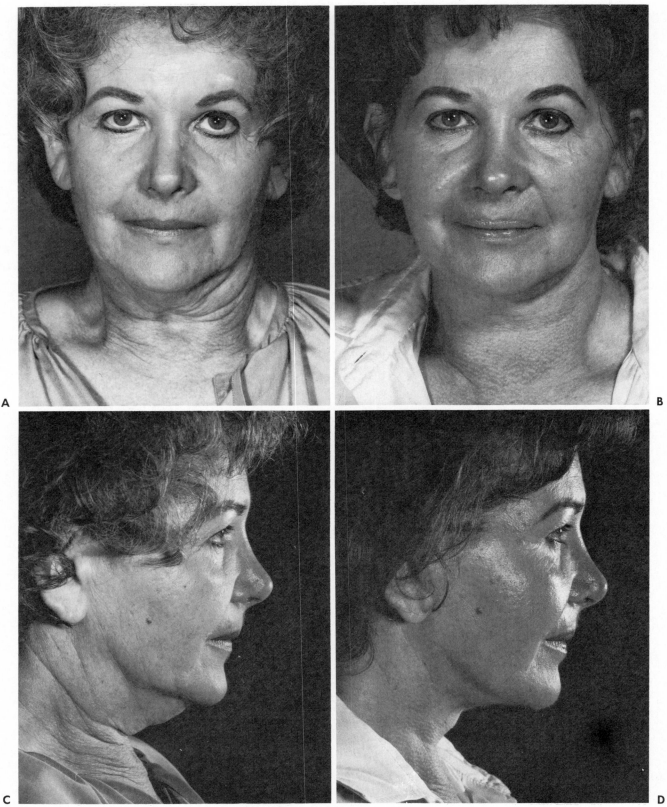

Figure 23–26. *See legend on the opposite page.*

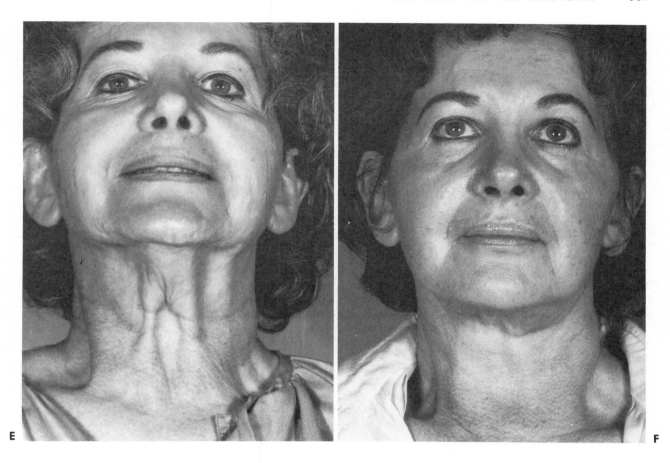

E   F

Figure 23–26. This patient had a very difficult neck problem that before the advent of wide exposure and direct surgical attack on the platysma and associated structures would have required two or perhaps three procedures to achieve a satisfactory result. The result was achieved in one operation according to the operative plan outlined on the worksheet drawing G). The author utilizes such worksheets for all patients in whom the need for platysma surgery is anticipated.

There was a loss of the natural cervicomental angle. This patient acknowledged that this angle had always been obtuse, even at a young age. Loss of a defined angle was the result not only of the aging process and redundancy of skin and fat, but also because the position of her anterior muscle had blunted naturally.

A wide approach with skin undermining, excision of fat, complete transection of the muscle, and plication of the muscle in the midline corrected the problem. A posterior SMAS flap, made according to the method of Skoog, helped to form a tight muscular sling of the upper portion of the platysma and to tighten the cheek and jawline.

Note the very strong anterior muscular platysma bands in E. Not only were these bands divided, but a strip of muscle measuring approximately 3 cm was removed.

See illustration on the opposite page.

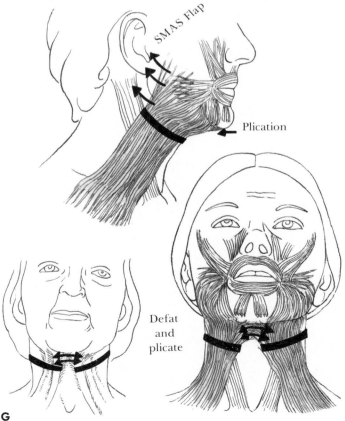

SMAS Flap

Plication

Defat and plicate

G

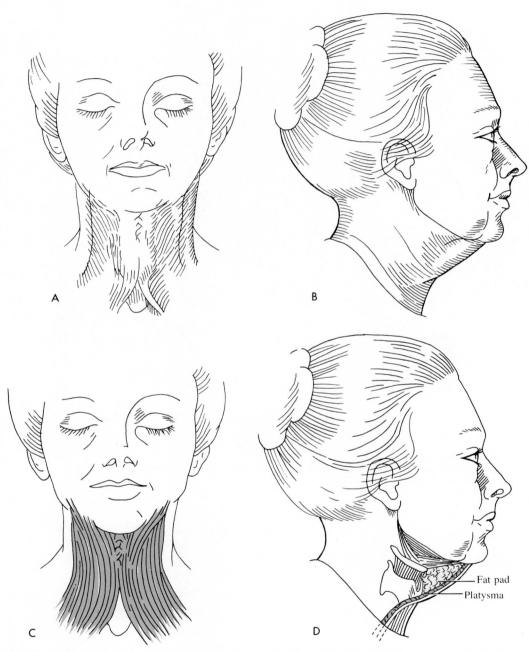

Figure 23–27. *A, B,* and *C,* Another important cause of "turkey gobbler" deformity that is often overlooked is the accumulation of a deep fat pad *beneath* the platysma and overlying the strap muscles of the upper neck. *D,* The fat pad is seen lying beneath the platysma.

Illustration and legend continued on the opposite page.

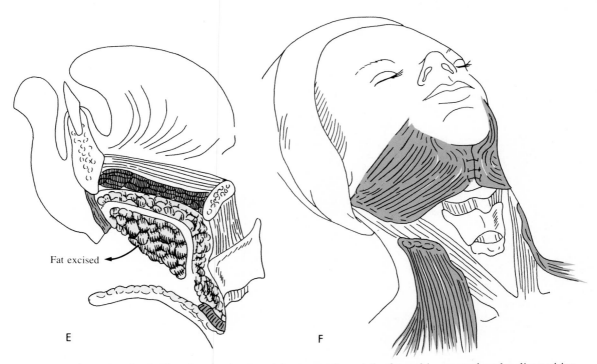

Figure 23–27 *Continued.* *E,* The platysma is opened (or resected), and the fat pad is removed under direct vision.

F, The platysma sling is then fashioned as previously described.

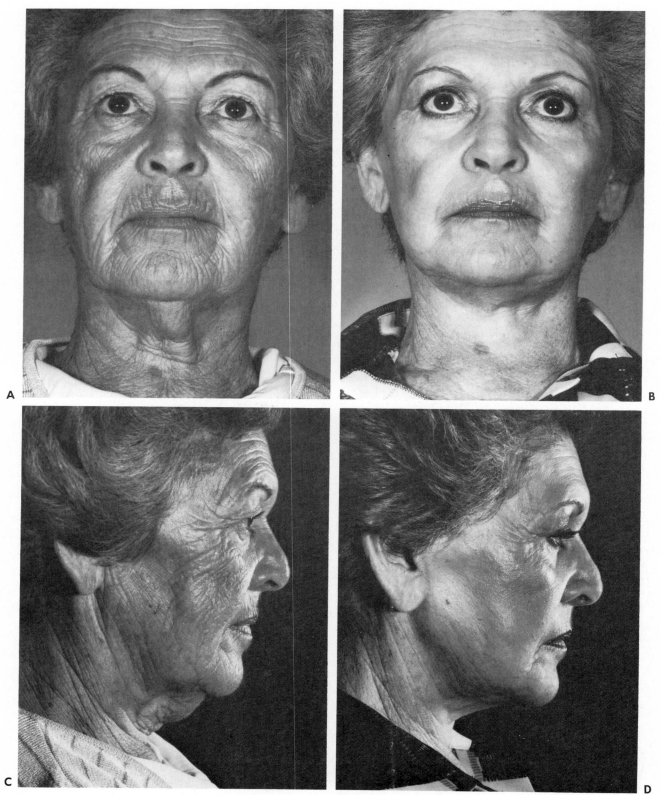

Figure 23–28.   *See legend on the opposite page.*

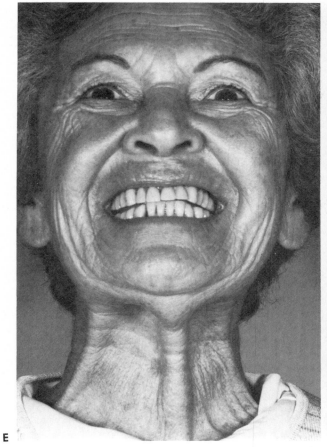

E

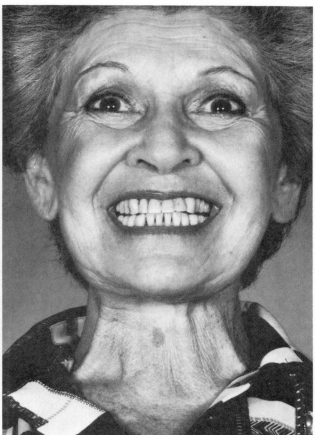

F

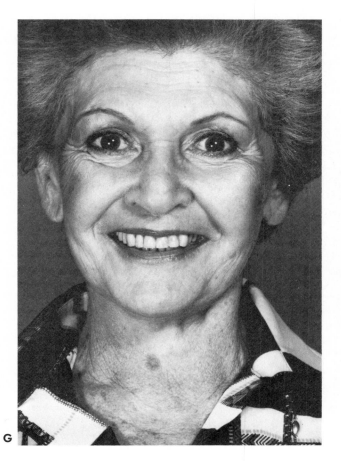

G

Figure 23–28. *A, C,* and *E,* Preoperative photographs showing a severe neck deformity that included a subplatysmal lipoma in the midline. Note the marked rhytidosis of the facial and neck skin. Such localized fat accumulations are true lipomas. They can often be removed through a small rent in the muscle, but it is usually preferable to open the midline between the medial borders of the platysma to gain sufficient exposure. Careful midline repair with suturing of the medial borders of the platysma is mandatory in such cases.

B, D, F, and *G,* The result after deep chemabrasion of the full face, excision of the subplatysmal fat pad, and complete transection of the muscle. Note the strong vertical bands in the preoperative animation ("jaw-clinch") photograph (*E*) and their attenuation in the postoperative animation photograph (*F*). The patient's pleasure at the result is clear (*G*).

Illustration continued on the following page.

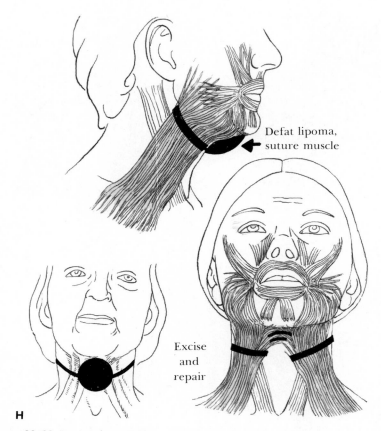

Figure 23–28 *Continued.   H,* The surgical plan is indicated on the platysma diagram.

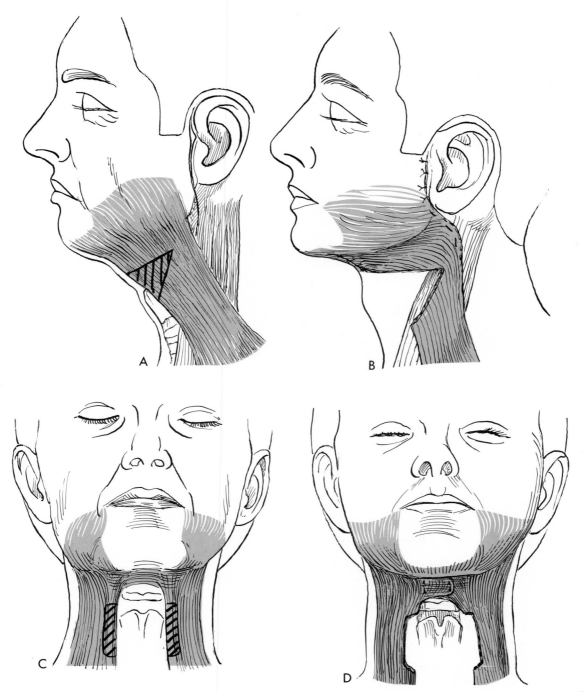

Figure 23–29. A limited and incomplete platysma resection suffices in some patients to correct the cervicomental angle. Such a partial transection of the platysma is particularly useful in patients with a thin, attenuated muscle and in patients with very thin neck structures in whom a complete transection of the muscle would likely result in an unsightly postoperative deformity in which all the structures deep to the platysma come into bas relief. This deformity resembles that seen after radical neck dissections. It is particularly distasteful to women. In cannot be overemphasized that careful preoperative evaluation of the individual anatomic problems that might be encountered is important in each patient.

A, An excisional triangle is indicated to divide the oblique anterior neck line.

B, The triangle is excised and a Skoog SMAS flap is sutured into the sternocleidomastoid and preauricular fascia.

C, Simple excision of the strong medial bands suffices in some patients.

D, Excision of the medial bands and plication of the muscle beneath the mentum suffices in other patients. Variability in the technique is urged after careful study of the patient.

Figure 23–30.   The surgical plan in this patient included defatting of the submental and submandibular regions in continuity after complete skin undermining. The midline "turkey gobbler," which included both fat and muscle, was resected along with a generous portion of the platysma muscle (indicated on the drawing insert).

See illustration on the opposite page.

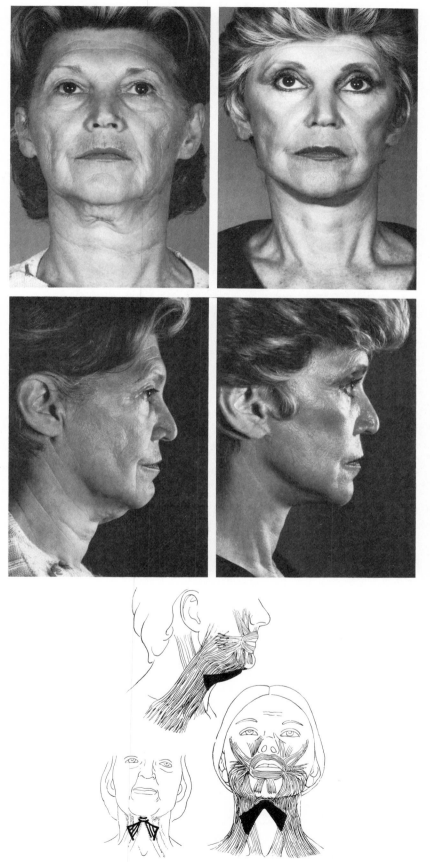

Figure 23–30. *See legend on the opposite page.*

Figure 23–31. The deep crease that occurs in some patients extending from the ala nasi to the lateral oral commissure and ending at the lateral aspect of the symphysis is usually hereditary and increases with age. It is caused by attachments of the muscles of facial expression and the SMAS into the dermis. The small skin pouches that occur along this line just lateral to the oral commissure are particularly distressing to patients. There is no complete solution to the problem short of total excison, and then there is a scar penalty to pay. Skin undermining to and just medial to the crease is the best solution (indicated in the drawing). A sub-SMAS dissection is also helpful in some cases. Other methods of treatment include liquid silicone injections, which can be a most helpful adjunct to surgery in some patients; however, this modality is still under investigation and is not available to most physicians. Subdermal liquid collagen may be of benefit. Methods of increasing the thickness of the subdermal collagen layer theoretically would be helpful.

See illustration on the opposite page.

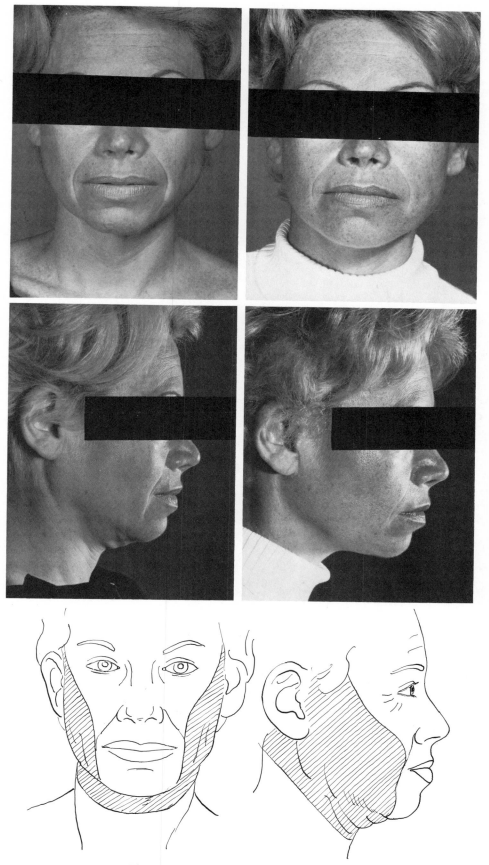

Figure 23–31. *See legend on the opposite page.*

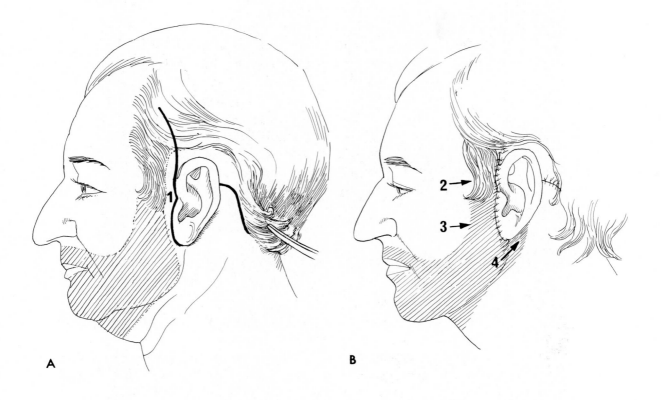

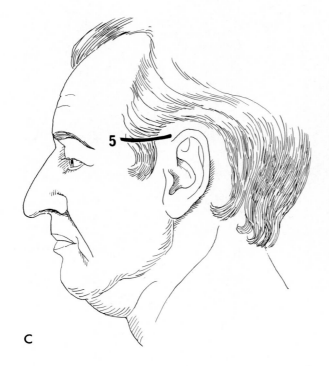

Figure 23–32. The male face lift. Face lifting for men presents certain unique features. Camouflaging scars behind the ears is more difficult because most men do not wear their hair long enough to comb it over the scars. The preauricular incision is much less of a problem, as most men naturally have rather deep creases in front of their ears in which the incisions can be placed. The sideburns (*B* 2) must be moved back in face lifting so that the beardless area (*A* 1) usually present between the posterior limit of the sideburn and the anterior helical and tragal margin will be obliterated. Moreover, the beard itself is moved posteriorly (*B* 3) and superiorly so as to lie behind the lobule of the ear (*B* 4), virtually to the mastoid skin, necessitating shaving of this region after surgery. Men should be advised of these eventualities prior to surgery. A horizontal incision through the hairline (*C* 5) is inadvisable in men. A staggered anterior hairline can result.

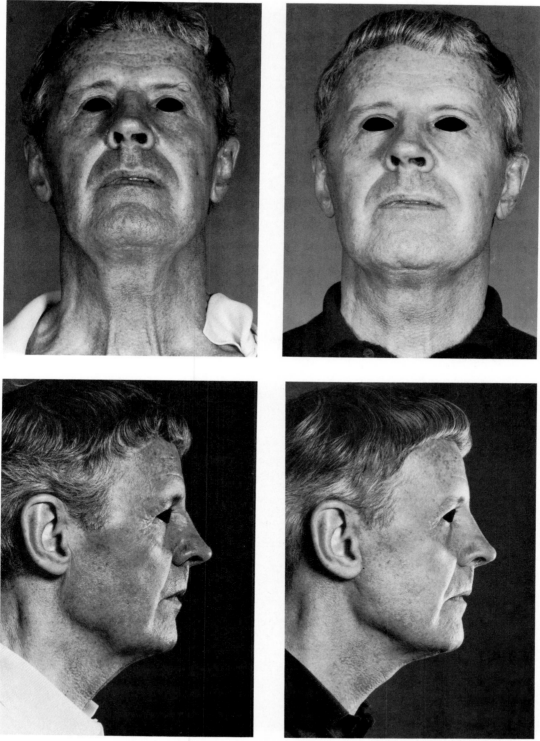

Figure 23–33. The face lift operation can be expected to accomplish the same result in men as in women — that is, a "cleaning up" of the jawline and upper neck, particularly in the early candidate such as this man. The same deficiencies are inherent in the operative technique too — namely, the nasolabial area is improved little or not at all by the operation. If great care is taken to avoid tension on the preauricular suture line, the resulting scar is virtually invisible. Most men have a deep natural skin crease at the exact site of the preauricular incision. Retrodisplacement of the hairline further camouflages the scar.

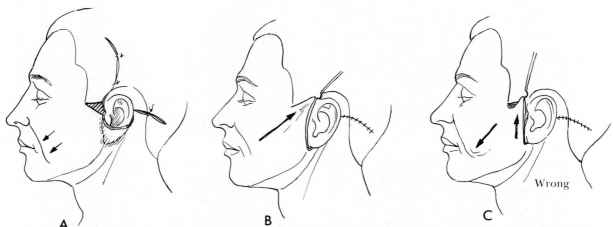

Figure 23–34.   Occasionally, a case can be made for a horizontal incision through the sideburn at the base of the temporal scalp line in men; however, in the author's opinion, such an incision should not extend further anteriorly (toward the midline) than the vertical temporal hairline.

A, If the main problem is a relaxed cheek with a heavy nasolabial fold (arrows), a small triangular incision similar to that described previously in this chapter can be used to achieve a rotation of the cheek flap.

B, The cheek flap is rotated in the direction of the arrow. The redundant triangle of skin is excised. The rotation should be posterosuperior.

C, The "wrong" direction of rotation is indicated as a cephalic pull without a posterior component. Such a direction of pull only accentuates the deformity.

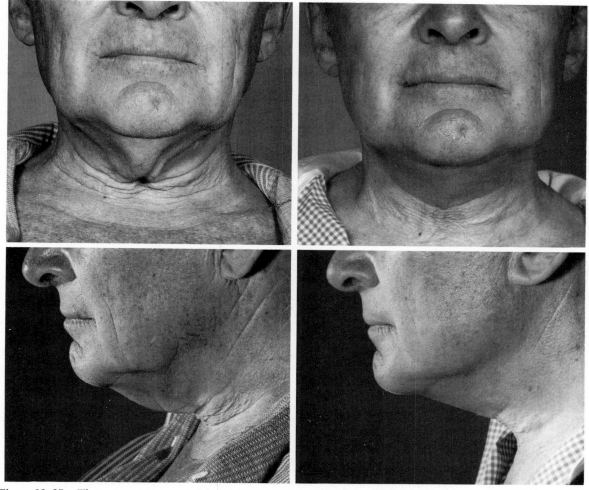

Figure 23–35. The most common complaint of men in middle age or older who seek facial plastic surgery is loose neck skin. A "wattle" of neck skin causes discomfort when shirts and ties are worn, is not attractive, and makes it difficult to wear turtle-neck shirts and other items of sportswear. In this patient, the problem was corrected by a two-stage operation. A rhytidectomy with very wide undermining of the skin around the midline of the neck was done first, followed after several weeks by a T-shaped incision of the front of the neck. A slightly longer hair style is helpful after surgery to hide the incisions. A sharp (acute) cervicomental angle could not be obtained in this patient because it had never been there. A hereditary neckline was related to a low position of the hyoid bone (see text).

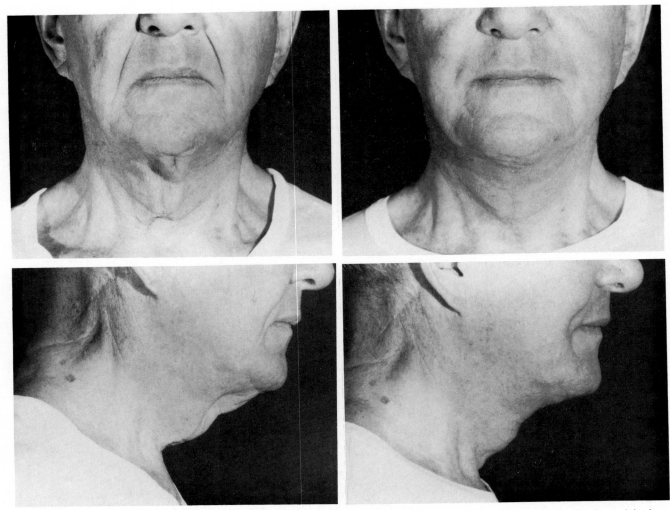

Figure 23–36. A "turkey gobbler" neck consisting of redundant skin of the upper neck region is apt to be the chief complaint in men. Some men are loath to undergo the standard rhytidectomy because of the difficulty in hiding the circumauricular incisions. In carefully selected cases, however, a Z-plasty of the lax skin with excision of the redundancy by direct approach to the anterior neck can be considered. This technique has been advocated by Carlin and Gurdin as well as by Cronin and Biggs. The resulting scar usually ages well. It is a necessary price to pay for a clean neckline. This "turkey gobbler" neck was corrected by the Z-plasty technique. Such a radical approach is rarely if ever indicated in women. (From Cronin, T. D., and Biggs, T. M.: Plast. Reconstr. Surg, *47*:534, 1971.)

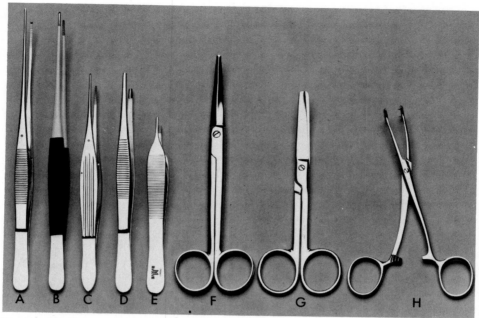

Figure 23–37.   *Rees Rhytidectomy-Platysma Set.**

A, Long forceps with single teeth for grasping the platysma at a distance beneath the skin flap.

B, Long, plain-tipped cautery forceps for pinpoint coagulation of bleeders beneath the skin flaps. Shank of forceps is insulated to protect the soft tissue from accidental burn.

C, McIndoe forceps with plain tips for electrocoagulation.

D, Medium length forceps with multiple teeth (Adson-Brown) for grasping edge of the SMAS during dissection.

E, Standard Adson-Brown forceps for skin suturing.

F, Rees double-edged face-lift scissors for dissection of the skin and platysma flap.

G, Stout, blunt-tipped scissors for skin trimming.

H, Semi-curve, mastoid skin flap forceps for traction and retraction of the postauricular skin flap.

*Available from Walter B. Lorenz Co.

lower flap was either ignored or also sutured in a posterior direction. This operation was a landmark in cervicofacial surgery. Guerrero-Santos was the first to publish on the platysma techniuqe (1974, 1978). Figure 23–21 shows platysma correction by the Guerrero-Santos method.

Platysma Transection

Complete transverse sectioning of the platysma was championed by Connell and Peterson. This maneuver was a natural extension of the Skoog subplatysmal dissection technique and permits a remarkable correction of an oblique cervicomental angle. Loss of an acute cervicomental angle has been attributed to a low positioning of the hyoid bone from which the strap muscles originate. Al-though a low hyoid position undoubtedly occurs, the best method for correcting this problem is platysma sectioning and fashioning of a muscle flap that can be pulled posteriorly and fixed to the stout fascia of the sternocleidomastoid muscle. This technique is continuous with tightening the SMAS and is shown in Figure 23–22. Midline fixation of the platysma completes the sling.

Connell formulated an important technique in correcting the ptotic neck muscle (Figure 23–23). It is reemphasized that the surgeon should determine preoperatively whether this full transection will result in an overly prominent larynx, particularly in women.

Figures 23–24 through 23–37 highlight some special problems and the methods used to correct them.

(For references, see pages 724 to 727.)

Chapter 24

Ancillary Techniques

THOMAS D. REES, M.D., F.A.C.S.

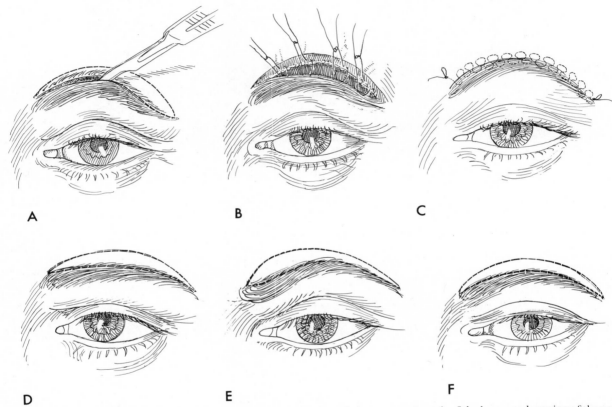

Figure 24-1. The temporal lift is most often used to correct (or to help to correct) ptosis of the brows and sagging of the upper face. Brow ptosis may be a prominent familial characteristic, in which case elevation can be achieved only by direct excision of a strip of skin immediately above the brow. This technique has been described by Castanares and others.

The design of the ellipse to be removed differs according to where the greatest amount of elevation is desired (*D, E,* and *F*). In most patients, the lateral third of the brow has dropped and cannot be corrected by upper eyelid plasty alone. In fact, repeated excision of excess skin from the upper eyelid can eventually result in bringing the brow closer to the lid margin, thereby increasing the brow deformity.

The principal objection to skin excisions over the eyebrows is the resulting scar, which can be obvious in the patient with few or no horizontal forehead wrinkles. When the surgeon decides that such excision would be helpful, he must advise the patient that after surgery it may be necessary to pluck and shape the brows, using an eyebrow pencil to create a new shape corresponding to the scar formed by the surgery.

It is important to place the incision just inside the superior row of hair follicles, as the final scar tends to migrate above the brow line (*A*). After the ellipse of skin is excised, it is not advisable to undermine the edges. The dermis should be approximated by several buried sutures of nonabsorbable material (*B*): the skin is closed with a subcuticular suture (*C*) and can be further sealed with sterile tape strips or interrupted sutures. Such sutures should be removed by the fourth or fifth postoperative day in order to prevent "cross hatches" on these incisions. The subcuticular suture is removed on the seventh day, after which the wound is supported by sterile tape strips for several more days.

684

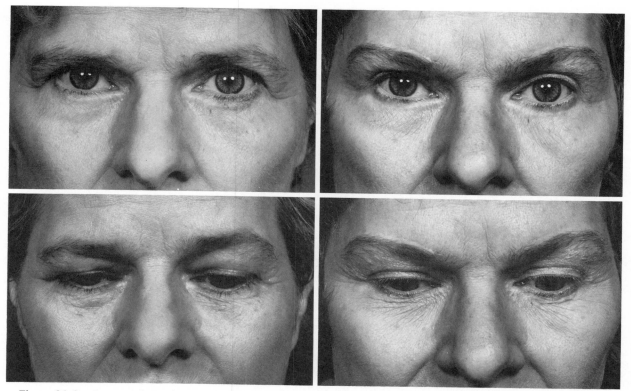

Figure 24–2.   Preoperative and postoperative photographs showing the result of direct suprabrow skin excision. The photographs on the right were taken one year postoperatively. Note the prominence of the postoperative scar—a detracting cosmetic result in almost all cases.

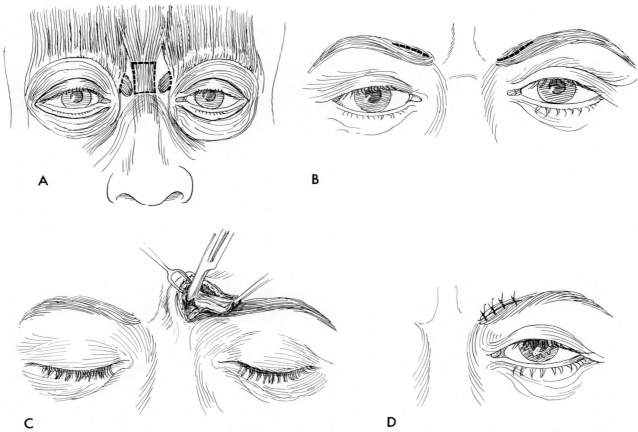

Figure 24–3.   Many different surgical techniques have been proposed for the correction of horizontal forehead wrinkles and vertical frown lines. None has been successful to the extent that it has been widely accepted and used. Temporary benefits may be achieved, but the cause of such wrinkles is the strong pull of the underlying muscles, which cannot be lessened without producing sequelae even less desirable than the original deformity. This illustration and Figure 24–4 show two methods in wide use for resecting portions of the procerus and corrugator muscles (A, C) to diminish muscle action as a cause of frown lines, whereby the muscles are resected through a small incision of the medial brow (B, D) as here or through a vertical incision in the natural frown line (Figure 24–4). A multiple Z- or W-plasty closure of this vertical line is advocated by some.

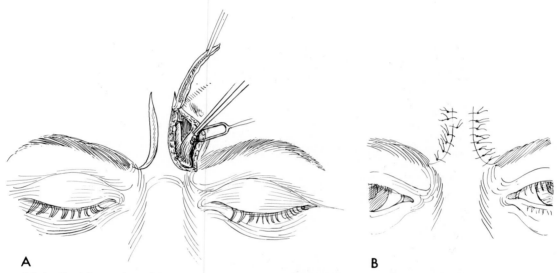

A   **B**

Figure 24–4.   Partial resection of the procerus and corrugator muscles (*A* and *B*) is sometimes thought to help to eliminate vertical frown lines, but the procedure affords only limited improvement, which is usually short-lived.

Purposeful paralysis of the temporal branches of the facial nerve to cause total relaxation of the forehead was advocated by Edwards. This is a rather drastic technique that the author considers rarely justified because it cannot be reversed and ultimately leads to marked ptosis of the brows.

Various implants of dermis and fat or of alloplastic sheet materials have been used to separate permanently the skin in the glabellar region from the underlying muscles, but this approach has also been largely unsuccessful; most of the alloplastic implants eventually require removal.

Unquestionably, the most promising technique to appear thus far has been the injection of silicone fluid, which has been under investigation in this country for several years but is readily available abroad. There seems to be little doubt that correction of vertical frown lines is one of the valid uses for this material in plastic surgery. Several injections are required, the silicone fluid being placed immediately beneath the dermis along the full length of the frown line. No more than 0.25 ml can be injected at a single site in one injection. Deep furrows are often eliminated entirely by this technique, and fine lines or creases are usually improved.

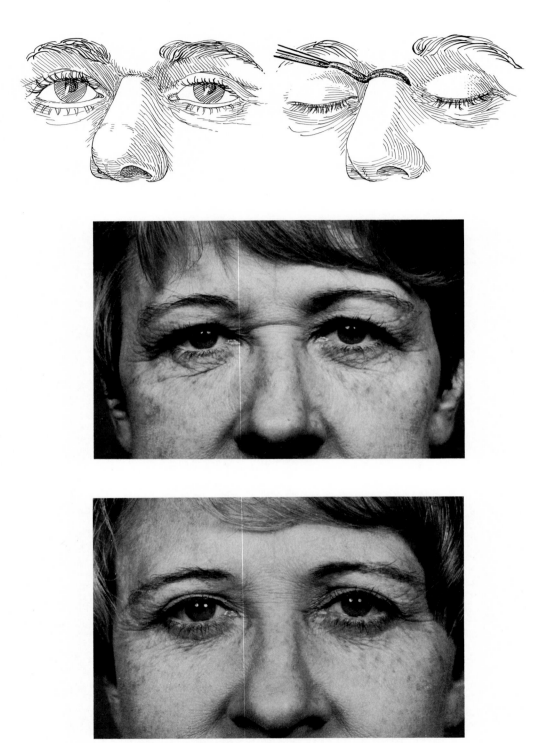

Figure 24–5. A deep wrinkle across the root of the nose, a very common problem, can be distressing to the patient. These are extremely difficult to eradicate. The only really effective method requires that the wrinkle be traded for a scar, a somewhat drastic technique that should obviously be used only when the patient fully understands the consequences. Simple excision and careful closure with fine sutures is the technique used. (Courtesy of Dr. Cary L. Guy.)

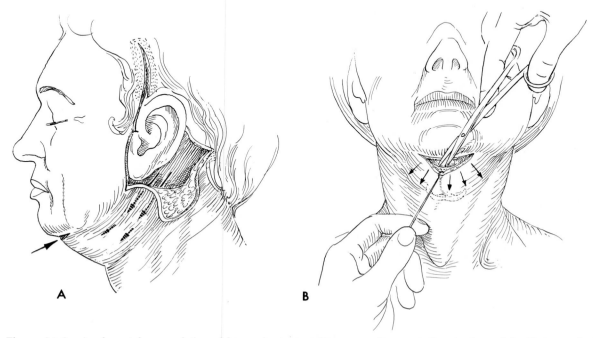

Figure 24–6.   A submental accumulation of fat, a subcutaneous lipoma, can be removed at the time of rhytidectomy. Such fat accumulations often extend around the neck and are continuous in the submental, submandibular, and supramandibular areas (jowls). The technique of sculpting and removing the excess fat is delicate. Sculpting should be contiguous and extend evenly around the neck, and it should include the preparotid areas. Some surgeons prefer to deal with the submental fat at a second operation — an acceptable choice. A certain number of patients require secondary procedures through a submental incision to correct small contour irregularities that result from either insufficient correction at primary operation or from the primary operation itself.

Since the skin flaps become adherent to the underlying fascia and muscle after undermining, it is important to leave a thin, smooth layer of fat on the flaps. It is also important to correct and adjust the platysma muscle to insure a smooth contour. (See section on platysma.)

The risk of hypertrophic scar or keloid formation in the submental incision is real; however, the benefit of clear access to the submental and submandibular regions far exceeds the risks in the author's opinion.

The submental incision is also of use in removing excessive skin beneath the jaw in patients in whom a standard lateral face lift approach is insufficient. With recent innovations in platysma surgery, and notably with reshaping of the cervicomental angle by muscle adjustment, there is less need for additional skin incision, since the redundant skin often is taken up in surfacing the newly deepened angle.

A, The arrows indicate the direction of undermining of the skin flaps and the submental incision, which is best located in the first natural submental crease.

B, The flaps are developed with the double-edged scissors, leaving an even layer of fat on the skin to prevent postoperative adherence to the fascia.

Illustration continued on the following page.

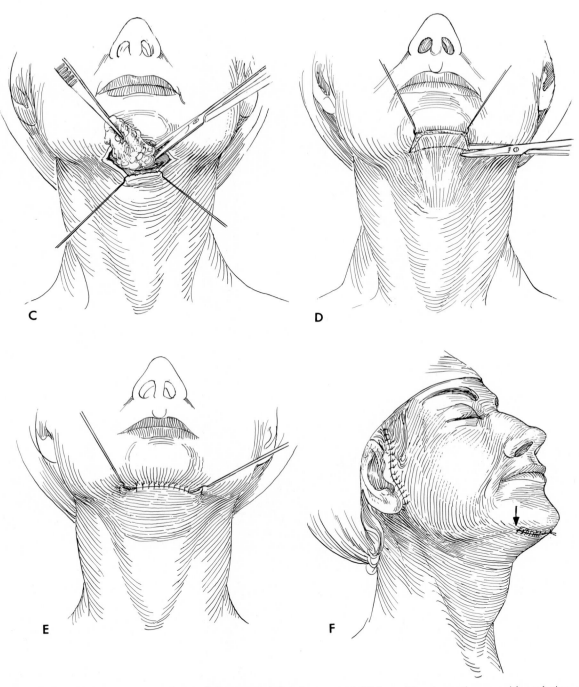

Figure 24–6 *Continued.* *C,* The submental fat accumulation is removed. This excision is contiguous with sculpting of the submandibular fat (Millard) and should extend as evenly as possible around the neck. Care must be exercised to avoid injuring the ramus mandibularis of nerve VII.

Adjustments of the platysma are facilitated by such a wide exposure. Transection, resection, suturing, or plicating the muscle is done as required. A fiberoptic retractor is of great help.

D, Redundant skin is draped over the wound edge and trimmed.

E, Suturing is carried out. Subcuticular sutures are best.

F, Small dog-ears may occur at the lateral edges of the wound. These can be trimmed by standard techniques. Dog-ears are best avoided by beginning the wound suturing from the lateral angles and working toward the middle.

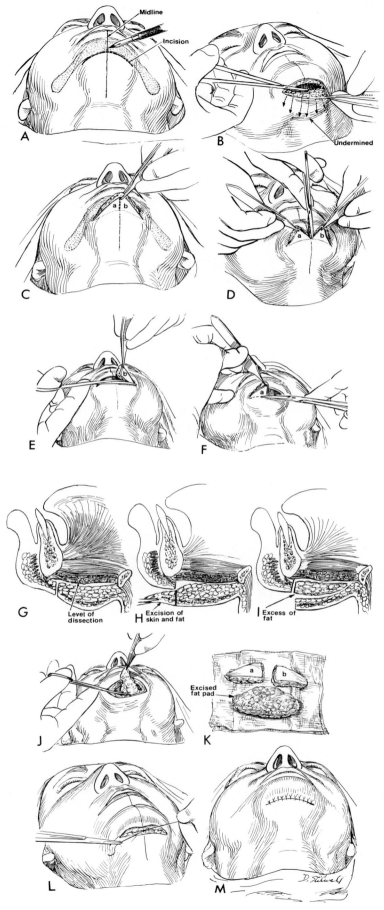

Figure 24–7. An excellent method for avoiding dog-ears is to split the redundant skin flap in the middle, forming two flaps that are then trimmed from side to middle. (From Guy, C. L.: *In* Converse, J. M.: *Reconstructive Plastic Surgery,* Vol. 3. Philadelphia, W. B. Saunders Co., 1977.)

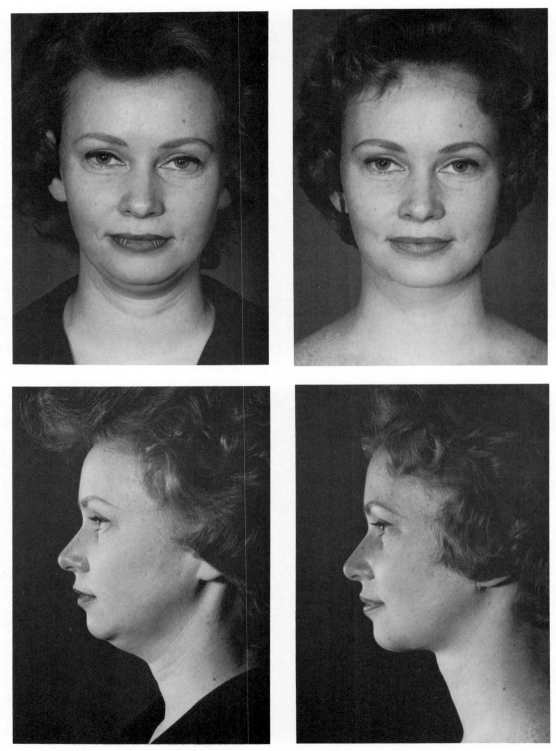

Figure 24–8.   This type of "double chin" is often familial and is a true submental lipoma. It occurs in patients who are not obese, and it may be the only evidence of excess fat accumulation. It is removed through a submental incision, but the patient will also probably need a face lift to take up the slack skin that may result from the incision.

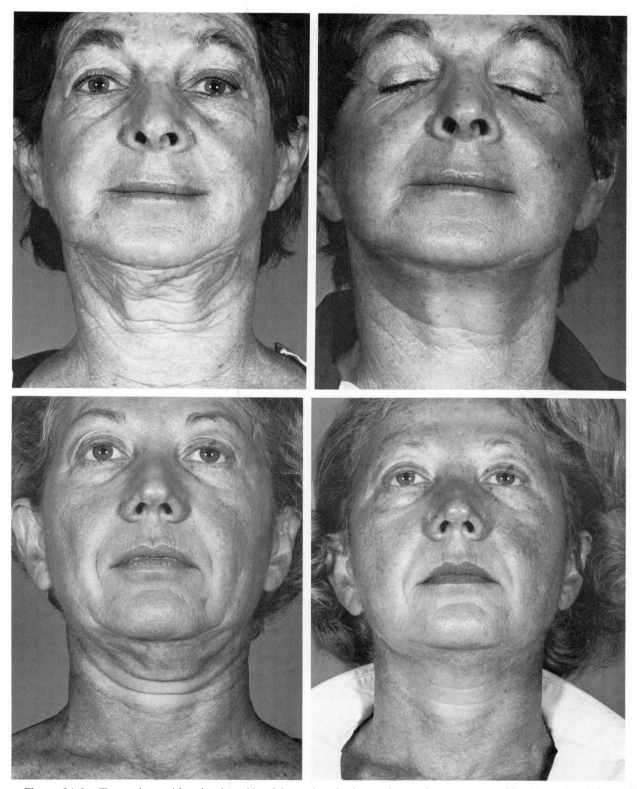

Figure 24–9. Two patients with redundant skin of the neck and submental areas that was corrected by skin undermining and excision by standard rhytidectomy and submental incisions. Muscle was not involved.

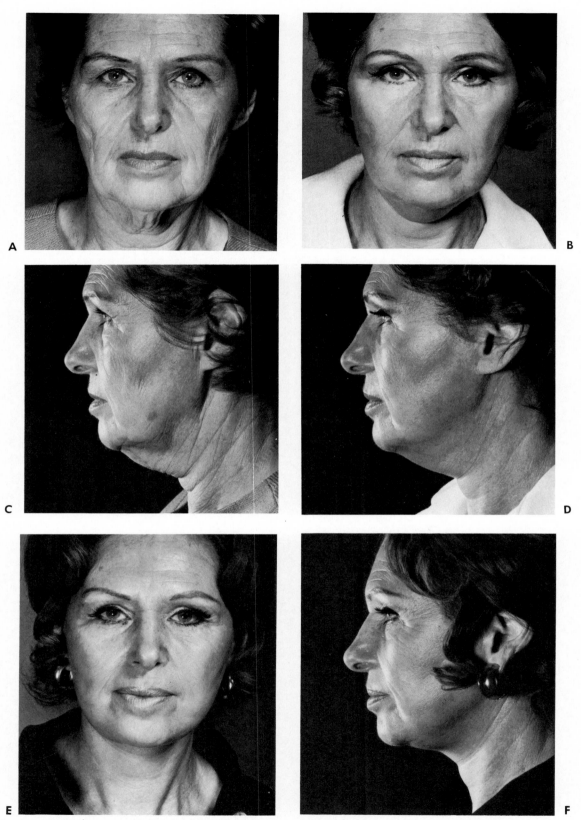

Figure 24–10. The very marked redundancy of the skin of the neck in this patient was corrected in two stages. In the preoperative pictures, note that the skin fold is essentially in the submental region (*A, C*). A thyroid type of incision in such a patient would be useless. The first operation consisted of a standard face lift procedure with complete undermining of the neck and a strong upward lift. The result was considerable improvement (*B, D*); however, as had been anticipated because of the degree of the deformity, it was not perfect. A second operation was done two months later. A submental T-shaped incision (as shown previously) achieved an almost perfect result (*E, F*).

(From Rees, T. D., and Guy, C. L.: Surg. Clin. North Am. *51*:353, 1971.)

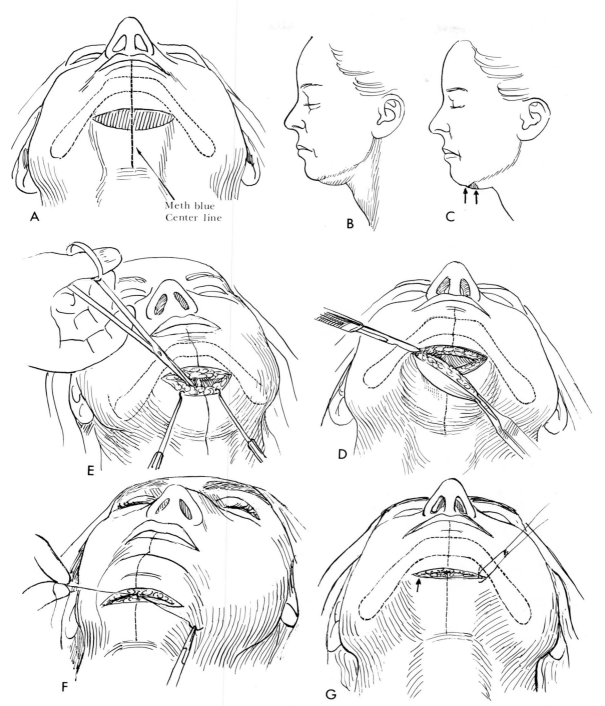

Figure 24–11. To avoid undermining of the skin flaps with some of the attendant problems of this maneuver, Castanares prefers direct excision of the double chin deformity. He argues that irregularities of contour, dog-ears, and so forth are the results of undermining of skin flaps and uneven fat excision. His technique avoids undermining and dog-ears. (See patient photographs in Figure 24–12.)

A, The midline of the mentum is indicated. The ellipse to be excised is located at the point of maximum "bulge."

B, Profile view of the problem.

C, The wedge excision is indicated at the maximum point of the deformity.

D and E, The redundant skin and fat are excised en bloc down to the fascia. The wound edges are not undermined, except minimally on the lower flap to afford closure.

F, A buried suture fixes the midline.

G, Closure is effected from the lateral angles of the wound toward the midline. This technique avoids chasing dog-ears.

Illustration continued on the following page.

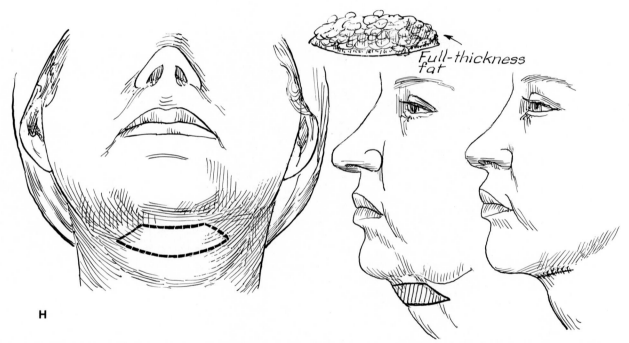

Figure 24–11 *Continued. H,* The design of the bloc to be excised is varied appropriately to conform to the problem at hand. The ultimate scar will fall in a natural crease or angle. It is to be emphasized that in this technique, minimal or no undermining of the flaps occurs.

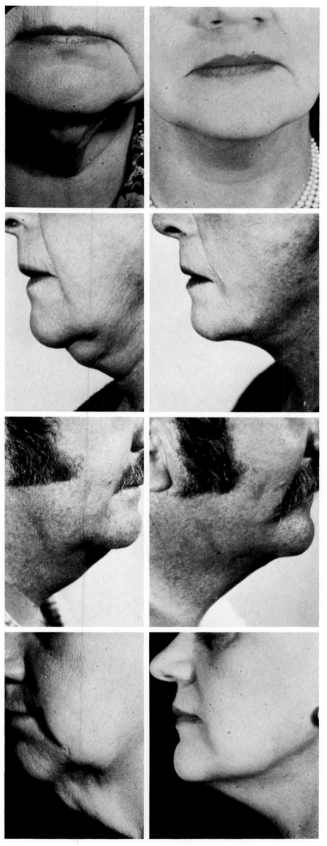

Figure 24–12.   Patients who underwent the Castanares technique for double-chin correction. (Courtesy of S. Castanares.)

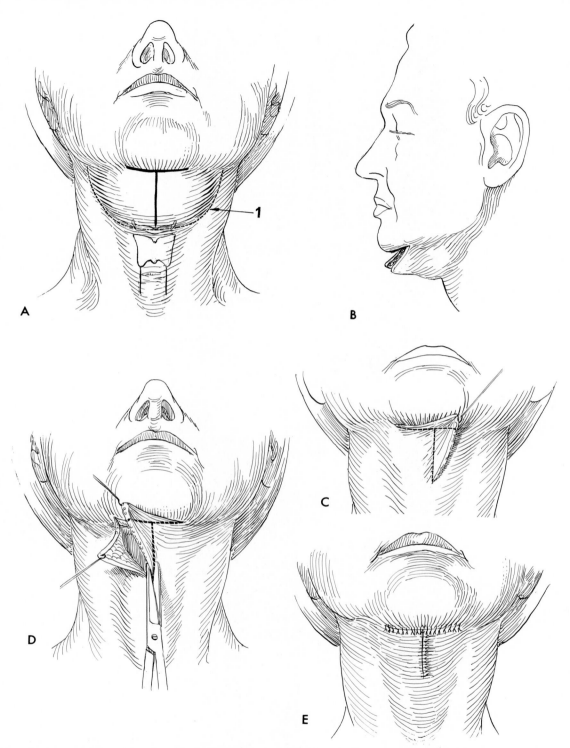

Figure 24–13. The use of a "T" incision to gain wide exposure of the upper neck is only *rarely* indicated in patients with extraordinary deformities requiring extensive dissection.

Vertical neck incisions in older patients heal surprisingly well if they do not extend inferior to the deep fold of skin at the cervicomental angle. They are apt to form hypertophic scars in younger patients.

The technique is as follows: *A* and *B,* A T-shaped incision is made and the flaps are undermined. The vertical limb of the "T" should not extend below the thyroid cartilage. Underlying fat and/or muscle dissection is carried out.

C and *D,* The redundant skin folds are treated as overlapping flaps. The excess is trimmed away.

E, The wound is sutured. When the redundant skin is excessive, as in severe turkey gobbler deformity, the vertical limb of the T can be converted into interlocking Z-plasties.

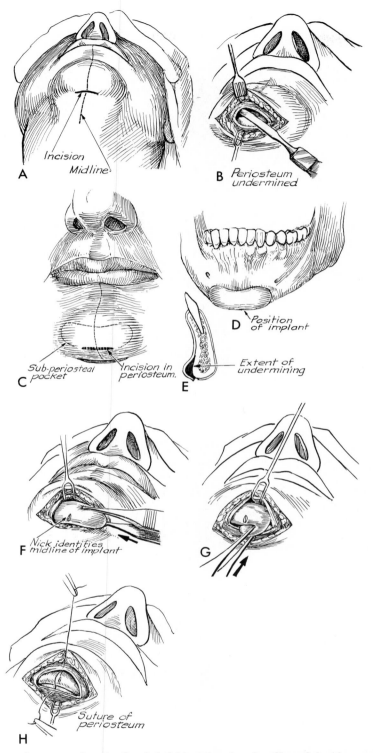

Figure 24–14. Augmentation mentoplasty is often helpful in enhancing the effect of rhytidectomy and submental lipectomy when microgenia or retrognathia is a component part of the problem. In fact, chin augmentation can make a startling improvement in some patients. The procedure must be understood by the patient, since many individuals are concerned about having "foreign implants" inserted into their bodies — a fear spread by magazine and newspaper propaganda.

The technique is simple and is not significantly different from that described in the chapter on mentoplasty. (From Converse, J. M.: *Reconstructive Plastic Surgery,* Vol. 3. Philadelphia, W. B. Saunders Co., 1977.)

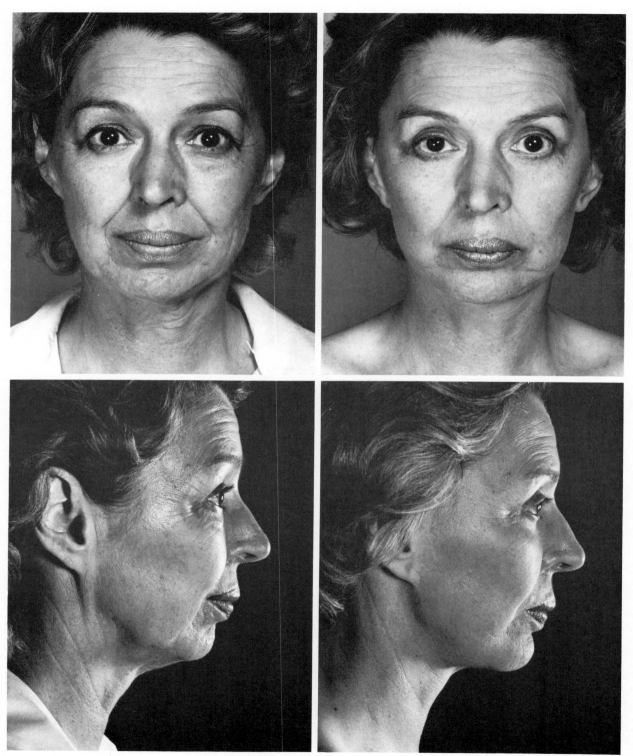

Figure 24–15. Rhytidectomy with chin implant.

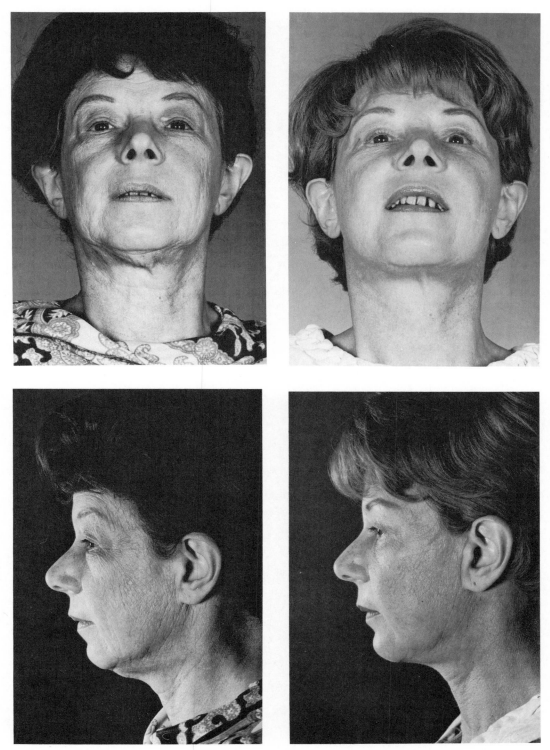

Figure 24–16. Minor degrees of "receding chin" often become more noticeable with age. Chin implants have a subtle enhancing effect on the face lift operation and are rarely conspicuous. This patient demonstrates such a result.

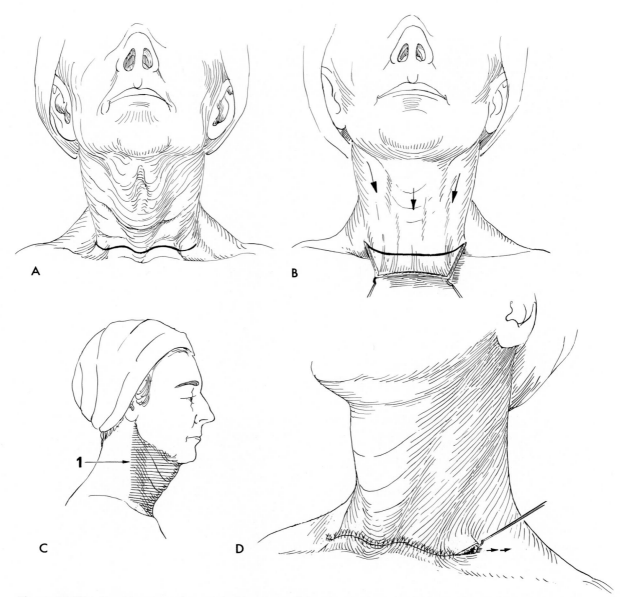

Figure 24–17.   Another approach to marked looseness of the skin of the lower neck below the cricoid cartilage ("turkey neck") that can be used as a secondary procedure when no satisfactory result can be achieved at the primary operation is the use of a thyroid incision (*A*), which permits undermining of the entire lower neck below the level of the larynx in the supraplatysmal plane. This technique was suggested by B.O. Rogers. The skin flap is then pulled inferiorly and the excess skin is resected (*B*). Just as with the submental incision, the disparity in length of the upper and lower skin flaps results in small dog-ears at both end of the closure. These can be trimmed so as to extend the line in a natural neck crease running laterally (*D*).

The lateral extent of the undermining is to the border of the sternocleidomastoid muscle (*C* 1), or further if necessary.

A thyroid incision should never be employed at the time of the primary face lift procedure. It will tend to migrate superiorly because of the upward pull on the face lift flaps. Several weeks should elapse between the two operations.

The author does not favor extension of face lift incisions to the posterior neck midline and removal of wedges of skin in this area as a means of improving the appearance of the neck.

Patients who present with extreme ptosis and excess skin folds of the neck or marked submental fat pads should be advised that two operations will probably be necessary. In extreme cases, a second face lift may be needed in as little as six months' time to achieve a satisfactory result, and a submental incision may be required as well.

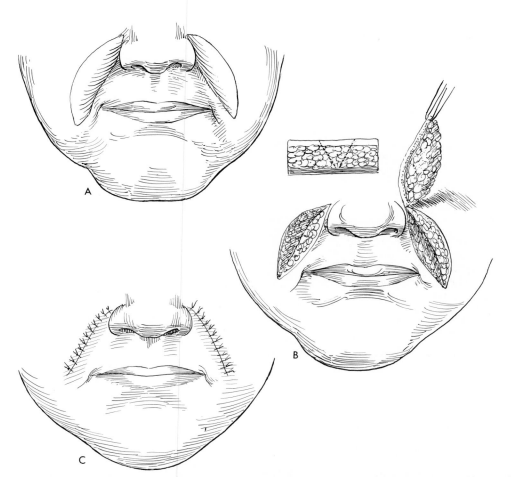

Figure 24–18. Some anatomic problems are difficult to overcome by standard rhytidectomy techniques without a direct surgical approach. The result is an external scar that is acceptable if it is concealed in a natural crease, such as the submental scar, or the brow. External scars of the face or anterior neck, however, are more difficult to conceal, but are an acceptable solution to the problem in highly selected patients. Castanares and Cronin as well as others have suggested direct surgical excision for cutaneous deformities of the nasolabial and oromental folds as well as for submental and cervical problems. The scars resulting from such procedures must be explained to the patient. Fortunately, in older individuals, cutaneous scarring is far less severe than in younger patients. Also, the appearance of wrinkles and folds of advancing age provide excellent camouflage for such scars. (See patient photographs in Figure 24–19.)

Correction of the cheek overhang deformity (Castanares).

Patients with strong cheek folds overhanging the nasolabial crease are candidates for direct surgical excision. Castanares recommends this technique in selected patients.

A, The problem. An elliptical excision is indicated.

B, The ellipses are excised en bloc. Note on the cross-cut of skin the V-shaped direction of the cut. No undermining is required.

C, The wound is closed in layers. The skin can be closed with interrupted or subcuticular sutures.

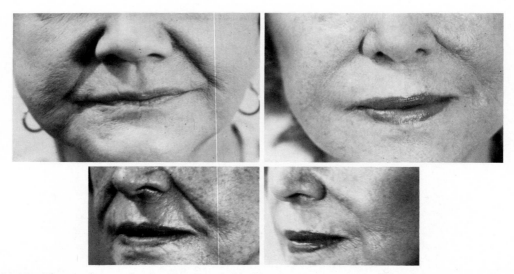

Figure 24–19.   These patients underwent direct surgical incision for correction of strong overhanging cheek folds. (Courtesy of S. Castanares.)

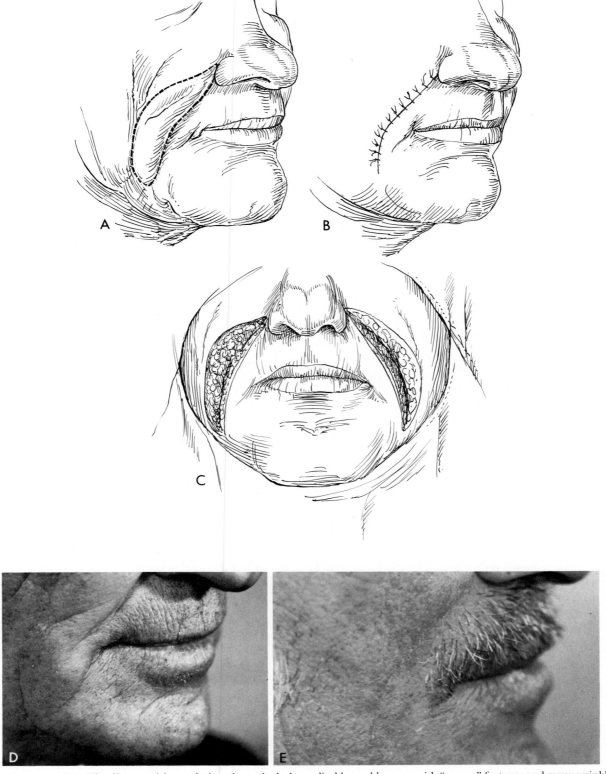

Figure 24–20. The direct excision technique is particularly applicable to older men with "craggy" features and many wrinkles and lines and where the redundant skin deformity extends to the jawline. Scars in such individuals are rarely troublesome.

A, The deformity.

B, Direct excision is carried out.

C, The wound sutured (after Castanares).

D and *E,* Preoperative and postoperative photographs of patient who underwent this technique. (Courtesy of S. Castanares.)

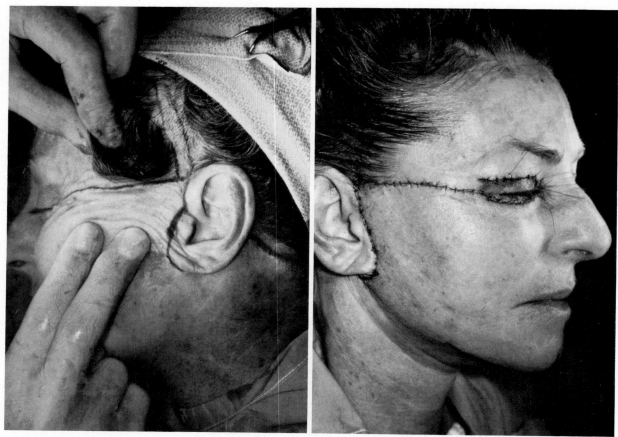

Figure 24–21.   Severe hypoelastic changes in the skin complicate the standard skin flap. Temporal rotation of the cheek flap in such a patient would move the hairline far too high. Preoperative manipulation of the skin with the index and long fingers as shown demonstrates that a more aggressive approach might be required. If the patient is willing to accept the transverse scar across the temple, such an incision is permissible. However, the author has found it necessary to utilize this technique only three times in 20 years. Despite preparation, two of the patients were not pleased with the end result.

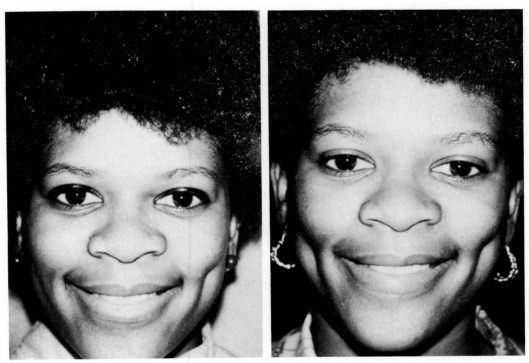

Figure 24–22.   Argamaso utilizes an 8-mm skin punch to create cheek dimples. The area to be excised is anesthetized, and a core of tissue is cut from the buccal mucosa to the dermis of the overlying cheek by a rotary motion of the punch biopsy from within. The wound is closed with one or two monofilament 4–0 nylon sutures that include a bite of the dermal base. (Courtesy of R. V. Argamaso.)

Chapter 25

Postoperative Considerations and Complications

Thomas D. Rees, M.D., F.A.C.S.

DRESSINGS AND DRAINS

A firm case cannot be made for the necessity of either dressings or drains after face lift surgery. Most surgeons prefer some form of dressing if for no other reason than to promote immobility of the head in the immediate postoperative period and to absorb serum or capillary bleeding from the wound edges. Moderately bulky occlusive dressings are all that are necessary, since very bulky dressings affixed with elastic bandages deliver pressure to the skin flaps but can be exceedingly uncomfortable for the patient (Figure 25–1). Complaints of pain or excessive constriction are an indication to cut the bandages beneath the chin to relieve the pressure and to inspect for possible hematoma formation.

Rubber drains or suction drains are preferred by many surgeons to siphon small accumulations of blood or serum beneath the skin flaps. They do not, however, either prevent or treat an expanding hematoma. The flat silicone drain with multiple perforations attached to a suction bulb designed by Jackson and Pratt is preferred by the author for those patients with excessive oozing (Figure 25–2). This type of drain remains functioning for 24 to 48 hours after surgery without becoming plugged with fibrin.

An increasing number of surgeons prefer not to use dressings or drains of any sort. It seems unnecessary to use both suction drainage and occlusive dressings.

POSTOPERATIVE CARE

Dressings are removed 24 or 48 hours after surgery. If soft rubber or suction drains were used,
708

these may also be removed at the same time or they may be left in place for an additional 24 hours. No additional dressings are required unless the patient wishes to cover the incisions in front of the ears.

After the dressings are removed, the patient's hair is usually matted and snarled. It may be gently combed out, using a comb with large teeth dipped in soapy water. The skin should also be gently cleansed of all caked blood, adhesive, and other debris. This cleansing, in combination with combing of the hair, tends to lift the patient's spirits at a time when they are apt to be at a low ebb. Most patients are shocked at their appearance in the mirror in this early postoperative period despite intensive preoperative attempts to describe the ecchymosis and edema that may occur and will surely be maximal at this time. Therefore, if it is at all possible, patients should be kept away from mirrors for a few days. This is obviously not always feasible, so patients should be cautioned as the dressings are being removed that what they see may be upsetting. If ecchymosis is minimal, however, patients may be pleasantly surprised. These immediate reactions, as well as the need to see what is going on, vary with the personality of the patient. Cautious ambulation begins immediately after the operation, but only with supervision and help. Hematoma is the greatest worry during the first few postoperative days. It therefore seems wisest to keep the patient's level of activity low. Excessive talking should be discouraged and it is often best to have the telephone disconnected. The upper body and head should be kept elevated at least 30 degrees in order to lower venous pressure and to decrease the likelihood of hematoma. A soft or liquid diet should also be prescribed until the

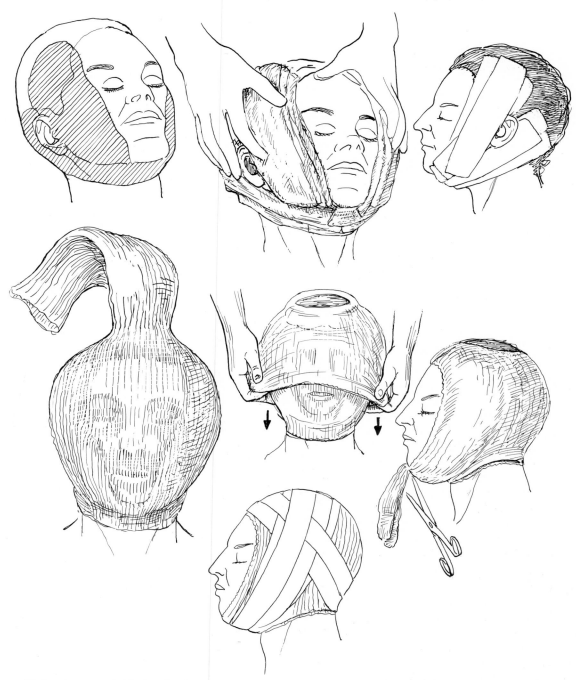

Figure 25–1. A snug and tidy dressing helps to immobilize the head and neck and deliver a certain amount of pressure to the skin flaps. Excessive pressure with embarrassment of the blood supply can result from winding elastic bandages too tightly. The dressing shown has proved satisfactory. The areas in front of and behind the ears are covered with layers of cotton wool soaked in sterile mineral oil. Sterile pads are used next, and the dressing is maintained in place with a surgical stockinette dressing as shown. The outer bandage is loose meshed gauze.

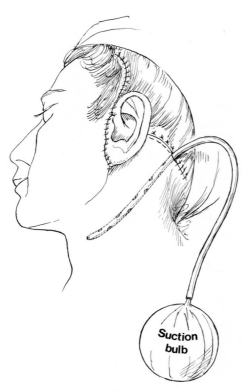

Suction bulb

Figure 25–2.

dressings are removed. Some surgeons prefer giving liquids through a straw only.

If suction drains are used, it is essential to maintain their patency. Attention must be paid to see that the suction is functioning and that the drains are not plugged. Gentle irrigation with a large-bore needle and saline solution at regular intervals is useful in keeping drains open. It is also worth noting that suction must be discontinued prior to removal of the drains. If this is not done, bleeding may be provoked by pulling away clots that are adherent to the holes in the tubing.

Postoperative medications are usually minimal. Appropriate drugs may be used to control pain, although pain per se is not a significant factor following facial plastic surgery. Routine prophylactic antibiotic therapy is preferred by many surgeons, but this is not essential since the rich blood supply of the facial and cervical tissues mitigates against infection. In apprehensive patients, diazepam (Valium) or other suitable tranquilizers may be helpful in allaying fear and in maintaining a relative degree of quiet during the immediate postoperative period. These are particularly helpful in high strung, exceedingly active individuals. Medications to prevent precipitous elevations of blood pressure, an important cause of hematoma, can be given postoperatively for 24 hours or more (see discussion in section on complications).

After 48 hours, the patient's activities need not be restricted, providing no hematoma is present. Bleeding after this initial 48-hour period is unusual. Hospitalized patients may be discharged on the second or third postoperative day and subsequently treated on an outpatient basis. Patients operated on in ambulatory units should be monitored by a responsible individual for the first 48 hours. Private nurses are often employed for this purpose. The surgeon or an experienced member of his staff should check on the patient's progress during this early period. A telephone call usually suffices, since the immediate complications of face lift surgery are usually clearly evident.

Suture removal begins on the fifth postoperative day with removal of all sutures in the preauricular incisions. These are normally the only incisions that are visible, and therefore it is important to prevent suture marks. The postauricular or temporal sutures are removed alternately from the 7th to the 10th or 12th postoperative days. Sutures that support the most tension in the temporal scalp and the posterior scalp are removed last.

The hair may be shampooed with a bland soap as soon as all sutures have been removed. Hair may be set, but it should be dried under warm — not hot — air. A hair dryer set on "hot" may burn the ears, which may still be hypesthetic at this time. Other routine postoperative instructions are provided in the "Letter to Patients." Patients should be encouraged to massage the final scars lightly with moisturizing creams or bland ointments to promote early softening and maturation of the scars.

THE DOCTOR-PATIENT RELATIONSHIP

Considering the highly emotional aspects of face lift surgery, the surgeon performing these operations should not be too surprised to find a high incidence of complaining and "niggling" from his patients in the immediate postoperative period. He should not be unduly distressed when a patient upon whom he has operated seems disappointed with what appears to be a superb result. No matter how completely the limitations and realities of surgical intervention are explained, the patient still may have unrealistic expectations. Anything short of complete restoration of youth by surgery engenders a degree of resentment against the surgeon (whose job it was to restore it), no matter how much he may have tried to make clear the limits of surgical reconstruction. This is not to say that the majority of patients undergoing rhytidectomy are not eventually pleased with the results. For the most part they are satisfied. This satisfaction increases as the months pass after operation, but it would be expecting too much of human emotions to anticipate immediate satisfaction with a result that is less than the preconceived "perfect."

A certain amount of minor complaining following facial cosmetic surgery must therefore be expected in most patients. The surgeon should not take personal offense at this but rather should attempt to understand the complicated motivations that give rise to these complaints so he can discuss them frankly, one by one, as they arise. Careful and thorough preoperative discussions accurate appraisal and frank opinions freely aired help to lessen postoperative disappointments. However, the education of the patient must be carried through the postoperative period as well. Unpleasant information that the patient does not want to hear may be psychologically blocked out during initial discussions. Apparent lapses of memory in reference to facts that were painstakingly imparted by the surgeon should not surprise him, nor should they try his patience. Pertinent information should be reiterated and reemphasized. This type of continuous calm outlook on the part of the surgeon and his staff often results in the transformation of what appeared at first to be a dissatisfied patient into a satisfied one. It is important that the surgeon's staff — nurses, assistants, secretaries, and others — have insights into those mechanisms at work in the patient undergoing cosmetic surgery so that they, too, can understand and deal with the myriad details of psychologic management as they occur during the course of treatment.

The author has found it useful to provide a letter of information to patients who are candidates for facial cosmetic surgery. Such a document can be read and reread before and after surgery. It reinforces the verbal information and instructions provided by the surgeon and his staff. Although it has not completely eliminated misunderstandings between patient and surgeon, it has been of great value in minimizing them. The letter is reproduced on pages 20 and 21. It can provide a guide for others who wish to prepare a similar document.

For cosmetic surgery, the doctor-patient relationship is a unique one and differs greatly from that between most patients and other surgical specialists. It is more in the nature of that between psychiatrist and patient, particularly in that a strong transference is often established. The cosmetic surgery patient frequently expects or hopes that the surgeon is going to be a prime force in providing the means for success, in recapturing lost youth, in gaining job opportunities, in re-kindling love life, and on and on. These attitudes are, of course, unrealistic, yet they do exist, particularly in the emotionally dependent patient. The relationship, even if of relatively short exposure and duration, can become strong during the course of most cosmetic operations. The patient may actually transfer to the surgeon the responsibility for opening the way to complete success or happiness — an impossible goal. When the impossible dream is not realized, the disappointment is then, quite logically in the patient's eyes, the fault of the surgeon. He is blamed for his inability to be a "miracle worker."

In certain severe mental disorders such as paranoia, this moment in the relationship between surgeon and patient can become dangerous for the surgeon. These episodes have been well documented, but fortunately they have rarely resulted in violence. All surgeons experienced in the practice of cosmetic surgery have encountered patients they recognize as being potentially dangerous. Such patients should be guided away from surgery into competent psychiatric hands.

In considering the average person, however, and not the psychotic or borderline psychotic, it is still not clear why many patients experience a period of depression following what appears to be highly successful cosmetic surgery. Such postoperative depressions do frequently occur and should therefore be anticipated by the surgeon. Unless the depression appears to be unduly severe, it can usually be handled by the surgeon on a day-to-day basis with tact, understanding, and discussion. It is natural for the surgeon to feel somewhat hostile toward a patient who complains about a result that the surgeon considers excellent. Such hostility obviously stems from a wounded ego. The clear realization that such feelings on the part of the patient, particularly the middle-aged patient, are frequently to be expected, and the knowledge that they will usually pass with time, patience, and understanding, should help the surgeon to survive in his relationship with the patient at this trying time. More importantly, it may prevent his precipitating a crisis or even permanent breach in the relationship by keeping his hostility from getting out of hand. Unresolved "transference" at this stage results in a permanently unhappy patient and possible legal trouble for the surgeon, much of which can be avoided by an understanding attitude.

Although the foregoing is true, it is not to be inferred that the cosmetic surgeon should not, at times, be quite firm and authoritative, particularly with the patient who appears to be getting aggressively out of hand. The patient who disrupts the surgeon's waiting room, patients, and office staff and who is generally a nuisance need not be tolerated. If communication on a meaningful level with such a patient cannot be established by gentle persuasion, the surgeon has every right to adopt a firm attitude.

Patients undergoing blepharoplasty are often less troublesome, in this regard, than are face lift patients. Usually the results of blepharoplasty are more immediately pleasing to the patient. Also, this is the most effective operation for actually restoring a "youthful look." It is usually the area around the eyes that ages first, and it is, of course, the eyes that are the center of expression of the face.

Patients undergoing rhytidectomy can be divided into three broad groups in regard to their postoperative reactions: (1) those who are exuberant and completely delighted with the results, (2) those who are initially somewhat disappointed that not all signs of age were removed but are generally pleased and become more so with the passage of time, and (3) those who are moderately to severely disappointed with the results and remain so. Fortunately, this last group is small, and most often patients in this category are there because of improper selection of candidates by the surgeon. However, such patients cannot always be weeded out, no matter how careful the selection process. Patients who are immediately pleased, even thrilled, with the results are usually people who are "up" and prone to look on the positive side of life anyway. Such patients are usually externalized types who easily overcome the minor setbacks of life without much difficulty. Their inner feelings, however, may sometimes be another matter, and if they are in any way disappointed in the results of surgery, they are careful not to show it. Sometimes, if such patients are followed over a long period, the surgeon may gain an inkling that all is not what it seems. However, it is often best not to probe too deeply.

Common causes for disappointment in the results of rhytidectomy are early recurrence of the so-called double chin and failure to ablate it at the time of the initial operation.

COMPLICATIONS

Complications following rhytidectomy can be divided into two distinct groups: true complications such as hematoma or infection and untoward results such as dissatisfaction on the part of the patient with the operative outcome.

HEMATOMA

Hematoma is the most significant and troublesome complication that can occur in facial cosmetic surgery. Hematomas may be very small or massive. They occur in 10 to 15 percent of all patients undergoing face lifting. However, minute hematomas are often ignored and thus not included in the general statistics (Tables 25–1 and 25–2).

Prevention is, of course, the ultimate goal. Every effort should be made to obtain adequate hemostasis at the time of operation. Vessels of large caliber should be ligated or coagulated with fine-pointed forceps and cautery. Drains, which are of questionable value in the prevention of hematoma, may be used if the surgeon questions the degree of hemostasis. Delayed bleeding under the skin flaps, resulting in hematoma, may occur for many reasons ranging from rebound bleeding following loss of epinephrine effect to blood dyscrasias.

Many studies have reported possible causes of hematoma following rhytidectomy. In a retrospective study of 23 hematomas among 806 rhytidectomy patients (Rees, Lee, and Coburn, 1973), we were unable to identify the hematoma-prone patient but did note an association between precipitous blood pressure elevation in the immediate postoperative period and the development of hematoma at that time. We also observed an association between the presence of upper respiratory infection or episodes of hyperkinesis, coughing, or retching and the development of hematoma later in the postoperative course. The use of general anesthesia with controlled hypotension has been suggested to help prevent hematoma (Stark, 1972, 1977). However, the usefulness of this technique was not borne out by our observations. In our series, general anesthesia was used for 20 of 23 rhytidectomy patients developing hematomas, and 12 of those 20 had controlled hypotension with systolic pressures of 60 to 80 mm Hg during surgery. Berner, Morian, and Noe (1976) evaluated 202 rhytidectomy patients and found that, in general, during the first two hours postoperatively, blood pressure recordings did not deviate greatly from preoperative levels, but that during the following three hours, when postoperative and intraoperative medications lose their effect, most patients had blood pressures well in excess of their preoperative level. Straith, Raju, and Hipps (1975) evaluated 500 rhytidectomy patients and found that patients with blood pressures above 150/100 mm Hg on admission developed hematomas 2.6 times more frequently than did normotensive patients. Berner's suggestion that chlorpromazine be

TABLE 25–1   HEMATOMAS FOLLOWING RHYTIDECTOMY
(Male and Female)

Authors	Year	Number Cases	Males	Large Hematomas	%
Serson and Neto	1964	170	?	2	1.2
Conway	1970	325	15 (5%)	21	6.6
McGregor and Greenberg	1971	524	21 (4%)	42	8.0
McDowell	1972	105	?	3	2.9
Galozzi, Blancato, and Stark	1972	100	?	3	3.0
Webster	1972	221	?	2	0.9
Pitanguy, Ramos, and Garcia	1972	1600	?	89	5.5
Morgan	1973	40	?	1	2.5
Rees, Lee, and Coburn	1973	806	?	23	2.9
Barker	1974	163	?	2	1.3
Black	1976	1804	?	48	2.7
Baker, Gordon, and Mosienko	1977	1500	61 (4%)	46	3.0
TOTALS		7358		282	3.7%

utilized routinely in the early postoperative course to reduce "reactive hypertension" seems logical.

The incidence of major hematomas — expanding, large hematomas requiring surgical evacuation — varies, but it has been reported to range from 0.9 percent (Webster, 1972) to 8 percent (MacGregor, 1972) when patients of both sexes are considered together. Baker, Aston, Guy, and Rees (1977) compiled statistics on 7358 rhytidectomy patients, about 4 to 5 percent of whom were male, and found the average incidence of major hematomas to be 3.7 percent. These reports were not analyzed according to sex, and since there is general agreement among plastic surgeons that males have more bleeding at the time of surgery as well as a higher incidence of postoperative hematomas than do females, the overall statistics may be somewhat misleading. Only two reports have attempted to evaluate complications in the male rhytidectomy patient statistically. The incidence of major hematomas in these reports was 7.7 percent (Pitanguy et al., 1973) and 8.7 percent (Baker et al., 1977). The higher incidence of hematomas in males may be related to the increased blood supply to the beard and sebaceous glands, although this concept is unproven.

There seems to be little correlation between the amount of intraoperative bleeding and postoperative hematoma. However, it is the author's clinical impression that rhytidectomy patients

TABLE 25–2   HEMATOMAS FOLLOWING RHYTIDECTOMY IN MALES

Authors	Year	Number Cases	Males	Large Hematomas	%	Small Hematomas	%
Pitanguy, Pinto Garcia, and Lessa	1973	52	52	4	7.7	2	3.3
Baker, Aston, Guy, and Rees	1977	137	137	12	8.7	14	10.2

bleed less and have a lower incidence of hematoma, since the patients have been instructed to discontinue aspirin and aspirin-containing products such as Alka-Seltzer, Anacin, Bufferin, Darvon compound, Empirin, Excedrin, Midol, and a host of other drugs for two weeks prior to surgery and one week postoperatively. Aspirin has been shown to inhibit the agglutination of platelets.

The vast majority of major hematomas occurs within the first 12 hours postoperatively. The single most important sign of an expanding hematoma is pain in the immediate postoperative period, as pain is exceedingly uncommon following an uncomplicated face lift. Ecchymosis of the buccal mucosa, swelling or bulging of the lips or cheeks, and unusual swelling or ecchymosis in the periorbital area should be considered as signs of hematoma until proven otherwise. Frequently, the patient becomes restless and develops a feeling of apprehension prior to the detection of the hematoma by the surgeon or the nursing staff.

If there is any question as to the existence of a major hematoma, the postoperative dressing must be removed immediately for inspection of the face. If a hematoma is present, there is usually tension on the skin flaps with circulatory compromise. The sutures should be clipped along the incision line to relieve tension on the skin flaps, and preparations should be made for returning the patient to the operating room. General anesthesia is preferable for evacuation of hematomas, but local anesthesia and sedation can suffice when necessary. All sutures should be removed, the facial flaps are elevated for visualization, and the hematoma is completely evacuated. A fiberoptic retractor provides a valuable light source for this procedure. After the gross clot is removed, vigorous irrigation with sterile saline will wash away clinging smaller clots and will aid in visualizing bleeding vessels. Rarely is only a single bleeding vessel detected. Hematomas are usually caused by the bleeding of multiple small vessels.

Small hematomas, varying from 2 to 30 cc, probably occur in about 10 to 15 percent of all patients undergoing rhytidectomy (Rees, 1972). Many hematomas are too small to be noted until the postoperative edema of the facial tissues begins to subside on the third to fifth day after surgery. Frequently, the initial indication is no more than an area of firmness that can be noticed on palpa-

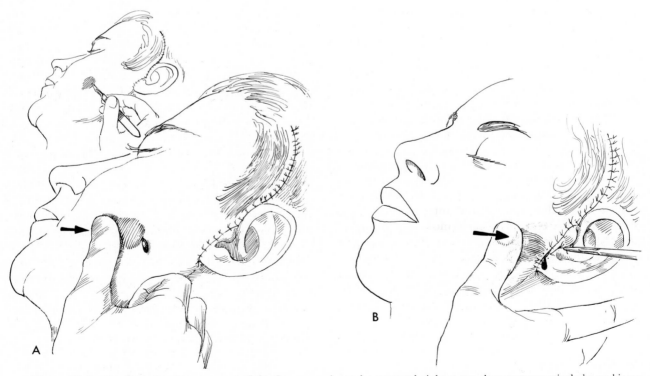

Figure 25–3. Small localized hematomas of the face or neck can be removed eight to ten days postoperatively by making a small stab incision tangentially through the skin and applying digital pressure. If the blood clot is near an incision line, removal of a few sutures allows evacuation.

A, Localized hematoma evacuated by thumb pressure through a stab wound.

B, Localized hematoma evacuated by thumb pressure through an adjacent incision. (Rees and Aston, 1978.)

tion, but after a few days, skin surface irregularity becomes obvious and ecchymosis may be visible. Small hematomas occur most frequently over the mastoid or periauricular areas but can occur anywhere in the operative region. Hematomas liquify between the seventh and fourteenth postoperative day. At this time, small hematomas can be expressed by gentle digital pressure through an adjacent incision or via a small stab wound made with a #11 knife blade directly through the skin over the accumulation (Figure 25–3). They can also sometimes be aspirated with a 15- or a 16-gauge needle. It may be necessary to repeat the procedure used on two to four successive days to assure removal of as much of the accumulated blood as possible.

Failure to evacuate small collections of blood at the proper time will result in organization of the clot with resultant discoloration, retraction, and puckering of the skin. If this occurs, it may take several months before the skin regains its normal texture and appearance. Hyperpigmentation may remain permanently after all other residual signs of the blood clot have disappeared. Intralesional injections of small doses of steroids help to dissolve residual organizing clots and minimize these complications. In late developing hematomas (after seven days), bleeding is usually caused by some trauma as simple as pulling the hair or bumping the cheek.

It should be noted that when a hematoma is being sought on one side of the face or neck, the surgeon and anesthesiologist should treat the opposite side with extreme care. It is not uncommon for a hematoma to develop on the opposite side during or shortly after exploration, probably as a result of manipulation. Massive hematomas that result from bleeding owing to occult blood dyscrasias are usually bilateral and associated with bleeding in the eyelid wounds and into other areas of the skin with extensive ecchymosis. Bleeding of this type is extremely rare and is difficult to diagnose by even the most sophisticated coagulation studies. A hematologist should be consulted at the slightest suggestion of such a problem, since control of the bleeding may require fresh whole blood or plasma transfusion.

PIGMENTATION

Hyperpigmentation owing to the formation of iron pigments may occur in the facial skin over sites of postoperative ecchymosis. The degree of pigmentation is apparently related more to skin type than to the amount of ecchymosis, as patients with darker complexions tend to have greater degrees of pigmentation. Patients with a preoperative history of unusual bruising have a greater tendency toward postoperative ecchymosis than do other patients, and hence they are more subject to hyperpigmentation.

Telangiectasia of the facial skin may be aggravated during face lift surgery by undermining of the skin flaps. An increase in the number of the small-vessel lesions, which are difficult to eradicate, occurs frequently. Lesions are particularly noticeable in the neck. In general, coverage with surface cosmetics is the most appropriate type of management, although the best treatment for larger lesions is electrocoagulation.

SKIN SLOUGH

Skin slough is the most feared complication of face lifting. In experienced hands, it is quite rare. Minor degrees of slough occur most often in the mastoid skin flap, where the tension is the greatest and where the blood supply is farthest from the tip of the flap. Fortunately, these sloughs are rarely extensive, and the resulting scar is behind the ear where it can easily be hidden by appropriate hairstyling. During the phase of necrosis, a black eschar forms. This should be treated conservatively and should be debrided at intervals, but only when separation of the edge occurs. Aggressive débridement has no place here, for the eschar is acting as a biologic dressing. If infection occurs beneath the slough, however, débridement is, of course, necessary.

Major skin sloughs are exceedingly rare. They are usually the result of massive hematoma that has been neglected. Occasionally, a large slough occurs for undetermined reasons. Such sloughs are undoubtedly the result of marginal circulation in the skin flap or localized thrombosis or ischemia. It is actually somewhat surprising that such problems are not encountered more often in face lifting, since the skin flaps are very thin and the undercutting is often extensive.

When these sloughs occur in the preauricular area, the resulting scar can be unsightly and may require secondary excision and repair as soon as the elasticity of the skin permits.

As with many of the complications that can follow rhytidectomy, preventive measures are of the utmost importance. Every effort should be made to prevent hematomas by adequate hemostasis at the time of surgery. Skin flaps must be handled as gently as possible, using skin hooks, т-clamps, or thimble hooks on the flap margins and avoiding traction with fingertips. Tension on retractors under a skin flap during dissection or while obtaining hemostasis should be carefully controlled, as excess tension can severely damage the flap. Care should be taken in the elevation of skin flaps not to let scissor tips cause damage.

Usually, the skin slough will contract and epithelialize, leaving a residual defect much smaller in appearance than the original. However, depending on the size of the slough area, scar excision and advancement of the facial skin may be indicated and can be performed after several months, as soon as skin elasticity permits. Occasionally, if the area of slough is excessively large, skin grafting of the area will be necessary.

SEQUELAE AND COMPLICATIONS OF SURGERY OF THE SMAS (SUPERFICIAL MUSCULAR APONEUROTIC SYSTEM OF THE FACE AND NECK)

Expanded use of dissection in face lift surgery has undoubtedly improved the results in certain patients. However, because the scope of this technique is far greater than that of the classical skin undermine, its risks are also greater.

Probably the most common sequelae of surgery of the SMAS are irregularities and depressions in the neck surface along the route of the platysma transection. These are magnified when the muscle is activated. The defect may disappear in a few months or it may be permanent. Minor contour deformities usually improve with time.

Failure to excise redundant fat superficial to the platysma muscle adequately can result in unsightly bulges along the course of the cut muscle and superior to it. This problem can be improved with secondary defatting procedures. In some patients, the platysma is extremely thick, and after transection, both the retracted upper and lower edges can be quite noticeable. When the muscle is thick, the edges can be bevelled in an effort to improve the condition.

The author believes midline suturing of the platysma is essential when this muscle is transected and drawn laterally, as in the Skoog maneuver (Figure 25–4). A midline suture buttresses the platysma in the submental region and mitigates against postoperative sagging of the muscle border along the jawline. Ptotic submandibular glands, particularly common in the elderly, accentuate the muscle bulge.

Patients with thin necks should be approached with caution when interruption of the platysma is considered, since complete transection of the muscle can result in a cadaveric or skeletonized look, much like that which occurs with radical neck dissection. In such thin patients, it might be wise to consider partially resecting the muscle along with excising, suturing, and plicating the offending medial bands, or tightening the muscle with a posterior sub-SMAS flap.

A prominent thyroid cartilage can be camouflaged by anterior platysma bands and/or fat in the midline. Removal of the fat and resection of the platysma bands can result in masculinizing the neck.

Since complete transverse section of the pla-

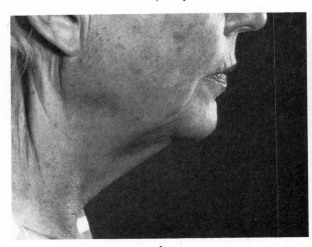
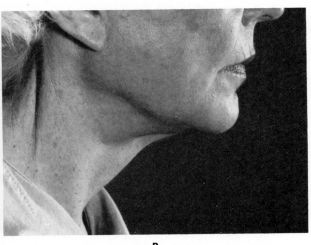

A   **B**

Figure 25–4. *A*, A difficult neck problem with loss of the cervicomental angle. The medial platysma bands are prominent and the submaxillary gland is ptotic.

B, The postoperative result after a full platysma flap. The muscle was completely transected and sutured in the midline, and the flap was sutured to the mastoid fascia. Note the only feature that mars the result is a fullness beneath the mandible and the depression below. In this instance, the flap was thick. The bulge created by the thick muscle flap was accentuated by the ptotic submaxillary gland.

tysma in the neck — theoretically, at least — interrupts the nerve supply to the muscle caudal to the transection, atrophy of this segment would be expected to occur. Aston (1978) tested reinnervation of this segment after one year in some of his patients. When reinnervation occurs, a selective neurectomy might be considered.

Paresis or paralysis of one of the branches of the facial nerve is obviously a risk in surgery of the SMAS. Injury to the ramus mandibularis is quite common in some series (Leman and Hamra, 1979). Fortunately, permanent loss of function seems to be quite rare. Causes of nerve injury may be related to trauma during surgery and variations in the direction of anatomic location of the nerve branches. The buccal branch is also prone to injury (1) if the cheek dissection is carried forward of the anterior border of the partoid gland, and (2) during attempts to remove the buccal fat pad of Bissot. Needless to say, great care should be taken during defatting of the submandibular and submental areas and transecting the platysma or dissecting beneath the muscle or aponeurosis. Some surgeons such as Owsley (1977) prefer to dissect with the aid of a nerve stimulator.

INFECTION

The face and hair cannot be "sterilized" with any known chemical agent used as a preoperative preparation. However, infection following face lift surgery is rare, probably because of the rich blood supply to the area. Small, localized pustules may occur along the suture lines if sutures are left in place too long. These are treated by suture removal and evacuation. More extensive infections such as cellulitis of localized abscess are treated by evacuation, open drainage of the involved area, and appropriate antibiotic therapy. There is little or no evidence to support the use of antibiotics prophylactically.

Rarely, chondritis of the ear cartilage associated with deep sutures of the postauricular wound occurs following facial plasty (Figure 25–5). Chondritis is an indication for hospitalization, wound drainage, and intensive antibiotic therapy to minimize cartilage destruction and subsequent ear deformity.

HAIR LOSS

Hair loss can occur in the temporal skin flap or adjacent to the incisions in the hair-bearing scalp. Such loss is most often found in patients with thinning hair and a tendency toward alopecia. It is most likely to occur following a second operation performed in the same area within a few weeks after the first procedure. Temporary hair loss is more common than permanent loss. Patients with healthy hair and scalp can be reasonably certain that the hair will grow back within a few weeks. However, this may take up to six months.

When hair loss appears unusually extensive, a dermatologic consultation should be obtained. Often, suitable medication such as topical or injectable steroids can reverse the trend. Localized hair loss adjacent to incisions or from spreading of scars can occasionally be improved by scar excision and revision.

Care must be taken in patients with a naturally

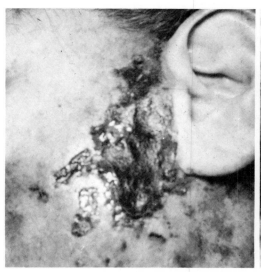
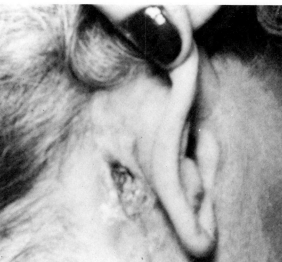

Figure 25–5. Chondritis of the ear cartilage.

high temporal hairline to prevent the hairline from being unduly elevated. Surgical incisions in such patients should be designed appropriately. A transverse incision just under the hairline allows rotation and elevation of the face flap without elevating the temporal hairline excessively. In males, alteration of the temporal hairline can be especially distressing, as a "step" in the anterior margin of that hairline is difficult to camouflage.

Reconstruction of the hairline in the mastoid area should also be carefully performed to prevent a significant "stair-step" effect. However, a small "step" is acceptable if necessary to obtain maximal rotation of the skin flap. Radical alteration of the postauricular or mastoid hairline in the male can and should be avoided by careful tailoring of the skin flaps and meticulous reconstruction of the hairline.

It should be explained to all male patients preoperatively that the hairless area of skin in front of the ear will be narrowed or obliterated, thus altering the beard pattern, since the incision for male rhytidectomy places the beard close to the anterior border of the ear. Only rarely is it possible to leave a strip of nonhair-bearing skin in the preauricular area. Furthermore, the bearded skin is frequently advanced to the retroauricular area, and shaving this area is somewhat difficult. An electric razor with a small shaving head is helpful in overcoming this difficulty.

SCARS

Conspicuous scarring following rhytidectomy is caused primarily by tension on suture lines and/or compromise of the vascular supply to the skin flaps. The most obvious and troublesome of such scarring is that which occurs in the preauricular area and extends to and around the earlobe. Skin flaps must approximate easily and must be sutured with minimal tension or the scar will widen during the postoperative course. All necessary tension should be exerted on the temporal and retroauricular suture lines only. If there is tension on the earlobe, the earlobe will be pulled downward, producing an unnatural appearance as well as a scar that is highly visible and difficult to camouflage.

Excessive tension in the temporal and mastoid areas, however, may result in wide scars that create bald spots that are difficult to hide if the hair is short or thin. Should such scarring occur, it may be possible after several months to revise these defects by approximating hair-growing follicles.

Hypertrophic scars, if they occur, usually ap-pear in the postauricular area within two to four months postoperatively. Small doses of intralesional steroids, such as 0.2 to 0.4 mg triamcinolone, will aid significantly in resolving such scars. Often, two or three injections spaced three to four weeks apart will be necessary. Hypertrophy of the preauricular or temporal scars is uncommon but can occur. True keloids are surprisingly rare. They are prone to occur in darkly pigmented skin. The treatment of keloids is excision and simultaneous injection of the dermal layers of the skin with steroids.

Submental incisions for excision of fat or skin should be carefully designed and placed in the natural skin creases of the submental area to minimize obvious scarring. The amount of skin to be excised must be carefully calculated, for excessive skin excision can result in marked wound tension, increasing the likelihood of scar hypertrophy or webbing of the vertical dimension of the neck flap. Overzealous resection of the submental fat pad, as well as insufficient undermining, can result in an unsightly depression of the submental area. Symmetrical defatting of the submandibular and submental areas helps prevent such a depression. Large submental excisions may result in "dog-ears" at each end of the incision. If uncorrected, these persist postoperatively as unsightly bumps. Extending the submental incision may correct dog-ears, but care must be taken to prevent the scars from extending beyond the border of the mandible or downward onto the neck where they are visible. Suturing submental wounds by beginning at the lateral angles and progressing toward the middle also helps to eliminate dogears.

Vertical scars in the anterior neck frequently produce unattractive, hypertrophic marks. Occasionally, a male patient with a severe "turkey gobbler" neck will require vertical excision with a z-plasty closure. A conspicuous, wide, beardless scar can result if excess tension is placed on the skin flaps. Fortunately, such incisions heal better in older patients, who are more likely to require such procedures. Vertical incisions on the anterior surface of a female neck — with or without z-plasty — are rarely indicated.

NERVE INJURY

The incidence of all intraoperative nerve injuries during rhytidectomy is reported in the literature to range between 0.53 (Baker, Gordon, and Mosienko, 1977) and 2.6 percent (MacGregor, 1972).

The most frequently injured nerve is a sensory

nerve, the greater auricular nerve. It is not infrequent for patients to have transient numbness in the preauricular areas, over the cheeks, and in the lower two thirds of the ear during the early postoperative course. However, as a result of the sectioning of small sensory nerves during surgery, transection of the greater auricular nerve can produce permanent loss of sensation and/or paresthesias over the lower portion of the ear. Injury to this nerve occurs when dissection is too deep over its course along the anterior border of the sternocleidomastoid muscle. When injury to this nerve is recognized during surgery, it should be immediately repaired in an attempt to restore sensory function and ideally to prevent the development of painful neuromas at the site of the nerve ends.

The problem of sensory nerve damage, however, is far less serious than is injury to the facial nerve. It is mandatory that the surgeon performing rhytidectomy be fully familiar with the usual course and common variations of the facial nerve. The surgical anatomy of this nerve has been extensively reviewed by Dingman and Grabb (1962), Pitanguy and Ramos (1966), Loeb (1970), and others. Keeping this knowledge in mind, and carefully dissecting just under the superficial subcutaneous tissue, the surgeon can minimize the incidence of facial nerve injury. Fortunately, permanent injury to a branch of the facial nerve, a catastrophe for both patient and surgeon, is very rare. Most patients recover full motor function following injury to a branch of the facial nerve within a few weeks to a year, although in an occasional patient it may take up to two and a half years for function to return to normal (Spira et al., 1968; Baker et al., 1977). The nerve branch injured most often varies according to report, but the temporal, marginal mandibular, and buccal branches are those usually involved.

Following infiltration of the face with anesthetic solution, temporary partial or total paralysis of muscles supplied by the facial nerve may occur. Complete return of muscular function occurs over the next four to eight hours as the anesthetic solution is metabolized and its effect on the nerve branches is resolved. Occasionally, a patient may have lingering paresis until the first morning after surgery. Weakness, as long as it is not complete paralysis, is little cause for alarm at this time, and full function generally returns within a few days to a few weeks. Possible causes of paresis of this nature are (1) injection of anesthetic solution into the immediate area of the nerve, (2) nerve trauma during blunt dissection, (3) edema within the nerve sheath, (4) trauma from cautery heat, and, rarely, (5) partial or complete transection of a nerve branch.

If it becomes obvious during the surgical procedure that a branch of the facial nerve has been transected, immediate surgical approximation of the nerve ends must be considered. When the skills of the surgeon permit and facilities are available, an operating microscope should be utilized. With present knowledge of microsurgical nerve repair, should such an injury be recognized, repair is indicated. Unfortunately, most often the surgeon will not be aware intraoperatively that a branch of the facial nerve has been injured because such injuries are rarely visible; furthermore, telltale twitching of the muscles at injury does not occur because the nerve has been rendered inactive by the anesthetic solution.

If injury to a temporal branch occurs, it is usually during subcutaneous dissection in front of the temporal hairline, midway between the outer canthus of the eye and the superior auricular angle, where the nerve crosses over the zygomatic arch, penetrates the fascia, and becomes superficial. Return of function may take up to two years following such injury. If an appropriate postoperative interval has passed and total paralysis of the frontalis muscle remains, transection of the temporal branch to the contralateral side will produce forehead symmetry. However, with the passage of time, the eyebrows will droop because of loss of muscle function. The innervation of the forehead area may be somewhat more involved than it may seem. Miller, Anstee, and Snell (1976) reported a patient who had the entire forehead avulsed but developed complete bilateral return of frontalis muscle function after the scalp was replaced as a free flap with anastomosis of blood vessels only. A buccal branch is most often injured in the loose areolar tissue anterior to the parotid gland. When such injury occurs, it is most often to a small peripheral branch arising after buccal branch arborization. Muscle function returns because of the multiple connections among buccal nerve branches and because of limited crossover with the fifth cranial nerve.

The marginal mandibular branch lies beneath the platysma muscle posteriorly from the angle of the mandible and anteriorly to its innervation of the depressors of the mouth, according to Dingman and Grabb (1962). Posterior to the facial artery, 19 percent of the marginal mandibular nerves course as much as 1 cm below the border of the mandible, whereas anterior to the facial artery, 100 percent course above the border of the mandible. Most often, it is at the anterior margin of the face lift dissection that this branch is injured.

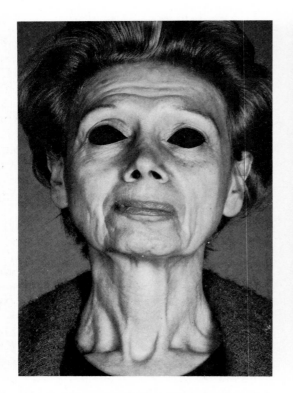

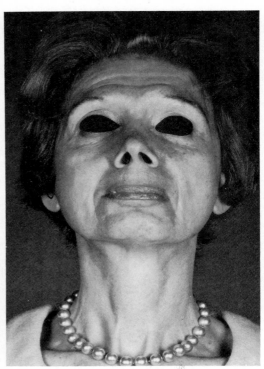

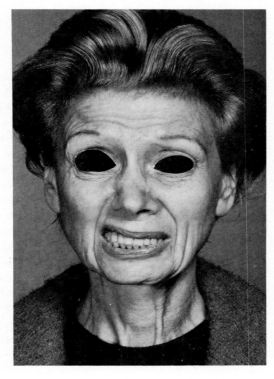

Figure 25–6. Preoperative examination of every patient who is a candidate for facial plastic surgery should include a careful inspection of the facial musculature for evidence of unilateral weakness or paralysis. If such a condition can be shown to exist preoperatively, it cannot later be ascribed to the surgery performed. This patient exhibited a left partial hemiparesis, the residual of an old Bell's palsy, that was hardly noticeable except with extreme animation. The same principle applies to facial asymmetry, which can be accentuated by surgery. Minor degrees of asymmetry or even paralysis can be missed in the initial examination unless the patient is instructed to display marked facial animation. Such minor deformities must obviously be pointed out to the patient before surgery in order to avoid postoperative repercussions.

Transection of the marginal mandibular branch renders a permanent deformity. Extreme caution is mandatory during subplatysmal and platysmal muscle flap operations. Subplatysmal dissection should be safe 2 to 3 cm below the border of the mandible. The author suggests an extra 2 cm margin of error anterior to the facial vessels.

Winging of the scapula owing to transection of the eleventh cranial nerve, the accessory nerve, has been reported by MacGregor (1972). The author has not seen this injury, but it can occur if dissection is too deep over the posterior margin of the sternocleidomastoid muscle.

Preoperative consultation and evaluation by the surgeon should include detailed inquiry concerning past facial nerve problems, especially any history of Bell's palsy, because a postoperative seventh nerve deficit in a patient with a history of Bell's palsy is quite likely due to a recurrence of this disorder. A careful examination of the face for seventh nerve motor function is mandatory (Figure 25–6). Any facial asymmetry or facial muscle weakness noticed during the preoperative examination should be pointed out to the patient before surgery so that it cannot later be ascribed to the operative procedure.

PAIN

Pain following rhytidectomy is very unusual, so during the immediate postoperative period, pain must be regarded as a warning of possible hematoma formation. Any pain at this time warrants thorough investigation.

Discomfort, such as a feeling of tightness when turning the head, is not uncommon during the first few days or even weeks after the operation. Anesthesia or hypesthesia of the skin flaps and earlobes may occur and last several months. Such loss of feeling, however, is always temporary, unless the greater auricular nerve has been sectioned during surgery and left unrepaired.

Small neuromas along the cervical sympathetic nerves or at the free ends of a transected greater auricular nerve can produce pain and discomfort in the late postoperative period. Pain along the area of sensory nerve distributions usually disappears by the third postoperative month. Frequent regional nerve blocks are helpful while the pain is present. Conway (1959) suggested an incidence of chronic pain following rhytidectomy of 2.5 percent. However, this figure is unconfirmed by others and seems high to the author. In general, chronic pain following rhytidectomy should en-

courage the surgeon to investigate possible psychologic causes.

With the recent adaptations of transecting and redirecting the platysma muscle in the neck, we have noted an increased incidence of transient postoperative discomfort. Such discomfort may often be relieved or lessened with muscle relaxants such as diazepam (Valium), as suggested by Guerro-Santos, Espaillat, and Morales (1974).

When prolonged pain occurs, the patient should be reassured that it is of a temporary nature. Regional sensory nerve blocks at weekly intervals may be of help as well as other supportive measures such as local applications of heat and ultrasound therapy.

SECONDARY RHYTIDECTOMY

It is not possible to predict with any reliable degree of accuracy when a secondary face lift operation will be required in any individual patient. This question is frequently posed by patients during the initial consultation. Certain generalities apply in guessing when a second operation may be required, but these are never definitive. The patient who shows marked premature aging of the skin with dehydration, loss of elasticity, rhytidosis, and so forth will probably require a second operation sooner than the patient with more youthful skin who may, for example, have only some excess skin of the neck or jawline as a complaint. Older patients with degenerative skin changes who have their first rhytidectomy in the sixth or seventh decade of life will require secondary surgery sooner than patients in their fourth decade with early evidence of skin aging. Weight fluctuation commonly hastens the date for secondary face lifts. For example, the patient who is slightly heavy before surgery and loses weight after primary rhytidectomy will quite obviously require a secondary operation sooner because of the skin sag resulting from loss of the subcutaneous adipose tissue.

Any changes in the patient's general health that would promote rapid or premature degeneration of the skin can also accelerate the need for secondary surgery. These include excess alcohol intake, loss of hormonal effect, certain systemic diseases (especially chronic cardiac and renal disorders), and severe emotional upsets. Heredity certainly plays a prominent role in the aging process in some families. Everyone knows of families in which people live to a ripe old age without a wrinkle in the facial skin, thus maintaining a surprisingly youthful appearance. Cessation of ovarian function after menopause or following oophorectomy can also rapidly and sometimes dramatically accentuate aging of the skin. This effect can often be minimized by the administration of conjugated estrogens.

Prolonged and repeated exposure to the elements, especially the wind and sun, accelerates skin aging more than any other environmental factor. This is particularly noticeable in fair-skinned blonds or redheads of Northern European descent. People with darkly pigmented skin can be remarkably deceptive about their age. For example, it is often very difficult to estimate the age of a black African. Maybe this is an explanation of why so many Caucasians spend so much time basking in the sun to darken their skin. Perhaps if they were aware of how much this practice hastened the aging process they would give it up. Instead, sun bathing flourishes because "everyone looks better with a tan."

It is unwise to make any predictions to patients as to when a second operation may be required, except under certain conditions. The patient with very marked sagging and skin folds might well require a second operation in six months to one year if a maximal operative result is to be obtained. The author advises such patients of this possibility. Likewise, if there is considerable skin and fat in the submental cervical area ("turkey gobbler" neck), it is sometimes necessary to do a second procedure within a few months using direct incisions in the submental region. These patients, too, are advised of the probable need for two operations within a relatively short time.

The current trend is more aggressive defatting of the submental and submandibular areas in continuity. Direct surgical attack on the platysma muscle along with extensive skin undermining may well prove to decrease the incidence of secondary rhytidectomy, at least in the first few years after primary surgery. Long-term, follow-up observations of this more radical approach to face lift surgery will clarify the situation.

Most patients should simply be told that a second operation can be done when and if it becomes necessary or desirable — usually somewhere within five to ten years. However, they can also be advised with reasonable assuredness that the results of the second operation will be more lasting than those of the first. Some patients may require a third or even a fourth operation.

The typical face lift patient today has the first operation in the early or mid-forties, the second in the fifties, and perhaps a third in the sixties. It could be conjectured that, with the increasing life span and the growing popularity of face lift surgery, these rules will no longer apply and that rehabilitative facial surgery will be continued for one or two decades past the sixties.

Many patients are of the opinion that once a face lift has been done, the second is a necessity because some sort of sudden collapse occurs requiring another operation. This is totally without fact, of course, and the patient should be so advised. It is interesting how such a rumor can create undue fear of a primary face lift in highly intelligent and otherwise well informed individuals.

Exactly when to do a second operation depends on the subjective feelings of the patient and the objective findings of the surgeon, just as the first one does. In general, the first indication that the aging process has again caught up and made itself evident is slight relaxation of the skin under the chin at the cervicomental angle and along the jawline (jowl). Surgery can then be undertaken for the second time or the situation can be allowed to progress further until the patient desires correction.

A word is in order about the patient who becomes obsessed with the idea that a second operation is indicated before objective evidence is present. The surgeon must tactfully prolong the waiting period and provide moral support to the patient. Often a divorce, death, or other personal tragedy will hasten the request for a second operation in a way similar to that in which such emotional traumas cause people to seek surgery in the first place. The patient hopes the operation will change his or her life or give the morale a boost. If such a patient was exceedingly happy with the first operation, it may be difficult to get him or her to wait. Even under such highly charged circumstances, however, the surgeon should not be coerced into operating again before he feels something can be accomplished, because the results of a secondary face lift are rarely as dramatic as the first, and the satisfied face lift patient may be turned into a disillusioned one. Such problems can be avoided by operating only when objective evidence indicates a second operation.

There is no doubt but that repeated facial operations associated with wide undermining and a certain amount of tension have an effect on the skin itself. Recent work has shown that repeated stretching under tension eventually elicits great and definite changes in the architecture of the skin, principally in the dermal collagen. Stretching of the skin, particularly repeated stretching, unquestionably causes a certain amount of ischemia because the tension is bound to have an effect on skin biology. This effect is probably less extensive following flap surgery on the face and neck skin than elsewhere because of the rich blood supply of this region.

Tension per se is apparently not as significant a fact as tension in the presence of wide undercutting. Myers (1964) utilized fluorescein dye injections to demonstrate the vascularity of wound edges in skin closures following radical mastectomy. His studies showed that tension was less a factor in postoperative skin slough than was devascularization owing to extensive undermining or undercutting of the skin.

Many studies on the biomechanical properties of skin have been conducted in both animals and man in recent years. These studies have shed light on the relationship between the structure of the skin—its thickness and so on—and the effects of edema, obesity, and other disease conditions, and, especially, the aging process that is thought to be essentially a process of atrophy and progressive dehydration. Interesting and provocative studies have been carried out along these lines by Rollhäuser (1950), Kirk and Chieffi (1962), Fry, Harkness, and Harkness (1964), Ridge and Wright (1965), Tregear (1966), Parot and Bourlière (1967), Graham and Holt (1969), and Gibson and Kenedi (1969). These studies, particularly those of Gibson and Kenedi, indicate that the skin owes much of its tensile properties to its dermal collagen and possibly its interstitial fluid. The physical relationship of the dermal collagen fibers is particularly of interest when considering repeated stretching of the skin such as occurs in face lifting. It has been shown that the collagen fibers tend to orient themselves perpendicularly to the stretch force when tension or a certain stretch load is applied to the skin.

The formation of natural wrinkles of the skin is unquestionably also a result of skin tension as well as of anchorage of the underlying muscles of facial expression to the integument. Most such creases are congenital and indicate the attachment of the skin to the tela subcutanea by connective tissue strands that extend from the epidermis through the dermis to the superficial aponeurosis. These wrinkles are often unrelated to the lines of Langer, making the Langer's lines of limited value to the surgeon in planning the effects of facial surgery. Cox (1941), and later Kraissl and Conway (1949), showed the discrepancies that exist between the classic Langer's lines and the normal skin folds and wrinkles in the face and neck that limit the value of the former in planning the incisions and scars.

Montandon (1967) carried out a series of very interesting experiments on the biomechanics of the thoracic esophagus of puppies, particularly on the effects of stretching the esophagus under tension. He did multiple excisions of esophageal segments with successive reanastomoses. He found that the esophagus not only stretched after each excision, but that a certain amount of tissue growth apparently took place so that the normal thickness and texture of the esophagus were restored. There was, however, a limit above which regeneration did not take place. Relating this experiment to stretching of the skin may not be valid, however, because of the anatomic differences of these two structures. Undoubtedly, the esophagus "gives" more easily because of its muscularis layer.

As the skin increases in age, its capacity to extend or stretch decreases. This same decrease in elasticity is observed in the presence of edema or obesity. It is well known that the skin of the younger patient will withstand repeated stretching with less effect than will that of the elderly or aged patient. This is probably true because the elastic fiber meshwork is more highly developed in the young and the collagen fibers are in a more active state of metabolism, so they are more easily able to adapt themselves to repeated stretch loads. More stretching is therefore needed in youthful skin (when stretching is desired) to overcome the natural resiliency of the elastic fibers or to cause perpendicular reorientation of the collagen bundles. An example of this is in the well known technique of serial excision of benign lesions such as hemangiomas, hairy nevi, or wide scars in the young.

The multiple-stage excision technique was first described by Morestin, who, in 1915, used it to remove a large benign lesion. He proposed serial excisions for many types of lesions, including nevi, hemangiomas, and scar tissue, but he cautioned against such excisions if they would produce tension on vital cosmetic areas such as the eyelids or the commissures of the mouth. In his early experimentations with this technique, he advised repetition of the serial excision every three to four days. However, in subsequent publications (1916), he allowed at least a month's interval between operations. Morestin's excisions were not accompanied by undermining or undercutting of the flaps, which was later recommended by Smith (1946, 1950, 1958), who was a strong advocate of the staged excision technique for the ablation of facial lesions.

The multiple-stage principle is applicable to both children and adults. However, it is noted that with repeated undercutting and stretching of the skin in adults, such as also occurs after several face lifts, the skin does seem to lose its natural elastic properties and can at times assume an unnatural appearance. This can result in a "mask look," which is considered most undesirable by both patient and surgeon. This most often occurs in patients who have repeated face lift operations at too frequent intervals. Such patients often travel from surgeon to surgeon until they find one who will accommodate their desires. It rarely occurs after judicious surgery, properly timed by a competent surgeon who varies his operative technique at each operation to meet the demands at that time.

Secondary operation is usually technically easier to perform than the first. The original incisions are used, sometimes with added innovations such as the horizontal temporal hairline incision or variations in the postauricular hairline incision. Such variations allow for changes in the direction of pull that may be required to correct secondary jowls or progressive loosening of the skin of the neck. All scar tissue at the previous incision site is excised. However, this should not be done until the undermining is completed, as it is frequently astonishing just how little skin margin can also be excised. In fact, the surgeon is usually surprised to find that despite extensive undermining of the skin, an unexpectedly small amount of tissue can be resected in secondary operations. Often, it is possible to excise no more than the previous scar itself. The improvement in results at secondary surgery is, therefore, probably more likely the result of redistribution of skin and whatever physical changes occur from undermining than from actual excision of excess skin, for, as just noted, there often is little or no excess. This may well be the result of the loss of the ability of the skin to stretch following previous surgery, which is probably related to the natural atrophy of the elastic fibers that occurs with age, dehydration of the skin (also a phenomenon of aging), and application of tension to the skin, which has caused a realignment of collagen fibers perpendicular to the direction of pull.

The undermining should proceed from the clearly visible scar plane left over from the primary surgery and should extend beyond the edge of this plane anteriorly over the jaw well into the neck. It is more often necessary in secondary than in primary surgery to undermine completely across the midline of the neck and to join up with the undermining of the opposite side. Contrary to what occurs in scar tissue planes elsewhere, as in the peritoneal cavity, bleeding from face lift scar planes is usually minimal or greatly reduced at secondary rhytidectomy. This significantly diminishes the operative time.

Secondary surgery may change the hairline by raising it or drawing the temporal hairline farther back. The patient should be advised of this, although it is rarely a significant problem.

Secondary facial surgery is frequently accompanied by submental incisions with excision of skin and fat as required, along with adjustments of the platysma muscle — which, like the skin with which it is intimately associated, loses much of its tone with increasing years. Platysma surgery is indicated more and more often with advancing age. The medial borders of this muscle in particular become more prominent as time passes, contributing to the "turkey gobbler" deformity so typical in later life. Resection of the medial border is frequently helpful in secondary rhytidectomy, but it should always be done in conjunction with reinforcement of the muscle in the midline beneath the chin by using sutures to "buttress" and strengthen the muscle sling. Transection of the muscle across its expanse in a horizontal direction, either partial or complete, is done, with the formation of muscle flaps as described elsewhere in this volume. In the secondary operation, it depends on the problem at hand.

The recovery period from secondary face lifting is also usually shorter than with the first, and the incidence of skin slough is less. The primary operation acts as a "delay."

REFERENCES

Adamson, J. E., Horton, C. E., and Crawford, H. H.: The surgical correction of "turkey gobbler" deformity. Plast. Reconstr. Surg. 34:598, 1964.

Alibert, J. L.: Monographie des Dermatoses ou Précis Théorique et Pratique des Maladies de la Peau. Paris, Daynac, 1832, p. 795.

Aufricht, G.: Surgery for excess skin of the face and neck. Transactions of the 2nd Congress of the International Society of Plastic Surgeons, edited by Wallace. Baltimore, Williams & Wilkins Co., 1960, pp. 495–502.

Baker, D. L., Aston, S. J., Guy, C. L., and Rees, T. D.: The male rhytidectomy. Plast. Reconstr. Surg. 4:514, 1977.

Baker, T. J.: Chemical face peeling and rhytidectomy. Plast. Reconstr. Surg. 29:199, 1962.

Baker, T. J., and Gordon, H. L.: Rhytidectomy in males. Plast. Reconstr. Surg. 44:219, 1969.

Baker, T. J., Gordon, H. L., and Mesienko, P.: Rhytidectomy, Plast. Reconstr. Surg. 59:24, 1977.

Bames, H.: Truth and fallacies of face peeling and face lifting . Med. J. & Rec. 126:86, 1927.

Bames, H.: Frown disfigurement and ptosis of the eyebrows. Plast. Reconstr. Surg. 19:337, 1957.

Barker, D. E.: Prevention of bleeding following a rhytidectomy. Plast. Reconstr. Surg. 54:651, 1974.

Barsky, A. J.: Plastic Surgery, Philadelphia, W. B. Saunders Company, 1938, p. 124.

Berner, R. E., Morian, W. D., and Noe, J. M.: Postoperative hypertension as an etiologic factor in hematoma after rhytidectomy, Plast. Reconstr. Surg. 57:314, 1976.

Bourguet, J.: La chirurgie esthétique de la face. Le Concours Médical, 1921, pp. 1657–1670.

Bourguet, J.: La chirurgie esthétique de l'oeil et des paupières. Monde Médical, 1929, pp. 725–731.

Castanares, S.: Forehead wrinkles, glabellar frown and ptosis of the eyebrows. Plast. Reconstr. Surg. *34*:406, 1964.

Castanares, S.; Facial nerve paralysis coincident with, or subsequent to, rhytidectomy, Plast. Reconstr. Surg. *54*:637, 1974.

Claoué, C.: Documents de Chirurgie Plastique et Esthétique. Compte Rendu des Séances de la Société Scientifique Francaise de Chirurgie Plastique et Esthétiques. Paris, Maloine, 1931, pp. 344–353.

Claoué, C.: La ridectomie cervico-faciale. Correction de la ptose cutanée cervico-faciale par accrochage parieto-temporo-occipital et résection cutanée. Acad. Nat. Méd. Bull. *109*:257, 1933.

Conley, J.: Face-lift Operation. Springfield, Ill., Charles C Thomas, Publisher, 1968.

Connell, B.: Cervical lift; Surgical correction of fat contour problems combined with full width platysma muscle flap. Aesth. Plast. Surg. *1*:355, 1978.

Connell, B. F.: Contouring the neck in rhytidectomy by lipectomy and a muscle sling. Plast. Reconstr. Surg. *61*:376, 1978.

Conway, H.: Factors underlying prolonged pain following rhytidectomy. Transactions of the 4th International Congress of Plastic and Reconstructive Surgery. Amsterdam, Excerpta Medica Foundation, 1969, pp. 1120–1122.

Conway, H.: The surgical face lift-rhytidectomy. Plast. Reconstr. Surg. *45*:124, 1970.

Correia, P. de C., and Zani, R.: Surgical anatomy of the facial nerve as related to ancillary operations in rhytidecomty. Plast. Reconstr. Surg. *52*:549, 1973.

Cox, H. T.: The cleavage lines of the skin. Br. J. Surg. *29*:234, 1941.

Cronin, T. D., and Biggs, T. M.: The T-Z-plasty for the male "turkey gobbler" neck. Plast. Reconstr. Surg. *47*:534, 1971.

Davis, A. D.: Obligations in the consideration of meloplasties. J. Int. Coll. Surg. *24*:568, 1955.

Dingman, R. O., and Grabb, W. C.: Surgical anatomy of the mandibular ramus of the facial nerve based on the dissection of 100 facial halves. Plast. Reconstr. Surg. *20*:266, 1962.

Dupuytren, G.: De l'oedéme chronique et des tumeurs enkystées des paupières. Lecons Orales de Clinique Chirurgicale. 2nd ed. Vol. III, pp. 377–378. Paris, Germer-Ballière, 1839.

Duverger, C., and Velter, E.: Thérapeutique Chirurgicale Ophthalmologique. Paris, Masson et Cie, 1926, p. 79.

Edgerton, M. T., Webb, W. L., Slaughter, R., and Meyer, E.: Surgical results and psychosocial changes following rhytidectomy. Plast. Reconstr. Surg. *33*:503, 1964.

Edwards, B. F.: Bilateral temporal neurotomy for frontalis hypermotility: Case report. Plast. Reconstr. Surg. *19*:341, 1957.

Elschnig, A.: Fetthernien, Sog. "Tränensacke" der Unterlieder. Klin. Mbl. Augenheilk. *84*:763, 1930.

Erich, J. B.: Surgical elimination of wrinkles, redundant skin and pouches about the eyelids. Proc. Mayo Clin. *36*:101, 1961.

Fomon, S.: Surgery of Injury and Plastic Repair. Baltimore, Williams & Wilkins Co., 1939, pp. 135–137.

Fomon, S.: Cosmetic Surgery, Principles and Practice. Philadelphia, J. B. Lippincott Company, 1960.

Fredericks, S.: The lower rhytidecomty. Plast. Reconstr. Surg. *54*:537, 1974.

Fry, P., Harkness, M. L., and Harkness, R. D.: Mechanical properties of the collagenous framework of skin in rats of different ages. Am. J. Physiol. *206*:1425, 1964.

Gibson, T., and Kenedi, R. M.: The significance and measurement of skin tensions in man. Transactions of the 3rd International Congress of Plastic Surgery. Amsterdam, Excerpta Medica Foundation, 1964, pp. 387–395.

Gibson, T., and Kenedi, R. M.: Biochemical properties of skin. Surg. Clin. North Amer. *47*:279, 1967.

Gibson, T., and Kenedi, R. M.: Factors affecting the mechanical characteristics of human skin. In Druphy, J. E., and Van Winkle, W., Jr. (eds): Repair and Regeneration. New York, McGraw-Hill Book Co., 1969, p. 87.

Gillies, H., and Millard, D. R.: Principles and Art of Plastic Surgery. Boston, Little, Brown and Company. 1957.

Ginester, G., Frézières, H., Dupuis, A., and Pons, J.: Chirurgie Plastique et Reconstructrice de la Face. Paris, Flammarison et Cie, 1967, pp. 184–187.

González-Ulloa, M.: Facial wrinkles. Plast. Reconstr. Surg. *29*:658, 1962.

González-Ulloa, M., and Stevens, E. F.: Senility of the face. Basic study to understand its causes and effects. Plast. Reconstr. Surg. *36*:239, 1965.

Gordon, H.: Rhytidectomy. Clin. Plast. Surg. *5*:97, 1978.

Graff, D.: Oertliche erbliche erschlaffung der Haut. Wschr. Ges. Heilk., 1836, pp. 225–227.

Grahame, R., and Holt, P. J.: The influence of aging on the in vivo elasticity of human skin. Gerontologia *15*:121, 1969.

Griffith, H.: The treatment of keloids with triamcinolone acetonide. Plast. Reconstr. Surg. *38*:202, 1966.

Geurrero-Santos, J.: Muscular lift in cervical rhytidoplasty. Plast. Reconstr. Surg. *54*:127, 1974.

Guerrero-Santos, J.: The role of the platysma muscle in rhytidoplasty. Clin. Plast. Surg. *5*:29, 1978.

Guerrero-Santos, J., Espaillat, L., and Morales, F.: Muscular lift in cervical rhytidoplasty. Plast. Reconstr. Surg. *54*:127, 1974.

Hamilton, J. M.: Rhytidectomy in the male. Plast. Reconstr. Surg. *53*:629, 1974.

Hoffman, S., and Simon, B. E.: Complications of submental lipectomy. Plast. Reconstr. Surg. *69*:889, 1977.

Hollander, M. M.: Rhytidectomy: Anatomical, physiological and surgical considerations. Plast. Reconstr. Surg. *20*:218, 1957.

Hunt, H. L.: Plastic Surgery of the Head, Face and Neck. Philadelphia, Lea & Febiger, 1926, p. 198.

Johnson, J. B., and Hadley, R. C.: The aging face. In Converse, J. M. (ed.): Reconstructive Plastic Surgery. Philadelphia, W. B. Saunders Company, 1964, pp. 1306–1342.

Joseph, J.: Plastic operation on protruding cheek. Dtsch. Med. Wochnschr. *47*:287, 1921.

Joseph, J.: Nasenplastik and Sonstige Gesichtsplastik nebst einen Anhang über Mammaplastik. Leipzig, Curt Kabitzsch, 1928, pp. 525–527.

Joseph, J.: Verbesserung meiner Hängemangenplastik (Melomioplastik). Dtsch. Med. Wochenschr. *54*:567, 1928.

Journal Universel et Hebdomadaire de Médecine et de Chirurgie Pratiques et des Institutions Médicales. Vol. 1–13, Oct. 1830–Dec. 1833.

Kapp, J. F. S.: Die Technik du Kosmetischen Enchieresen. Beih. Med. Klin. *3*:65, 1913.

Kapp, J. F. S.: Premature Old Age in Women; A Study in the Tragedy of the Middle Aged. New York, P. L. Baruch, 1925.

Kirk, J. E., and Chieffi, M.: Variation with age in elasticity of skin and subcutaneous tissue in human individuals. J. Gerontol. *17*:373, 1962.

Knorr, N. J., Edgerton, M. T., and Hoopes, J. E.: The "insatiable" cosmetic surgery patient. Plast. Reconstr. Surg. *40*:285, 1967.

Kolle, F. S.: Plastic and Cosmetic Surgery. New York, Appleton, 1911, pp. 116–117.

Kraissl, C. J., and Conway, H.: Excision of small tumors of skin and face. Surgery *25*:592, 1949.

Lagarde, M.: Nouvelles techniques pour le traitement des rides de la face et du cou. Arch. Franco-Belg. Chir. *31*:154, 1928.

Leist, F., Macksson, J., and Erich, J. B.: A review of 324 rhytidectomies emphasizing complications and patient dissatisfaction. Plast. Reconstr. Surg. *59*:525, 1977.

Lemon, M., and Hamra, S.: Evaluation of the Skoog subplatysmal dissection. Paper presented at the annual meeting of the American Society of Aesthetic Plastic Surgery, San Francisco, May, 1978.

Lewis, G. K.: Surgical treatment of wrinkles. Arch. Otolaryngol. *60*:334, 1954.

Lexer, E.: Zur Gesichtsplastik. Arch. Klin. Chir. 92:749, 1910.

Lindgren, V. V., and Carlin, G. A.: Preventing a pulled-down or deformed earlobe in rhytidectomies. Plast. Reconstr. Surg. 51:598, 1973.

Litton, C.: Chemical face lifting. Plast. Reconstr. Surg. 29:371, 1962.

Loeb, R.: Technique for preservation of the temporal branches of the facial nerve during face-lift operations, Br. J. Plast. Surg. 23:390, 1970.

Macgregor, F. C.: Some psychological hazards of plastic surgery of the face. Plast. Reconstr. Surg. 12:123, 1953.

Macgregor, F. C.: Selection of cosmetic surgery patients; Social and psychological considerations. Surg. Clin. North Am. 51:289, 1970.

Macgregor, F. C., and Schaffner, B.: Screening patients for nasal plastic operations: Sociologic and psychiatric considerations. Psychosom. Med. 12:277, 1950.

MacGregor, M. W., and Greenberg, R. L.: Rhytidectomy. In Goldwyn, R. M. (ed.): The Unfavorable Result in Plastic Surgery. Boston, Little, Brown & Co., 1972.

Maliniac, J. W.: Is the surgical restoration of the aging face justified? Med. J. & Rec. 135:321, 1932.

Marino, H.: Frontal rhytidectomy. Bol. Soc. Cirug. B. Aires 47:93, 1963.

Marino, H., Galeano, E. J., and Gandolfo, E. A.: Plastic correction of double chin. Plast. Reconstr. Surg. 31:45, 1963.

May, H.: Reconstructive and Reparative Surgery. Philadelphia, F. A. Davis Co., 1947, pp. 325–326.

Mayer, D. M., and Swanker, W. A.: Rhytidoplasty. Plast. Reconstr. Surg. 6:255, 1950.

McDowell, A. J.: Effective practical steps to avoid complications in face lifting. Plast. Reconstr. Surg. 50:563, 1972.

Millard, D. R., Jr., Garst, W. P., and Beck, R. L.: Submental and submandibular lipectomy in conjunction with a face lift, in the male or female. Plast. Reconstr. Surg. 49:385, 1972.

Millard, D. R., Pigott, R. W., and Hedo, A.: Submandibular lipectomy. Plast. Reconstr. Surg. 41:513, 1968.

Miller, C. C.: Semilunar excision of the skin at the outer canthus for the eradication of crow's feet. Am. J. Dermatol. 11:483, 1907a.

Miller, C. C.: Subcutaneous section of local muscles to eradicate expression lines. Am. J. Surg. 21:235, 1907b.

Miller, C. C.: The eradication by surgical means of the nasolabial line. Therap. Gaz. 23:676, 1907c.

Miller C. C.: Cosmetic Surgery. The Correction of Featural Imperfections. Chicago, Oak Printing Co., 1908, pp. 40–42.

Miller, C. C.: Cosmetic Surgery. Philadelphia, F. A. Davis Co., 1924, pp. 30–32.

Miller, C. C.: Facial bands as supports to relaxed facial tissue. Ann. Surg. 82:603, 1925.

Miller, G. D., Anstee, E. J., and Snell, J. A.: Successful replantation of an avulsed scalp by microvascular anastomoses. Plast. Reconstr. Surg. 58:133, 1976.

Mitz, V., and Peyronie, M: The superficial musculoaponeurotic system (SMAS) in the parotid and cheek area. Plast. Reconstr. Surg. 58:80, 1976.

Montandon, D.: Quelques aspects des techniques du traitement chirurgical de l'astéside de l'oesophage. Thèse No. 3079, Geneva, Editions Médecine et Hygiène, 1967.

Montandon, D.: Personal communication, 1970.

Morel-Fatio, D.: Cosmetic surgery of the face. In Gibson, T. (ed.): Modern Trends in Plastic Surgery. London, Butterworth & Co., Ltd., 1964, pp. 221–222.

Morestin, H.: La réduction graduelle des déformités tégumentaires. Bull. Mém. Soc. Chir. Paris 41:1233, 1915.

Morestin, H.: Cicatrice trés étendue du crâne réduite par des excisions successives. Bull. Mém. Soc. Chir. Paris 42:2052, 1916.

Myers, M. B.: Wound tension and vascularity in the etiology and prevention of skin sloughs. Surgery 56:945, 1964.

Noël, A.: La Chirurgie Esthétique. Son Role Social. Paris, Masson et Cie, 1926, pp. 62–66.

Noël, A.: La Chirurgie Esthétique. Clermont (Oise), Thiron et Cie, 1928.

Owsley, J. Q.: Platysma-fascial rhytidectomy. Plast. Reconstr. Surg. 59:843, 1977.

Padgett E. C., and Stevenson, K. C.: Plastic and Reconstructive Surgery. Springfield, Ill., Charles C Thomas, Publisher, 1948, p.514.

Pangman, W. J., II, and Wallace, R. M.: Cosmetic surgery of the face and neck. Plast. Reconstr. Surg. 27:544, 1961.

Panneton, P.: Mémoire sur le blepharochalazis. 51 cas dans la mete famille. Un. Med. Canada 65:725, 1936b.

Parot, S., and Bourlière. F.: Une nouvelle technique de mesure de la compressibilité de la peau et du tissu sous-cutane. Influence du sexe, de l'âge et du site de mesure sur les résultats. Gerontologia 13:95, 1967.

Passot, R.: La chirurgie esthétique des rides du visage. Presse Méd. 27:258, 1919

Passot, R.: La Chirurgie Esthétique Pure (Technique et Résultats). Paris, Gaston Doin et Cie, 1931, pp. 176–180.

Peterson, R.: Cervical Rhytidoplasty Presented at the Aesthetic Society Symposia on The Aging Face, Denver, October 1976.

Peterson, R. A.: Cervical Rhytidoplasty—A personal approach. From presentations given at the Annual Symposium of Aesthetic Plastic Surgery, Guadalajara, 1974.

Pitanguy, I.: Personal communication, 1970.

Pitanguy, I., Pinto, A. R., Garcia, L. C., and Lessa. S. F.: Ritodoplastia em homens. Rev. Bras. Cir. 63:209, 1973.

Pitanguy, I., and Ramos, A. S.: The frontal branch of the facial nerve: The importance of its variations in face lifting. Plast. Reconstr. Surg. 38:352, 1966.

Rees, T. D.: Rhytidectomy: some observations on variations in technique. In Masters, F. W., and Lewis, J. R. (eds.): Symposium on Aesthetic Surgery of the Face, Eyelid, and Breast. St. Louis, C. V. Mosby Co., 1972, p. 37.

Rees, T. D., and Wood-Smith, D.: Cosmetic Facial Surgery. Philadelphia, W. B. Saunders Company, 1973.

Rees, T. D.: Question, Is there a place for the staple gun in plastic surgery? Ann. Plast. Surg. 1:2, 1978.

Rees, T. D., and Aston, S. J.: Clinical evaluation of submuculoaponeurotic dissection (Skoog) in face lift surgery Plast. Reconstr. Surg. 6:851, 1977.

Rees, T. D., and Aston, S. J.: Complications of rhytidectomy. Clin. Plast. Surg. 5:1, 1978.

Rees, T. D., Lee, Y. C., and Coburn, R. J.: Expanding hematoma after rhytidectomy. Plast. Reconstr. Surg. 51:149, 1973.

Ridge, M. D., and Wright, V.: The rheology of skin: A bioengineering study of the mechanical properties of human skin in relation to its structure. Br. J. Dermatol. 77:639, 1965.

Robertson, J. G.: Chin augmentation by means of rotation of double chin fat flap. Plast. Reconstr. Surg. 36:471, 1965.

Rollhäuser, H.: Die Zugfestigheit der menschlichen Haut. Gegenbaur. Morph. Jahrb. 90:249, 1950.

Sheehan, J. E.: In McIndoe, A. H.: Personal communication, 1955.

Skoog, T.: Rhytidectomy—A personal experience and technique. Presented and demonstrated on live television at the Seventh Annual Symposium on Cosmetic Surgery at Cedars of Lebanon Hospital, Miami, Florida, February 1973.

Skoog, T.: Plastic Surgery—New Methods and Refinements. Philadelphia, W. B. Saunders Company, 1974.

Smith, F.: Multiple excision and Z-plasties in surface reconstruction. Plast. Reconstr. Surg. 1:170, 1946.

Smith, F.: Plastic and Reconstructive Surgery. Philadelphia, W. B. Saunders Company, 1950.

Smith, F.: Multiple excision with occasional Z-plasty for correction of disabilities of exposed surfaces. Am. J. Surg. 95:173, 1958.

Spira, M., Gerow, F. J., and Hardy, S. B.: Cervicofacial rhytidectomy. Plast. Reconstr. Surg. 40:551, 1967.

Stark, R. B.: Plastic Surgery. New York, Paul B. Hoeber, 1962, p. 229.

Stark, R. B.: Follow-up clinic on deliberate hypotension for blepharoplasty and rhytidectomy Plast. Reconstr. Surg. 49:453, 1972.

Stark, R. B.: A rhytidectomy series. Plast. Reconstr. Surg. *59*:373, 1977.

Stephenson, K. L.: The "mini-lift," an old wrinkle in face lifting. Plast. Reconst. Surg. *46*:226, 1970.

Straith, R. E., Raju, D., and Hipps, C.: The study of hematomas in 500 consecutive face lifts. Plast. Reconstr. Surg. *59*:694, 1977.

Thompson, D. P., and Ashley, F. L.: Face-lift complications. Plast. Reconstr. Surg. *61*:40, 1978.

Tipton, J. B.: Should the subcutaneous tissue be plicated in a face lift? Plast. Reconstr. Surg. *54*:1, 1974.

Tregear, R. T.: Physical Functions of Skin. New York, Academic Press, Inc., 1966.

Uchida, J. I.: A method of frontal rhytidectomy. Plast. Reconstr. Surg. *35*:218, 1965.

Vogt, A.: Die senile determination des Keimplasmas, bedbachtet an eineigen Zwillinges des 55–81 jahres. Schweiz. Med. Wschr. *16*:576, 1935.

Webster, G. V.: The ischemic face lift. Plast Reconstr. Surg. *50*:560, 1972.

Part 5

ASSOCIATED
PROCEDURES

Chapter 26

Forehead and Brow

BERNARD L. KAYE, M.D., F.A.C.S.

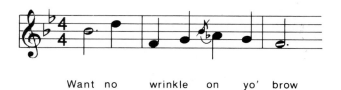

Want no   wrinkle   on   yo' brow

GEORGE GERSHWIN, DUBOSE HAYWARD, AND IRA GERSHWIN
"Bess, You Is My Woman Now"
Porgy and Bess*

HISTORY

The usual facial rhytidectomy is thought of as a procedure designed to rejuvenate the lower two thirds of the face and the neck. Although the upper third of the face may be more resistant to aging than the lower two thirds (Fredricks, 1971), it is not immune to the ravages of time and gravity. Both clinically and in the plastic surgical literature, good results have been observed from rhytidectomy in the lower two thirds of the face and neck without improvement in the upper third. Many times the untreated upper third, in contrast, may give the patient a sad, tired, or angry look (Connell, 1978; Ortiz-Monasterio, Barrera, and Olmedo, 1978).

The forehead lift is not a new concept in surgery for the aging face. Lexer discussed it in 1910, Hunt described a coronal skin resection in 1926, and Joseph described forehead excisions both within and anterior to the frontal hairline in 1931. In the same year, Passot described excision of skin posterior to the hairline for correction of forehead wrinkles, adding denervation of the temporal branch of the facial nerve to the procedure in 1933. A temporal nerve neurotomy was described again 14 years later in a case report by Edwards (1957). In the same year, Bames described a direct eyebrow lift in which he excised the corrugators, undermined up to the hairline, and bluntly crosshatched the frontalis.

In 1961, Pangman and Wallace described a forehead lift employing an incision either along the hairline or 1 cm posterior to the hairline for treatment of deep forehead lines and lowered eyebrows. In 1962, González-Ulloa described a complete forehead lift as part of his extended face lift procedure.

The coronal forehead lift lost favor because its results were thought to be temporary (Castanares, 1964; Johnson, 1964; Marino, 1971; Rees and Wood-Smith, 1973). Earlier forehead lifts involved excision of portions of forehead or scalp skin and underlying tissue, with or without undermining, but *without interrupting the action of the frontalis muscle.*

The importance of interrupting the frontalis muscle was recognized by a number of authors, and various methods were described to accomplish this. Bames (1957) bluntly crosshatched the frontalis through a superciliary excision. Others incised the frontalis (Eitner, 1935; González-Ulloa, 1974; Regnault, 1972). Uchida (1965) described a technique for isolation of the frontalis and reinsertion of its lower cut edge to a lower level on the forehead. Partial excision of the frontalis has been advocated by Griffiths (1974), Hinderer (1974), Marino (1964, 1971), Skoog (1974), and Viñas, Caviglia, and Cortinas, (1976). Viñas et al. stated that excision of a strip of frontalis muscle eliminated the dynamic factor that caused formation of the horizontal wrinkles and also permitted more stretching of the superficial layers of skin and subcutaneous tissue. Washio (1975) studied the transverse septa between frontalis and skin in cadaver foreheads. He concluded that it was necessary to remove a transverse segment of muscle, including some fibrous septa, in order to allow significant passive elevation of the forehead. Tessier (1968) and LeRoux and Jones (1974) advocated complete removal of the frontalis muscle. The author agrees with Marino, Viñas et al., and others about the necessity of interrupting the vertical pull of the frontalis muscle in order to produce a forehead rhytidectomy with lasting results.

The author occasionally uses the forehead lift as an isolated procedure, but more often it is combined with blepharoplasty and/or rhytidectomy. When used as an adjunct to these procedures, it does not add much additional operating time. The results have been pleasing and lasting, and complications have been few and minor.

INDICATIONS FOR FOREHEAD LIFT

The primary indication for a forehead lift is ptosis of the forehead and eyebrows, with concomitant ptosis of the upper lids, especially in their lateral portions. Frequently, such patients present themselves for upper lid blepharoplasty, thinking their problem is entirely due to excess upper lid skin (Figure 26–1). Clinical evaluation will readily demonstrate that any attempt to remove all the apparent excess eyelid skin surgically would attach the eyelids close to the eyebrows and would require long lateral extensions of the incisions to eliminate dogears and reduce lateral upper lid fullness. Such incisions would extend considerably beyond the border of the lateral orbital rim, a situation that is best avoided (Pitanguy, 1978). If, during initial evaluation, the surgeon manually raises the patient's forehead and eyebrows to a normal level in relation to the superior orbital rim, the excess eyelid fullness that is due to eyebrow and forehead ptosis becomes immediately obvious, and the apparent excess of upper eyelid skin is reduced considerably. Sometimes, this maneuver will reveal that a forehead lift will be sufficient to accomplish the desired objectives without performing an upper lid blepharoplasty (Kaye, 1977; Ortiz-Monasterio, Barrera, and Olmedo, 1978).

Some patients come to the plastic surgeon with complaints of drooping of their upper eyelid skin to the point of interference with upper visual fields, plus eyelid fatigue owing to the eyelid skin resting on the upper eyelashes. Most of these patients are found to have a significant degree of forehead and brow ptosis that contributes to their disability (Fig. 26–2). Upper lid blepharoplasty alone is considered to be insufficient to correct this problem, and in most of these cases, a forehead lift is also indicated.

In younger patients, apparent upper lid ptosis may actually be due to congenitally low position of the forehead and eyebrows, sometimes giving them a sad or frowning look. Correction of this condition can usually be obtained from a forehead lift alone without upper lid blepharoplasty (Fig. 26–3). The surgeon can determine this preoperatively by manually elevating the forehead and eyebrows and seeing what this does for the eyelid ptosis.

Secondary indications for forehead lift include (1) transverse forehead wrinkles, (2) vertical glabellar frown lines, (3) transverse wrinkles at the root of the nose (exaggerated when the forehead is manually drawn inferiorly), and (4) a drooping nose. (Since the soft tissue covering of the nose is suspended from the forehead, it is reasonable to postulate that at least some of the nasal droop associated with aging may be associated with ptosis of the forehead. On the other hand, an extensive amount of nasal droop would also require a rhinoplasty for its correction.)

PREOPERATIVE PREPARATION

Preoperative preparation is the same as that for a face lift. To avoid bleeding problems associated with aspirin, patients are instructed to avoid aspirin and aspirin-containing compounds* for four weeks prior to surgery. Because of the large number of aspirin-containing compounds available, we find it simpler to limit patients to acetaminophen-containing medications only (e.g.,

Text continued on page 736.

---

*A partial list of aspirin-containing compounds includes:

Alka Seltzer	Fiorinal
Anacin	Dristan
Ascriptin	Empirin
BC	Excedrin
Bufferin	Midol
Cheracol Capsules	Sine-Aid
Cope	Sine-Off
Coricidin	Percodan
Darvon Compound	Stendin
Vanquish	Triaminicin

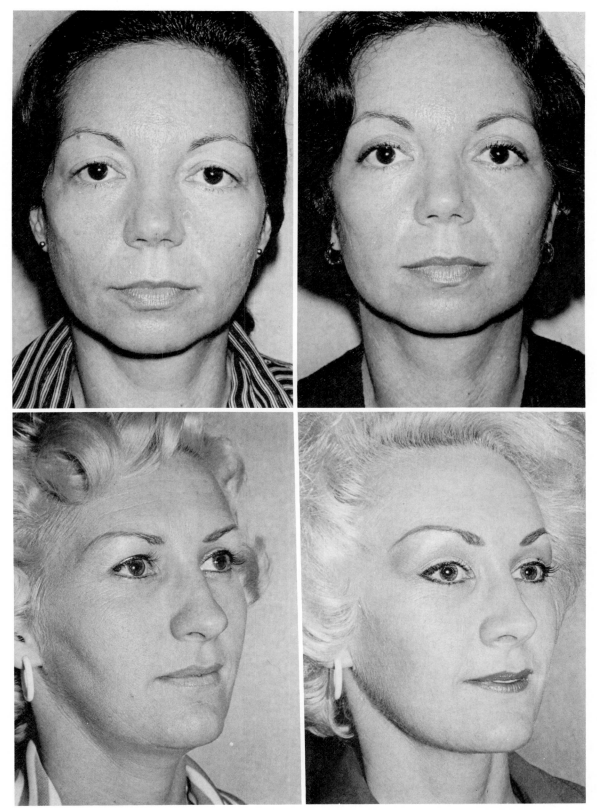

Figure 26–1. Patients presenting with upper lid fullness. *Above:* Result with combined forehead lift and upper lid blepharoplasty. *Below:* Result with forehead lift without blepharoplasty. Patient also had rhinoplasty and face lift.

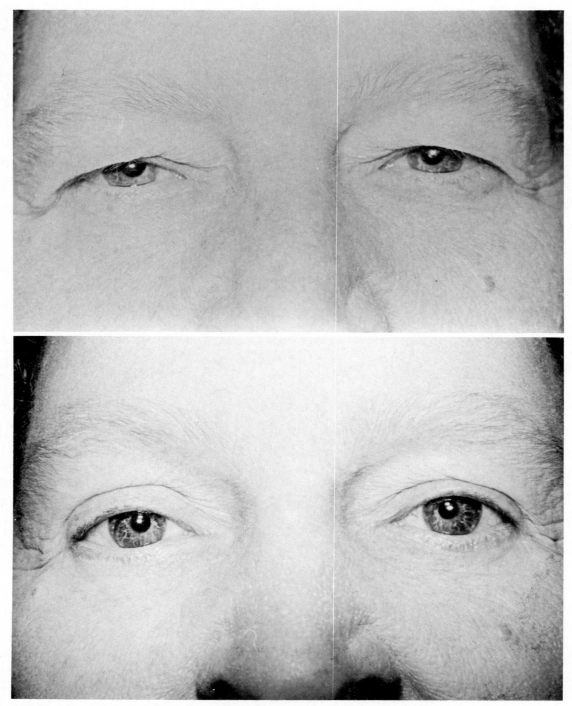

Figure 26–2. *Above:* Limitation of upper visual fields due to severe ptosis of upper lids and brows. *Below:* Correction by combined forehead lift and upper lid blepharoplasty. Blepharoplasty alone would have been insufficient to correct deformity.

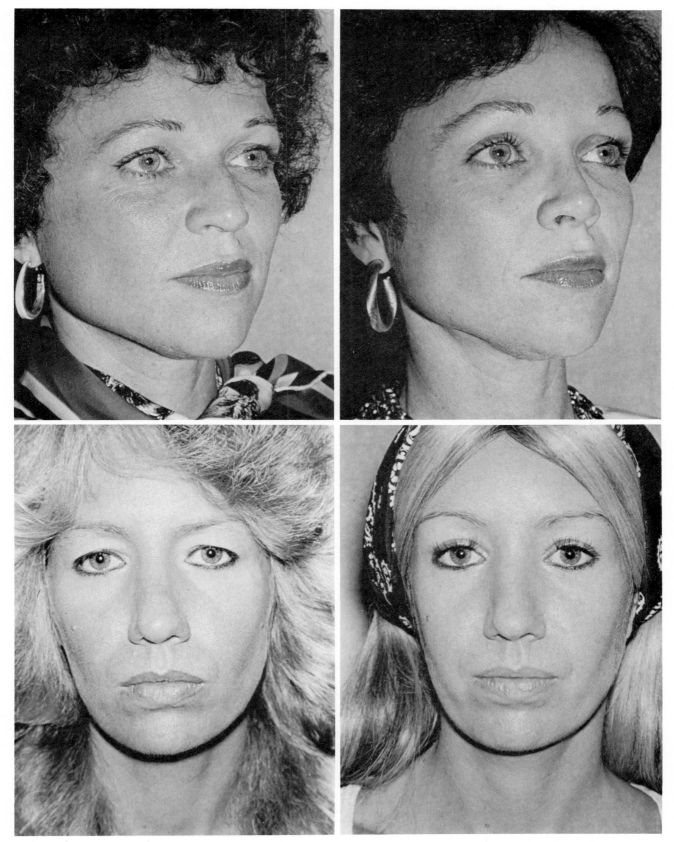

Figure 26–3. Younger patients with congenitally low foreheads and brows, improved with forehead lifts without upper lid blepharoplasties. Patient above also had rhinoplasty.

Tylenol). Vitamin E preparations are empirically discontinued for two weeks prior to surgery because of suspicion that this compound may also interfere with blood coagulation (Vinnick, 1977). The author avoids scheduling surgery during the interval from five days prior to a menstrual period to five days afterward because of increased bleeding believed to occur during this time.

Patients are instructed to shampoo their hair with pHisoHex for ten minutes the evening before surgery. The author favors the use of "preventive" antibiotics and starts patients on antibiotics the evening prior to surgery. Hair is prepared prior to surgery. Hair anterior to the planned incision is tied with rubber bands. Although many surgeons do not cut any hair, some prefer to clip a pathway along the course of the proposed incision approximately 1.5 to 2 cm in width. Since most or all of this clipped strip is removed during the operation, patients who are apprehensive about having some hair cut can be assured that they will have hair abutting hair at the completion of the procedure.

SURGICAL TECHNIQUE

The operation can be carried out under local or general anesthesia. In either case, local anesthetic solution (Xylocaine, 0.5 percent with epinephrine 1:200,000) is infiltrated across the lower forehead at the level of the eyebrows, blocking the supraorbital and supratrochlear nerves plus any additional branches that course superiorly. The proposed incision line is also infiltrated superficial to the galea for anesthesia as well as additional hemostasis.

The incision begins at the root of the helix of the ear and extends superiorly and slightly posteriorly (Figure 26–4). The incision then turns medially, paralleling the frontal hair line to meet a similar incision from the opposite side. A gull wing incision is thereby created anteriorly, which allows for more precise adjustment of the elevation levels of various portions of the brows and obviates the need for a central wedge excision. The author tries to place the central portion of the incision sufficiently far behind the frontal hairline so that the resulting scar will be at least 3 to 4 cm posterior to the hairline. If the forehead lift is to be done together with a face lift, the preauricular face lift incision is made continuous with the forehead lift incision.

To reduce bleeding, the incision is made in segments, with the surgeon's and assistant's fingers compressing the skin on either side of the incision. The incision, beveled to parallel the hair follicles

in order to avoid injury to them, is carried down through the galea to the skull periosteum centrally and to (but not through) the temporalis fascia laterally. The anterior edge, which will be excised, is clamped with a series of Raney clips for hemostasis. Bleeding from the posterior edge is controlled by clamping curved hemostats (or Dandy clamps) to the cut edge of the galea and letting them hang downward.

The forehead flap can be elevated by very rapid scissor dissection in the areolar and almost bloodless subgaleal plane immediately above the periosteum (Figure 26–5). Subperiosteal dissection appears to offer no advantages and could have some theoretical disadvantages such as denuding the frontal bone of part of its blood supply and the possibility of creating adhesions between the flap and underlying bone (Marino, 1977). Moreover, it is easy to slip inadvertently below the periosteum with overly vigorous blunt dissection as one nears the supraorbital ridges.

The eyes are protected with a sponge as the forehead flap is reflected downward. Lateral to the supraorbital neurovascular bundles, the flap is elevated to the supraorbital ridges by sharp dissection. The author sees no need to enter the orbital cavities. Also, as long as the dissection is kept immediately superficial to the periosteum and in the natural areolar plane, there is no danger of injury to the temporal branches of the facial nerve. In order to allow for more elevation of the brows laterally, the author deliberately incises the periosteum over the supraorbital ridges lateral to the supraorbital neurovascular bundles (Figure 26–6).

Gentle, blunt dissection with a "peanut" dissector readily exposes the supraorbital neurovascular bundles, the corrugators, and the root of the nose (Figure 26–7). If indicated for nasal droop, the undermining may include the entire nasal covering down to the nasal spine (González-Ulloa, 1962; Kaye, 1977; Pitanguy, 1978) (Figure 26–8). Laterally, the dissection is carried down over the temporalis fascia, almost to the level of the zygomatic arches.

The corrugator supercilii muscles are separated from the supraorbital neurovascular bundles, and approximately 0.5 cm of muscle is excised from each bony origin. The stumps are electrocoagulated. (The author has not encountered any postoperative skin depressions from this excision.)

A transverse strip of frontalis muscle, approximately 1 cm in width, is excised from beneath the flap extending to but not beneath the hair-bearing portions of the temporal scalp (Figure 26–9). The author prefers to excise this strip in three separate

Text continued on page 741.

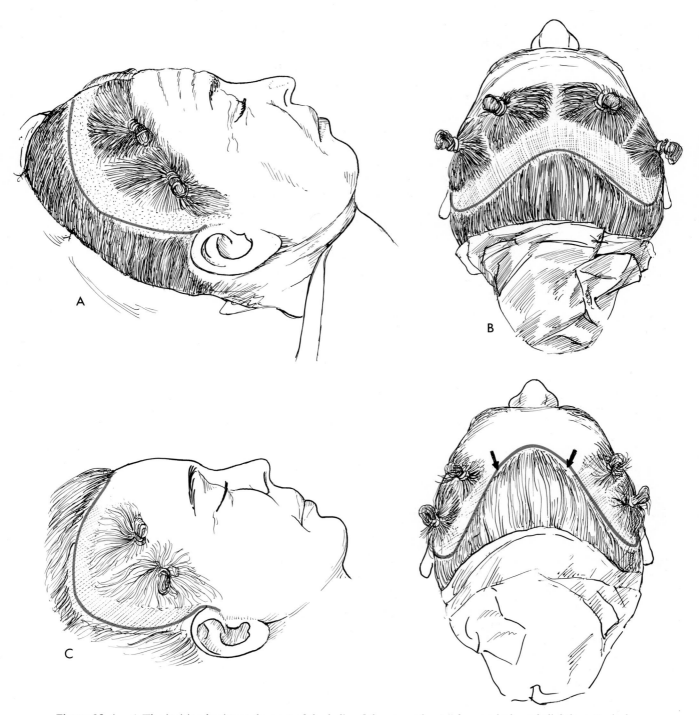

Figure 26-4.   *A,* The incision begins at the root of the helix of the ear and extends superiorly and slightly posteriorly.

B, The incision turns medially, paralleling the frontal hairline to meet a similar incision from the opposite side. A gull wing incision is thereby created anteriorly, which allows for more precise adjustment of the elevation levels of various portions of the brows and obviates the need for a central wedge excision. The resulting scar of the coronal incision lies at least 3 to 4 cm posterior to the hairline.

C, An alternative design of the incision to be considered in a limited number of patients who have a high hairline to begin with and who are willing to accept the scar at the hairline.

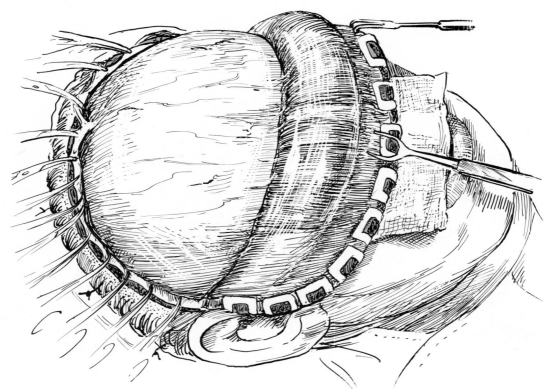

Figure 26–5.   The forehead flap is turned down after having been dissected in the areolar, supraperiosteal plane. Bleeding has been controlled by application of Raney clips to the anterior cut edge of the flap and by grasping the posterior cut edge of the galea with hemostats, which are allowed to hang downward.

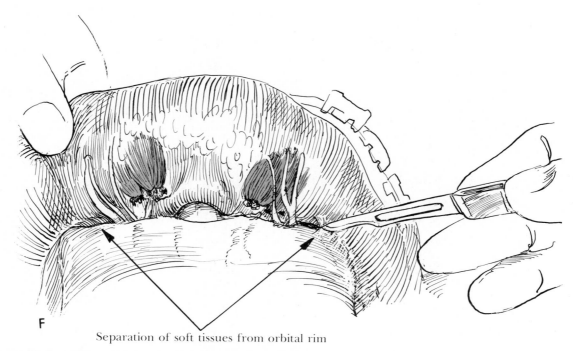

F

Separation of soft tissues from orbital rim

Figure 26–6.   Incision of the periosteum over the supraorbital ridges to allow for more elevation of the brows laterally. (If the supraorbital ridges are excessively prominent, they may be reduced conservatively at this point with an osteotome or rasp or both.)

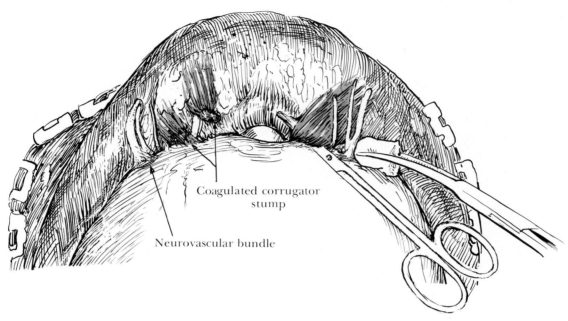

Figure 26–7. The neurovascular bundles, corrugator muscles, and root of the nose are best dissected bluntly with a "peanut" dissector. Scissors indicate the separation of the origin of the right corrugator from the right supratrochlear neurovascular bundle.

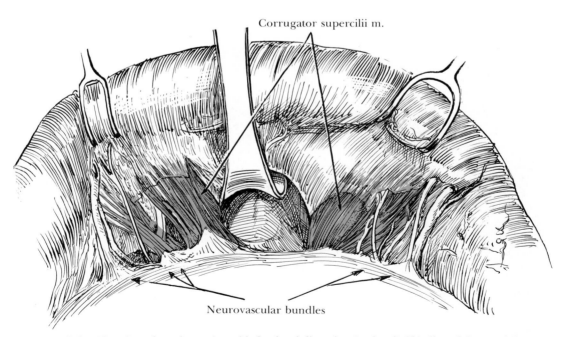

Figure 26–8. Elevation of nasal covering with forehead dissection (optional), if indicated for nasal droop.

Markings for muscle excision

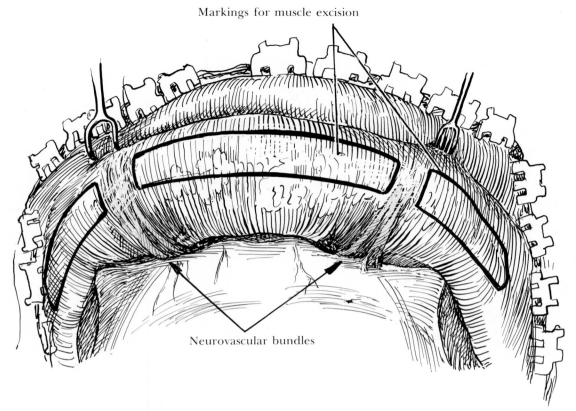

Neurovascular bundles

Figure 26–9.   Transverse strips of frontalis muscle to be excised, marked in three separate segments, with intact bridges over the courses of the supraorbital nerves, to avoid injury to the nerves. Laterally, the lower borders of the strip excisions should be at least 3 cm superior to the supraorbital ridges to avoid possible injury to the frontal branches of the facial nerves.

Frontalis m.

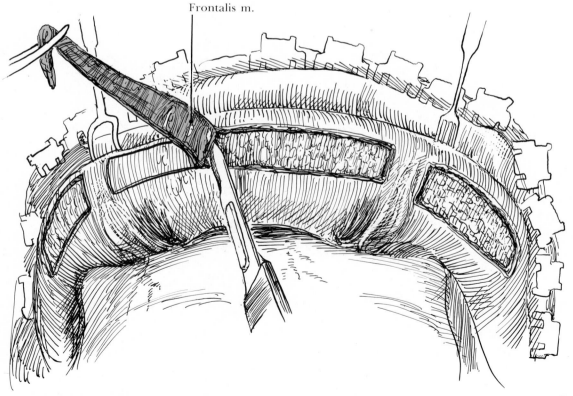

Figure 26–10.   Excision of strips of frontalis muscle, leaving intact bridges over the courses of the supraorbital nerves and avoiding injury to larger vessels wherever possible.

segments, leaving a small bridge of muscle intact over the course of the supraorbital nerves, in order to avoid injury to them (Figure 26–10). Laterally, the lower border of the strip excision should be at least 3 cm superior to the supraorbital ridges in order to avoid possible injury to the frontal branches of the facial nerves. Also, during excision of this strip, it is prudent to avoid injury to underlying blood vessels in the flap as much as possible (Ortiz-Monasterio et al., 1978). In most patients, the frontalis muscle is quite thin and contributes relatively little to the thickness of the forehead flap. Recently, there has been renewed interest in merely interrupting muscle fibers by transverse incisions (Marino, 1977) or cross hatching (Pitanguy, 1978).

If the forehead lift is done as an independent procedure, it can be trimmed and sutured at this point. If it is being done together with a face lift, the author prefers simply to clip the edges together with a towel clip while proceeding with the incising and undermining for the face lift operation.

For the rhytidectomy, the face is undermined in the usual superficial plane, with or without separate treatment of the superficial musculoaponeurotic systems (SMAS) (Mitz and Peyronie, 1976; Owsley, 1977). The forehead flap has been elevated in a deep, subgaleal, and submuscular plane. The two planes are reconciled by creating a musculoaponeurotic pedicle or web ("mesotemporalis") (Marino, 1971), containing the frontal branches of the facial nerve medially and the superficial temporal vessels at its lateral border (Figure 26–11, top).

So as not to injure the motor nerve branches, avoid knives or scissors and use blunt dissection medially in the region over which the nerves are located. Nerves have more tensile strength than does connective tissue, and therefore they can tolerate gentle blunt dissection better than sharp dissection. The author uses a finger wrapped in two single layers of gauze, gently peeling the pedicle away from the overlying skin and subcutaneous tissue (see Figure 26–11) or pressing down on the pedicle while gently lifting the overlying tissues off it. Occasionally, a hole is inadvertently poked in the thin pedicle, but no injury to the frontal branches of the facial nerve results, presumably because the nerve filaments are merely pushed aside rather than divided, an indication of their relative strength compared with the connective tissue they lie in.

Despite the creation of this pedicle, the forehead flap may be tethered down by the superficial temporal vessels located at its lateral edge. To gain more upward mobility of the forehead flap, the author usually ligates the superficial temporal vessels and transects the lateral portion of the pedicle for a distance of 1 to 2 cm near its most superior point, where it attaches to the forehead flap, to avoid possible injury to the frontal branches of the facial nerve (Figure 26–12). There is no significant circulatory compromise from doing this, and the brisk bleeding that results when the forehead flap is trimmed later is evidence of its excellent blood supply.

At this point, the forehead flap is trimmed and sutured. This is done in small segments to reduce bleeding. Trimming is begun with a series of segmental, perpendicular "pilot" incisions and sutures, starting in the midline and continuing laterally in each direction at selected key points 3 or 4 cm apart (Figure 26–13). The D'Assumpçao rhytidectomy instrument* (D'Assumpçao, 1970) is very helpful in making these pilot incisions. The most important precaution at this point is to avoid excess tension. If, after making a pilot incision and inserting a pilot suture, the flap anterior to it blanches, it is best to back off a few millimeters, partially close the pilot cut, and replace the pilot suture.

The scalp strips are then trimmed segmentally, beveling the incisions in the direction of the hair follicles. Scalp strips are rarely excised wider than 2.5 cm; most are 1 to 1.5 cm in width. Each trimmed segment is rapidly sutured with continuous, through-and-through 3-0 monofilament Prolene to minimize bleeding from the cut edge. Adjacent segments are trimmed and sutured individually until the entire forehead incision flap has been closed. Surgical staples may be used to advantage here.

If the forehead lift is being done in conjunction with a face lift, it is preferable to close the entire forehead flap first, then trim and suture the facial flaps. If an upper lid blepharoplasty is planned along with a forehead lift, *it is essential to complete the forehead lift before doing the blepharoplasty.* The forehead lift will always reduce the quantity of redundant upper lid skin, and, as mentioned, may sometimes make the upper lid blepharoplasty unnecessary.

At the completion of the operation, the author blocks the supraorbital and supratrochlear nerves by injecting Marcaine, 0.5 percent (without epinephrine) near the points at which they emerge from their foramina to reduce postoperative discomfort. The incision is dressed with cotton soaked in sterile mineral oil to absorb blood and serum, and a well padded forehead bandage is applied

---

*Available from Padgett Instruments, 2838 Warwick Traffic Way, Kansas City, Missouri 64108.

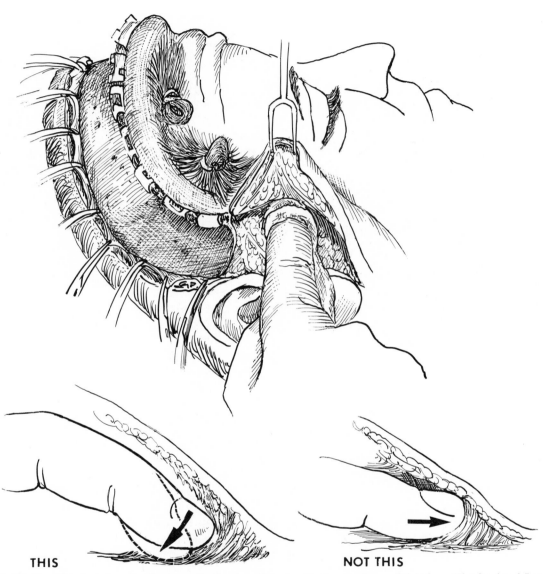

Figure 26–11. For the lower rhytidectomy, the face is undermined in the usual superficial plane. The forehead flap has been elevated in a deep, subgaleal and submuscular plane. The two planes are reconciled by creating a musculoaponeurotic pedicle containing the frontal branches of the facial nerve medially and the superficial temporal vessels laterally. To avoid injuring these structures, blunt dissection with a gauze-wrapped finger is utilized, using a peeling rather than a pushing motion.

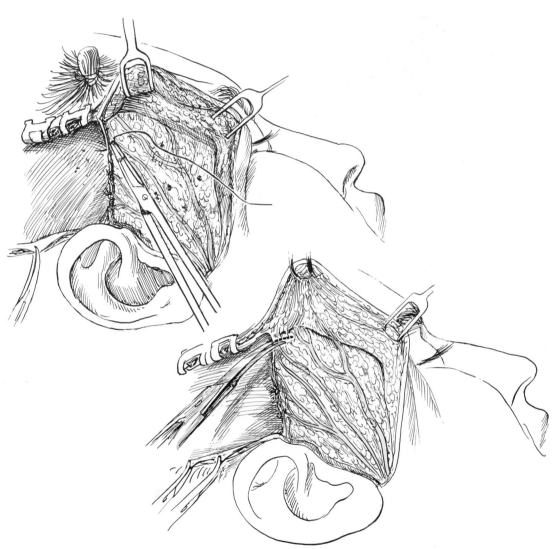

Figure 26–12.   To gain more mobility of the forehead flap, the superficial temporal vessels may be ligated, and the lateral 1 to 2 cm of the edge of the pedicle may be transected superiorly near its insertion into the forehead flap, where there is no danger of harm to the frontal nerves.

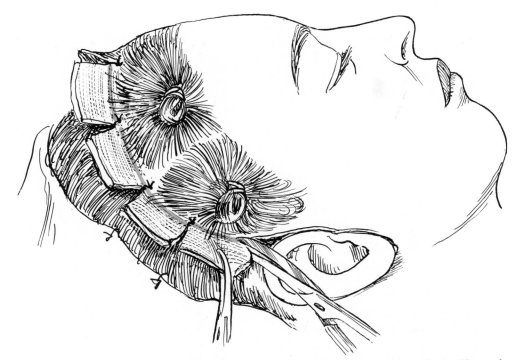

Figure 26–13.   To minimize bleeding, the forehead flap is trimmed and closed in segments after making and suturing several "pilot" incisions. The segments are best trimmed with a scalpel (rather than scissors as illustrated), beveling the incisions in the direction of the hair follicles.

with very light compression. The author does not use drains.

POSTOPERATIVE CARE

Analgesics are used as needed following a forehead lift. Most patients can get along very well on oral medication. Frontal headache, probably owing to stretching of the supraorbital and supratrochlear nerves, can be relieved quickly by injections of plain Marcaine around their sites of origin.

The author empirically continues antibiotics for two days postoperatively. The dressing is removed in 24 hours. Patients are told to expect significant swelling of their eyelids, often worse on the second or third postoperative day, but they are assured that such swelling will subside. They may wash their hair on the second postoperative day and thereafter as often as they wish. Patients are cautioned against using a hot dryer, however. Sutures are left in place for at least fourteen days.

Patients are almost invariably pleased with the results of forehead lifts. We believe they last as long as, if not longer than, facial rhytidectomies (Figures 26–14, 26–15). Although the forehead regains motion, transverse wrinkling is generally reduced. Many patients report that friends tell

them they look rested or that they have a pleasant look of well-being.

COMPLICATIONS

Complications of the forehead lift operation are infrequent and mild. As might be expected, they are similar to complications seen in the temporal portions of a facial rhytidectomy.

Hematoma.   Because of the relative avascularity of the plane of dissection, bleeding is easy to control in the forehead lift. Moreover, after the forehead flap is trimmed and sutured into place, the underside of the flap lying on the skull and periosteum is under some degree of compression, which may further tamponade small bleeders. Hematomas are rare and are usually small and treated easily by aspiration.

Necrosis.   The author has not seen any cases of extensive skin necrosis. Initially, occasional small areas of spot necrosis were noted where pilot sutures had been tied tightly to control the brisk bleeding from the pilot incisions. Since these are no longer tied tightly, regardless of the amount of bleeding in pilot incisions, such spot necrosis no longer occurs. If such areas were to occur and the resulting hairless scars interfered with hair styling, they could be excised secondarily.

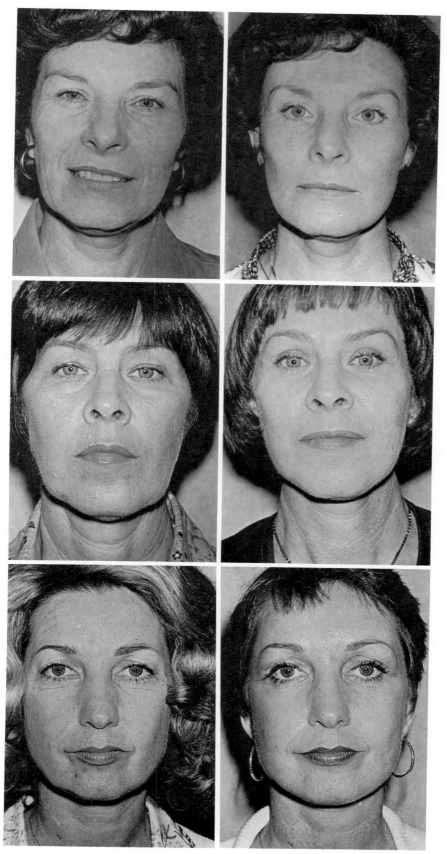

Figure 26–14. Two year results for forehead lift, face lift, and upper and lower blepharoplasties. (Above left, from Plast. Reconstr. Surg. *60*:161, 1977.)

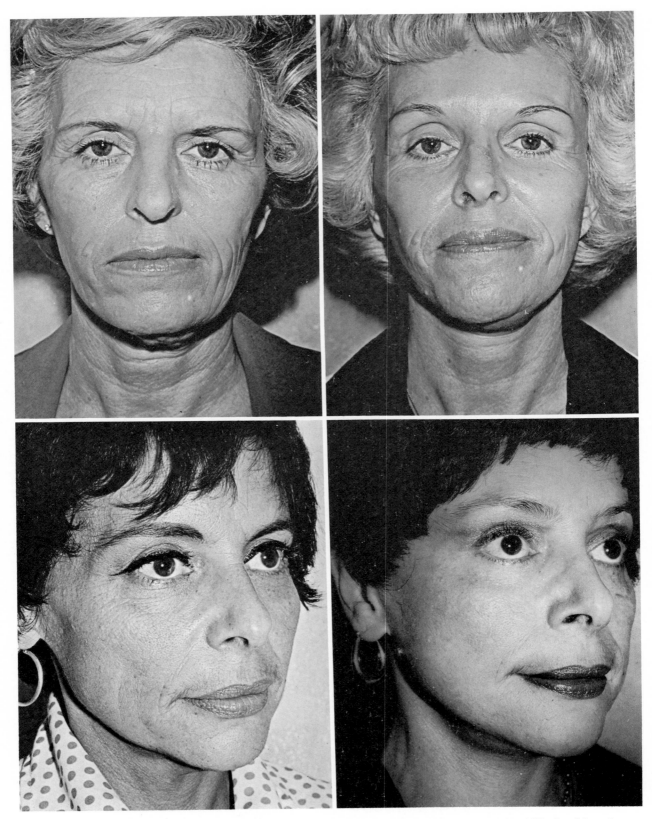

Figure 26–15.   Patients in whom forehead lifts *outlasted* initial face lifts. Each patient had a forehead lift, face lift, and upper and lower blepharoplasty. Each subsequently had a secondary face lift for recurrent facial laxity. Forehead lifts, performed at time of initial procedures, have lasted. *Above:* Two year result. *Below:* Three year result. (Above left, from Plast. Reconstr. Surg. *60*:161, 1977.)

Hair Loss. The author has seen two cases of temporary hair thinning anterior to the incision. Treatment consisted of reassurance and watchful waiting for return of normal growth.

Motor Nerve Injury. In an initial series of cases, there were no instances of injury to the frontal branches of the facial nerve. The author started seeing occasional temporary forehead lag while making the transverse strip of frontalis excision more inferiorly. Subsequently, the inferior margins of the lateral muscle strip excisions were made at least 3 cm superior to the orbital ridges, and thereafter, no additional cases of temporary forehead lag were seen.

The course of the temporal branch of the facial nerve should be kept in mind during this operation (Correia and Zani, 1973; Furnas, 1965; Loeb, 1970; Pitanguy and Silveira Ramos, 1966). When the forehead lift is combined with a face lift, gentle, blunt dissection over the medial portion of the musculoaponeurotic pedicle has been a significant factor in helping to avoid permanent injury to these branches.

Sensory Changes: Numbness and Itching. Numbness of the anterior scalp results from division of the supraorbital and supratrochlear nerves when making the coronal incision. Sensation usually returns, although there may be instances where numbness could be permanent. Patients should be informed of this possibility preoperatively.

As the nerves heal, patients often experience itching, and they are also informed of this probability preoperatively. If itching becomes severe, it can be helped by use of Temaril, 2.5 mg QID, or Periactin, 4 mg QID.

Forehead Lift in Patient with Previous Upper Lid Blepharoplasty. Surgeons should evaluate patients who have had previous upper lid blepharoplasties very carefully before undertaking to perform forehead lifts on them. Following upper lid blepharoplasty, there is a paucity of upper lid skin, which, when combined with the upward pull of the forehead lift, could make these patients unable to close their eyes. Obviously, complications from this problem could be serious. During the preoperative evaluation, one should determine that the patient can close his or her eyes completely without straining when the forehead is held up in its proposed new position. A second observation should be made immediately before surgery, when the patient's eyelids have relaxed under sedation or general anesthesia. Under these conditions, if the eyes remain open enough to expose the corneas to any significant extent, it is safer to abandon the forehead lift.

FOREHEAD LIFT VERSUS DIRECT EYEBROW LIFT

The forehead lift seems to have several advantages over the direct eyebrow lift.

Absence of Visible Scars. The forehead lift incision is hidden within the hairline, or immediately in front of the hairline if a frontal approach is used.

Natural Elevation of Eyebrows. By lifting the eyebrows and glabellar areas as a unit, a more natural elevation is produced. In contrast, occasionally a Mephistophelian look results from a direct eyebrow lift when proportionately more skin was removed above the lateral portion of the eyebrow than above the medial part.

Treatment of Root of Nose. Transverse nasal wrinkles are often seen with ptosis of the brow and glabellar region. The forehead lift also elevates this area, resulting in a rhytidectomy of the skin at the nasofrontal angle.

Exposure for Other Ancillary Procedures. (A) The forehead lift provides excellent exposure for partial resection of corrugator muscles for glabellar frown. (B) It helps to reduce or eliminate forehead wrinkles by permitting the surgeon to perform a partial resection of the frontalis muscle. (C) It can help to correct nasal drooping if the undermining is extended to include the dorsum of the nose — down to the nasal spine if necessary. (On occasion, it is convenient to rasp down a bony nasal hump through the forehead lift approach; after completing the forehead operation, the rest of the rhinoplasty can be done from below.)

ALTERNATIVE INCISIONS

Some authors (González-Ulloa, 1962; Viñas et al., 1976; and Ortiz-Monasterio et al., 1978) prefer a straight coronal incision for their standard forehead lifts. Excision of such a straight, uniform strip of scalp undoubtedly saves time, but it may necessitate excision of a central compensatory wedge of scalp. The author prefers an angled or gull wing-type incision, approximately paralleling the frontal hairline, as also used by Connell (1978) and Pitanguy (1978). This type of incision enables the surgeon to vary the width of the excision in different portions of the forehead. It also eliminates the need for a central wedge excision.

If the frontal hairline is high, an incision and scalp resection posterior to the hairline would make the forehead even higher. In such cases, the patient can be offered the alternative of having the central part of the incision made immediately in front of the hairline. (Over the temporal regions, the incision would curve back into the hair-bearing scalp.) These patients usually wear their hair down over their foreheads to compensate for their high hairlines, and an incision line just anterior to their frontal hairlines would not change their lifestyles. If an anterior incision is chosen, it should be closed with half buried 3–0 Prolene or Nylon vertical mattress sutures, tied on the hair-bearing posterior side of the incision and left in place for at least 14 days. Fine adjustments can be made with 5–0 or 6–0 sutures, which are removed before the fifth postoperative day. One advantage of this approach is that additional forehead lifts can be done using the same incision, without raising the central frontal hairline.

Regnault (1972) described a standard face lift incision combined with a discontinuous higher forehead incision separated by a bridge of scalp about 2 cm wide. She believed this bridge contributed to the vascularization of the flap and also permitted two different directions of traction. Ortiz-Monasterio and co-workers (1978) also described discontinuous face lift and forehead lift incisions, with the lower face lift incision following the sideburn and contour of the hairline for 2 or 3 cm, in order to preserve the position of the hair at the sideburns.

THE FOREHEAD LIFT IN THE MALE

The male who has reached middle age or beyond and still has adequate hair coverage in the frontal area as well as a favorable family history of male hair retention will probably continue to have good hair coverage, subject to the usual additional thinning that occurs in both males and females as they get older. In this type of patient, the forehead lift incision may be made posterior to the frontal hairline, as in the female patient.

Although the incisions described so far are not applicable in cases of male pattern baldness, alternative approaches have been used. Connell (1978) described excision of a transverse strip of forehead skin and subcutaneous tissue, located so that the resulting incision line will fall into one of the transverse forehead wrinkle lines. A direct eyebrow lift as described by Bames (1957) and Castanares (1964) could also be used. González-Ulloa and Flores (1971) described posterior extensions of preauricular rhytidectomy incisions that meet in the midline of the occipital region, thereby creating an almost total scalp flap, based anteriorly, which is undermined to the supraorbital ridges and over the nose, in the same way as the usual forehead lift. When the flap is trimmed, the resulting incision line is hidden in the occipital hair.

CONCLUSIONS

The forehead lift is a useful procedure to rejuvenate the upper third of the face. It can be used as an isolated procedure, but more frequently it can be a useful adjunct to face lift and blepharoplasty. The procedure is not overly time consuming, so it can be combined with other facial operations. Complications have been relatively few and minor. Furthermore, the forehead lift, when combined with a procedure to interrupt the pull of the frontalis muscle, is lasting; in fact, it appears to last as long as a face lift (sometimes even longer).

(For references, see pages 859 and 860.)

Chapter 27

Chemabrasion and Dermabrasion

Thomas D. Rees, M.D., F.A.C.S.

There are two effective methods for removing layers of skin to improve dermatologic defects: chemabrasion (chemical peeling) and dermabrasion (surgical removal). Chemabrasion, generally performed with a phenol solution, is most useful for the removal of fine facial wrinkles and abnormal pigmentation. Dermabrasion, which can be performed by using abrasive substances such as wire brushes or by dermatome excision, is more useful in smoothing surface irregularities produced by acne pits or scars.

CHEMICAL FACE PEEL

Today, chemabrasion is a generally accepted plastic surgery procedure, although it was not until 1960 that it came to prominence in the plastic surgery literature (Brown et al., 1960).

For many years before that, however, Sir Harrold Gillies, without publishing his procedure, was using pure carbolic acid in a painting and taping technique for correction of "slight laxity of lid" (Gillies and Millard, 1957; Batstone and Millard, 1968). Also before that time, dermatologists had used phenol peels for removal of superficial blemishes, and beauty operators had given the chemical face peel a somewhat patchy notoriety. Nonetheless, it fell to Brown and the surgeons and dermatologists who followed him to popularize the technique among plastic surgeons and to refine it (Baker et al., 1961, 1962, 1963, 1966, 1974; Litton et al., 1962, 1966, 1973; Ayres, 1962, 1964; Sperber, 1963, 1965 a and b; Spira et al., 1974).

Indications

Chemical face peeling, as a *sole* procedure, is indicated for the eradication of fine wrinkles in the absence of gross sagging of the facial skin. Although dermabrasion will also produce temporary improvement in such cases, chemical peel achieves a more prolonged effect. Moderate tightening of the forehead skin may also be achieved by chemabrasion in some patients, without the risks of hair loss or obvious scars that may be encountered with more radical approaches to forehead wrinkling.

Chemabrasion can also be useful as an *adjunctive* procedure if facial wrinkling is accompanied by sufficient laxity of skin to warrant blepharoplasty and/or rhytidectomy — removing fine rhytides, especially those in the periorbital and perioral region, which would be unaffected by the usual techniques of eyelid or facial plasties (Figures 27–1 through 27–3). If peeling is limited to the lips and/or forehead, it may be done at the same time as the eyelid or facial surgery. If a full face peel is indicated, the eyelid or facial plasty should be done first, and the chemical peel should be deferred for a period of three or more weeks to allow for recovery of the skin from the operative insult. Chemabrasion may also be used in conjunction with other techniques for the removal of deep wrinkles, since their removal is only partially effected by chemical peeling.

Chemabrasion is also indicated for telangiectasia, superficial keratosis, hyperpigmentation, and areas of diffuse, patchy pigmentation such as that which may occur in chloasma or following episodes of certain types of dermatitis (Figures 27–4, 27–5, and 27–6). Chemical peel appears to offer a prolonged if not permanent cure for these problems.

Patient Selection

Generally, the ideal candidate for chemabrasion is the patient with a minimal facial sag and finely wrinkled skin that has been constantly exposed to the elements — a patient who desires improvement but is not quite a candidate for face lift.

Patients with fair complexions are better candidates than are those with olive-toned skin, for the latter tend to show an obvious line of demarca-

Text continued on page 756.

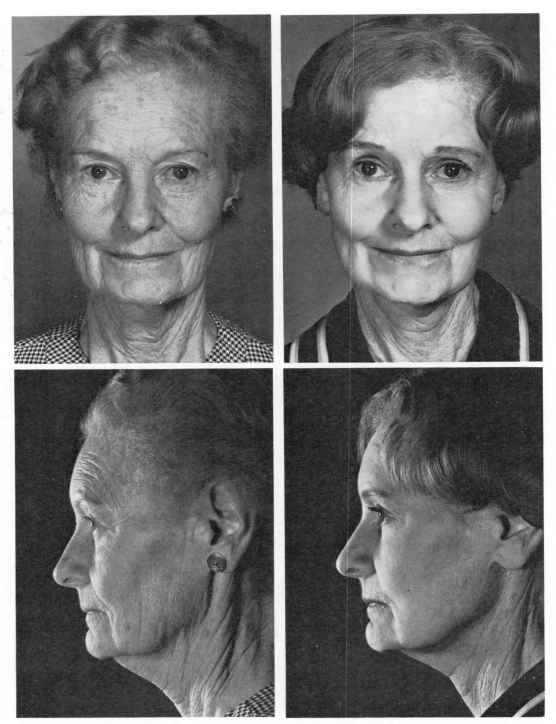

Figure 27–1.   Full-face chemabrasion was done for this patient several weeks after facial plastic surgery. Although the improvement shown here may be regarded as typical, the results of chemical abrasion are not consistent. It is not possible to promise any particular degree of improvement in attempts to ablate fine rhytides. Chemical peeling is better done after facial and cervical rhytidectomy, although the sequence can be reversed if necessary. Notice the neck is still wrinkled after peeling because the chemical cannot be applied to this area with complete safety.

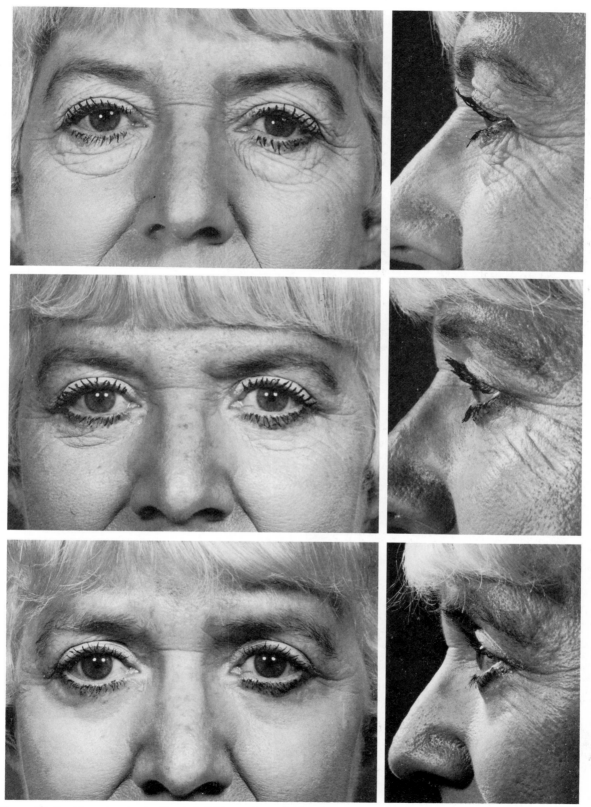

Figure 27–2.   Chemabrasion is often helpful in erasing wrinkles of the eyelid skin which cannot be removed—and which may even be accentuated—by blepharoplasty. The photographs at the top of the page show the preoperative condition; note the unusual thickness of the skin and the deep wrinkling. The middle set of photographs show the results after a complete blepharoplasty. The palpebral bags are gone, but much of the wrinkling remains. The final result after deep chemical peeling, shown in the lower photographs, is long lasting. Chemabrasion for this purpose is better and safer than dermabrasion.

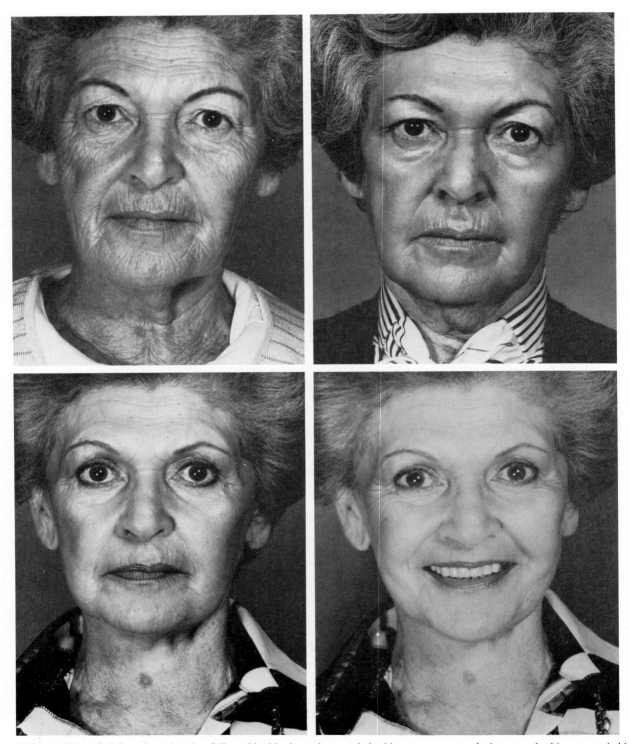

Figure 27–3. Full-face chemabrasion followed by blepharoplasty and rhytidectomy two months later resulted in a remarkable improvement in this patient with severe familial rhytidosis.

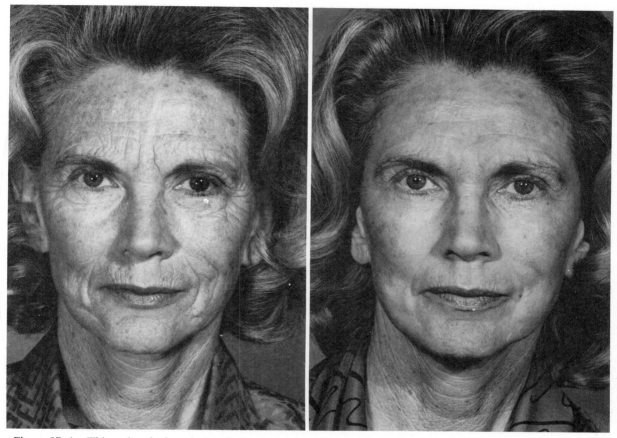

Figure 27–4.   This patient had marked and premature rhytidosis of the facial skin. Her facial bone structure is excellent and her facial features are striking. Prolonged actinic exposure resulted in innumerable keratotic lesions of the face.

The postpeel photograph shows not only the improvement of the rhytides that can occur, but also the removal of many of the superficial keratotic lesions. In this respect, chemabrasion is much like treatment with radioactive materials such as 5-fluorouracil. This patient was also ideal to treat, since her skin was dry and very fair.

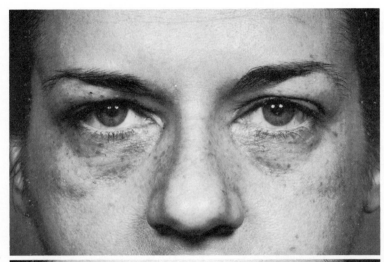

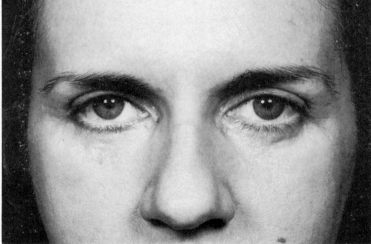

Figure 27–5. In certain types of pigmentation, the pigment is quite superficial and responds to chemabrasion. The irregular and unsightly pattern of pigmentation seen in this patient had been present since her childhood. Blepharoplasty followed in six weeks by deep chemical peel achieved the result shown in the postoperative view, which has persisted for two years.

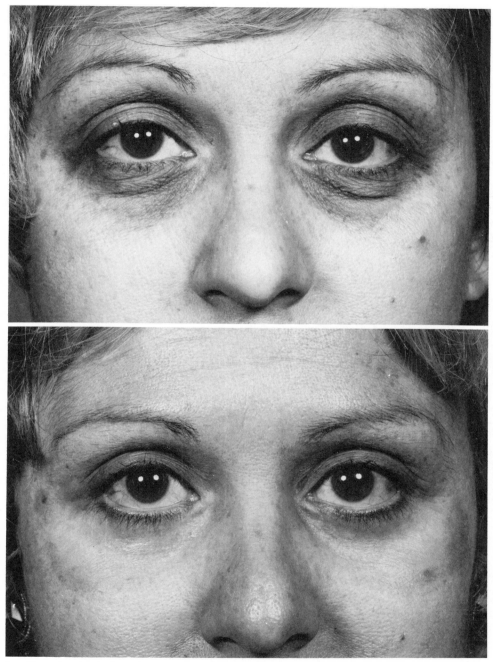

Figure 27–6.   Chemabrasion is the *only* technique available to treat dark-pigmented eyelids of hereditary origin. The degree of success achieved is related to the depth of the pigmentation. Success is also achieved because the eyelid skin is so thin that the depth of the burn probably extends almost full thickness in many instances.

This patient obtained an excellent result from chemabrasion of the eyelids following blepharoplasty. The dark circles under her eyes had been present since childhood and distressed her more than the redundant skin and fat. The condition is frequently hereditary and is often found in peoples of Mediterranean origin.

tion between treated and untreated areas, having a tendency toward a permanent blotchiness of skin color in the chemabraded areas as well. For similar reasons, blacks and other dark-skinned patients should be accepted for chemabrasion only with great caution.

Chemical Agents

The chemical most often used as the primary irritant in chemabrasion is phenol (C_6H_5OH) in a solution with distilled water, croton oil, and liquid soap based on Baker's formula. The phenol itself produces an immediate reaction of keratolysis and coagulation, probably caused by disruption of the sulfur bridges of keratoprotein and aided by denaturation owing to its acid nature. No greater concentration than 80 per cent phenol should be used, since stronger solutions produce keratocoagulation to such an extent as to form a barrier to further penetration of phenol into the dermis (Rothman, 1945). Schwartz and Peck (1946) emphasized the importance of the passage of absorbable material via the skin appendages as a prime route to the site of action on dermal collagen.

The croton oil acts as an additional irritant and speeds the destruction of the epidermis. It is also thought to facilitate the penetration of the phenol to the dermis, although no definite proof of this action has been found. Certainly, however, omission of this substance from the solution does appear to reduce its overall efficacy.

Liquid soap, on the other hand, acts to retard penetration and absorption of phenol by increasing surface tension. It is added to the formula to balance the desired macerative and irritant effects of any given concentration of phenol against the tendency of that concentration of phenol to limit its own penetrating ability by excessive keratocoagulation.

The action of the phenol can be prolonged and therefore deepened by use of a vapor barrier, usually waterproof tape. The tape acts to confine the active ingredients to the region of application and, by preventing evaporation of the phenol, to promote maceration and, in turn, further phenol penetration. When indicated, especially in patients with thin, fair skin, this prolonged, deeper action of phenol can be modified by delaying the application of tape and waiting for the solution to dry, providing time for some of the phenol to evaporate.

Changes in the Skin

The inflammatory reaction that immediately follows phenol application to the skin is characterized by keratocoagulation, epidermolysis, a zone of cellular destruction in the upper dermis, and the subsequent formation of a crust of keratin, necrotic epidermis, and proteinaceous precipitate. This response passes its peak by 48 hours and is gone by the third month. Epidermal regeneration begins the second day following the chemical peel and is complete by the end of ten days or two weeks. Dermal thickening occurs at about two weeks as a consequence of the subsiding of the inflammatory reaction.

Long-term changes in microscopic anatomy of the skin, as demonstrated by biopsy techniques, also follow chemabrasion (Brown et al., 1960; Baker, 1962; Baker et al., 1966, 1974; Spira et al., 1970).

First, dermal collagen is reorganized with a change from its usual wavy shape to a straight pattern lying parallel to the skin surface (Figure 27–7). This is accompanied by an increase in the density of associated fibroblasts. These changes appear to be the basis for the clinical benefits of the procedure. Such changes do not occur to the same extent following dermabrasion, which may explain the relative inefficiency of dermabrasion in the long-term eradication of fine facial wrinkles.

Secondly, there is a marked decrease in the number of melanin-producing cells in the basal layer of the epidermis, which is demonstrable using the Fontana-Masson silver stain. Thirdly, there is an increase in elastic tissue in the dermis as can be demonstrated with special stains.

Follow-up studies of up to 13 years (Baker et al., 1974) have shown that these three basic histologic changes follow chemical peel with consistency, predictability, and apparent permanency. Baker and associates (1974) feel that there has been no evidence, clinically or histologically, that these effects are deleterious in any way.

Systemic Reaction

Following chemabrasion, a certain amount of phenol is absorbed into the systemic circulation. Resultant blood levels are easily determined using spectrophotometry. Following the application of 3 ml of 50 percent phenol to the entire face, Litton (1962) observed blood levels of 0.68 mg/100 ml after one hour, 0.19 mg/100 ml two hours after exposure, and 0.10 mg/100 ml four hours after the procedure. Since blood levels of phenol as high as 23 mg/100 ml after ingestion of phenol have been associated with survival, it seems logical to assume that careful application of a reasonable volume of phenol to a restricted area poses little risk of phenol toxicity (Litton, 1966). It should be noted, however, that chemical peeling of extensive areas (face, neck, and upper thorax) by lay operators has resulted in death owing to the absorption of large volumes of phenol. Such a case was reported by Brown et al. (1960).

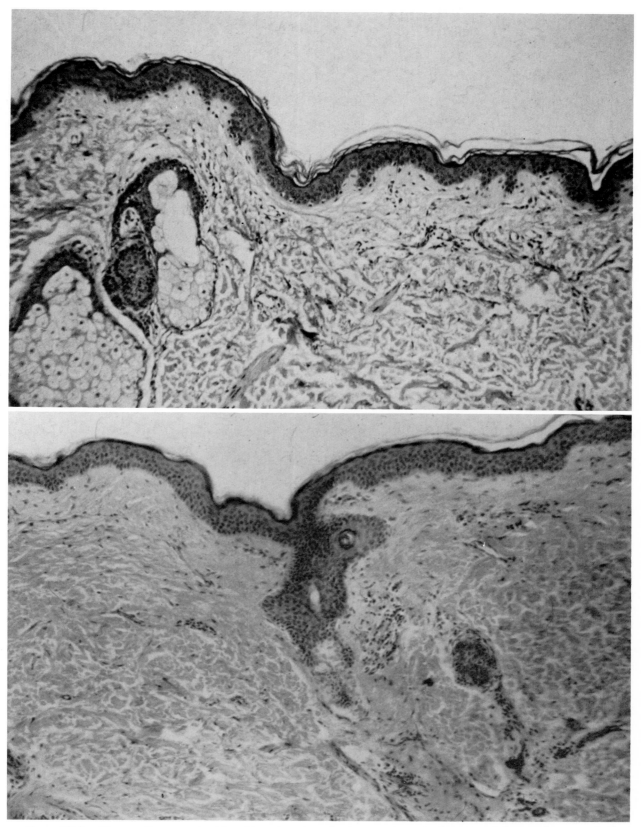

Figure 27–7.   Changes that occur in skin subjected to chemabrasion are shown in these photomicrographs. Normal skin is shown in the top figure, while the postchemabrasion picture at the bottom demonstrates a marked increased in collagen, in a lamellar distribution. (Courtesy of Dr. Tom Baker.)

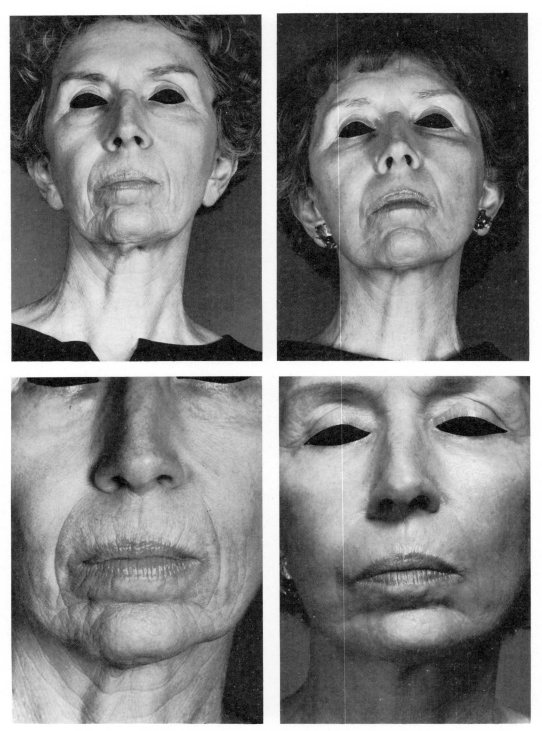

Figure 27–8.   Loose skin along the mandibular border and of the neck is not improved to a significant degree by chemical peel. But chemical abrasion following a standard face lift procedure will aid the final result quite considerably because it will improve the rhytides around the mouth.

The minimal volumes of phenol absorbed following carefully performed chemical face peel are excreted by the kidney. The phenol may first be conjugated with glycuronic and sulfuric acids or detoxified to hydroquinones and pyrocatechnin. However, some free phenol is also excreted.

Truppman and associates (1978) found that cardiac irregularities are not uncommon after application of phenol solution to large areas of the face. Their findings were the result of continuous monitoring of patients during chemabrasion. Such a disturbance in cardiac muscle irritability is likely to be the result of absorption of the drug; therefore, it is recommended that only limited areas of the face be treated, with intervals of several minutes between applications. No serious problems were reported, and only temporary disturbances in the electrical activity of the cardiac conduction system occurred.

Precautions

To assure the most successful possible results from chemical face peels, certain precautions should be taken by the surgeon.

Patients should be carefully selected according to both the criteria mentioned earlier in this chapter and the criteria discussed in Chapters 1 and 2. Chemabrasion and its discomforts and usual sequelae should be carefully explained to the patient, especially since the postoperative appearance is, to say the least, frightening.

A complete history and physical examination should precede the chemabrasion. Special attention should be given to the hepatorenal system. Any history of drug sensitivity or prior chemabrasion by another surgeon should warrant a test of a small area of skin, usually performed most conveniently in the preauricular area. Routine blood analysis should also be obtained prior to chemical peel, and preoperative photographs, ideally both in black and white and in color, should be taken.

The surgeon must be aware of the limitations of the procedure. For example, chemical peel of the neck should be approached with caution since attempts to peel neck skin have resulted in hypertrophic scarring because of the difficulty in controlling the depth of the "burn" and the paucity of skin appendages (Figure 27–8).

Attempts to peel the arms and the thorax have been quite unsuccessful and are not without potential danger from phenol toxicity because of the large areas to be treated. The skin of the hands does not respond as well as the skin of the face does, although certain surgeons are performing hand peels (Litton et al., 1973). Should hand peeling be attempted, patients must keep their hands out of water for a minimum of five to seven days, since water tends to convert a second degree peel to a third degree peel and to retard healing and cause scarring and hyperpigmentation (Litton et al., 1973).

No attempt should be made to do a blepharoplasty and an eyelid peel at the same time because ectropion may result, and certainly the presence of a tight lower lid postblepharoplasty is a reason for considerable delay of an eyelid peel. Furthermore, because of the marked inflammatory reaction that follows chemical peeling, it is not always wise to peel both upper and lower lids at the same time because the resultant swelling will leave the patient temporarily without vision.

Extensive malformations such as strawberry hemangioma or nevus flammeus do not respond to chemabrasion, even though lesions such as telangiectases and superficial keratoses are amenable to improvement by this technique.

PROCEDURE (Figure 27–9)

Chemabrasion can be performed either in the hospital or on an ambulatory basis. In either instance, however, appropriate precautions listed in the preceding section should be taken. The skin is washed on the evening prior to the procedure to remove all cosmetics and again the next morning. Although no anesthesia is necessary, the patient should be well premedicated.

Premedication is a matter of personal preference. The author prefers intravenous premedication at the time of or just prior to peeling. Demerol, 50 to 100 mg, given slowly, intravenously along with titrated amounts of valium, usually 10 to 20 mg, also given very slowly until speech is slurred, has proved effective in most paients to promote amnesia and provide analgesia. Other narcotics and sedatives are equally effective.

The patient is placed on the operating table with the head slightly elevated. Skin oils and residual soap are removed with ether. Phenol solutions should be freshly mixed for each use following the formula below:

Phenol 88 per cent U.S.P.: 3 ml
Croton oil: 3 drops
Septisol soap: 8 drops
Distilled water: 2 ml

This volume will suffice for a full face application.

The solution is applied by means of a cotton-tipped applicator stick with the tip well wrung out so as to avoid any chance of dripping or splashing

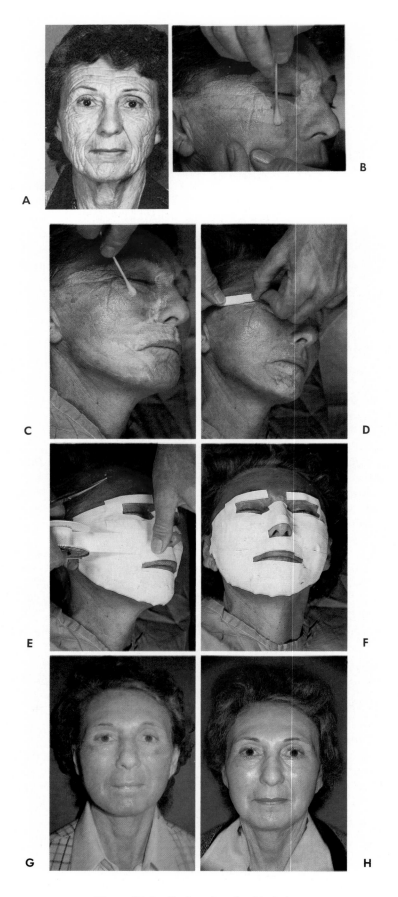

Figure 27–9. *See legend on the opposite page.*

760

Figure 27–9. Technique of chemabrasion of the skin. The patient is an excellent candidate for the technique. Her skin is dry and fair. She has many fine wrinkles that are partly hereditary in origin but exacerbated greatly by over-exposure to sun and wind. A face lift operation in this patient without chemabrasion would be a great disappointment, since the wrinkling would not be relieved.

A, The preoperative condition of the patient. *B* and *C,* The phenol solution is applied sparingly with cotton-tipped applicators to one area at a time. Several minutes are allowed between area applications to permit the patient to adjust to any absorption of phenol that may occur through the skin.

D, E, and *F,* The tape mask is applied to one area at a time. Waterproof adhesive tape is used. In this patient, the forehead had been treated previously and so was not treated on this occasion.

G, Appearance of the face on the eleventh day after peeling.

H, Appearance of the facial skin six months after chemabrasion. This patient had an unusually prolonged erythema. During this period, it is unwise for the patient to be exposed to direct sunlight without the use of an excellent sun screen.

I, Postpeel appearance at 10 months.

J, and *K,* Pre- and postpeel photographs of the forehead area. Chemabrasion is satisfactory in many patients as a modality of treatment for forehead rhytides.

See illustration on the opposite page.

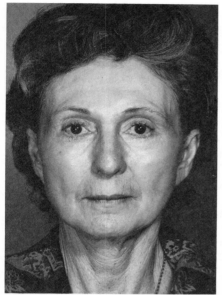

I

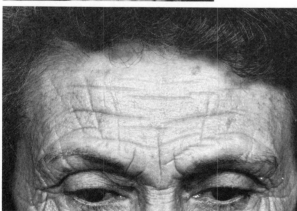

J

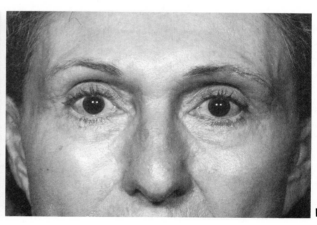

K

the solution. Throughout the procedure, the solution should be stirred frequently, as phenol and water tend to "layer," which could cause unequal concentrations of phenol to be applied at different times.

The application should be made evenly to produce a smooth white surface. When an area of greater penetration is desired, a more vigorous rubbing of the applicator will achieve this result, although care should be taken in so doing. Gentle stretching of the skin will enable the fluid to coat the depths of wrinkles evenly, an important point to observe. Application of phenol solution should encroach slightly on the hairline to avoid a visible margin of untreated skin. No permanent damage to the hair will result.

It is necessary to come right to the vermilion border of the lips. If in doubt, a margin of vermilion may be included. The vermilion will blister and be somewhat painful, but a thin band of obviously untreated skin will not occur. The ciliary margins should be skirted by 2 mm to avoid any chance of corneal or conjunctival burns. The treated area should extend just below the mandibular margin, but no further.

When treating the whole face, application should be made section by section, and in patients with the average type of skin, tape should be applied to each completed section before treating the next. Suitably sized sections for treatment are the left cheek (with lower lid, if planned), the right cheek, the nose and upper lip, the chin and lower lip, and the forehead (and upper lids, if planned). Upper and lower lids should not be peeled during any one procedure.

Many varieties of occlusive covers exist, the most elegant of which is a custom-made rubber mask. However, for all practical purposes, a standard one half inch zinc oxide adhesive tape applied in two or three layers, with great care being taken to avoid skin creases underneath, is both the easiest and the best means of occlusion. As mentioned earlier in this chapter, in patients with thin, fair, and delicate skin, the solution should be allowed to dry, with partial evaporation of phenol, before the tape is applied.

Various authors have described different methods of tape application. For the first layer, the author has found it satisfactory to butt short strips edge to edge with care being taken not to wrinkle the skin below. The second and third layers, if needed, can be laid in any convenient fashion over the first layer, again taking care not to produce creases in the underlying skin.

A transient stinging sensation, replaced by anesthesia, is often a complaint of the patient during application of phenol solution. Occasionally, it is necessary to administer further analgesic medication during the course of the procedure.

POSTOPERATIVE CARE

After returning to the room, the patient will often complain of a fiery, itching sensation that requires narcotic relief. The patient is best left well sedated for the first 48 hours after the procedure, with relatively free access to narcotic analgesics.

If the lips have been treated, it is advisable to keep the patient from speaking and to administer a fluid diet by straw for the first 48 hours. This is necessary to avoid lifting of the adhesive from the skin, which would lessen the desired effect. Bed rest is usually desirable for at least the first 24 hours, and preferably 48 hours, when a large area of the face has been treated.

After 48 hours have elapsed, the patient is given another dose of narcotic, and the adhesive mask, with its adherent necrotic superficial skin layers, is gently peeled off the face. The raw, moist surface is dusted with thymol iodide powder, U.S.P., to produce a thin coagulum. Other coagulating powders have been used, particularly antibiotic-based powders, but these appear to offer no advantage and, in fact, they may carry a risk of producing hypersensitivity. The use of the powder two or three times a day on any moist areas is helpful for the next 72 hours, after which time it may be discontinued. Coincident with the removal of the adhesive mask, the diet may be liberalized, but chewing should still be kept to a minimum, as should talking. General activity is to be encouraged, but overexertion and sweating must be avoided.

On the fifth day after the removal of the adhesive mask, the patient is instructed to apply a liberal coating of bland cold cream, polymyxin B (Neosporin) or petrolatum jel to the coagulum. On the following day, the powder mask is usually easily removed to reveal a layer of delicate pink new skin. In a patient with a relatively hairy face, it is occasionally advisable to wait another day to remove the coagulum, as the added time loosens the grip of the hair on the crust. The face is then cared for by daily washing with a mild soap and water. The new skin should be kept moist with cold cream or moisturizing cream. After the passage of a week to allow for maturation of the new skin, a light makeup may be applied. Regular makeup use may be resumed after two to three weeks.

The intense pink color will fade rapidly, but an excess pink coloration will remain for six to eight weeks. The skin will be somewhat tense and smooth, with the finer rhytides gone and the deeper groves much less evident. Care should be taken to protect the area from exposure to sun for a minimal period of three to six months, and use of a sun screen such as Uval or A-Fil should be advised in any sunny region.

COMPLICATIONS

The complication that arises most often after chemical peel is a bleaching of skin color in treated portions of the face, resulting in a noticeable line of demarcation surrounding the peeled areas. This problem is virtually impossible to avoid entirely in a darker-skinned patient, but special precautions to counter this effect can make it less of a postoperative problem. Careful preoperative explanation of post-peeling results will help the patient adjust more easily to minor irregularities in color. Feathering the depth of the peel at the margins is helpful. Baker and Gordon (1972) as well as Spira and associates (1974) recommend extending the peel beyond the tape mask to decrease the depth of the peel in the area immediately surrounding the treated site. Treatment of complete aesthetic units of the face, rather than small segments, also aids in camouflaging disparities in coloration. The use of natural boundaries minimizes the visibility of color differences. For example, if the peel is carried just below the mandibular margin to the "shadow area," skin color differences will be largely hidden. If the peel stops at, before, or more than 1 or 2 cm below that margin, the junction between peeled and unpeeled skin may become much more apparent.

Blotchy hyperpigmentation is most often seen postoperatively in darker-skinned patients who often have a degree of blotchiness preoperatively. Any such pigmentation present before surgery should be pointed out to the patient at that time, with the explanation that it may be intensified. Prevention of this complication involves removal of all soap and skin oils with ether before application of phenol, continuous stirring of the phenol solution to assure equal concentrations of phenol being applied to all treated areas, and making sure the tape mask is of equal thickness over the entire face. If the peel is being performed to correct abnormal skin hyperpigmentation as in chloasma, a tape mask should not be used at all (Spira et al., 1974). Should hyperpigmentation problems occur postoperatively, the one effective method of dealing with the problem thus far has been repeeling of the entire face without using a tape mask.

Other postoperative sequelae involving pigment defects include the darkening of preexisting nevi, the appearance of new nevi, and the increased prominence of telangiectases present before surgery because of the bleaching of the skin. These are less of a problem if the patient who is predisposed to them is amply forewarned. Spira and associates (1974) suggest removal of any large nevi prior to, and not simultaneously with, peeling, as removal of these nevi at the time of chemabrasion may lead to more visible residual scars.

Persistent erythema is more of an annoyance to the patient than a true complication. Erythema is initially present in all chemabrasion patients. In some, it resolves in a matter of weeks; in others, it may take months. A temporary increase in erythema following chemabrasion has been associated by some surgeons with ingestion of even small amounts of alcohol. Spira and associates (1974) recommend the use of topical steroids twice daily to attempt to hasten the resolution of persistent erythema.

Hypertrophic scarring and a tight "postburn" appearance can generally be prevented by regulating the depth of the peel. The peel should be kept superficial by careful, light painting of the area to be treated and by delaying the taping procedure in patients with thin, delicate skin to permit evaporation of some of the phenol. Baker and Gordon (1972) feel that limiting the patient's talking immediately postoperatively may also be helpful in reducing the incidence of scarring and contractures following perioral peel.

The author has found no specific therapy to be effective in treating scars or tightness except the passage of time or excision with consequent surgical defects. Spira and associates (1974) report one case with deep perioral scarring in which multiple steroid injections helped loosen the scar, with improvement taking place slowly over 8 to 12 months.

Ectropion has followed peeling of the lower lids in some cases. If adhesive support over a period of time does not alleviate this problem, corrective surgery may become necessary.

Full-thickness skin loss has been reported following chemabrasion performed at the same time as face lifting (Litton et al., 1973; Spira et al., 1974). It is considered very unwise to undermine the skin and apply peeling solution at the same time. Such a defect, should it occur, should be allowed to epithelialize spontaneously. The results of such healing can be acceptable and surgical revision is thus avoided.

Milia may be found up to three months after the peel owing to temporary blockage of sebaceous gland orifices. Small milia usually resolve spontaneously. Larger milia may have to be opened with an 18-gauge needle and their contents must be expressed.

An increase in the size of skin pores is seen so frequently after chemabrasion deep enough to remove wrinkles that patients should be forewarned that this will occur.

Phenol intoxication should not be a problem if the peel is carefully performed and the limitations previously discussed are observed. Nevertheless, as recently as 1966, Litton advised a two hour wait before completion of the second section of the face to allow for phenol detoxification. This view is not, however, shared by the majority of surgeons who perform this procedure.

REPEAT CHEMICAL PEELING

Chemabrasion may be cautiously repeated, but this is rarely indicated (Baker et al., 1962, 1966). Should a repeat peel be necessary, the author feels a wait of 12 to 18 months is optimal, despite the suggestion of Litton (1962) that this therapy may be repeated in six weeks to two months or the advice of Spira and his associates (1974) that it may be repeated after three months.

DERMABRASION

The first efforts at mechanical or surgical abrasion of the skin for the purpose of treating dermatologic lesions were performed by Kromayer as early as 1905. He initially used cylindrical knives and later progressed to the use of dental burs on skin made firm and anesthetic by ethyl chloride spray.

Janson (1935) first reported the use of the wire brush as an abrading instrument, but dermabrasion enjoyed only limited acceptance until Iverson (1947) published his success with sandpaper abrasion in the removal of traumatic tatoos of the face. McEvitt (1950) and Kurtin (1953) further popularized the procedure by reporting successful results with electrically driven, waterproof carbide abrasive paper cylinders and diamond impregnated burs. The latter are capable of producing a very fine and easily controllable depth of abrasive therapy and have proved particularly advantageous where very superficial abrasion is required.

In 1962, DaSilva added further dimension to the procedure with the introduction of a miniature electric dermatome with a suction attachment to stabilize the skin for cutting split-skin grafts from

blemished areas. In 1971, Malherbe and Davies introduced the narrow Davies electric dermatome for planing the central portions of the cheek and forehead, the areas where the greatest incidence of acne pits and scars occur. They also concurrently introduced a motor-driven sandpaper cylinder that leveled the edges of the planed area.

Today, dermabrasion is an accepted method of treatment for the removal of acne pits and scars, just as chemabrasion is accepted as effective in the eradication of facial wrinkles and certain types of hyperpigmentation.

Indications

Dermabrasion is primarily indicated for smoothing of surface irregularities produced by scars and acne pits (Figure 27–10). It can also be used to aid in the preparation of a recipient site for a skin graft. A layer of deep dermis is left intact and a split-thickness graft is placed on this dermal bed — a so-called overgraft (Webster, 1954; Hynes, 1957; Rees and Casson, 1966). This technique not only results in a greater skin thickness than can be obtained with a single thick-skin graft, but postoperative contraction does not occur. Furthermore, overgrafts rarely fail (Figures 27–11 and 27–12).

Skin Changes in the Dermabraded Area

Immediately following dermabrasion, the serum from the wound forms a coagulum across the abraded surface, trapping much cellular detritus. This is followed by a period of intense proliferation of squamous epithelium from the adnexal elements as soon as three to four days after the operative procedure (Eisen et al., 1955).

By the fifth day after dermabrasion, a thin epidermis has usually regenerated, lacking rete pegs but possessing developing hair follicles and sebaceous glands. On the third day after the procedure, a cell-free layer arises under the new epidermis. Evidence of dermal regeneration appears by the fifth postoperative day, and by the seventh day, some loose attachment of the new epidermis to the dermis may be observed.

During the first two weeks following dermabrasion, many young fibroblasts lying with axes in a horizontal plane can be found in the newly regenerated dermis. Luikart and associates (1959) noted a persistence of this horizontal striated collagenous pattern for at least four years following abrasive therapy, and they attributed the smoothness of the skin following the procedure at least in part to the presence of this newly formed collagen. A further factor in the smoothness and tautness of abraded skin is the phenomenon of interisland contraction described by Converse and Robb-Smith (1944). Interisland contraction not only is a

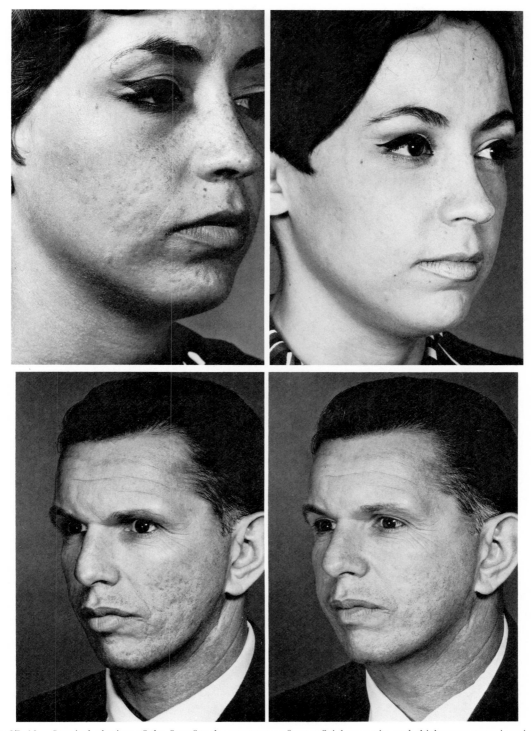

Figure 27–10.   Surgical planing of the face for the treatment of superficial acne pits and chickenpox scars is quite adequate when the pits are shallow and the scarring does not extend deeply into the dermis, as in this patient (top). The results of surgical planing when deep dermal scarring is present, as in this patient (bottom), are an improvement but are not so dramatic as when scarring is superficial. Such patients should be advised of the limitations of the procedure before surgery.

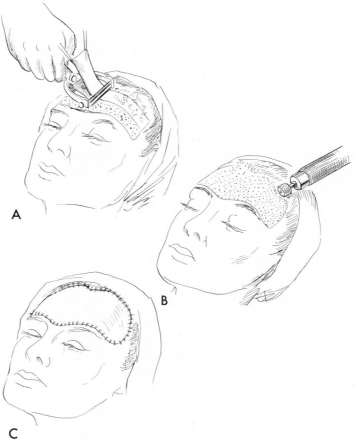

Figure 27–11.   Another excellent adaptation of the use of dermabrasion is in the surgical preparation of the recipient bed for the overgrafting technique, which is of particular importance in resurfacing burn scars so that an optimal cosmetic result can be achieved. Dermabrasion and overgrafting also constitute an effective technique for the treatment of decorative tattoos.

A scarred area, such as the forehead, is denuded of epithelium by use of a dermatome or by dermabrasion, or both (*A* and *B*). A split-thickness skin graft is applied to the abraded dermal bed (*C*). A complete "take" of the graft is practically assured because of the rich blood supply entering the undersurface of the dermis from the subdermal plexus. The cosmetic results of such unit grafts are superior to those of full-thickness excisions, because the integrity of the deep dermis is maintained and contraction is therefore minimal. (From Rees, T. D., and Casson, P. R.: Plast. Reconstr. Surg. *38*:522, 1966. Reproduced with permission.)

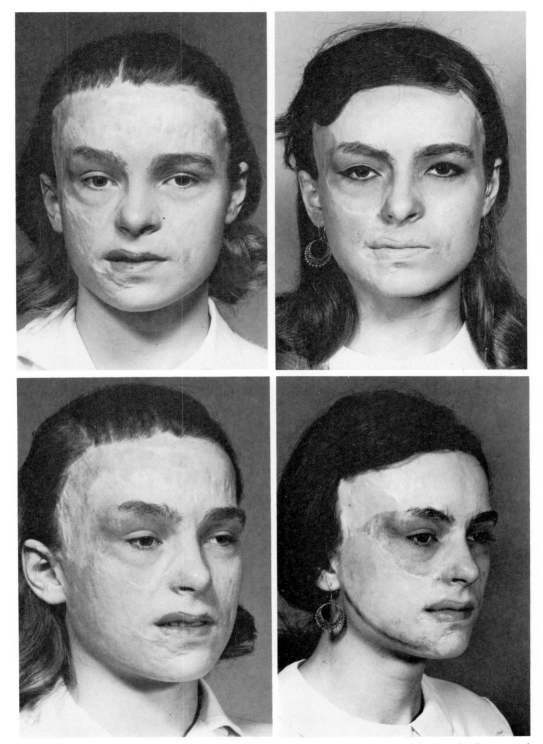

Figure 27–12.   Results of overgrafting of the forehead and cheek in a young patient with extensive burn scarring. Note the improved texture of the overgrafted areas in the postoperative views. The application of camouflaging makeup is facilitated. (From Rees, T. D., and Casson, P. R.: Plast. Reconstr. Surg. *38*:522, 1966. Reproduced with permission.)

probable factor in smoothing the skin following abrasion for acne scars, but it also probably aids the collapse and constriction of some of the deeper acne pits.

For the first three or four weeks after dermabrasion, there is little evidence of pigment formation, but this appears to progress from that time on. During this vital period of pigment reformation, it is essential that the skin be protected from exposure to the sun, since the complication of hyperpigmentation appears to be directly related to careless exposure to actinic rays. Effective sunscreens and avoidance of direct sun or sunglare exposure is as mandatory for two to four months following the procedure as it is for postchemabrasion skin.

Success of dermabrasion is dependent on the ability of the skin to rebuild a new epidermal layer from epithelial elements in the deep skin adnexa. Scarred areas, where there is a loss of skin adnexa from either thermal, direct, or irradiation injuries, heal slowly or incompletely following abrasive therapy. The same, of course, holds true for regions of the body such as the eyelids, the skin of the lower anterior neck, the inner aspect of the arm, the dorsum of the hand, and other areas relatively deficient in pilosebaceous adnexa. The risk of delayed healing and/or increased scarring is higher in such regions.

OPERATIVE PROCEDURE

The author prefers general anesthesia for all but the most minor dermabrasion procedures. The use of topical sprays and local anesthesia infiltration has proved to be lacking in sufficient anesthetic effect and thus frequently leads to a compromise in the extent of procedure performed because of patient discomfort.

The depths of the pits can be pinpointed by application of ink, Bonney's blue, or gentian violet dye so as to be readily visible following dermabrasion if complete obliteration of the depths of the sulci has not been achieved. However, the depth of abrasion is best confined to superficial or intermediate thickness, as abrasion to deeper levels may result in hypertrophic scarring and increase the likelihood of irregular pigmentation. Therefore, it is the author's preference to reabrade on one or two occasions rather than to attempt to obliterate the scar irregularities completely at a single session. A rest period between abrasions of three to six months is sufficient for the skin to return to more or less normal activity and for pigmentation to approach normal.

Hemostasis is achieved by the application of gauze sponges soaked in 1:50,000 epinephrine solution or topical thrombin. Final hemostasis is achieved by blowing warm air from a hairdryer over the dermabraded area. This helps not only with hemostasis but with the formation of a dressing eschar as well.

A thick paste of topical thrombin mixed with saline also aids in promoting an early eschar across the abraded area. The author does not routinely apply dressings.

POSTOPERATIVE CARE

Patients are discharged on the day following dermabrasion and are instructed to use the hairdryer daily to dry all exudate and maintain the eschar. On the sixth or seventh day, the patient applies a generous layer of cold cream or vegetable oil to the eschar. These applications, performed several times daily, begin the separation of the coagulum. The patient is told not to peel the coagulum from the abraded area forcibly except in hairy regions.

Exposure to direct or reflected sunlight must be avoided for at least six months following treatment, so an effective sun screen must be properly applied during this period. In patients in whom full pigmentary return has not occurred by this time, use of sun screen should be even more prolonged.

In the rare instance in which hyperpigmentation occurs, it usually undergoes spontaneous regression over a period of 3 to 18 months. When regression does not occur, secondary chemabrasion may help to establish uniform color match. In the author's experience, most problems of hyperpigmentation or irregular pigmentation have been associated wtih excessive exposure to actinic radiation.

DERMABRASION WITH CHEMABRASION

Because it is often necessary to dermabrade the periphery of an acne-scarred area, carrying the abrasive therapy into the thinner and frequently uninvolved skin of the infraorbital, lateral nasal, temporal, or submandibular area in order to secure an acceptable color match and avoid demarcation lines, Spira (1977) suggests a combination of dermabrasion for scarred areas and chemabrasion for thin, uninvolved border areas. First, the area to be chemabraded is peeled in the usual manner.

The phenol solution is applied well into the areas of scarring to insure a good overlap between the peeled area and the dermatome excision site. Then several strips of split-skin graft are removed using a Davol disposable-head, battery-powered dermatome and carefully planing parallel to the lines of least skin tension. In areas of deepest scarring, two or even three successive grafts may be removed from the same site. The peeled areas are then covered with waterproof tape, and a fine, mesh gauze, impregnated with antibiotic ointment, is placed over the dermabraded regions. A bulky, saline-moistened gauze roll dressing is used as an overlay, held in place with a light elastic bandage. The following day, with the patient under heavy premedication, all tape, fine mesh gauze, and gauze roll are removed. Warm air from a hair-dryer is then used to encourage drying of the superficial eschar, and antibiotic ointment is applied to the dried eschar twice daily.

(For references, see page 860.)

Chapter 28

Mentoplasty

RICHARD J. COBURN, D.M.D., M.D.
THOMAS D. REES, M.D., F.A.C.S.
SIDNEY HOROWITZ, D.D.S.

The basic facial contour is genetically determined. Intrauterine birth and postnatal trauma can of course act to modify hereditary intentions. In a like manner, the surgeon can intervene if genetics and/or physical forces have resulted in facial imbalance or disharmony. The scope of this chapter will be limited to the mild to moderate deviations in facial contours that are of common concern to the surgeon. The major disjunctures, hypertelorism, midfacial retrusion, or craniofacial dysostoses will not be included. Consideration will be given to mensuration and analysis of the normal and the standard methods for determining the degree of the abnormality. Diagnostic criteria once formulated must then be interpreted in terms of the patient's aesthetic desires and objectives, the fundamentals of all cosmetic surgery.

The concept of facial contouring is the major focus of this text. Recontouring the deformed nose and excising ptotic skin contributes to restoring facial harmony. In the context of this chapter, the surgeon needs to develop the vision and touch of a sculptor. In no other area of aesthetics can one exercise his ability more to envision existing facial dimensions and project a meaningful change. The skill can be natural or learned; the first is easier, but this chapter will help in achieving the latter.

Patient expectations must be the common denominator of any treatment plan. To ignore this and to pursue a sophisticated cephalometric analysis pinpointing major disharmony is courting failure. As in all aesthetic considerations, the initial focus must be on the concern of the patient.

The Framework and Integument of the Face

The chin, the nose, and the forehead are the three important balancing masses of the face. A well proportioned nose cannot reach its fullest aesthetic impact without a chin that is in a proportionate and normal relationship. An understanding of the normal physical balance of these facial structures and of their position to each other are keys to the diagnosis and to the selection of an appropriate operative technique. Many patients seeking rhinoplasty are not aware that a small chin is also contributing to their physical defect and that this also should be corrected in order to achieve the optimal operative result — a balanced face. The role of the chin has been emphasized as a balancing feature of the face by Converse (1950), Millard (1965), González-Ulloa (1968), and others.

Deformities involving the chin are most apparent when normal maxillomandibular and dental relationships are disturbed. Thus, the relationship of the jaws to each other and the occlusion of the upper and lower teeth may contribute importantly to the total appearance of the face. Minor deviations — e.g., a slightly "weak chin" (microgenia) — can often be corrected quite easily by insertion of a prosthetic implant. In contrast, major malrelationships of the jaw such as marked recession (micrognathia, retrognathia) or asymmetry may require corrective bone surgery to improve the skeletal framework. This may involve the upper or lower jaw or both, in order to establish not only an a esthetically acceptable result but also to provide sound occlusion. Such severe deformities may be the result of hypoplasia, hypertrophy, or malposition from developmental or traumatic causes.

Corrective jaw surgery, including the treatment of the small or recessive chin is divided into two main categories: those that can be corrected with camouflaging techniques (implant, onlays) and those requiring major surgery upon the jaws themselves — i.e., osteotomy or bone graft. Most patients present with deformities of the first type.

Only those procedures in which osteotomies on the mandible can be performed without interruption of the dentition, such as horizontal, sagittal, or vertical osteotomy (or ostectomy of the rim of the mandible), will be described, since they are of greatest interest to the aesthetic surgeon. Description of the more complicated techniques can be found in works devoted to reconstructive jaw surgery.

DIAGNOSIS AND TREATMENT PLANNING

ANALYSIS OF THE FACE

The methods readily available to the practicing surgeon for facial analysis are medical photography, dental study models, moulage, and radiographs, including cephalometrics. Add to this the patient's and surgeon's objective analysis, and there is sufficient data to dissect facial disharmony and formulate a treatment plan.

The artist or sculptor looking at the face divides the structure into anatomic thirds: the upper face or brow area, the midface or maxillary region, and the lower face or mandible. Classical proportions suggest equal thirds. Deficiencies in a given area can either be augmented to equal the normal or reduced to achieve a balance. The concept is limited by the availability of tried surgical procedures, but the basic premise is valid for most instances of body disharmony.

Patients with facial imbalance manifested by lip hypertrophy, microgenia, or prognathism will need graduated degrees of facial analysis. An uncomplicated candidate for a chin implant is best evaluated with lateral, three quarter, and full face medical photography. Using the matte finish, a simple augmented sketch of the chin profile line and the full face contour is sufficient to measure patient needs and expectations aesthetically. The prognathic patient, on the other hand, will benefit from the full complement of facial analysis technique.

Radiographs

The aesthetic surgeon is not likely to be prepared to take his own x-rays for analysis. Therefore, the basic films are requested from an interested radiologist or orthodontist. A panoramic view of the teeth or a standard intraoral study is useful to assess the health of the dental structures, the quality and quantity of bony support, and the presence of serious dental pathology. Any signifi-

cant deviations from normal should be corrected before embarking on osteotomies and arch segment mobilization.

Facial harmony and balance involve complex relationships between the hard and soft tissues that are not always easily evaluated either clinically or from photographs. Orthodontists who have a special interest in the dental-skeletal-integumental balance of the lower face have evolved the cephalometric roentgenogram as a diagnostic aid for this purpose.

The technique of cephalometric roentgenography was first described about 40 years ago and is now well standardized. The apparatus consists of two elements: an x-ray source and a head holder. The latter is used to fixate the patient's head by means of ear posts that enter the right and left external auditory meatus for a short distance. The source of radiation is similarly fixed so that the central beam is lined up with the ear posts. Enlargement and distortion are minimized for practical purposes by using a tube-midsagittal plane distance of five feet, which is now standard in cephalometric installations in this country.

The advantage of the cephalogram for the aesthetic surgeon stems from the standardized technique, since the device makes it possible to obtain comparably oriented preoperative and postoperative views of both the hard and soft facial tissues. The widespread use of standardized roentgenography by orthodontists led inevitably to the development of numerous schemes for analysis. Almost all of these are based on measurements of various angles and dimensions of the face and cranium. Although the diagnostic validity of such precise numbers may be questioned, the cephalogram does provide important information regarding the *relative* size and position of various facial structures. In this way, it assists the clinician in making judgments and in evaluating the changes that occur with treatment, whether surgical or orthodontic (Figure 28–1).

Accurate description of the human face has presented a challenge to artists, scientists, and mathematicians for centuries. Attempts to establish basic mathematical or statistical rules for facial aesthetics have all proved inadequate, which is simply a reflection of the variability among individuals that is the rule and not the exception. It is not surprising, therefore, that cephalometric research studies of people with pleasing facial aesthetics (actresses and beauty queens, for example) confirm this observation. In these individuals, the dimensions and angular relations of the hard and soft tissues of the face, as measured on the cephalogram, fall within the ranges previously estab-

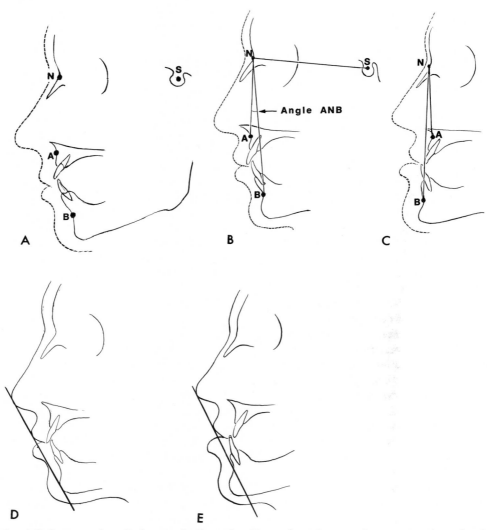

Figure 28–1. *A,* Reference points: S: Center of sella turcica; N: nasofrontal suture; A: most posterior point along junction of maxillary basal bone and alveolar process; B: most posterior point along junction of alveolar process and mandibular basal bone.

B, Reference planes: S-N: Plane through sella turcica and nasion; N-A: Plane through nasion and most posterior point along maxillary alveolus; N-B; plane through nasion and most posterior point along mandibular alveolus; Angle ANB: angle developed between planes N-A and N-B, normal range being 5 to −2 degrees.

C, Reverse, or minus, angle in prognathism of the mandible.

D, The esthetic line, a plane between the nasal tip and the upper lip, passes on or near pogonion, the most anterior bony chin point, when the lower and middle face are balanced.

E, The esthetic line falls behind pogonion in a prognathism.

lished as population norms, but they show wide variability. It is apparent that even the most pleasing examples of facial harmony involve skeletal and integumental relationships that cannot be conveniently and simply reduced to average measurements that have any clinically useful meaning in diagnosis and treatment planning.

Soft Tissue Balance

The cephalometric x-ray is particularly helpful in visualizing relationships between the skeletal framework and three curves within the facial profile that are of the greatest significance esthetically.

Calvin Case, a physician turned orthodontist, described these facial curves in detail in his textbook published in 1921, and little needs to be added to his observations (Figure 28–2).

The lowest curve of the face shapes the character of the chin and should form (as Case said) a "graceful and concurve" arc from the chin to the border of the lower lip with the profile in repose. Below the nose, the curve of the upper lip should be slightly concave, "gracefully curving with a light deepening of the naso-labial lines where it joins the cheek." The uppermost curve in the facial profile, the frontonasal, is as important as this lower curve. It is essential to recognize that the facial curves described by Case occur normally when the lips are

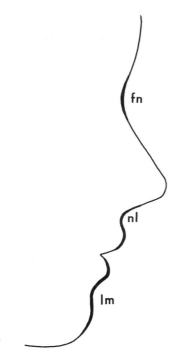

Figure 28–2. Curves of the face (after C. S. Case, see text): *fn*—frontonasal; *nl*—nasolabial; *lm*—labiomental.

closed with ease *in repose* and that the mandible is in "rest" position; i.e., with some distance between the upper and lower jaws so that the teeth are *not* in contact. Under normal conditions, therefore, the features are in unconscious repose when the lips are closed and the teeth are slightly apart. In a well balanced face, the lips thus close without strain, and the curves of the face are neither abnormally deep nor straight.

The drapery of the facial musculature of the lower one third of the face also controls lip seal (lip competency). Rest position is established relatively early and involves not only the masticatory musculature but the muscles of facial expression as well (Ballard, 1967). The orofacial pattern is characteristic of the individual and, under normal conditions, it is instinctive for each individual to produce a lip seal of the soft tissues around the mouth in the rest position. If this does *not* occur, adaptive postures are used and the muscles around the mouth are almost continually contracted and maintained in that position in order to accomplish lip seal. *Competent* lip posture implies adequate lip seal, with the lips able to contact one another without strain when the mandible is in rest position. *Incompetent* lip posture occurs when the lips are unable to form an adequate seal under similar unstrained conditions (Figure 28–3). Most importantly, competent lip posture is functionally related to the soft tissue contour of the chin. Attempts to achieve adequate lip seal when there is lip incompetency often result in unsightly strain of the perioral musculature (Figure 28–4).

Cephalometric and Occlusal Analysis

A cephalogram is taken to assess the relationship of the mandibular basal bone to the maxilla. To achieve this, a soft tissue outline must be incorporated in the cephalometric technique as described. The considerable attention focused on the cephalogram is justified, since this parameter, in conjunction with the dental study models, permits simultaneous manipulation of function and aesthetics. Thus, a balance can be sought between the optimal occlusal alignment that will yield the maximal correction of facial contour.

Cryptic cephalometric formulas, although impressive in growth and development studies, have not proved meaningful in the management of facial deformity. The twofold purpose of analysis, the study of basal bone relationships and mensuration, can be obtained with a minimum of geometric tracing. Our cephalometric analysis is determined by construction of standard reference planes and angles. The sella-nasion plane is used to identify the stable cranial base. The lines Na and Nb permit calculation of angles SNA and SNB (see Figure

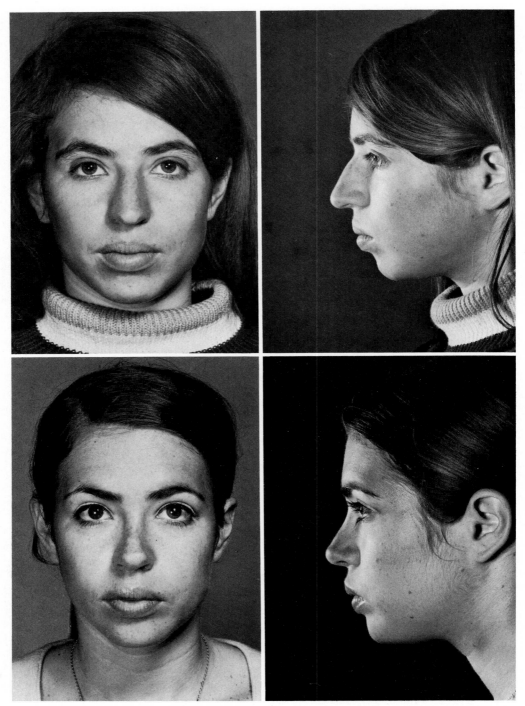

Figure 28–3. Protrusion of the lips is often caused by bimaxillary protrusion of the teeth or macrocheilia, or both. Chin augmentation cannot alter either of these basic deformities, but it can soften the effect and promote an altogether more pleasant facial appearance. This patient demonstrates the marked improvement that can be effected by augmentation mentoplasty combined with rhinoplasty in the presence of bimaxillary protrusion.

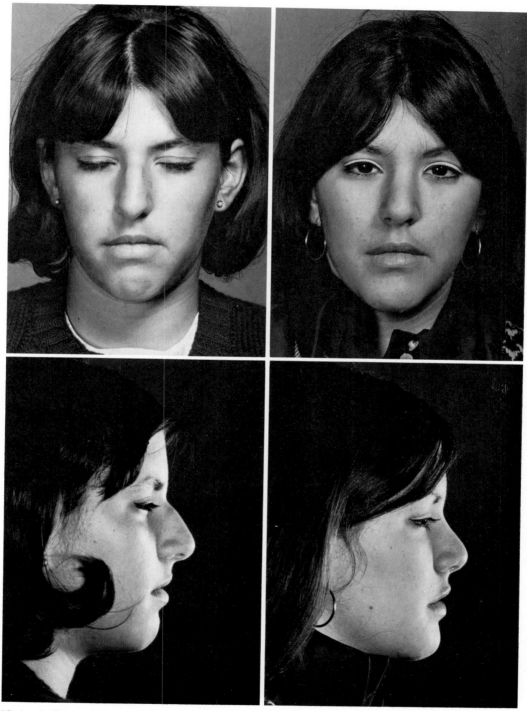

Figure 28–4.   A silicone chin implant in this young lady successfully eliminated unsightly wrinkling or bunching of the muscle mass anterior to the mentum, at the same time achieving a slight but effective augmentation of the chin. The muscle mass at the front of the chin is a complicated interlacing network, and its action can be cosmetically unattractive. Making the pocket for an implant and stripping the soft tissue mass and periosteum from the anterior mandible, as well as positioning the implant itself, seems to eliminate or at least ameliorate this problem in most patients.

28–1). The difference between the two, the ANB angle, is a measure of the basal bone alignment and is used to confirm the diagnosis of a prognathism. A negative value of ANB (SNA−SNB) is characteristic of the prognathic deformity. To eliminate underdevelopment or retrusion of the maxilla as in a relative prognathism conclusively, one further observation is required: the value of SNA and SNB must be compared with the norms.

A final adjunct is the Panorex radiograph or complete set of dental films. These are used to exclude nonassociated pathology, to locate the level of the mandibular canal, and to appreciate the bony configuration of the mandibular rami. It is axiomatic that dental caries, periodontal disease, and related oral pathology be stabilized prior to operation.

Evaluating the Cephalogram. Reference points and lines useful in basic cephalometrics are detailed in Table 28–1. To analyze, fix the radiograph on a viewing box, cover with thin tracing paper, and plot the following points — (N-)nasion, the most anterior point on the nasofrontal suture; (A) the most posterior or the deepest point along the maxillary alveolar process; (B) the most posterior point along the mandible and alveolar process; (S) center of sella turcica. With a compass, measure angles SNA, SNB, and ANB. Referring to Table 28–1 for norms, it is easy to define the mandible and maxilla in relation to each other and the cranial base. A negative angle suggests a prognathism. If doubt exists after routine cephalometric tracing, a more detailed study can be undertaken using a number of standard texts.

Nonmetric techniques for using the cephalogram depend upon the evaluation of relationships between the underlying skeletal and dental structures and the integument that are judged subjectively. Despite the subjectivity involved, these methods have been helpful in (1) rapid evaluation of the initial discrepancy and (2) stimulating pro-file changes that might result from surgical-orthodontic procedures. The cephalogram also makes it possible to evaluate the surgical result objectively by comparison of the preoperative and postoperative films.

Cut-Out Technique

This technique is particularly useful in evaluating nose-chin balance and in determining the site and extent of change required for improvement (Figure 28–5). When the maxillary anterior teeth are protrusive, for example, the chin may appear underdeveloped. Two possible treatment strategies for changing the profile must be considered in such cases: surgical-orthodontic setback of the anterior maxillary dentoalveolar segment or advancement of the chin point by implant or by horizontal osteotomy. In either instance, the anticipated result can be reasonably predicted by (1) moving the maxillary cutout posteriorly or (2) moving the mandibular cutout anteriorly. The appearance of many such patients may also be improved by routine orthodontic therapy.

FACIAL PLANE

When the curves of the lower face are distorted in an attempt to obtain lip seal over a procumbent upper and lower dentition, the "facial plane" used by orthodontists is an excellent guide in planning treatment. In these conditions, "bimaxillary protrusion," the chin also appears to be underdeveloped because of the facial convexity.

The facial plane connects the points *nasion* — the most anterior point on the x-ray outline of the frontonasal suture — and *pogonion* — the most anterior point on the mental symphysis (Figure 28–6). In faces with acceptable dentofacial balance, this line usually intersects (or closely approximates) the outline of the lower central incisor crown.

The process of constructing this line is reversed in bimaxillary protrusion cases in order to obtain a guide to the amount of chin advancement required; that is, a line is drawn on the cephalogram tracing from *nasion through the lower incisor crown outline*. The line indicates the new position of the *pogonion* point that will provide an aesthetically satisfactory lower face contour, and the result may be achieved either by horizontal osteotomy with chin point advancement or, in less severe cases, with an implant.

Dental Models

The use of plaster models, long thought to be the prerogative only of the dentally oriented, should be familiar to aesthetic surgeons interested

TABLE 28–1. CEPHALOGRAM NORMS
NORTHWESTERN ANALYSIS*

Angle	Adult Measurement (degrees)	Standard Deviation
SNA	82.01	3.89
SNB	79.97	3.60
ANB (relation of maxilla to mandible)	+2.04	1.81

*Riedel, R.: The relation of maxillary structures to cranium in malocclusion and in normal occlusion. Am. J. Orthod. 22:142, 1952.

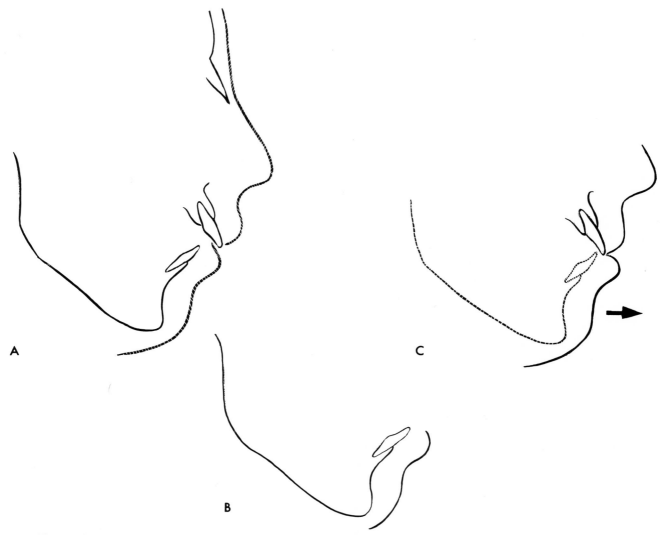

Figure 28–5. The cutout technique in cephalometric evaluation. *A,* The original cephalometric tracing of a patient with maxillary protrusion. *B,* Cutout tracing of the mandible. *C,* The cutout moved anteriorly into correct occlusal relationship, showing the hypothetical improvement in soft tissue contour to be expected as the result of chin point advancement.

Illustration continued on the following page.

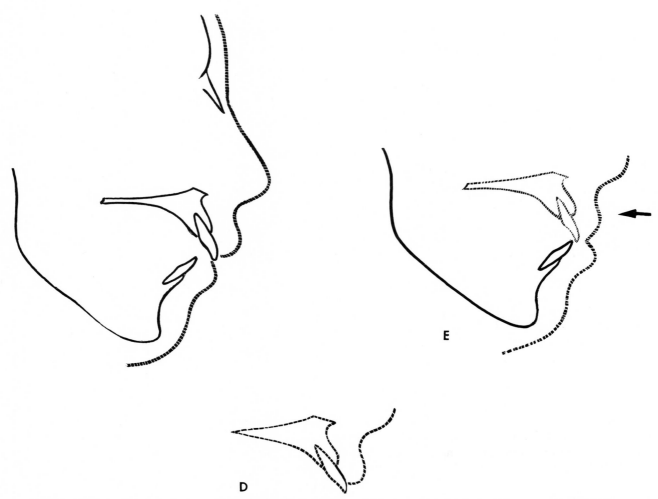

Figure 28–5 *Continued.*   *D,* Cutout tracing of the maxilla. *E,* The cutout moved posteriorly into the correct occlusal relationship, again showing the hypothetical improvement that could be achieved by anterior maxillary dentoalveolar setback.

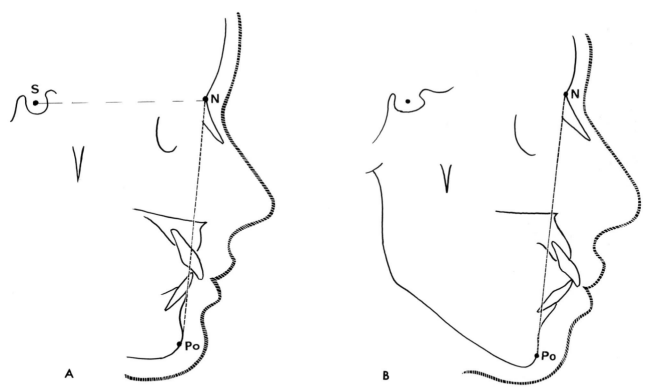

Figure 28–6. The facial plane. A line drawn on the cephalometric tracing connecting the points marked *N* ("nasion") and *Po* ("pogonion") usually intersects the crown outline of the lower incisors in a well-balanced face (*A*). When the dentoalveolar area is procumbent relative to other facial structures (that is, when there is bimaxillary protrusion), the lower third of the face appears convex in profile and the facial plane falls posterior to the lower incisor crown outline (*B*).

in jaw contouring. The mechanics of taking impressions are simple. Obtain from a dental supply house a mixing bowl, a spatula, impression materials, a set of impression trays, white plaster, and model formers (Fig. 28–7). Select an impression tray that fits the arch; they can be bent slightly to conform to minor irregularities. Mix the impression materials following instructions, work rapidly, fill the tray to three quarters full, and insert it into the mouth. Remove it in approximately 90 seconds or when it has hardened to touch. Pour the plaster immediately, using a thin mix, and vibrate to remove trapped air. Undertake a second mix for a base and use the rubber molds.

Models have three main uses: they provide a permanent record of the unoperated occlusion, they act as a final guide to the patient's occlusion (i.e., the relationship of the maxillary to the mandibular teeth), and they serve as a workbench for planning tooth removal and movement in jaw repositioning. Basic occlusal relationships are described in terms of the relationship between the first upper and lower molars. An Angle Class I relationship exists when the mesial buccal cusp of the maxillary first molar rests in the buccal

groove of the mandibular tooth. This mesial buccal cusp is forward in a Class II relationship and back in a Class III relationship. (These categories are explained later in this chapter.) These basic positions are then subdivided by crossbites in which a segment of the lower arch may be shifted to fall inside or outside its normal relation to the opposite arch. For example, the upper right molars may be displaced towards the palate. This disharmony is called a right maxillary posterior lingual crossbite. Another important occlusal characteristic obtained from the models is the degree of overbite and overjet of the anterior teeth. These distances can be measured in millimeters.

The measurements derived from the cephalometric tracing are tested on the dental study models. Casts are obtained by taking an alginate impression of the dental arches and pouring in plaster. A bite registration is recorded in soft wax and the models are articulated, preferably on a simple articulator or by hand.

The models are used to identify associated malocclusions, particularly an anterior open bite that might only be aggravated by indiscriminate surgery. Gross malalignments or disproportionate

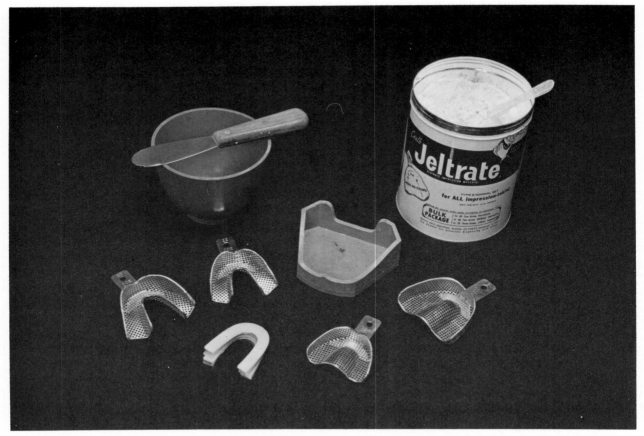

Figure 28–7.   The equipment necessary for taking and pouring impressions; obtainable from any dental supply house.

occlusal planes should be treated orthodontically prior to surgery. Minor single tooth and cuspal irregularities can be ground into occlusion, but severe disharmony warrants an orthodontic evaluation.

The dental casts are duplicated and the working models are juggled into a posterior occlusion where cuspal interdigitation is maximal (Figure 28–8). To facilitate this registration, the mandibular model is sectioned across the base, worked into the proposed articulation and fixed with soft wax. If the models are accurately trimmed, the amount of displacement can be directly measured. The millimeters of bony recession permitted for functional occlusion can then be compared with that required to improve the soft tissue profile. Usually a balance between the two is adopted, and satisfactory aesthetic and functional results can be anticipated. Nevertheless, an occasional patient with marked prognathism, or prognathism in conjunction with macrogenia, is found, and despite well planned mathematical correction of the malocclusion, a chin prominence persists. This is best appreciated on the working cephalogram using the profile analysis and must be anticipated preoperatively so that the patient may be forewarned that subsequent genioplasty may be required to realize complete correction.

With the discovery of a reasonably functional occlusion on the study models, areas of obvious cuspal interference are identified and ground out preoperatively in the mouth to permit the establishment of a stable occlusion at surgery. Fixation is thereby facilitated and maintained. Postoperative adjustments are routine, but skilled planning before operation will reduce needless sacrifice of tooth structure. When a body osteotomy is planned, the models are sectioned to determine the limits of bony excision required for correction. Teeth in the lines of resection are similarly removed. Templates, fashioned to duplicate the desired excision, are useful intraorally in mapping the osteotomy lines.

Using the dental models as a planning board involves the secondary preparation of working models. Repeat the described impression technique, but on the original model, and pour in a soft stone obtained from the dental supply house. With a hand plaster saw, an alcohol burner, and soft wax also obtained from the supply house, the models

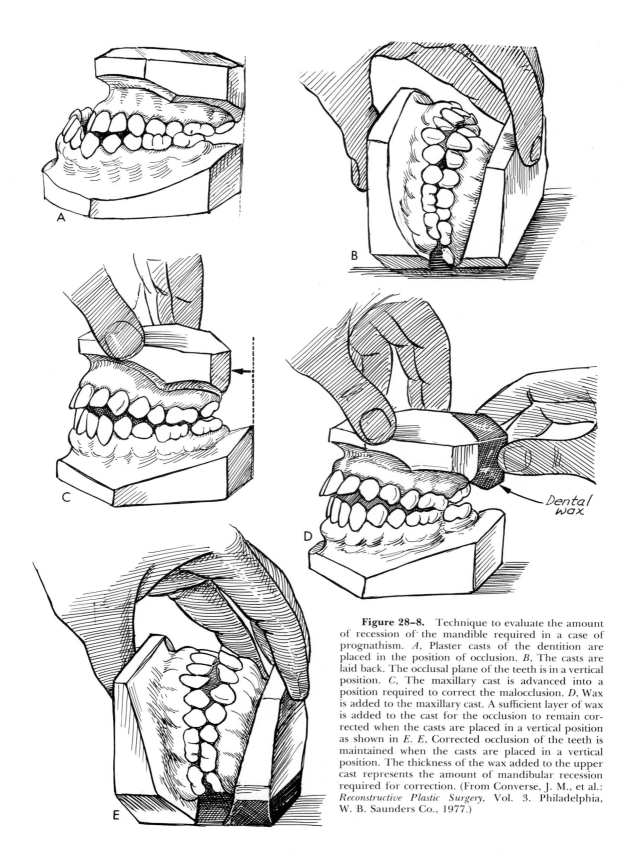

Figure 28–8. Technique to evaluate the amount of recession of the mandible required in a case of prognathism. *A*, Plaster casts of the dentition are placed in the position of occlusion. *B*, The casts are laid back. The occlusal plane of the teeth is in a vertical position. *C*, The maxillary cast is advanced into a position required to correct the malocclusion. *D*, Wax is added to the maxillary cast. A sufficient layer of wax is added to the cast for the occlusion to remain corrected when the casts are placed in a vertical position as shown in *E*. *E*, Corrected occlusion of the teeth is maintained when the casts are placed in a vertical position. The thickness of the wax added to the upper cast represents the amount of mandibular recession required for correction. (From Converse, J. M., et al.: *Reconstructive Plastic Surgery*, Vol. 3. Philadelphia, W. B. Saunders Co., 1977.)

are then cut to plan the approximate tooth removal or bone graft to achieve the desired reduction or lengthening. The wax is melted and used to reassemble the divided models. Lastly, the original models are kept as a permanent preoperative patient record.

Medical Photography. The standard 5″ x 7″ black and white glossy and matte finished photographs are the most useful of all the mensuration methods available to the plastic surgeon — not because of their degree of sophistication but because as aesthetic surgeons, we are most familiar with their use. It also gives us maximal insight into what looks aesthetically pleasing. To add and subtract contours on the matte finished photograph is also the most effective form of patient education.

Bimaxillary Protrusion

This common condition involves anterior displacement of the maxillary and mandibular components. It is characterized by an anterior inclination of the incisor teeth, often associated with an open bite. This forward displacement results in unusual bulging and fullness of the lips, a bimaxillary prognathism. It is more common in blacks than in caucasians. The molar teeth are often in Class I occlusion.

Evaluation necessitates the entire spectrum of radiographs, models, and photographs. Working models are used to plan tooth extraction and movement necessary to correct the protrusion bilaterally. If the molars are in a satisfactory relationship, the best approach is a segmental section of the maxilla and mandible. If there is an associated molar disharmony, consideration is given to the previously described procedures for mandibular ramus, body or sagittal osteotomy.

The method of segmental maxillary osteotomy is described under maxillary prognathism. Usually a first or second bicuspid is removed and the segment is moved posteriorly. If there is an associated open bite, it can be relieved by inserting a bone graft between the nasal floor and the mobilized maxillary segment.

The technique of mandibular osteotomy is that of Schuchardt. The anterior mandible is exposed through a Converse degloving procedure. The mental nerve must then be identified. The first premolar is extracted and an osteotomy is developed from this socket inferiorly and anteriorly below the apices of the incisor teeth. The nerve must be protected, since the osteotomy should pass just anterior to the foramen. The maxillary and mandibular segment are retrodisplaced and wired both within and between the arches. The inter-

maxillary fixation can be relaxed at three weeks. The interdental fixation should remain for eight weeks.

The most common complication is mental nerve damage. There will usually be an element of transitory numbness and occasionally it will be permanent, despite maximal efforts to protect the trunk. Recurrence of the protrusion can occur; the risk is minimized by adequate bone resection at surgery and absolute fixation. If a tendency for relapse is noted, the surgeon should check for faulty occlusion and reapply the fixation. Nonunion, infection, bleeding, and tooth loss are reported but are uncommon.

Wedge Removal. One type of bimaxillary protrusion occurs in extremely long faces. The mandible is characteristically deformed in such cases, showing an overdevelopment in height that results in distortion of the labiomental curve. The face must be shortened and the chin point must be advanced to gain profile improvement in these conditions. The facial plane line is again used to determine the new and more prominent position of pogonion, as just described. In addition, a wedge of bone is removed from beneath the tooth roots in order to reduce face height (Figures 28–9 and 28–10).

Prognathism

Mandibular overgrowth is a hereditary condition of low penetrance. It is characterized by an anterior prominence of the jaw both in full face and profile, a Class III malocclusion with an anterior end-on or crossbite and, more rarely, a speech impediment.

When diagnosed early, the orthodontist may be able to guide forward growth of the mandible or at least to mask the occlusal disharmony. Patients 18 or older are candidates for surgery. The condition appears slightly more often in males and in blacks than in caucasians.

The scope of this book does not permit an exhaustive treatise on prognathism. Indeed, it was specifically not the author's purpose to discuss this complicated subject except as it pertains to most aesthetic surgeons; nevertheless, most patients with true prognathism who do not have open bite or strong potential for developing open bite after surgery, as attested by cephalogram, x-ray, and dental casts, can be corrected by one or two current techniques that are quite simple and in wide use. The collaboration of an orthodontist knowledgeable of the diagnostic and surgical planning techniques of jaw surgery is mandatory to good results.

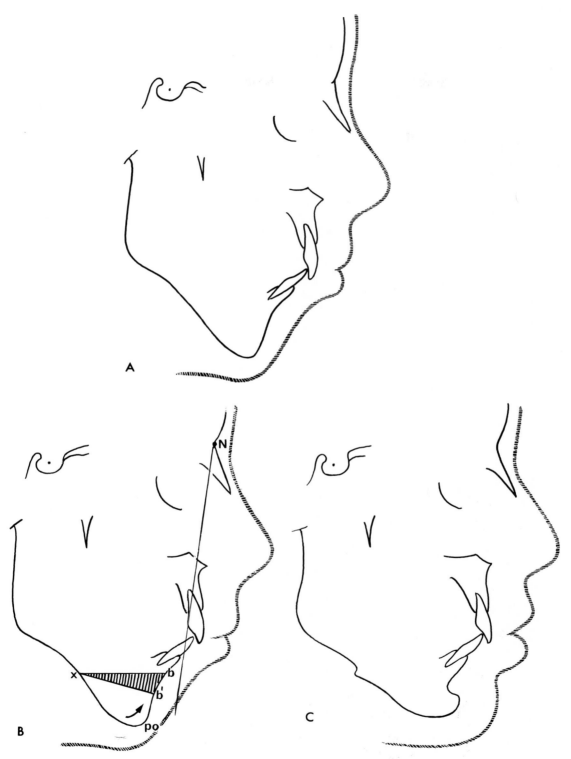

Figure 28–9.   *A*, Preoperative cephalometric tracing of a young woman with bimaxillary protrusion, facial convexity, excessive facial height, and loss of the labiomental curve. *B*, Cephalometric planning involves determination of the facial plane and the desired new position of "pogonion." Wedge removal to reduce facial height involves elimination of the shaded area and elevation of the mobilized fragment. *C*, Postoperative tracing, showing the improvement in soft tissue contour resulting from wedge removal and advancement of "pogonion." Preoperative and postoperative photographs appear in Figure 28–10.

Mandibular prognathism, although seen less frequently than microgenia or maxillary protrusion, requires especially careful attention both in planning and in the surgical correction procedure. In order to understand this deformity fully it is necessary first to describe briefly some intermaxillary relationships as they are classified by orthodontists.

When the teeth make maximal occlusal contact under unstrained conditions, the interdigitation of teeth provides a guide to the *relative* positions of the maxillary and mandibular alveolar arches. Three broad classes of occlusion are categorized as follows: Class I, "normal" maxillomandibular relationship; Class II, the maxillary dentoalveolar arch *relatively* anterior to the mandibular

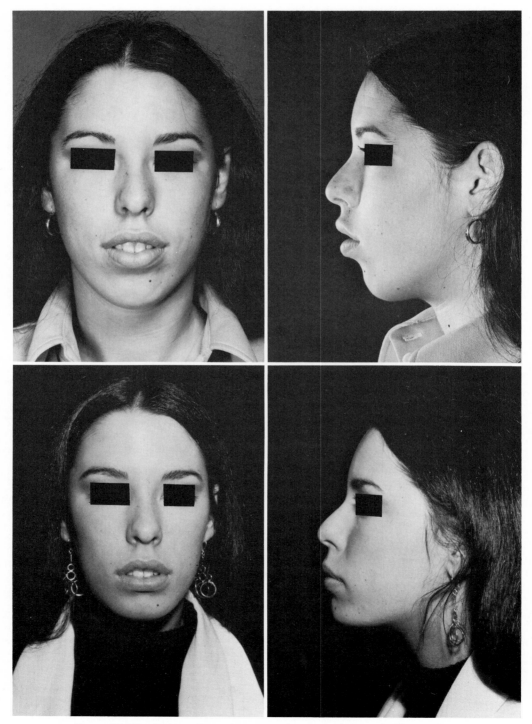

Figure 28–10.   Patient who underwent wedge removal shown in Figure 28–9.

arch; and Class III, the mandibular teeth and alveolar arch *relatively* anterior to the corresponding maxillary structures.

Mandibular prognathism may be defined by two criteria: (1) Class III malocclusion of the teeth and (2) an unsightly appearance of the lower third of the face, with loss of the labiomental curve. It is, therefore, a dentofacial deformity, and although it is possible in many cases to correct the dental malocclusion by orthodontic treatment, aesthetic improvement in facial contours usually requires a combined surgical-orthodontic approach.

Numerous surgical procedures have been proposed for the correction of mandibular prognathism (Converse and associates, 1977) and each has its champions. The surgeon is well advised to master one or two approaches. Indications may suggest one procedure over another, but they are not absolute, and unless the volume of prognathism patients is unusually high, the surgeon's opportunity to master and understand all the available procedures is unlikely.

Clinical Assessment of Prognathism. The surgeon confronted with the Hapsburg jaw (Grabb, 1968) problem must analyze the characteristics of the deformity and select an appropriate operative plan based on this assessment. Some considerations may be resolved in part by clinical inspection. Does the patient indeed suffer a forward overgrowth of the mandible, or is there an associated defect masquerading as a prognathism? Maxillary hypoplasia (or retrusion) often associated with trauma or cleft deformities must be identified to avoid a misdirected operative procedure. Careful clinical observation of the profile, coupled with study of the photographs, will aid in diagnosis and in establishing a treatment plan. Nevertheless, cephalometric and occlusal analyses are mandatory to confirm the diagnosis and to arrive at the correct modality of treatment. A prominent chin secondary to a posteriorly positioned or underdeveloped maxilla is referred to as a relative prognathism.

It is important to determine if the jaw prominence is associated with Class III malocclusion (a true prognathism) or if it is due to an overgrowth of the chin (macrogenia). Such cases are rare, but they do occur. True prognathism connotes an anterior displacement of the mandible in relation to a normally positioned maxilla, with the lower teeth in mesioocclusion to the uppers. The question is resolved by clinical examination of the teeth and alveolar arches and examination of the study models. Pseudoprognathism is a clinically meaningless term referring to cases when patients can bring the lower anterior teeth into end-on occlusion with the maxillary incisors.

When maxillary hypoplasia and macrogenia have been eliminated from the differential diagnosis, it must be determined whether the prognathism is surgically correctable. Mandibular growth should have ceased prior to operative intervention. Failure to await growth maturation invites the possibility of a relapse. A minimum age of 16 can be justified by the evidence that condylar and ramus growth are virtually completed in most patients by this period. Should doubt exist, such guides as bone age, secondary sexual development, and sibling and parent size can be used as a crude index of the remaining growth potential, yet delay could hardly be criticized. We have defined no maximum age limitation, but common sense must prevail in considering patients over 35 years old.

Secondary or associated disease entities must be excluded in an exacting differential diagnosis. The most emphasized and yet the least common is acromegaly. Hemangioma can produce bony overgrowth and occasionally a prognathism; failure to recognize an occult lesion has led to massive hemorrhage at surgery.

FIXATION

INTRA- AND INTERMAXILLARY FIXATION

Osteotomy procedures on the maxilla and mandible usually necessitate intra- and inter-arch fixation. The method selected and the duration depend upon needs, experience, and facilities available. Most contouring procedures on the maxilla or mandible require some form of fixation. The surgeon performing an occasional procedure will be well served by simple Kazanjian loops or arch bars. A surgeon oriented more toward maxillofacial surgery with access to an orthodontist or prosthodontist may elect to use bands or cast splints. The choices available will be discussed.

The simplist fixation is the fashioning of a circumferential loop and twisted bracket using 20 to 24 thousandth orthodontic wire; the figure eight loop is made around the adjacent teeth and a bracket is fashioned. This will serve for short-term fixation but tends to loosen as the wire fatigues and it is noxious to the gingiva.

The most common method of fixation is the arch bar. There are numerous varieties; however, the appliance is wired to the individual tooth using 20 thousandth wire. It serves well for inter- and intra-oral fixation. It can accommodate elastics or wire fixation between the arches and is excellent for use within the arch stabilization. It is also unkind to the gingiva, and the circumdental wires will need tightening periodically.

Orthodontic bands and the new spot brackets are excellent means of intermaxillary fixation. They can also be used to attach an arch bar for intra-arch immobilization. They are more time consuming to prepare and generally require the services of an orthodontist. The new spot welded brackets are infinitely simpler to apply than the old bands. Both are well tolerated by the gingiva.

Acrylic and cast splints are very useful in intra-arch fixation. They require precise preparation and planning. The splints must be prepared from working dental models, and at surgery, the planned occlusion must be accurately obtained. This forces the surgeon to think of occlusion as well as aesthetics. Acrylic and cast splints are also very kind to the gingival tissues.

The selected method of fixation is not as critical as excellent skill in mastering whichever technique is chosen. Therefore, select a procedure with which you are comfortable and avoid trying each new appliance that is presented.

VERTICAL OSTEOTOMY OF THE RAMUS

This procedure, advocated by many, can be employed in most prognathic patients and is the single most useful procedure for the plastic surgeon. It is contraindicated for an open bite. It is distinguished by the opportunity it affords to alter the gonial angle and thereby improve the contour of the lateral profile. It permits unrestricted exposure and avoids wound contamination by oral flora. The ramus mandibularis of the seventh nerve must be carefully protected; otherwise, few anatomic structures are jeopardized.

Under general nasotracheal anesthesia, an incision is begun just below the gonial angle in a prominent skin fold (Figure 28–11). With experience, a wound of 2 to 3 cm will suffice. The dissection is carried bluntly upward and medially to expose the lower border and angle of the mandible. The lip is observed throughout this phase, as proximity to the mandibular branch of the seventh nerve will be signaled by muscular twitching at the commissure. A nerve stimulator is most useful in identifying possible nerve branches. The periosteum at the angle is scored, and with a curved 2 cm periosteal elevator, the masseter is freed along the lateral ramus from the sigmoid notch posteriorly, anterior dissection being unwarranted. The posterior border is freed and the medial pterygoid is similarly elevated to the notch. Dissection here is confined to the posterior medial ramus to avoid injuring the dental nerve and vessels. A hook is next placed in the sigmoid notch and the line of resection, extending from the notch 1 cm anterior to the angle, is plotted. Using the hook as a guide, the osteotomy line is scored with a tapered bur. The resection is completed using the bur for the outer two thirds and a saw for the medial plate.

A similar procedure is performed on the opposite side and the mandible is displaced posteriorly. It is critical to position the posterior fragment to achieve an overlap with the anterior fragment on the lateral side; the pull of the lateral pterygoid will then insure firm bony contact. The wounds are closed with fine sutures; intermaxillary fixation, usually accomplished with ligatures through edgewise arch appliances, is secured and maintained for eight weeks (Figures 28–12 through 28–14).

Other more complicated procedures for the treatment of prognathism are described in standard textbooks. (Converse, 1977).

SAGITTAL SPLIT

This method advocated, modified and reintroduced by Obwegeser (1957) can be used in all cases of prognathism, except those in which alterations of the gonial angle is desired. Advantages include exposure and preservation of the inferior

Text continued on page 791.

Figure 28–11. The technique of vertical osteotomy for correction of prognathism. *A,* A small incision is made in a natural neck crease below the angle of the jaw. *B* and *C,* Dissection is carried down to the inferior margin of the mandible at the angle. A nerve stimulator is employed. The periosteum is incised and elevated. *D,* A fiberoptic retractor is an invaluable aid in any such tunnelling procedure. *E,* The osteotomy is performed with an oscillating saw, aided by an air drill and osteotomes. *F,* The bone is cut posterior to the entrance of the neurovascular bundle (the lingula). *G,* The anterior fragments are retropositioned and placed medial to the posterior fragments in order to prevent medial displacement as a result of the action of the pterygoid muscles. *H,* The final position of the jaws; immobilization is by intermaxillary fixation, and the bone fragments themselves are not wired.

See illustration on the opposite page.

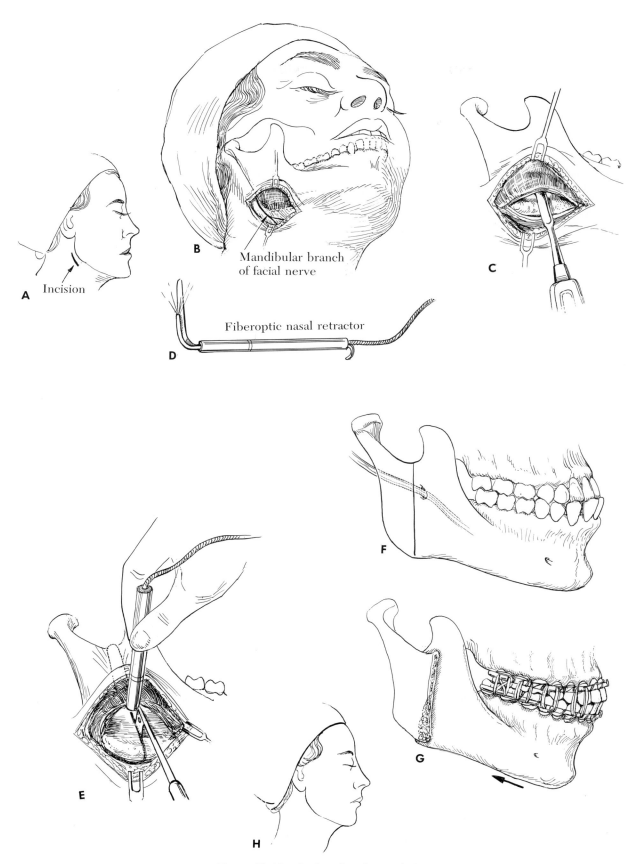

A Incision

B Mandibular branch
of facial nerve

C

D Fiberoptic nasal retractor

E

F

G

H

Figure 28–11. *See legend on the opposite page.*

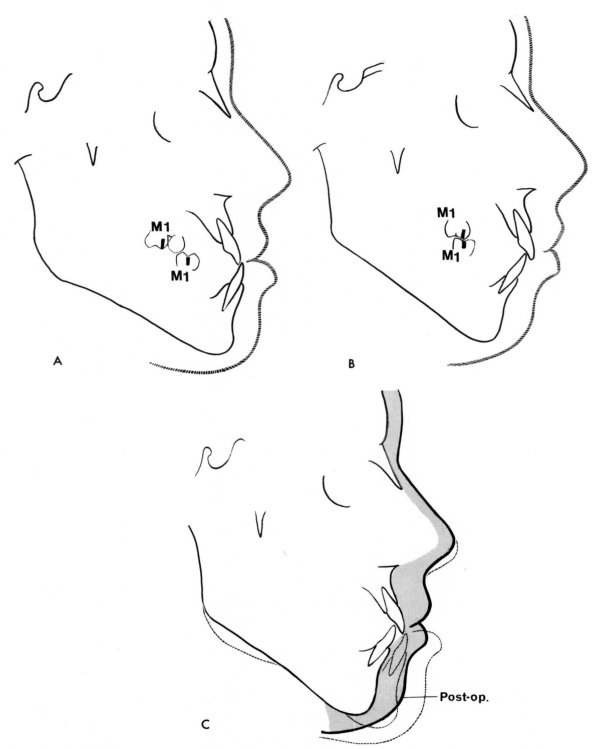

Figure 28–12. Results of vertical osteotomy; *A*, Preoperative cephalogram tracing, showing typical prognathism with loss of the labiomental curve and Class III (Angle) malocclusion. Note the position of the molars (M_1). *B*, Postoperative cephalogram. *C*, Superimposed cephalograms, showing advancement of the bone and soft tissues. Preoperative and postoperative photographs are shown in Figure 28–13.

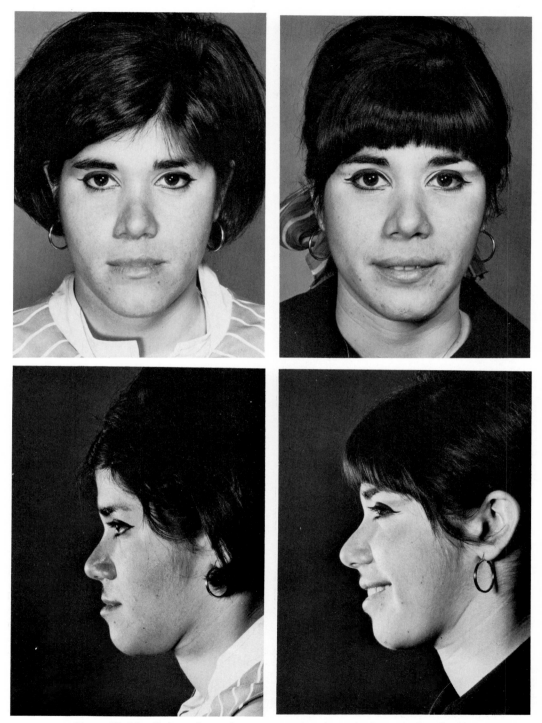

Figure 28–13.   Patient who underwent operation shown in the preceding figure.

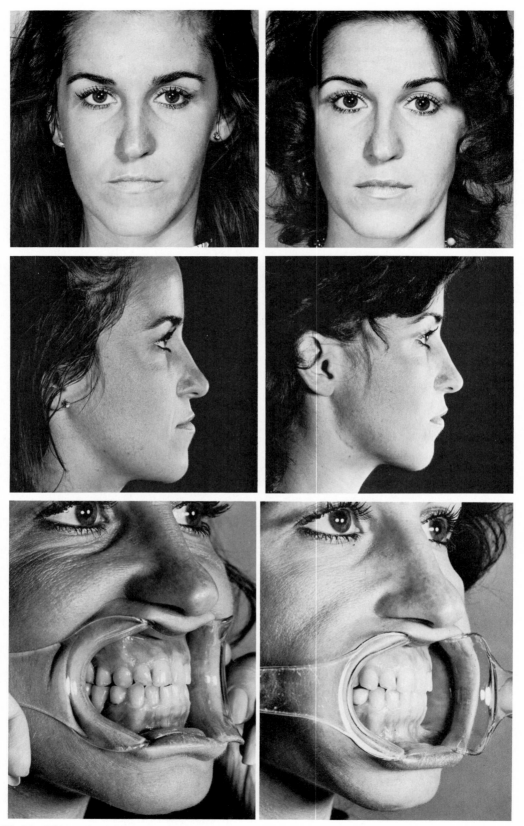

Figure 28–14. This patient's photographs demonstrate the subtle but effective change in facial appearance that can result from even a slight retropositioning of the mandible after vertical osteotomy. In this patient the mandible was moved back only about 3 mm, according to the tracing and as evidenced by the occlusion photographs, but the facial appearance was markedly softened and improved.

alveolar nerve, absence of an external scar, sparing of the mandibular branch of the seventh nerve, and the opportunity for maximal bony contact following retrodisplacement.

The procedure as performed by Obwegeser is begun under general anesthesia with nasal intubation. An intraoral incision is made along the anterior border of the ramus and extends from the level of the maxillary tuberosity forward to the bicuspid region of the buccal sulcus (Figure 28–15 and 28–16). The masseter and internal pterygoid muscles are reflected from the ramus with a flat periosteal elevator. An angular elevator is used to free the muscular and ligamentous attachments along the posterior border. The linguala is exposed and, using a curve channel retractor, the soft tissues and dental nerve are displaced medially while a flame bur is then used to score the anterior medial bony cortex just above the mandibular foramen. With this improved exposure, a straight bur is then used to deepen the initial groove through the medial cortex. Next, a vertical cut is fashioned through the lateral plate of the mandibular body opposite the second molar. The two cuts are then joined and the split is completed with the gentle tap of a straight splitting osteotome. The dental nerve is readily exposed and protected by the periosteum. It usually separates with the medial fragment. The procedure is duplicated on the opposite side and the jaw is retruded into the new occlusion. A buried circumferential wire is introduced externally at the angle with an awl and the excess buccal bone of the lateral fragment, the overlap, is excised. Intermaxillary fixation is obtained by passing wire ligatures through the previously placed Obwegeser continuous loops. Fixation is maintained for six to eight weeks.

Complications are infrequent but include recurrence of the prognathism, bleeding from the pterygoid plexus or internal maxillary vessels, nerve entrapment, and, more rarely, infection.

OSTEOTOMY OF THE MANDIBULAR BODY

The procedure described by Dingman and modified by Converse and others is particularly indicated in patients with anterior open bites or missing teeth in the molar or premolar region. Because the edentulous areas permit osteotomy without sacrificing teeth, advocates of the procedure also champion the simplicity, the opportunity to modify localized anterior or lateral crossbites, and the absence of visible scarring. It is least disturbing to the masticatory musculature and in this regard may be less susceptible to relapse.

The intraoral approach is made through an L-shaped incision in the buccal mucosa extending from the mandibular canine posteriorly and inferiorly, and a distally based subperiosteal flap is elevated. The dissection is continued in the area of the proposed osteotomy, either an edentulous space or through the socket of a previously extracted bicuspid or molar, to expose the inferior border of the mandible. With a straight bur, a step osteotomy is performed in the lateral plate and carried across the lower border. The direction of the step is fashioned to permit the upward muscular pull on the posterior fragment to assist in abutting the anterior segment. Predetermined models depicting the bony excision are needed in plotting the lines of osteotomy. On the lingual side, a simple tunnel is elevated exposing the medial plate, and the osteotomy is completed. Final separation is accomplished with an osteotome with regard for the dental nerve. The bone wedge is removed and the procedure is repeated contralaterally. The mandible is displaced posteriorly and fixed in the previously programmed occlusion with both interosseous wires and intermaxillary fixation for eight weeks.

Several variations of the procedure have been described, including a combined intraoral and extraoral approach and an external submandibular technique. The use of local anesthesia has also been advocated. The osteotomy may be stepped as described or straight. The first, although more demanding, provides a firmer wedge of bone.

The most frequent complication is trauma to the dental nerve, but fortunately, spontaneous repair nearly always ensues. Transient hypoesthesia can be minimized by appreciating the level of the mandibular canal on the radiograph and proceeding cautiously with the final split.

Complications

The treatment of prognathism should be accomplished with minimal morbidity. Ambulation, nutrition and freedom from pain can be anticipated within 24 hours. Nevertheless, patients must be well orientated to the possibility of transient hypoesthesia, occasional swelling secondary to hematoma formation, and the general inconvenience of eight weeks or more of intermaxillary fixation.

Hypoesthesia of the mental distribution secondary to the injury of the inferior alveolar nerve results from direct trauma, compression, or

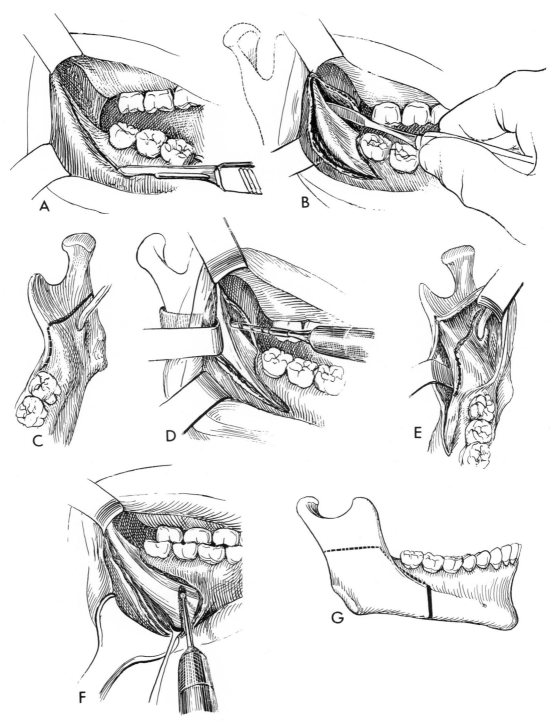

Figure 28–15.   Technique of Obwegeser-Dal Pont sagittal osteotomy of the ramus. *A,* An incision is made along the anterior border of the ramus following the oblique line. *B,* Subperiosteal elevation of both the medial and lateral surfaces is begun. *C,* The medial cortical osteotomy is placed above the level of the mandibular foramen and is continued anteriorly along the oblique line. *D,* Bone can be removed from the medial aspect of the anterior border of the ramus to permit a better view of the lingula and the mandibular foramen region. The Lindemann spiral bur cuts the medial cortex above the foramen. *E,* The medial section of the cortex is completed. *F,* A vertical cut through the lateral cortex in the region of the second molar tooth is made with a small round bur. *G,* The cortical line of section is indicated by the broken line over the medial aspect of the ramus and along the anterior border. The solid line represents the vertical cut through the lateral cortex of the body of the mandible. (From Converse, J. M., et al.: *Reconstructive Plastic Surgery.* Philadelphia, W. B. Saunders Co., 1977.)

Illustration continued on the opposite page.

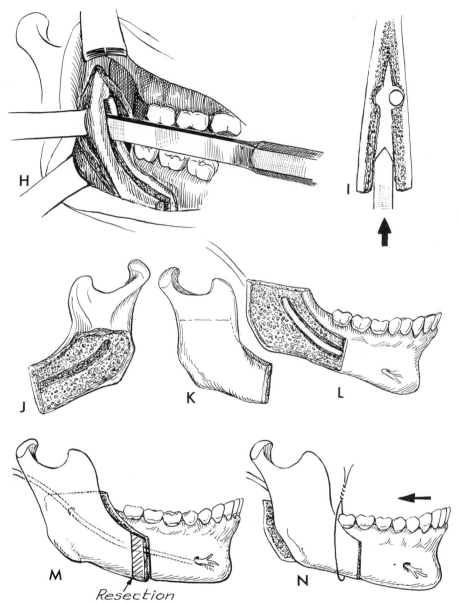

Figure 28–15 *Continued.* H, The sagittal splitting of the ramus is performed with a thick osteotome. I, The thick osteotome also acts as a wedge as it splits the ramus. J, View of the medial aspect of the lateral (condylar) fragment. K, The lateral aspect of the lateral (condylar) fragment. I, The medial (tooth-bearing) fragment. M, Excess bone (shaded area) must be resected from the anterior portion of the lateral fragment to allow for bony apposition after posterior displacement of the tooth-bearing fragment. N, Final position of the tooth-bearing portion of the mandible. A buried circumferential wire around the fragments or an interosseous wire is placed to approximate the fragments. (After Obwegeser, 1957.) (From Converse, J. M., et al.: *Reconstructive Plastic Surgery*, Philadelphia, W. B. Saunders Co., 1977.)

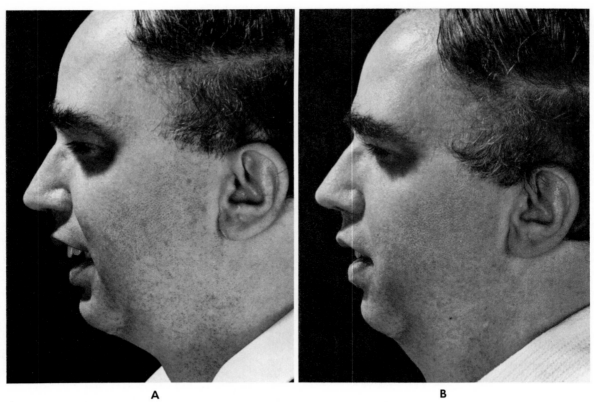

A   **B**

Figure 28–16. *A,* A 39-year-old man with mandibular retrognathia including 10 mm of overjet. Patient underwent an Obwegeser advancement osteotomy. *B,* Correction of occlusal disharmony and improvement in the facial esthetics.

stretching. Functional return varies directly with the degree of insult, but patients can be advised that chin sensibility will be near normal within three months. Longer periods suggest partial or complete interruption, more common with body than with ramus osteotomies.

Delayed hemorrhage with hematoma formation is unusual. Treatment is conservative with maintenance of the compressing dressing, analgesics, and heat as required. Infection, also rare regardless of the approach, is treated with incision, drainage, and appropriate antibiotics.

Nonunion or fibrous union infrequently complicates prognathic surgery. Early removal or mobility of the fixation is the principal cause. In cases in which bony apposition is known to be decreased as a result of the method—the horizontal ramus section being the worst offender—or because the fragments were malpositioned, the fixation should be extended to 10 or even 12 weeks. A fibrous union may be without clinical symptomatology; however, nonunion requires a second course of fixation. Should this fail, reexploration with direct wiring or bone grafting is indicated.

The tendency to revert to the prognathic state is frequently discussed but infrequently observed.

Nevertheless, correction prior to mandibular growth maturation invites this complication. Fortunately, the most minimal shift can be immediately detected by the patient as an occlusal prematurity or shift from centric. Should this occur, a cephalogram is taken for documentation and a chin cap is prescribed for nightwear to maintain the mandible posteriorly. Recurrence, or worse — the development of an anterior open bite — may result from the ramus osteotomy. Two mechanisms are responsible: (1) the pull of the temporalis muscle on the anterior fragment following an oblique or vertical osteotomy may rotate the mandible into an anterior open bite and (2) with all ramus procedures, but particularly the horizontal section, overlapping can occur with resultant shortening of the ramus height. This loss of intermaxillary space, reflected in the molar area, results in an anterior open bite. Treatment of the temporalis pull by resection of the insertion along the anterior ramus and coronoid is reserved for patients with existing anterior open bites who are being corrected by ramus section. Attention to operative technique and selection will minimize this complication, yet it is prudent to employ the body osteotomy in all cases of apterognathia.

CHIN REDUCTION

Correction of macrogenia not in conjunction with prognathism is an uncommon but sometimes rewarding surgical exercise. The operation generally involves major bone recontouring and thereby is associated with measurable morbidity. It is not a casual undertaking.

Patients presenting with macrogenia require an entire battery of analytic tests, excluding the dental study models, to properly evaluate need, expectation, and results. The necessity of ruling out a true prognathism is obvious.

Several surgical methods for chin reduction exist: simple shaving of the bony enlargement, excision of a pie-shaped wedge of bone, the horizontal osteotomy, and an adjustment of the inferior fragment to compensate for isolated deficiencies or excess.

Medical photographs, especially with matte finish, can be useful to fashion a graphic assessment of the surgical objectives for the patient and surgeon. Cephalometric and panorex radiographs will be useful in assessing an associated prognathism and the depth of the tooth roots.

Simple bone contouring with a round bur through a submental approach is limited to minor bony excesses or exostoses. The surgical approach for the local shaving and the horizontal osteotomy begins with a degloving procedure exposing the anterior, inferior, mandibular segment. Extreme caution must be exerted in the area of the mental foramen. Dissection is necessary here to gain maximal exposure. Ideally, the nerve is exposed and protected. Practically speaking, caution is usually sufficient. Inadvertent divisions should be sutured.

Using a reciprocating saw or multiple bur holes, a wedge is resected from the lower segment of the anterior mandible. The inferior portion is then manipulated into position to achieve a desired goal. It can be recessed to minimize anterior mental projections, it can be rotated to improve a hemi-atrophy, or it can be advanced if necessary. Fixation is by internal wire or external pullout wires anchored to the lower anterior teeth.

Postoperatively, a Barton's dressing and soft diet are considered essential for the first 96 hours.

Complications. These include asymmetry, infection, bleeding, and numbness. Temporary numbness is very common, secondary to swelling or traction on the mental nerve. Permanent anesthesia warrants reexploration. Asymmetry is also common, secondary to inadequate immobilization and inability to appreciate subtle soft tissue contours at the surgical table. If significant and persistant, secondary contouring may be indicated. Bleeding and infection are rare.

MANDIBULAR RETROGNATHIA

This deformity is aesthetically and functionally more of a handicap than prognathism, especially in the male. The absence of a strong cervicomental angle weakens the entire lower third of the face. The occlusal relationship resulting from the mandibular retrodisplacement, a Class II malocclusion, with an anterior overbite and overjet often results in an unattractive smile and premature periodontal disease. The normal spill ways and self-cleansing characteristics of a more normal alignment are lost, and the lower anterior teeth are particularly susceptible to early bone loss.

Diagnosis is readily made by clinical observation and an intraoral examination of the occlusal relationship. Confirmation with study models and cephalograms is more for treatment than for diagnosis. A forward displacement of the maxilla on the cranial base could present as a mandibular retrognathia and is ruled out by calculation of the SNA angle.

Formulation of a treatment plan begins with the dental models, photographs, and x-rays. Sketching on the matte finish profile photographs will give some aesthetic index of the required advancement of the anterior chin point. Manipulation of the study models will permit a millimeter estimate of the allowable anterior displacement. A satisfactory occlusion must be found, and this will determine the degree of forward movement. If the allowed occlusal advancement does not appear to correct the aesthetic disharmony, a chin implant, horizontal osteotomy, or maxillary adjustment can be introduced in conjunction with the mandibular surgery. It is an absolute necessity to formulate and present to the patient the final surgical program that will accomplish the required functional and aesthetic improvement. Often, several options should be reviewed so that a mutual decision can be reached. This is very common in dental therapeutics but not in surgery.

Surgical approaches to the mandible have been reviewed in the prognathic section and will only be considered in terms of specific modifications for retrognathia.

Sagittal Split Operation. This versatile procedure permits either forward or backward movement of the mandible once this split is accomplished. Technique is similar to that described for a prognathism. No bone grafting is required, since there is bony contact between the lateral and the medial sections of the ramus.

Vertical or Oblique Osteotomy. The external approach is the same as for the prognathism except that a bone graft from the hip or rib must be inserted into the resulting defect following advancement of the anterior fragment.

Body Osteotomy. This is a little used procedure for advancement, since it would leave a dentureless area in the oral cavity requiring a bridge or prosthesis. The technique is as described except for the necessity of a bone graft.

Complications. Complications are similar to those occurring with prognatic surgery. With the intraoral osteotomy, there is a strong tendency for a relapse. A slight overcorrection is recommended if possible. Careful monitoring and reestablishment of fixation will minimize this tendency when diagnosed.

AUGMENTATION MENTOPLASTY

For many years, while the search for an acceptable prosthetic implant material went on, chin augmentation was accomplished mainly with homologous or autogenous cartilage or bone grafts. Foreign implants were criticized by most plastic surgeons because of their unnatural consistency and tendency to extrude. However, the necessity of obtaining autogenous grafts from the rib cage or the ileum required a second surgical wound, which sometimes was more troublesome to the patient than the operation on the chin itself. Furthermore, it was found that autogenous bone grafts to the chin region had a marked tendency to resorb because of the strong molding forces placed on such grafts by the constant mobility and pressure of the soft tissues. Cartilage grafts particularly, whether autogenous or homologous, tended to absorb or warp. Secondary or tertiary operations on the chin were not uncommon following mentoplasty with bone or cartilage, each succeeding operation becoming more difficult through the scar tissue.

The first prosthetic materials that seemed to have some of the desirable properties for chin augmentation were polyethylene and methylmethacrolate. They were used extensively by Rubin, Robertson, and Shapiro (1948), González-Ulloa and Stevens (1968), and others. Unfortunately, these substances are difficult to fabricate and shape and they require molding and sizing prior to the operative procedure, although minor adjustments may be made at surgery. They are also extremely hard in consistency, a major objection. Although

tissue reaction to polyethylene and acrylic is not excessive, it has become evident that other materials developed subsequently (silicone, Teflon, and Dacron) are better tolerated and generally less reactive.

With the development of the silicone rubber compounds, augmentation mentoplasty became simplified. During the past two decades, the use of such implants for genioplasty has become almost universally accepted. Most of the "die-hard" bone graft and cartilage graft proponents have abandoned these more complicated techniques for the use of alloplasts in simple chin augmentation.

Silicone rubber (Silastic*) is available in several degrees of firmness or as a fine-celled sponge. Carefully carved and shaped silicone implants seem superior to sponge because immediate shaping and sizing is possible. When sponge is used, the final result cannot be assessed for months because of pressure on the implant by the natural fibrous capsule, with subsequent contraction of the sponge.

Millard (1965) pointed out that there are few operations in the field of cosmetic surgery other than genioplasty in which almost 100 percent of the patients are pleased with the results. In his series, 15 percent of patients having rhinoplasty also received chin augmentation. Seventy-five percent of these patients were not directly conscious of the original chin discrepancy, but all of them were pleased with the final chin implant improvement. The author's experience, as well as that of many other surgeons, certainly confirms these findings.

As a general precept, it is unwise for the surgeon to suggest an operation to correct a defect of which the patient is not aware. Chin augmentation is, in our opinion, an exception to this rule. Many patients seeking rhinoplasty are not aware that their chin is small (microgenic) or out of balance with the rest of the face until this fact is pointed out to them. Profile photographs can graphically demonstrate the point, and oriented lateral x-rays (cephalograms) provide further substantiation.

Parents often are aware of a slight "weakness" of the chin in their children but are hesitant to call this fact to the attention of their child or the surgeon. In such instances, it behooves the surgeon to point out that augmentation mentoplasty can be almost as important to the result as is the nasal plastic operation (Figure 28–17). In some instances, an augmentation mentoplasty may supersede the rhinoplasty in importance. Admittedly this occurs in a very small percentage of cases, but

*Product of Dow-Corning Corporation.

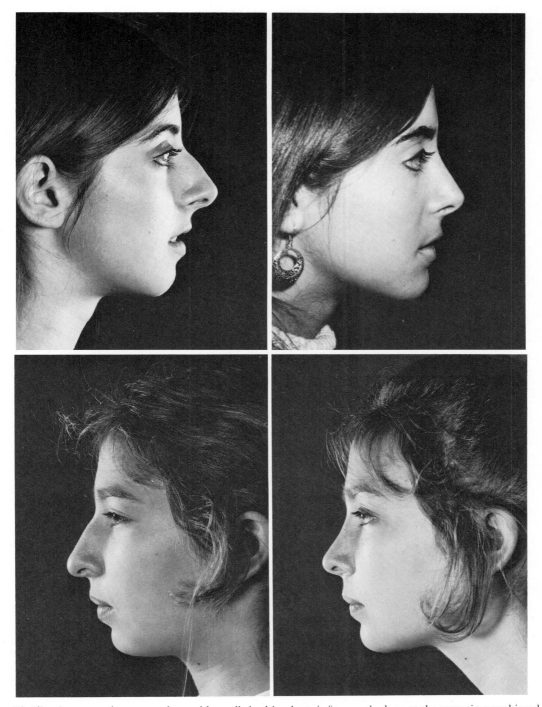

Figure 28–17.   Augmentation mentoplasty with small-sized implants is frequently done at the same time as rhinoplasty. Such implants are easily inserted via the intra-oral approach with little added morbidity. The effect of even such a minor chin build-up is to add measurably to the final result by improving facial balance. Since genioplasty and rhinoplasty are so commonly carried out at the same operation, the surgeon should not hesitate to point out a weak chin to the patient and family during consultation for rhinoplasty. These photographs illustrate typical improvements; note in particular the improvement in lip posture.

the reservation applies in particular to those patients in whom a rhinoplasty might be fraught with problems and unpredictable results.

Whether it is advisable to do the nasal plastic first followed by mentoplasty, or the reverse, depends upon the type and severity of the deformities of the nose and chin. Both procedures are usually done at the same operative session. However, if the chin is markedly underdeveloped or retruded, it is advisable to operate on this structure first since this change in profile may be helpful in guiding the surgeon in planning nasal reduction. Too often, patients are seen who have had simultaneous nasal plastics and chin augmentation in which too much has been removed from the nose and too much added to the chin. This overcorrection of both structures can result in a facial disharmony that is as unbecoming as the original condition.

Horizontal osteotomy and other types of direct bony surgery must be done as a separate operation. Horizontal osteotomy usually requires general anesthesia and a longer operating session. Both factors militate against concomitant rhinoplasty.

The author employs two techniques for mentoplasty. When augmentation with implants is considered the technique of choice, prefabricated, commercially available silicone rubber implants are used. The implants need not impose a specific size or shape upon the surgeon, as they can be trimmed

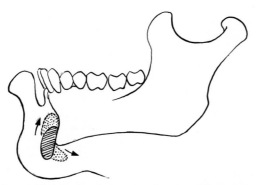

Figure 28–18. Implants must be placed into sockets of exact size over the anterior surface of the mandible, so that displacement and resulting malposition, and sometimes extrusion, cannot occur. It is difficult to increase the length of the chin vertically with prosthetic implants, because they cannot be readily fixed to bone. Attempts to gain length without positive fixation tend to place the implant so that it projects inferiorly beyond the mandibular border, which then acts as a fulcrum to the implant's lever, facilitating displacement. When increased vertical length is desired, bone grafts are more suitable, because they can be fixed into position with interosseous wires. Development of a suitable "glue" to fix prosthetic implants to bone would be a great help in alleviating this technical problem.

at the operating table with scissors or scalpel to whatever dimension and shape is desired. The preformed implants reduce operating time and do not impose the nuisance of sculpting an implant from raw blocks.

Close-celled silicone sponges and gel-filled prostheses provide acceptable results in chin augmentation. If used, the sponge should be slightly oversized to allow for shrinkage from and contraction of the scar capsule and compression of the sponge.

Evaluation is best accomplished with medical photographs using the matte finish to sketch the planned profile. This will provide the surgeon with an estimate of the anterior, posterior dimension of the planned implant (Figures 28–18 and 28–19). It is best to err on a larger size, as it is easy to trim at surgery. Radiographs including cephalograms are helpful for more exacting determinations.

TECHNIQUE

Surgery is done under location anesthesia following light sedation in the office or the hospital. A bilateral mental nerve block is useful, as it provides profound anesthesia and limits the volume required that may mask needed augmentation. Anatomically, the nerve exits between the first and second lower bicuspid, and it can be approached intraorally or pericutaneously. The two standard surgical approaches are intraoral or submental. It is the surgeon's and patient's choice.

Intraoral Approach

Since Converse (1950) demonstrated the safety and feasibility of introducing autogenous bone grafts through intraoral incisions, this approach has been widely used. Synthetic implants can also be placed via the intraoral approach with a surprisingly low complication rate. It is most helpful to prepare the mouth preoperatively by attending to dental hygiene. The teeth should be scaled and cleansed well. Brushing the teeth with pHisoHex for two or three days before surgery is also of benefit in decreasing wound contamination. Antibiotic coverage is best started in full therapeutic doses 48 hours before surgery and is continued for 10 days postoperatively.

The intraoral approach described by Converse (1950) (Figure 28–20) is an incision made superiorly on the labial side of the lower labiogingival sulcus. It may be made as long as required, leaving a cuff of mucosa on the oral surface of the

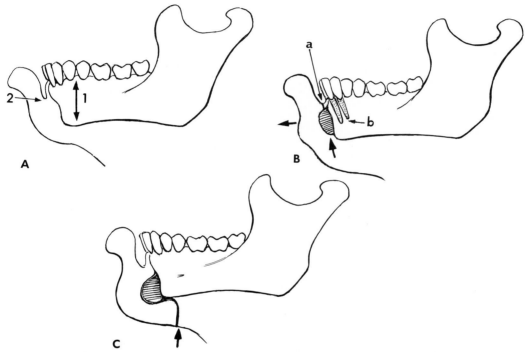

Figure 28–19. Augmentation mentoplasty is difficult in the presence of certain anatomical variations of the lower jaw, such as decreased vertical height at the symphysis (1 in *A*) and the shallowness of the gingivolabial sulcus (2 in *A*). An implant placed too high (*B*) would elevate the sulcus (*a*), creating an uncomfortable bulge and an unnatural chin shape (arrows). Horizontal osteotomy is also difficult in such patients because the roots of the teeth may extend into the customary plane of section (b). The proper placement of an implant in such a circumstance is shown in *C*. The pocket should not be dissected as high as the gingivolabial sulcus. The implant must be placed on the exact tip of the chin and not permitted to slip down. A two-layer soft tissue closure helps to maintain this position.

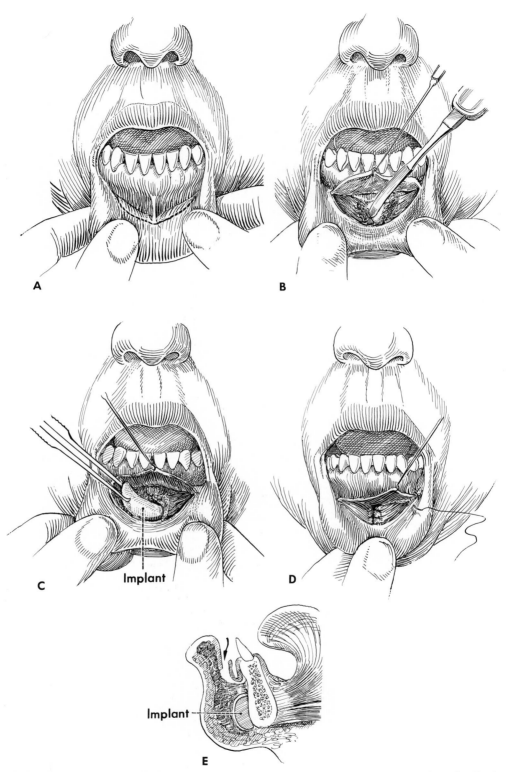

Implant

Implant

Figure 28–20.   A useful variation of the intra-oral approach for augmentation mentoplasty is that of Millard, who advocates incising the labial mucosa along the sulcus (*A*), but splitting the musculature in a vertical direction (*B*). Closure, therefore, places the deep muscle layer at right angles to the mucosa, which decreases the likelihood of wound breakdown over the implant resulting in extrusion. The implant is shown in its proper position in *E*.

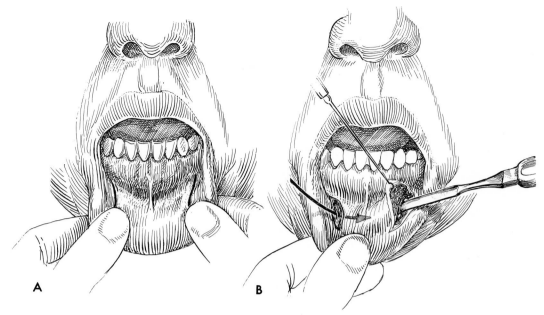

Figure 28–21. Augmentation mentoplasty by insertion of an alloplastic implant using two incisions placed laterally. The periosteum is raised and a socket is created by a tunnelling procedure. This technique avoids a long horizontal incision directly over the implant, which would increase the likelihood of exposure and extrusion.

lip to provide sufficient soft tissue for a tensionless closure. This incision is carried down to bone, and a subperiosteal pocket of suitable size is developed to accept the implant. Pitanguy (1968) favors this basic approach, but he emphasizes utilization of the median raphé of the chin musculature to fix the implant in position. He dissects this "ligament" free from its inferior insertion, turns it 180 degrees, and passes it through a notch in the center of the implant for fixation. He believes the notch aids in the formation of a chin dimple. Millard (1971) favors a horizontal incision in the labial mucosa and a vertical separation of the musculature of the lip by blunt dissection extending to the bone, where he fashions lateral extensions of a pocket by blunt dissection. Such a technique has the distinct advantage of providing a mucosal incision of minimal length, well-buttressed from beneath by a muscle closure at right angles. The authors favor this approach for implants of smaller size. Larger implants require wide exposure, however, and these are best inserted through the submental or external approach.

A useful variation of the intraoral exposure is the use of two incisions placed at the lateral extensions of the pocket. The implant is placed by "tunneling" between these two incisions (Figure 28–21).

Submental (External) Approach

Certain factors militate against optimal results from the intraoral approach. A short mandibular body (micrognathia) associated with a shallow labial sulcus may cause the implant to be placed in too high a position if placed intraorally. This results in loss of the natural lip-chin crease (labiomental fold). In addition, the implant is an annoying mass in the labial sulcus, which the patient is able to feel with his tongue.

Such a combination of circumstances (a short mandible and shallow sulcus) usually requires the implant to be placed from below (submental incision) (Figure 28–22). This approach permits the surgeon to elevate the periosteum only as high as required for the implant and thus to preserve the integrity of the sulcus. In this way, the implant can also be placed at a lower level or even along the inferior mandibular margin if desired. As previously stated, large implants are best inserted from an incision in the submental crease so as to prevent excessive tension on the intraoral suture line, which can lead to wound breakdown and extrusion (Figure 28–23). Accurate positioning of large implants is also facilitated by the external approach.

It is timely to discuss here the oft repeated
Text continued on page 806.

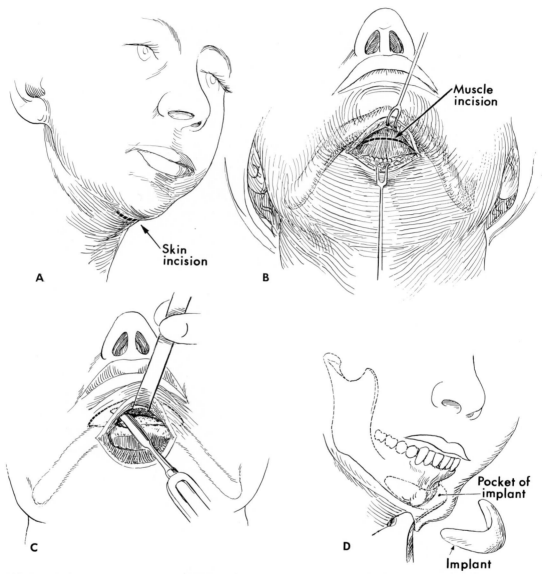

Figure 28–22.   Insertion of a prosthetic chin implant for augmentation by the submental (external) approach. *A,* An incision is placed in the submental crease. *B* and *C,* An exactly sized socket is dissected subperiosteally after the muscle is split. *D, E, F* and *G,* The socket should be so made that the implant rides along the border of the mandible but does not extend higher than the natural labiomental sulcus (*F*). *H,* The periosteum should not be cut free along the lower border of the mandible except over the symphysis, so that the implant cannot slide caudally by a rocking action. *J,* Redundant soft tissue of the submental region is excised. *K* and *L,* The wound is closed in layers.

Illustration continued on the opposite page.

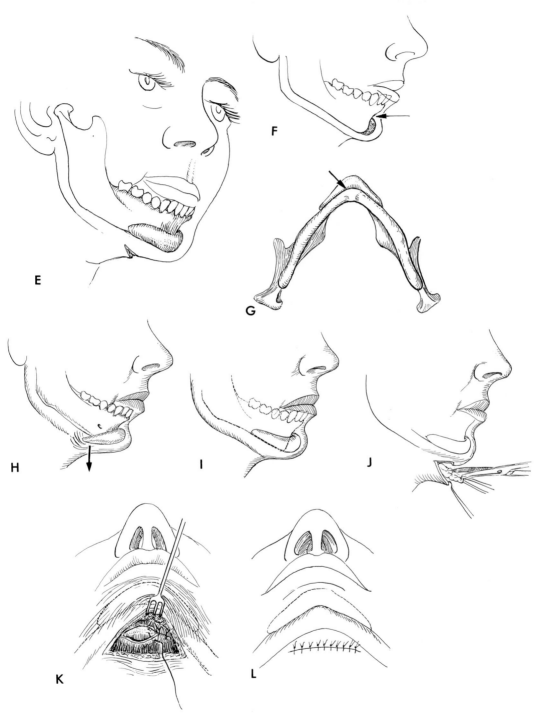

Figure 28–22. *See legend on the opposite page.*

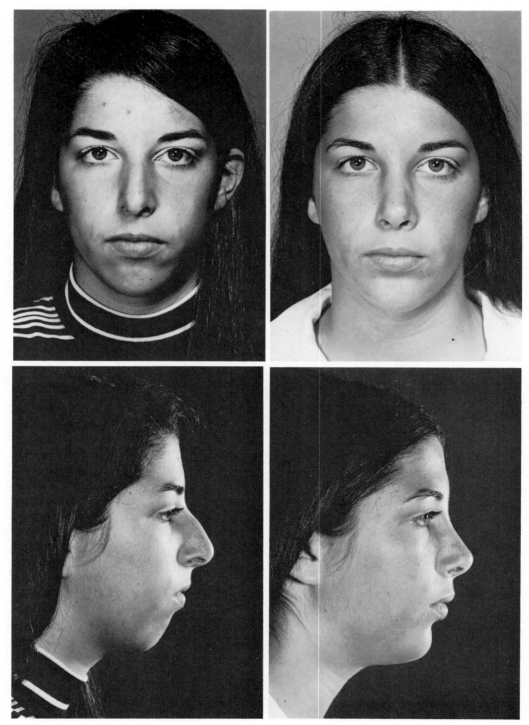

Figure 28–23.   When retrusion of the chin is marked, and particularly in the absence of a Class 2 occlusion, substantial correction can still be achieved at the time of rhinoplasty by the use of larger chin implants. However, these are best inserted through a submental incision, because it is easier to dissect a socket that is properly sized and positioned. It is subsequently easier to place the implant in the proper position.

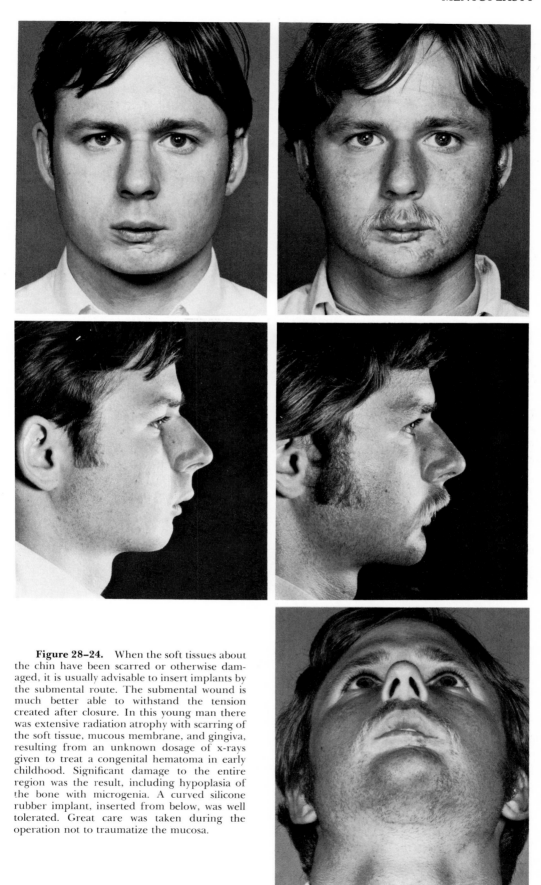

Figure 28–24. When the soft tissues about the chin have been scarred or otherwise damaged, it is usually advisable to insert implants by the submental route. The submental wound is much better able to withstand the tension created after closure. In this young man there was extensive radiation atrophy with scarring of the soft tissue, mucous membrane, and gingiva, resulting from an unknown dosage of x-rays given to treat a congenital hematoma in early childhood. Significant damage to the entire region was the result, including hypoplasia of the bone with microgenia. A curved silicone rubber implant, inserted from below, was well tolerated. Great care was taken during the operation not to traumatize the mucosa.

assumption that implants or grafts can be placed subperiosteally. In the author's experience, they cannot. One need only examine the nonyielding and inelastic nature of periosteum to realize that it cannot be made to stretch and to cover completely an implant of appreciable size. The periosteum can certainly be elevated and an implant can be placed beneath it on the bone, but then only rarely is it possible to close the periosteum over the implant.

Implants may be placed directly on cortical bone or overlying the periosteum, and this makes little difference in the final result. However, they should *not* be placed in a subcutaneous or intramuscular pocket where they can be readily palpated. Close to the bone will suffice. If the submental approach is used, the surgeon should close the wound in two layers. The deep closure that brings muscles together is most helpful in fixing the implants and protects the skin incision from dehiscence. The danger of extrusion is thus minimized (Figure 28–24).

DRESSINGS AND POSTOPERATIVE CARE

Elastoplast and adhesive tape splinting are usually applied as a "basket weave" pattern and maintained for two to four days. All dressings are then removed and none are replaced. Wide spectrum antibiotic coverage is maintained for 10 days postoperatively.

When the intraoral approach is used, only a liquid diet is permitted for three days postoperatively, until the wound is healed.

COMPLICATIONS

Extrusion, malposition, bone absorption, infection, bleeding, and *hypoesthesia of the lip* are the main complications of augmentation mentoplasty when solid implants are used (Friedland, Coccaro, and Converse, 1976). Infection can occur, but this is rare. When infection does occur, extrusion of the implant is almost certain, although on occasion prompt and vigorous treatment with wide spectrum antibiotics can save implants.

Sponge implants can change in size. This is more of an inconvenience than a complication. Initially sponges fill with serum or fluid, causing swelling of the chin. As the fibrous capsule forms around the implant, the sponge contracts slowly, so that the chin size also diminishes. The degree of change is usually not significant and does not contraindicate the use of fine-celled sponge.

Extrusion can occur with any implant, al-though perhaps not for many months or years after the surgery. Adequate-sized pockets and careful anatomic placement of the implant are the best prophylaxis. Nevertheless, even the most carefully placed implant can shift in position and present as a pressure point either within the mouth or externally at the chin. If the implant becomes extruded, it can be replaced. This may not always be necessary, because the residual scar capsule may preserve enough augmentation to please the patient. Malpositioned implants can be repositioned by adjusting the size and shape of the pocket.

Erosion of bone by onlay implants was reported by Robinson and Shuken (1969), Robinson (1972), and Jobe, Iverson, and Vistnes (1973) (Figure 28–25). The bone responds to the pressure of the implant by osteolytic activity. Such erosion does not appear to represent a significant contraindication for implants, since apparently it is self-limiting (Rees, 1973).

HORIZONTAL OSTEOTOMY

The chin can be brought forward surgically by sectioning the mandible in a horizontal plane beneath the alveolar canal (Figure 28–26). The severed segment of the mandible with or without muscular attachments is then advanced as far forward as necessary and wired in position to the lower teeth until consolidation has taken place. This technique is an excellent one in solving certain problems such as increased vertical heights or asymmetry.

Horizontal osteotomy of the chin was probably first practiced in Germany during or shortly after World War II, according to references cited by Converse and Wood-Smith (1964) and Hinds and Kent (1969). The operative technique was first reported by Obwegeser (1957) in the English literature in conjunction with a paper on the surgical correction of mandibular deformities of different types. Converse and Wood-Smith (1964) discussed variations of the technique and defined five possibilities. These variations and the technique were subsequently strongly endorsed by Hinds and Kent, who recommended it for correction of almost all deformities of the chin to the complete exclusion of the implant technique.

The operation is one of considerably more magnitude than augmentation by implants and carries a significantly higher morbidity, healing time, and complication rate. It is also much more inconvenient to the patient. It is, however, the unquestioned operation of choice in patients who have retrognathia in association with increased

Text continued on page 816.

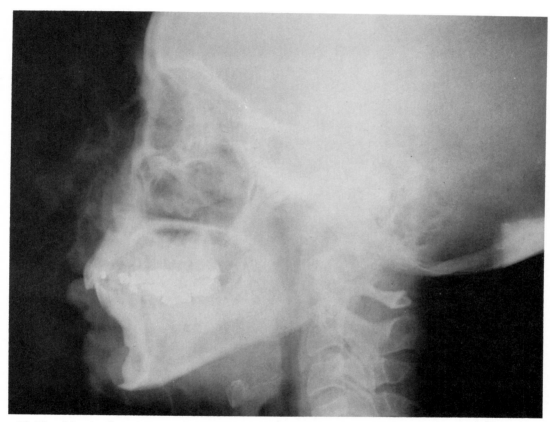

Figure 28–25. After implantation, most implants on the mentum "settle" into the bone. Such erosion is a well-known phenomenon in orthopedic surgery. It can occur whether or not the implant is positioned directly on the bone or on top of the periosteum in the soft tissue. The bony erosion is probably self-limiting. The tooth roots are very rarely encroached upon.

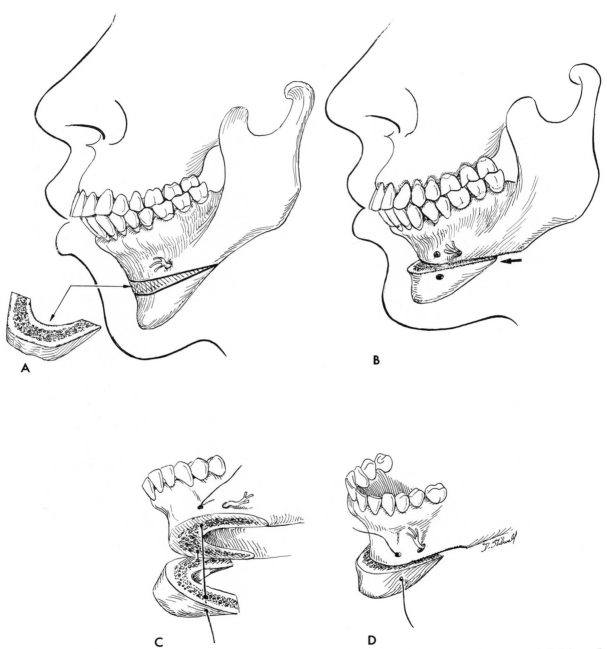

Figure 28–26.   Patients with increased vertical height of the chin benefit most from horizontal osteotomy. *A*, A "piece of pie," of a size predetermined by cephalograms, is resected. *B*, The mandibular segment is set forward into the desired position. *C* and *D*, Interosseous wiring is used for fixation.

Illustration continued on the opposite page.

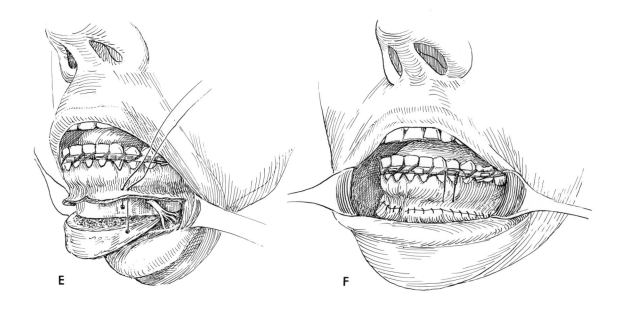

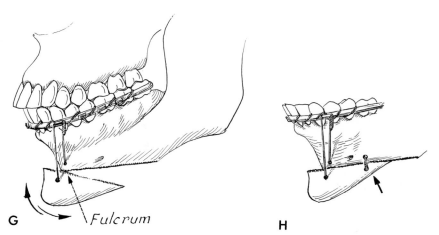

Figure 28–26 *Continued.*   *E*, It is best to extend the wires through the mucosa as a pull-out. *F*, The pull-out is tightened around the dental appliance. *G* and *H*, Care must be taken to prevent a lever type of action which will displace the fragment. It may be necessary to apply additional wiring (arrow in *H*) to prevent displacement.

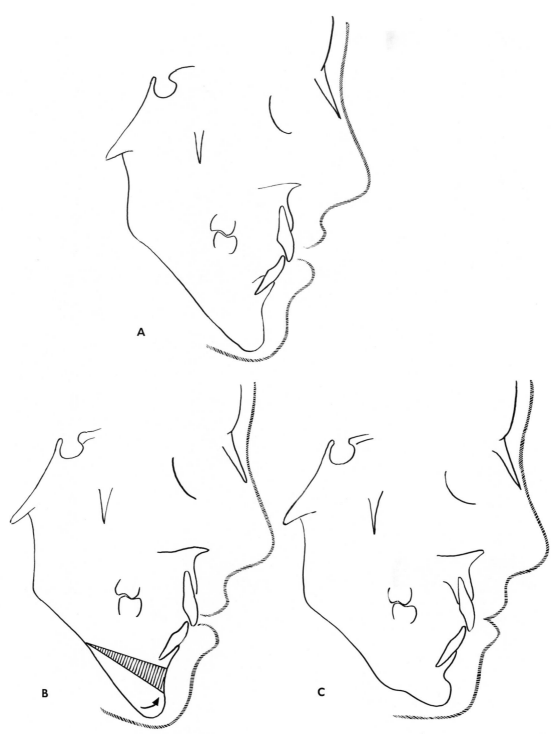

Figure 28–27.   *A*, Preoperative cephalometric tracing of a patient with excessive facial height and loss of lip competency. Note the loss of the labiomental curve in the preoperative profile photograph on the next page. *B*, Plan for wedge removal and elevation of the mobilized fragment. *C*, Postoperative tracing. Preoperative and postoperative photographs appear in Figure 28–28.

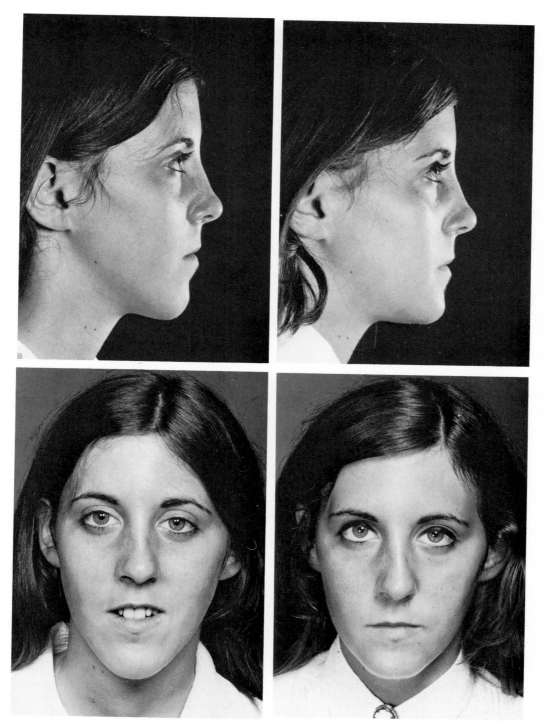

Figure 28–28. Patient who underwent the operation shown in Figure 28–27.

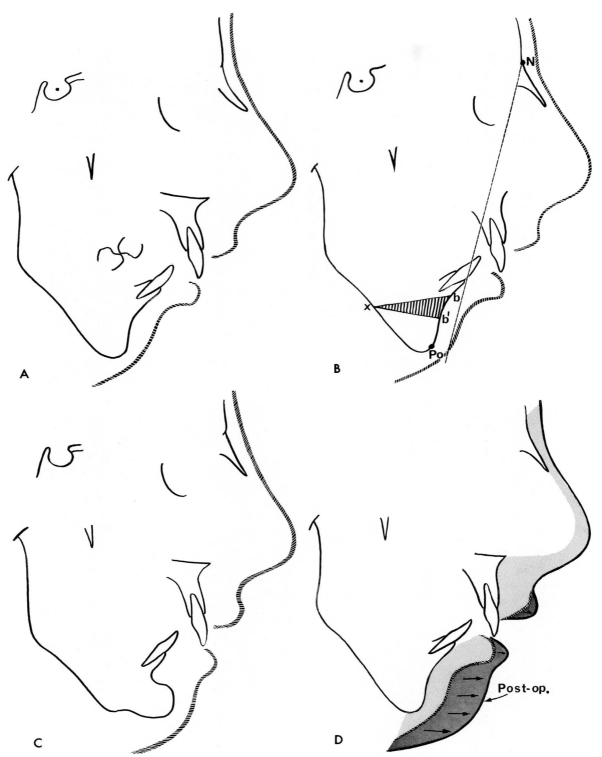

Figure 28–29.   *A,* Preoperative cephalometric tracing of a young man with micrognathia, a severe maxillomandibular dentoalveolar discrepancy, maxillary hypoplasia, and a nasal deformity. *B,* The operative plan was removal of a wedge (shaded), elevation of the fragment, and consequent advancement of "pogonion" to the facial plane. *C,* Postoperative tracing. *D,* Preoperative and postoperative tracings are superimposed to show the improvement in soft tissue contours. In addition, the patient underwent vertical osteotomy, rhinoplasty, and otoplasty, with the results shown in Figure 28–30.

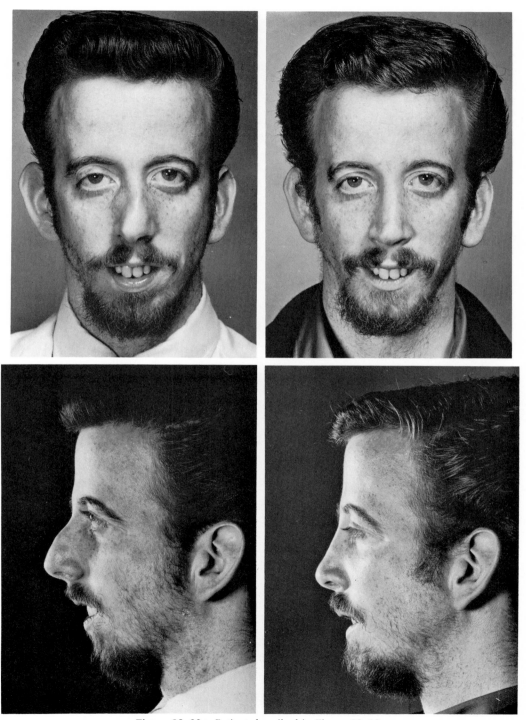

Figure 28–30.   Patient described in Figure 28–29.

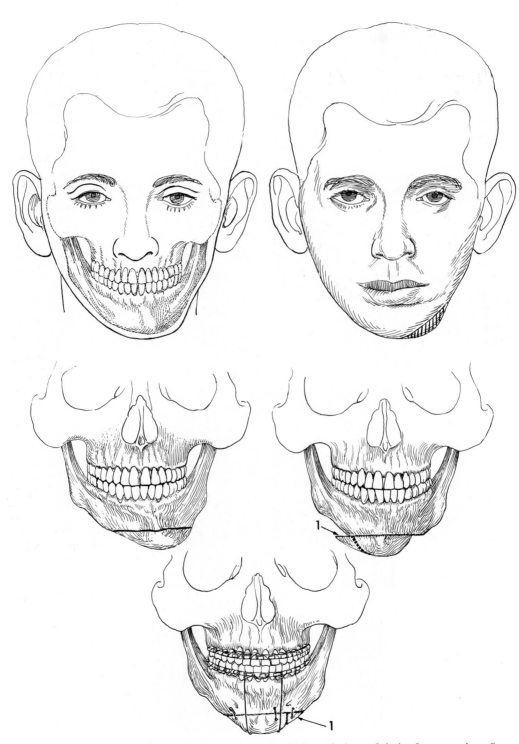

Figure 28–31. Horizontal osteotomy with lateral repositioning is the technique of choice for correction of severe asymmetry. The extra bone (1) can be resected and transferred as a free graft to fill in the opposite side.

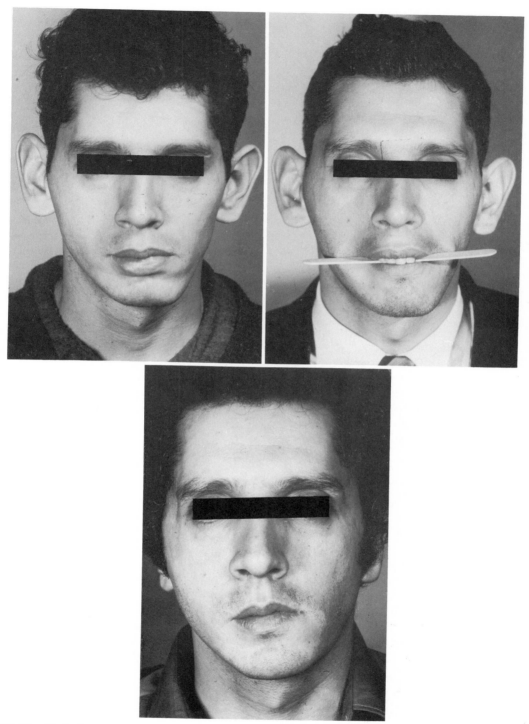

Figure 28–32.   Marked asymmetry of the mandible involving the body and the rami, considerably improved by horizontal osteotomy and a lateral shift.

vertical height of the mandibular body at the symphysis, aptly demonstrated in the patients shown in Figures 28–27 and 28–28. Such a deformity requires not only horizontal sectioning of the mandible but, in addition, a "piece of pie" (or wedge) resection from the body and the lower fragment is then brought forward and upward to a position in front of the cut border, where it is fixed in position by wiring to a simple orthodontic appliance. The chin prominence is augmented by this procedure while at the same time the height of the mandible is foreshortened. The amount of bone to be resected, as well as the amount of advancement of the lower fragment, can be almost exactly planned from preoperative cephalometric studies. Horizontal osteotomy can also be used in certain patients with more complicated jaw deformities such as micrognathia, moderately severe retrognathia with severe maxillomandibular dentoalveolar discrepancy, maxillary hypoplasia, and so forth, *provided* other options are ruled out after a thorough discussion of the problem between surgeon and patient has occurred. Such complicated problems may require a combination of techniques in which horizontal osteotomy is only one of the procedures used. The patient in Figures 28–29 and 28–30 presents just such a problem.

Horizontal osteotomy is also clearly the technique of choice in asymmetry of the chin (Figures 28–31 and 28–32). Implants in such cases are difficult or impossible to position.

In severe retrusion, both horizontal osteotomy and subsequent prosthetic implant may be necessary for optimal results.

TECHNIQUE

The anterior mandible is "degloved" by making an incision on the labial side of the lower sulcus, leaving a sufficient cuff of mucous membrane. The incision is made as far laterally as necessary on either side to gain sufficient exposure of the bone and mental foramen. The mental nerves on either side are carefully dissected clear of investing tissues and guarded from trauma at all times during the procedure.

The subperiosteal dissection continues to the lower border of the mandible, where it is often necessary to divide some of the muscular attachments to allow sufficient mobility for forward displacement. The design of the bone cuts is then made by drawing on the bone with blue dye. The osteotomies are done with a Stryker saw and the air-driven drill. If a segment of bone (the "piece of pie") is to be removed, all pieces of bone are saved.

These may be used as chips to fill gaps between the mobile fragment and the bone of the mandible (see Figure 28–31).

It may be necessary, when the fragment is to be advanced forward for a considerable distance, to strip the fragment of most of its anterior soft tissue attachments so that it becomes virtually a free bone graft. Only lingual attachments remain — those of the digastric and genial muscles. This presents surprisingly few difficulties, and such "grafts" seem to take readily.

Rough bone edges are polished with a bur, and the upper surface of the lower fragment is fitted to the lower edge of the cut mandible in the desired position and relationship. Permanent direct interosseous wiring is rarely necessary, since the mandibular fragment is readily immobilized by wire suspension to prefixed orthodontic appliances previously placed in the lower teeth. Drill holes strategically placed in the fragment are required and usually three to four such cable wires are used.

The intraoral mucosal incision is sutured with interrupted sutures of 4–0 chromic catgut, and a simple Barton's bandage is applied. Intermaxillary fixation is not necessary in such patients.

POSTOPERATIVE CARE

Consolidation occurs within six weeks, during which time the suture line is kept clean with saline, weak peroxide irrigation, or mouthwashes. Wide spectrum antibiotics are given for about ten days postoperatively. The cable wires are removed six to seven weeks postoperatively.

COMPLICATIONS

Temporary hypoesthesia or anesthesia of the chin and lower lip can occur if the mental nerves are excessively stretched or otherwise traumatized. This is usually temporary, but it may persist for several weeks or even months. If the nerve is cut or otherwise irreversibly injured at the time of operation, permanent anesthesia results. Protection of the nerve and its branches during surgery is of prime importance. Should the mental nerve be cut during surgery, it should be repaired before closure.

Infection of the wound can be serious, particularly when the mobilized fragment consists of a free piece of bone with only minimal muscular attachments. Sequestration is then a possibility. However, infection is uncommon and has not been a significant problem in our experience. Antibiotic coverage and the establishment of adequate preoperative oral hygiene undoubtedly account for the low incidence of infection.

Irregularities of the mandibular margin are sometimes palpable at the ends of the fragment, but these are more of a nuisance than a complication and in time tend to become molded.

MAXILLARY PROGNATHISM

Overdevelopment or anterior displacement of the maxilla not associated with a major craniofacial disjuncture is not a common deformity for which the patient seeks treatment. Patients who do present are often concerned with the relatively underdeveloped mandible and may initially be interested in a mandibular correction. A clinical inspection will reveal a balanced mandible with a prominent upper lip and excessive anterior overjet of the maxillary teeth, often with an open bite (Figure 28–33). Evaluation necessitates the entire complex of radiographs, dental study models, bite registration, and medical photographs. The differential diagnosis is a mandibular retrognathia, and this can be excluded by cephalometric tracings.

The treatment plan is based on the amount of retrocorrection required for aesthetic and occlusal balance. The former is determined by clinical examination and photographic retouching. Occlusal relationships are balanced after study of the cephalogram and the models. The millimeters of retrusion are limited by the space resulting from tooth extraction or existing edentulous areas. The osteotomy site is usually at the second or first premolar, unless there is an established posterior space. On the working models, the teeth to be extracted are cut out and the model is reconstructed using dental wax. This upper restored working model is reworked over the mandibular model, and the occlusal relationship is established. Certain cusps may require grinding to achieve a preliminary working occlusion. All patients will need an element of occlusal equilibrasion postoperatively, but the surgeon needs to have a planned occlusion that will be established at surgery. The surgical procedure is done under nasotracheal anesthesia. The first step is development of the posterior osteotomy site. An L-shaped flap is developed just anterior to the planned tooth extraction and the maxillary alveolus is exposed. The tooth is extracted using appropriate forceps. Often, the premolar will have two roots and the surgeon who is performing his own extraction must be certain the entire root is removed (Figures 28–34 and 28–35).

The procedure is repeated on the opposite side, and a horseshoe tunnel is elevated across the hard palate. Using a motorized drill with a straight fissure bur, the bone of the buccal and lingual tooth socket is removed and a bony channel is created across the palate. Injury to adjacent teeth and the soft tissue of the nasal and sinus floor is avoided by using good lighting, suction, irrigation, and slow dissection during the final stage. Absolute full thickness, bony removal is required to allow the anterior fragments to move posteriorly. Next, a 2 cm incision is made on the alveolar mucosa below or outside the depth of the labial sulcus opposite the anterior frenulum or maxillary incisors. The mucosa is elevated again in a tunnel fashion posteriorly on each side to the osteotomy site. Using a narrow fissure bur, a horizontal cut is made above the apices of the teeth below the sinus. Review of the dental x-rays is helpful to approximate root length. A 4 mm osteotome can be used to encourage separation. On completion, the anterior maxillary segment is free and can be displaced into the planned occlusion. Resistance is usually secondary to a bony spur in a difficult section of the posterior osteotomy.

Intramaxillary fixation is achieved first by whatever method is planned. Most surgeons add intermaxillary fixation for three weeks, but some operators feel it is unnecessary (Fig. 28–36). A Barton dressing, liquid diet, and inactivity begin the postoperative period. With graduation based on experience, maxillary fixation should be maintained for eight weeks.

Complications are few. Bleeding and infection are treated as they present. Prophylactic antibiotics are suggested. Devitalization of the teeth should be common, but fortunately this is unusual according to the literature.

MANDIBULAR AND MAXILLARY CONTOURING

The surgical treatment of bony growth or underdevelopment of the jaws is an exciting facet of maxillofacial surgery that belongs in the armamentarium of the aesthetic surgeon. It is not a procedure likely to be used daily, weekly, or even monthly but one that is reserved for exacting indications. On the other hand, once mastered, it is reasonable for the surgeon to be comfortable performing limited numbers of such operations.

Indications for this type of bony contouring procedures are 25 percent technical and 75 percent personal motivation of the patient. Many patients have true underdevelopment of the man-

Text continued on page 822.

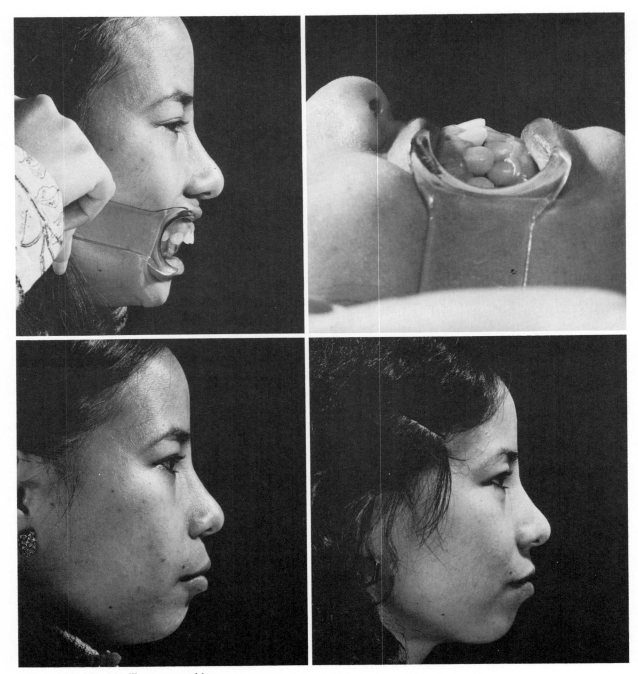

Figure 28–33. Maxillary prognathism.

Profile and dental views of patient with maxillary prognathism. Patient had 5 mm of overjet and 4 mm of overbite on the dental study model. Cephalometric evaluation revealed anterior displacement of the maxilla in relation to the mandible. A maxillary pushback was undertaken with removal of the second bicuspids bilaterally.

Profile and dental views of patient six months after maxillary pushback show that an esthetic and functional result has been accomplished.

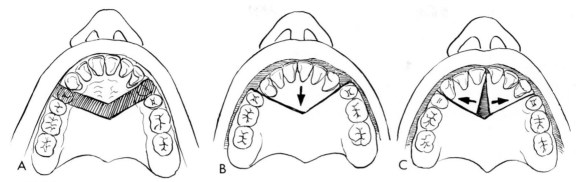

Figure 28–34. *A,* V-shaped osteotomy to prevent rotation of the recessed anterior maxillary segment. *B,* Loss of alignment of the dental arch after the set-back. *C,* A midline palatal osteotomy realigns the dental arch. A triangular bone graft fills the gap. (From Converse, J. M., et al.: *Reconstructive Plastic Surgery.* Philadelphia, W. B. Saunders Co., 1977.)

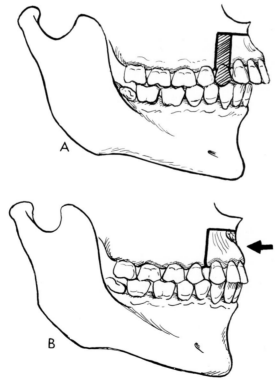

Figure 28–35. The subnasal premolar maxillary set-back osteotomy. *A,* The subnasal line of osteotomy. The bone to be resected is indicated by the shaded area. *B,* Relationships after completion of the procedure. (From Converse, J. M., et al.: *Reconstructive Plastic Surgery.* Philadelphia, W. B. Saunders Co., 1977.)

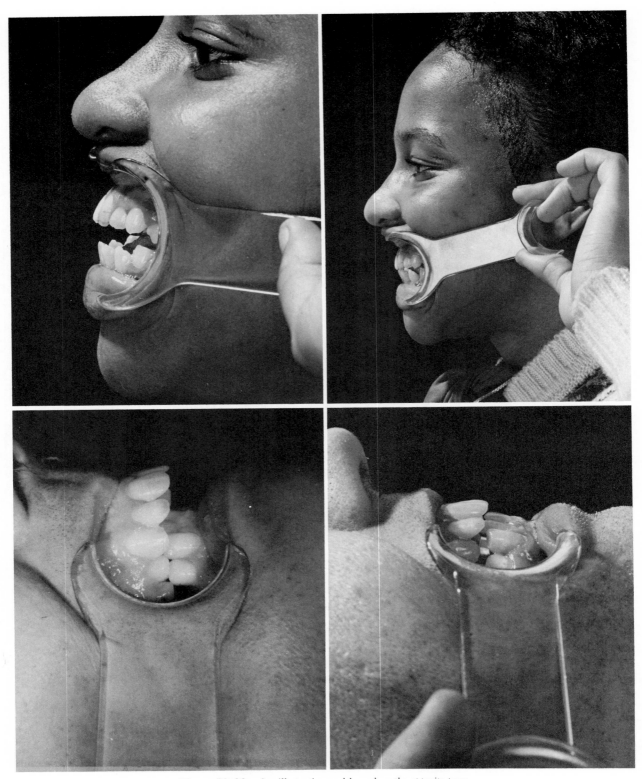

Figure 28–36.   *See illustration and legend on the opposite page.*

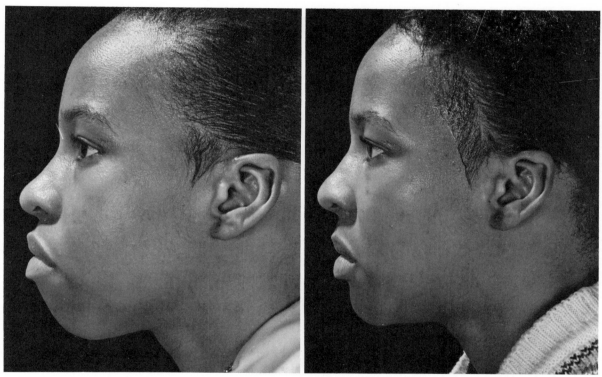

Figure 28–36.   A 19-year-old female was operated on for correction of occlusal and esthetic deformities associated with bimaxillary protrusion and anterior open bite. A maxillary pushback and bone graft corrected the upper jaw malalignment. The mandible was repositioned by extracting the lower second premolars and mobilizing the anterior segment. The mental nerve remained with the posterior segment. The mandible was secured with internal fixation, the maxilla with intermaxillary fixation. Postoperative results show good esthetic and occlusal alignment.

See illustration on the opposite page.

dible with an "Andy Gump" appearance, a deep overbite and overjet, Class II malocclusion, and the rest of the characteristics of this facial complex and would never consider surgical contouring. No matter how appealing the end result, these operations have built-in morbidity without complications, and with complications, they can be extremely inconvenient. Patient education must be maximal and should include interviews with previously operated patients whenever possible. Only a few of us surgeons can know first hand the trials and tribulations of 12 weeks of intermaxillary fixation.

MALARPLASTY

A chapter on facial contouring would be incomplete without a discussion of the highly prized full cheekbone. It has become a trademark of numerous public celebrities.

Evaluation is readily accomplished with facial photographs. A moulage is useful if there is asymmetry or related abnormality suggesting an unusual circumstance. Surgery is facilitated by careful preoperative planning and marking the position of the implant. Using marking dye, the upper, lower, and medial limits of the malar bones are carefully outlined, preferably in the sitting position. A pocket is then developed using the preauricular or intraoral approach. A well carved prefabricated or silicone block implant is then inserted. No fixation is required if pocket development is conservative. Complications are those involving nerve damage, bleeding, infection, and failure to achieve a mirror image. Careful technique will minimize their magnitude and frequency.

SOFT TISSUE CONSIDERATIONS

Lip posture and the location of the soft tissue mass of the chin are extremely important elements in the total facial appearance. They are largely dependent upon jaw form and the relative position of the mandible and the teeth, as noted previously.

The chin mass is of particular importance to the surgeon planning an operative procedure on the mental symphysis. Mandibular osteotomies of various types and implant augmentations have a direct effect on the soft tissues of the anterior muscle mass of the chin and the submental area (Figure 28–37).

Chin augmentation often has a dramatic effect on the submental soft tissue. A "double chin" (or early "turkey gobbler" effect), which is the result of skin excess only, is sometimes eliminated by simple augmentation as shown in Figures 28–38 and 28–39. A salutary effect is achieved when this procedure is done in conjunction with rhytidectomy (Figures 28–40 and 28–41). Chin augmentation is being suggested more and more frequently to rhytidectomy candidates.

In patients with an excessive submental fat pad, the excess fat, as well as some skin, can be excised at the time a chin implant is introduced through the submental approach.

The anterior soft tissue mass or "chin pad" can be profoundly affected, and the location of this structure and the possible effects of the surgery should be taken into consideration preoperatively. For example, in the "backward divergent" face, the mandible may show increased vertical height and a retruded chin point. The chin pad then often rides high and appears most unnatural when the circumoral musculature is brought into action. In such a patient, augmentation by implantation alone would increase the forward projection of the chin, but it would also exaggerate the unnatural appearance of the chin pad and might possibly elevate it even further.

A reduction osteotomy by horizontal section, combined with wedge removal and advancement of the lower segment, usually puts the chin pad in a more normal anatomic relationship. This results in a much more natural facial expression by relaxing the soft tissues of the chin pad.

CHIN DIMPLE

A central chin "dimple" is considered to be an attractive beauty mark by many. Some prominent personalities in the entertainment industry have been identified by such an indentation. Chin dimples are usually hereditary in nature, but attempts to create them have been made by surgeons (Figures 28–42 and 28–43). These techniques provide a cicatricial union between the undersurface of the dermis and the underlying bone or periosteum. Alternatively, an implant that has a carved indent in its center to which the overlying soft tissues conform may be inserted (Pitanguy, 1968). These methods can be successful, but the results are inconsistent and thus not predictable.

The method based on producing a scar contracture of dermal adhesion can be disappointing, because even with meticulous attention to anatomic location and detail, such dimples are frequently asymmetrical and unnatural in appearance; they do not move with facial animation.

Natural chin dimples occur almost exactly in

Text continued on page 828.

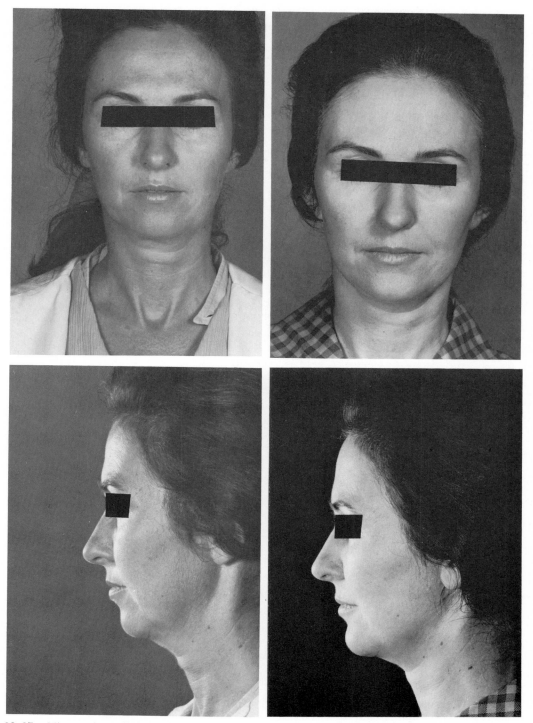

Figure 28–37.   Microgenia can limit face lift results, and the effect of a cervicofacial rhytidectomy is often enhanced by augmentation mentoplasty. Some patients have never been aware that microgenia is a part of the problem, so that suggesting a chin implant to improve the face lift result is usually welcomed. Other patients are hesitant to inquire about chin correction even though they may have been conscious of a weak chin for many years. In addition, chin implants improve the mentocervical angle.

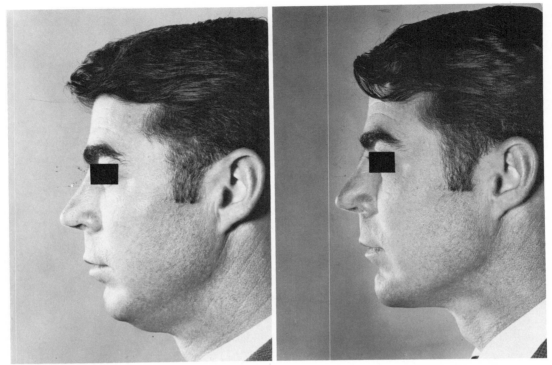

Figure 28–38.   A chin implant is sometimes all that is required to correct a "double chin" caused by an excess of skin without any excess fat. A curved silicone implant inserted by the intra-oral route accomplished such a correction in this 36-year-old man, in whom rhytidectomy was not required.

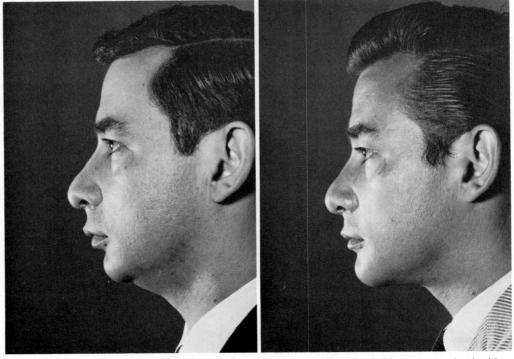

Figure 28–39.   Note the improvement in the cervicomental angle that resulted from chin augmentation in this patient. Minor degrees of double chin are often improved in this way, though this patient posed a difficult problem because the vertical height of his mandible was quite small. The pocket to accommodate the implant must be dissected to exactly the correct size in such a patient, and the implant must be so shaped that it cannot be easily displaced. Bony fixation in such a situation would be highly desirable, but is not as yet possible.

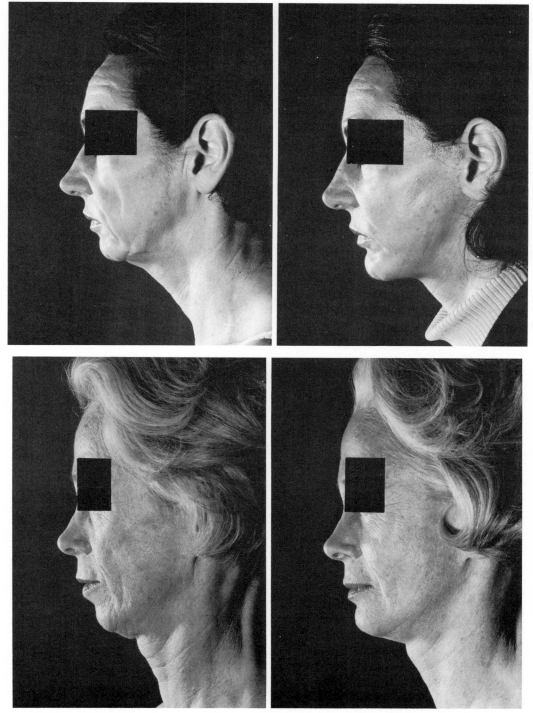

Figure 28–40. A combination of microgenia (or retrognathia) with marked redundancy and ptosis of the skin along the jaw and upper neck can be adequately corrected only by cervicofacial rhytidectomy and augmentation mentoplasty. Patients in this age group are not good candidates for extensive jaw surgery to restore contour and occlusion. They have often had malocclusion for most of their lives and need extensive dental attention. Inasmuch as direct procedures on the mandible are contraindicated, the choice comes down to only implants, which can be placed with ease and which provide excellent contour correction, as seen in these two patients.

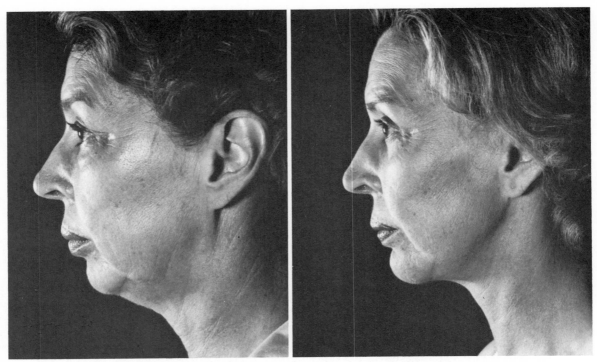

Figure 28–41.   Patient who underwent a combination of chin implant and rhytidectomy.

Figure 28–42.   Many people consider dimples to be attractive. Natural dimples are thought to be the result of connection of integumentary fibers with attachments from the dermis to underlying muscle. They are most common in the mobile areas of the cheeks, lower lip, or chin.

Several methods to produce dimples have been tried, but most have been lacking in naturalness of effect because the methods rely on the formation of scar adhesions. The recent technique described by Argamaso seems to be the most promising method so far devised to produce a natural cheek dimple; the method of creating a natural appearing chin dimple still eludes us.

See illustration on the opposite page.

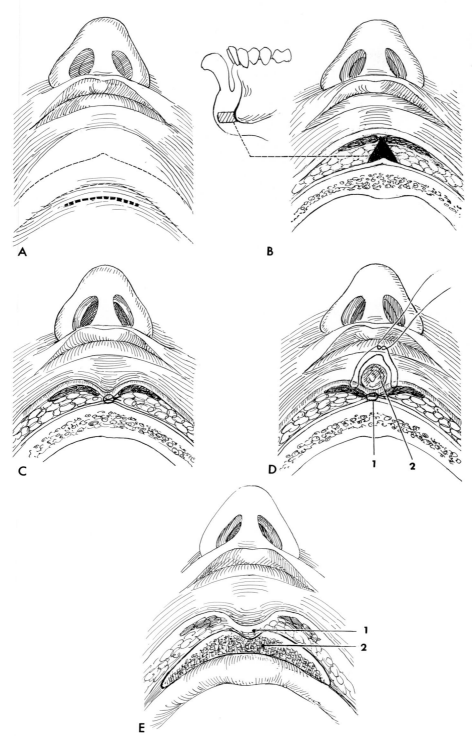

Figure 28–42. This demonstrates a method of creating a chin dimple by cicatricial adhesions. Through a submental incision (A), a wedge of tissue with the base of the periosteum of the anterior surface of the mandible is excised (B). This wedge includes muscle of the midline and subcutaneous tissue. A buried suture fixes the dermis to the periosteum of the midline (C). A tie-over roll or bolus dressing is used to maintain the depression (C).

Another method of forming a dimple advocated by many is shown in E. A notched chin implant is inserted, which theoretically imposes a notching or dimple on the overlying soft tissue. This method is usually far less effective in practice than it seems in principle.

See legend on the opposite page.

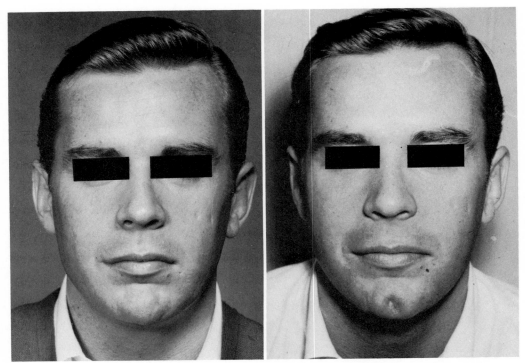

Figure 28–43.   The surgical formation of a chin dimple by the technique illustrated in Figure 28–42. The preoperative appearance (*A*) and the postoperative result (*B*) show the disadvantage of this technique, which is the unnatural appearance of the dimple as a result of scar adhesions.

the midline and take the shape of a vertical furrow. This symmetry of nature may be most difficult to duplicate by surgery. It is also somewhat risky to attempt to excise musculature and subcutaneous tissue from the dermis in the midline in an attempt to obtain adherence of the dermis to a prosthetic implant. This violates the main safety rule relating to implants — that of adequate soft tissue cover. Local pressure necrosis and the possibility of exposure and extrusion of the implant are possible complications.

The risk of such complications or imperfect results notwithstanding, a chin dimple is frequently demanded by certain patients. The surgeon is then justified in attemping to form one.

When simultaneous augmentation is not required, the simplest technique is to make a submental incision in the natural skin fold and to undermine the soft tissues of the chin just above the periosteum. A Y-shaped segment of soft tissue, including muscle and subcutaneous tissue, is then excised from the midline of the chin (which, of course, must be carefully marked beforehand), where the desired indentation is planned. This resection extends superficially to the dermis. One or two buried sutures of nylon or chromic catgut are than placed through the undersurface of the

dermis and the periosteum of the mandible directly beneath and tied, thus approximating the dermis to the periosteum. Several trial sutures are usually placed until the desired effect is obtained. This manufactured depression can be reinforced by tying a rolled bolus of dry or greased gauze into the external indenture with mattress sutures.

If augmentation mentoplasty is required in addition to a dimple, the technique of Pitanguy (1968) can be used. A suitable prosthesis is carved with a notch in its center. The notch must be placed exactly in the midline over it to fill the contour depression. Some soft tissues can be excised, however, but with great caution and conservativism. When compression bandages are applied over the implant too vigorously, the blood supply may be compromised and pressure necrosis of the skin may result.

CHEILOPLASTY

Lip contouring is a patient pleasing, underutilized procedure that can modify abnormalities of a highly visible facial characteristic. It is generally an office or outpatient procedure with low morbidity (Figure 28–44).

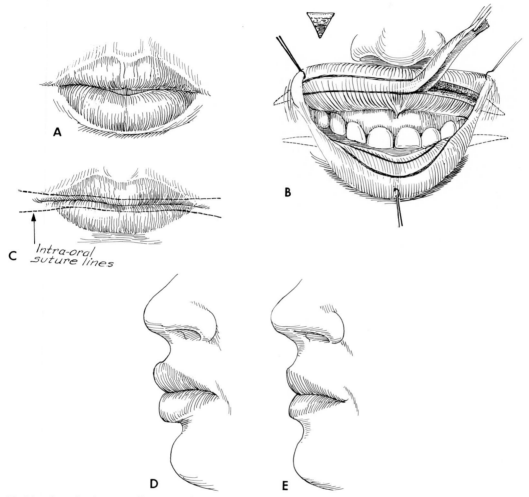

Figure 28–44. Oversized, protruding, or malpositioned lips can be a distressing facial deformity for many patients. Etiologies include obscure types of low-grade inflammatory reactions, congenital lesions such as hemangiomas or lymphangiomas, and racial characteristics, and many cases are of unknown cause. Protruding lips can also result from protruding teeth, and surgical trimming of the lips will not achieve improvement without correction of the malocclusion.

Many patients have enlarged lips that can be significantly improved by excision of large wedges of soft tissue. If such an excision is done on the mucosal side of the lip, the scar will be invisible. It is often necessary to extend the incision past the commissures on both sides and well into the buccal mucosa, but care must be taken not to interfere with or cross the commissure, because a constricting band may result. Excisions of soft tissue are sometimes carried down to (and may even include) muscle. Undermining is not necessary. Simple interrupted sutures are used for closure.

A and *D* show the extent of a typical problem. The operative plan for lip reduction is quite simple, but certain points are worthy of note. The wedges of tissue (*B*) will vary in width according to the amount of reduction required. *C*, The intra-oral sutures are indicated by the dotted lines and are seen to extend well beyond the commissures. *E*, The postoperative result.

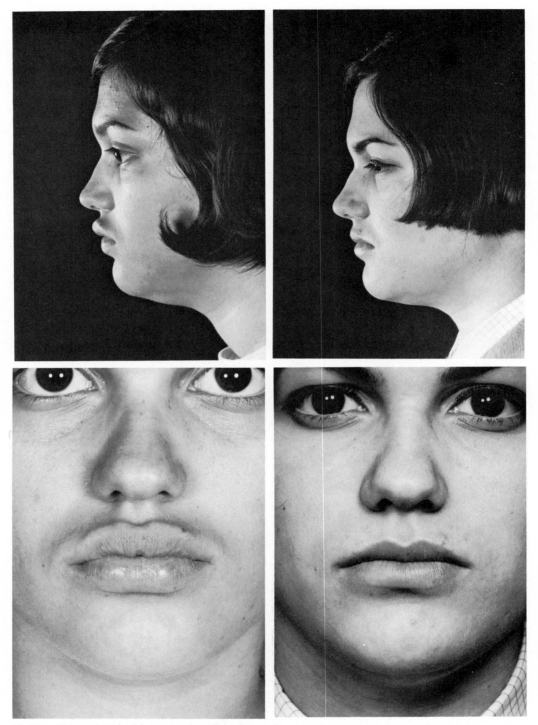

Figure 28–45. This patient had hypertrophy of the lips with protrusion, present since early adolescence. Excess tissue was excised in the form of a long ellipse from the mucosal surfaces of both lips, down to and including a small strip of muscle. The biopsy was unremarkable except for the equivocal presence of extra mucus glands. The postoperative result has endured for five years without recurrence of the protrusion.

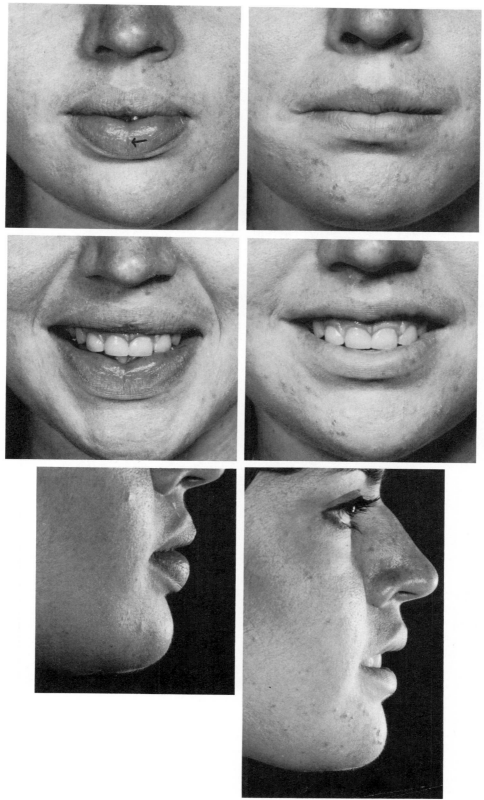

Figure 28–46.   In addition to some hypertrophy of the lips, this patient also had a small midline pit surrounded by a tubercle on the lower lip (arrow in first preoperative photograph). After surgical paring and excision of the pit, the patient was able to achieve normal lip seal more easily than had been the case, although in the relaxed position she still exhibited some gingival "show." See the text for a discussion of lip posture.

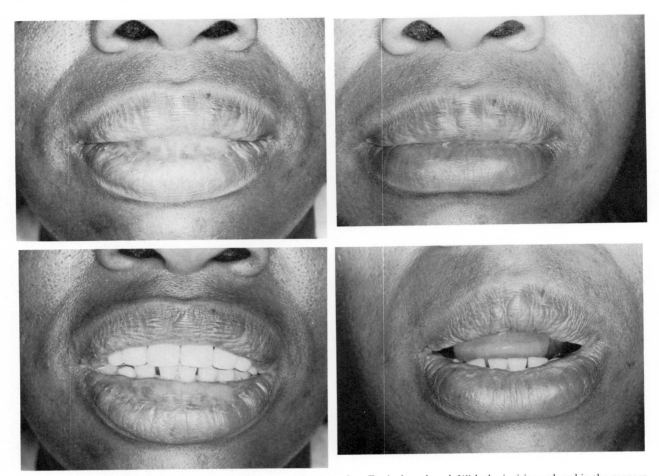

Figure 28–47. Large lips characteristic of Negro patients can be effectively reduced. With the incisions placed in the mucosa, there is virtually no danger of keloid formation. The excision should not be excessive or the closure too tight, because the lips might not seal.

Preoperative planning is best accomplished by thorough patient observation and photographs. The condition can be unilateral or bilateral with the lower lip being affected more often. Sketching on the matte finish photograph will give an impression of the needed reduction, or in rare cases, of augmentation.

Lip Reduction

Before the injection of local anesthesia, the anterior incision is drawn just behind the margin of the wet line — the area of lip mucosa behind the lip seal region. The posterior limit of excision is determined by the amount of lip mucosa to be removed. Use a tenacious marking ink such as tincture of Bonnie Blue and add a few cross hatchings to permit ease of realignment. Following introduction of the local anesthesia, a conservative strip of mucosa, underlying glands, and thin ribbon of muscle is excised. After careful hemostasis, closure is begun with buried catgut and finished with 5–0 silk. A soft diet and elevation are advised to reduce the swelling, which is often excessive (Figures 28–45 through 28–47).

Lip Augmentation

A y-v muscle flap can be used to fill local defects in lip fullness. In patients with hemiatrophy or traumatic loss of lip bulk, a tongue flap procedure can be used to add desired volume. Jackson (1972) described the use of an anteriorly based tongue flap to recontour a lip compromised by an electrical burn.

(For references, see pages 860 and 861.)

Chapter 29

Otoplasty

Donald Wood-Smith, M.D.

The protruding or lop ear deformity is a common malformation with a frequent concomitant psychologic disturbance. Children thus afflicted are often the object of misguided ridicule from others, and for this reason, we prefer to correct the problem in the four- to six-year age span. At this time, the ear growth has neared completion, and we do not find growth deficit to be a problem. In the older patient who has achieved adulthood, the lop ear is rarely a problem as he has usually adjusted to his appearance or learned to camouflage the ears by hair styling.

HISTORY

Dieffenbach (1845) first attempted to correct the protruding ear by simple excision of skin from the postauricular sulcus combined with suture fixation of the ear cartilage to the periosteum of the mastoid region. This method is still employed, with variations, by some surgeons; it forms, in part, the basis of the technique revitalized by Furnas (1968).

Although many authors credit Morestin (1903) with the first attempts at modification of the cartilage, Ely (1881), Keen (1890), Monks (1891), and Cocheril (1894) had all modified the Dieffenbach technique by both incision and excision of the segments of the conchal cartilage. The foundation of the modern techniques of otoplasty was laid by Luckett, who in 1910 first recognized the importance of the unfurling of the antihelix and the need for correction of this flattening to produce a satisfactory ear contour. This combination of antihelix and conchal correction that is the basis of most modern techniques was decribed by Mac-Collum in 1938 and later refined by Young (1944), who excised segments of the scapha and concha and incised the cartilage along the line of the inferior crus of the antihelix.

Although early results of all these procedures

were satisfactory, the sharp margins in the cartilage formed by the simple incisions soon became quite evident as the operative edema regressed; this marred the final result. Many varied methods were devised in an attempt to correct this technical deficiency. Significant contributions were made by McEvitt (1947), who used multiple parallel incisions along the line of the antihelix; variations of his method were described by Pierce, Klabunde, and Bergeron (1947) and Dufourmentel (1958). Holmes (1959) attempted to achieve a similar weakening of the antihelix and correction of contour by the use of multiple incisions in the scalp aspect of the antihelix cartilage to produce a fishscale-like appearance. The use of surgical abrasion to weaken the antihelix was described by Farrior in 1947 and subsequently championed by Stark and Saunders in 1962. In his improvement of the procedure described by Barsky in 1938, Becker (1952) emphasized the need for removal of the cauda helicus to reduce the cartilaginous protrusion in this region.

These techniques were integrated and refined by Converse, Nigro, Wilson, and Johnson in 1956 and were more recently modified by Converse and Wood-Smith in 1963 and 1971.

Mustardé (1963, 1967, 1971) popularized Owen's method of nonabsorbable suture fixation of the cartilage in its corrected position. This technique has gained a wide acceptance because of its simplicity. Furnas (1968) reemphasized the importance of fixation of the conchal cartilage to the underlying mastoid periosteum in patients with a relatively well formed antihelix and in whom the primary problem is protrusion of the conchal cartilage. Like the Mustardé method, the Furnas technique is popular because of its simplicity; however, indications for its usage are more limited than either the Converse — Wood-Smith or Mustardé techniques.

Modification of the cartilage by surgical weakening of its anterolateral aspect was described by

833

Stenstrom (1963), who utilized multiple incisions combined with excision of a postauricular segment of skin. The anterolateral aspect of the cartilage is approached from the postauricular incision, and the procedure is completed with the aid of a special scoring instrument. Ju, Li, and Crikelair (1963) exposed the cartilage from its lateral aspect, excising and modifying the contour of the cartilage under direct vision. This latter method appears to carry an unwarranted risk of visible scarring.

ANATOMY (Figures 29–1 and 29–2)

The auricle usually meets the adjacent scalp at an angle of approximately 30 degrees; the basic structure is a delicate, intricately shaped elastic cartilage with a thin, closely adherent skin covering on its anterolateral aspect. The skin cover is somewhat thicker and less adherent on the scalp aspect of the cartilage and may be readily stripped on this surface. The helix rim arises anteriorly and inferiorly from a crus extending horizontally above the external auditory meatus. The helix continues superiorly and then inferiorly to merge to the cauda helicus and join the lobule of the ear. The antihelix rises superiorly where the anterosuperior and anteroinferior crura join to form the antihelix body. This separates the helix posteriorly from the conchal rim and concha proper. A low shallow fossa of varying prominence, the scapha, lies between the antihelix crura. Enclosed between the two crura is the fossa triangularis.

The conchal cavity composed of cavum below and cymba conchi above meets the antihelix at the conchal rim and is bounded anteriorly by the tragus and the external auditory meatus, and posteriorly and inferiorly by the antitragus, which is separated from the tragus by the intertragal notch. The lobule exhibits varying degrees of development and attachment to the adjacent scalp and cheek.

The auricle is principally supplied by the superficial temporal and posterior auricular arteries. Sensation is supplied by anterior and posterior branches of the greater auricular nerve, reinforced by the auriculotemporal and lesser occipital nerves. A portion of the posterior wall of the external auditory meatus is supplied by auricular branches of the vagus nerve.

PATHOLOGY

Intelligent planning of the best method of correction of the lop ear deformity requires careful evaluation and analysis of the component parts of the deformity in comparison with the "normal" anatomy. The main characteristics of the lop ear deformity, which may occur singly or in all combinations, are (1) poorly developed antihelix, (2) overdevelopment of the conchal cartilage, and (3) an increased angle between the lobule and the scalp (Figure 29–3). The surgeon should carefully analyze these elements in each patient under consideration.

Analysis of the component parts should include these aspects:

A. The antihelix is unfurled in:
   1. The body of the helix
   2. The posterior-superior crus
   3. The body and posterior-superior crus
B. The concha shows excess cartilage:
   1. As uniform excess
   2. In the upper third to upper half
   3. In the lower third to lower half
   4. In both upper and lower thirds
C. The helix rim and conchal rim show size disparity (the cup or shell ear deformity)
D. The lobule shows:
   1. An increased angle of protrusion
   2. An excess size
E. The Machiavellian ear shows:
   1. Poor definition of the helix rim
   2. Usually an excessive ear size
   3. An excess of conchal cartilage
   4. A weak auricular cartilaginous framework
F. The auricle shows a left side to right side size disparity
G. Associated anomalies are:
   1. Darwin's tubercle
   2. Preauricular tubercle
   3. Miscellaneous

The antihelix is commonly unfurled (Figure 29–4). The superior crus is poorly defined and passed imperceptibly into both the scapha and the triangular fossa, which may appear as a flattened area in contrast to the inferior crus, which is usually well developed. The body of the antihelix is often flattened. Correction requires a partial tubing, with the tube wider superiorly, of the body and the superior crus to form a smooth convexity between the helix and the conchal rim.

Excess of conchal cartilage is found throughout, or the excess may be confined only to the upper third or half or to the lower third or half (Figure 29–5). Cartilage may also be in excess above and below, being of normal contour in the intermediary portion. This variable component must be evaluated before any surgical removal of conchal rim, as it governs the conchoscaphal angle and the vertical angle made by the ear with the skull. The importance of adequate removal of conchal rim in the upper and lower thirds cannot be overemphasized to prevent the relatively common postoperative deformity noted in Figure 29–6. Frequently there is a relative disparity of conchal rim size to helix rim, giving a "cup" or "shell" appearance. The cause of this disparity may be either an excessive size of conchal rim or a relative shortage of helix. In its fully developed state, this deformity is that of a microtic ear. However, lesser degrees of the deformity are amenable to correction by removal of an adequate amount of conchal cartilage and reshaping of the ear framework.

The lobule may meet the mastoid process at an excessive angle. Correction is achieved by removal of both lobule and mastoid skin and not by an excision of lobule skin alone, which may result in a deformity of the lobule.

The Machiavellian ear represents a total distortion of the auricular anatomy and demonstrates failure of definition of the helix rim, unfurling of crura and the body of the antihelix, excess of conchal cartilage, and a general weakness of the whole auricular cartilage (Figure 29–7).

Disparity in size as well as shape may exist between the two ears. If marked, wedge excision of auricular skin and cartilage in the region of the scapha can correct the asymmetry (Tanzer, 1962).

Embryonic vestiges, such as an excessively large Darwin's tubercle or preauricular tags, can be removed at the time of correction of the lop ear deformity (Figure 29–8).

The three commonly employed operative techniques are described and illustrated in Figures 29–9 through 29–17.

COMPLICATIONS AND UNTOWARD RESULTS

Hematoma

Hematoma is the most immediate problem, and when it occurs, it requires immediate and vigorous treatment. Presence of persistent pain under the dressing heralds this complication and demands immediate removal of the dressing and inspection of the ears. The presence of a hematoma is indicated by a tense and bluish swelling of the retroauricular space; if bleeding has persisted for some time, there will be ecchymosis of the surrounding tissues. The skin sutures should be removed, the blood clot evacuated and all bleeding points coagulated, and the wound closed and a pressure dressing reapplied with great care. Large doses of antibiotics are indicated at this time, as this problem is a common precursor of perichondritis.

Perichondritis

Perichondritis may occur in the early postoperative phase and usually is a sequel to an undetected and/or inadequately treated hematoma, although this is by no means an essential etiologic factor. Large doses of the appropriate antibiotics are indicated, and the wound should be cultured for a later confirmation of the efficacy of the antibiotic. Adequate drainage is achieved by opening all sutures and carefully irrigating necrotic debris from the wound with hydrogen peroxide solution. Even in the face of such active therapy, a massive destruction of cartilage with severe deformity can result in an ear whose appearance may mimic that of a microtic ear.

Inadequate Correction

Inadequate correction is perhaps the most common untoward result of otoplasty; it is, however, often more evident to the surgeon than to the patient and, indeed, it is quite unusual for the patient to be dissatisfied with the result. Contour distortions or asymmetric correction may require secondary operation. The surgeon should approach every procedure with great care, since difficult to control distortions are easy to produce but troublesome to correct. The "telephone" ear deformity is particularly unpleasant since correction will require a "plastering" of the ear to the side of the patient's head, which is a quite unsatisfactory compromise (Figure 29–18).

Hypertrophic Scars

Hypertrophic scars in the line of skin incision are frequently seen in the younger patient and are more common in the patient with deeply pigmented skin. Such hypertrophy often resolves with conservative treatment, although intralesional steroid injections may dramatically increase the rate of resolution of the scars in many patients.

We have utilized triamcinolone acetonide, 40 mm per ml strength, injecting approximately 0.25 ml into the hypertrophic scar. The treatment is repeated at weekly intervals when signs of regression appear and we continued for at least four weeks, at which time the time interval may be

Text continued on page 859.

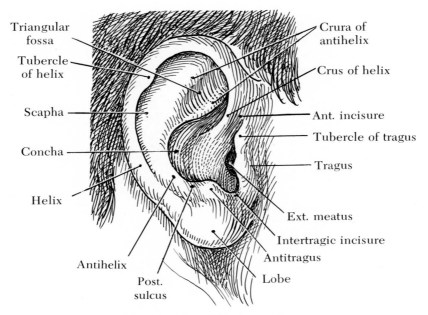

The anatomy of the external ear.

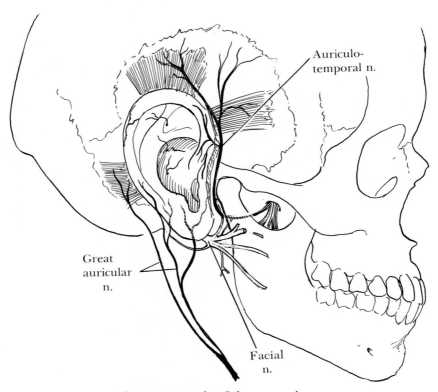

The nerve supply of the external ear.

Figure 29–1.   The anatomy and nerve supply of the external ear.

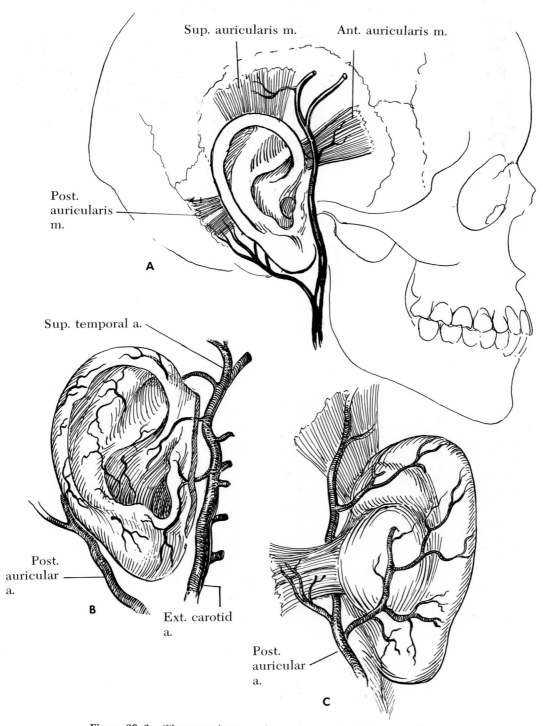

Figure 29–2. The musculature and vascular supply of the external ear.

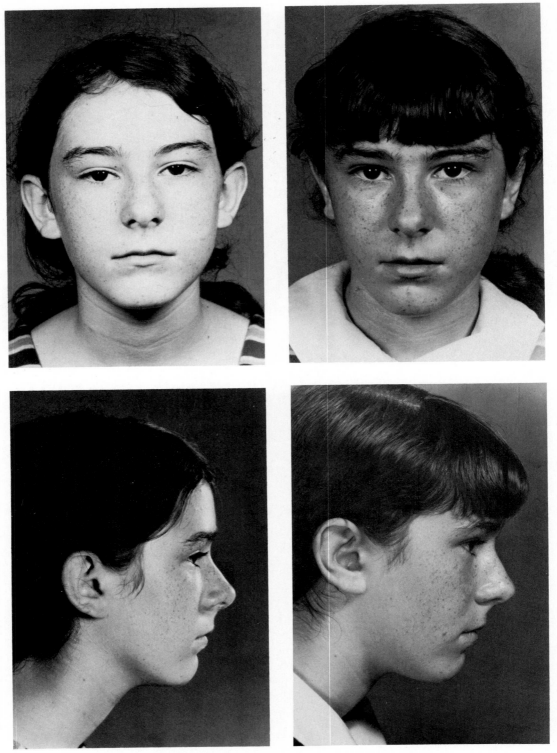

Figure 29–3. *See legend on the opposite page.*

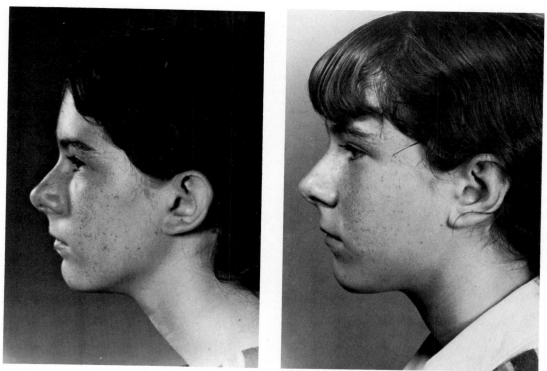

Figure 29–3.   A typical example of lop ear deformity. The postoperative views were taken 12 months after correction by the Converse–Wood-Smith technique.

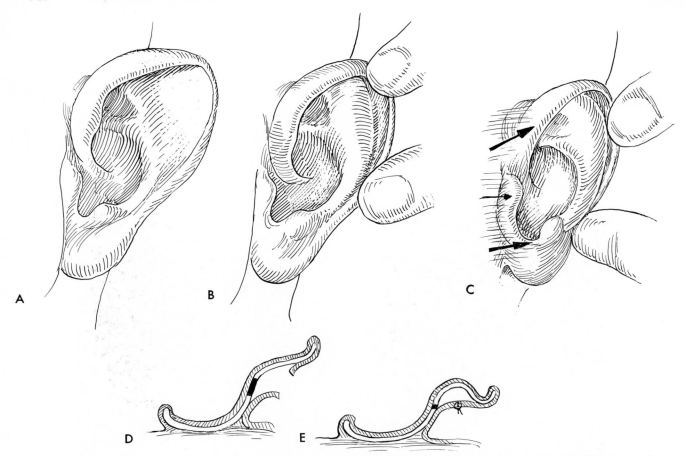

Figure 29–4. *A*, Unfurled antihelix with conchal rim excess. *B*, Pressure in the scaphal region forms the antihelix and superior crus. *C*, Further increase of pressure throws the conchal rim into prominence and emphasizes the anterior superior and inferior conchal excess. *D*, The excess conchal rim cartilage and skin. *E*, Representation of the corrected ear.

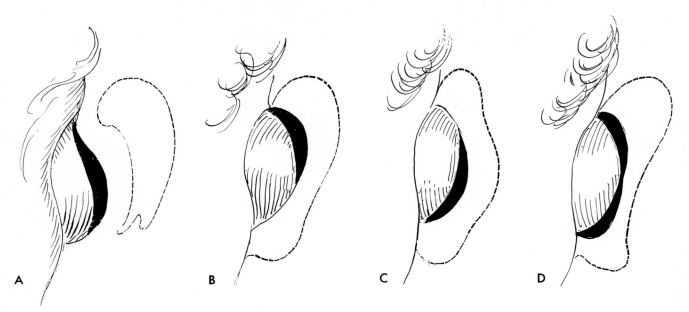

Figure 29–5. *A*, Uniform excess of conchal cartilage (black). *B*, Upper third to upper half conchal cartilage excess. *C*, Lower third to lower half excess. *D*, Upper third and lower third excess.

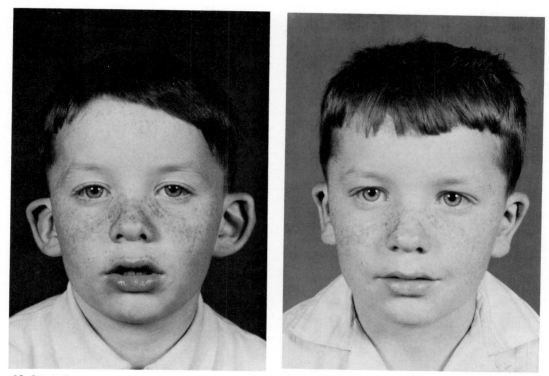

Figure 29–6.   A four-year-old boy with lop ear deformity corrected by the Converse–Wood-Smith technique, but with inadequate excision of the superior and inferior conchal rim excess.

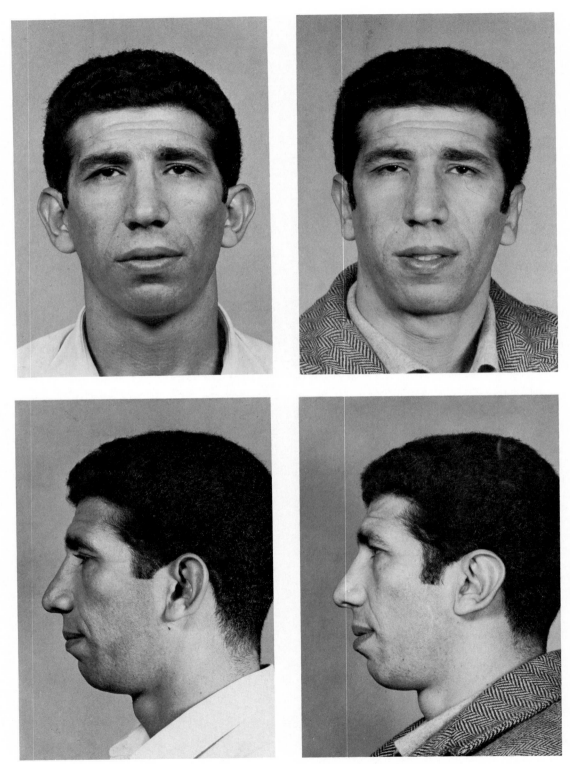

Figure 29–7.   The machiavellian ear, preoperatively and postoperatively.

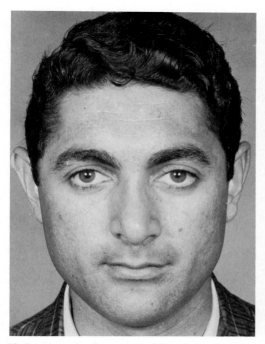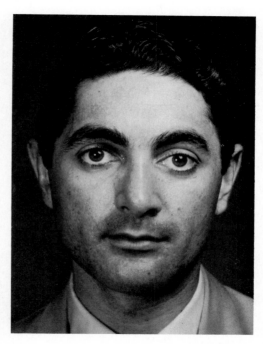

Figure 29–8.   Excessive formation of Darwin's tubercle and mild lop deformity of the right ear, corrected by the Converse–Wood-Smith technique. (From Converse, J. M., and Wood-Smith, D.: Plast. Reconstr. Surg. *43*:118, 1963. Reproduced with permission.)

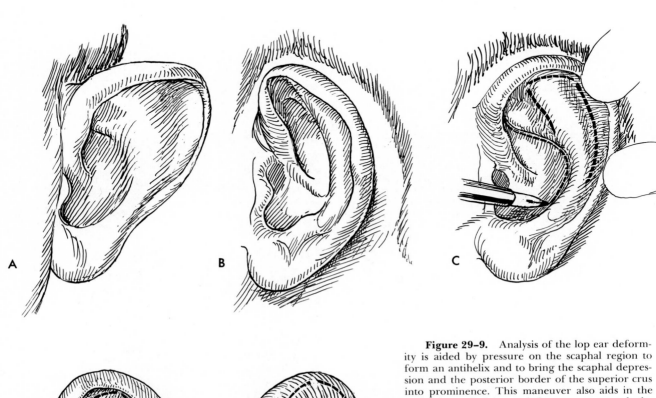

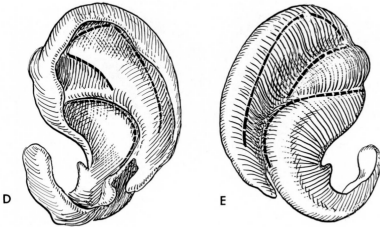

Figure 29–9. Analysis of the lop ear deformity is aided by pressure on the scaphal region to form an antihelix and to bring the scaphal depression and the posterior border of the superior crus into prominence. This maneuver also aids in the evaluation of the conchal component and the amount of skin to be removed from the scalp aspect of the ear.

Local anesthesia is preferred for cooperative patients over the age of six or seven years. However, we do not hesitate to use a general anesthesia in the uncooperative or unduly apprehensive patient. Local anesthesia is achieved by blocking the auricle at its base. Dissection of the postauricular skin and anesthesia of the postauricular area are further aided by the "hydraulic" dissection afforded by local anesthetic infiltration.

The operative field is prepared and draped, and then the procedure outlined above is repeated. The patient's hair is neither clipped nor shaved. The ear is folded back by gentle pressure in the region of the scapha to produce a tubing of the body of the antihelix and the superior crus of the antihelix. The posterior border of the antihelix and its superior crus are outlined in ink on the anterolateral aspect of the auricle, together with the anterior border of the superior crus, which is thrown into prominence by gentle pressure between the finger and thumb in the region of the junction between the superior and inferior crura (A to C). A third line is marked, parallel and immediately adjacent to the superior helical rim between the two previously marked lines but joining neither. The conchal rim is marked on the anterolateral aspect of the auricle, extending superiorly into the region of the cymba conchae and inferiorly to the external auditory meatus (D and E).

Figure 29–10.   The ear is infiltrated with local anesthetic and an ellipse of postauricular skin is removed. The perichondrium is exposed and, after modification of the shape of the cartilage and resection of excess cartilage, suturing of the edges of the skin under some tension will aid as a splint to hold the auricle in its corrected position. The center line of the ellipse to be removed is determined by passing needles from the anterolateral aspect of the auricle through the center line of the body of the antihelix and the superior crus (A and B).

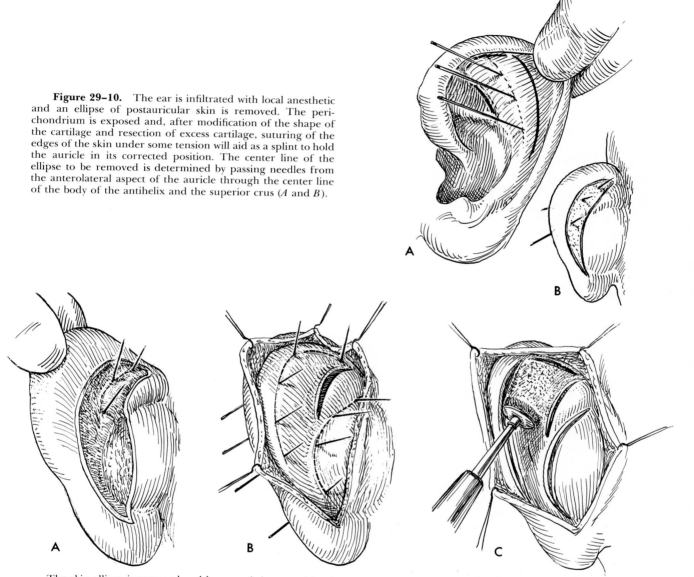

The skin ellipse is removed and hemostasis is secured by electrocoagulation of the bleeding vessels. Skin and subcutaneous tissues are elevated to expose the posterior aspect of the helical rim. Exposure of the perichondrium must extend to the anterosuperior and inferior limits of the conchal rim. The entire posterior aspect of the concha is thus exposed down to its junction with the mastoid process.

By passing straight cutting needles (Keith) from the lateral aspect of the auricle through the postauricular aspect, the posterior border of the antihelix, the superior crus, the superior border of the superior crus, the anterior border of the superior crus, and the conchal rim are outlined. The needles may be left in place and the incisions made to join them, or small ink spots may be placed where the needle points perforate the auricular cartilage.

Incisions are made through the cartilage up to but not including the perichondrium over the anterolateral aspect of the auricular cartilage (A and B). The incisions should not join one another; a gap of a few millimeters is maintained between the ends. The cartilage of the body of the antihelix and the superior crus may require thinning to facilitate folding. An electrically driven rotating wire brush is employed for this purpose (C). The brush removes perichondrium and a layer of cartilage, allowing for its easy folding into a tube. The use of the brush is not always necessary, for the cartilage is often sufficiently weak to permit tubing without such weakening.

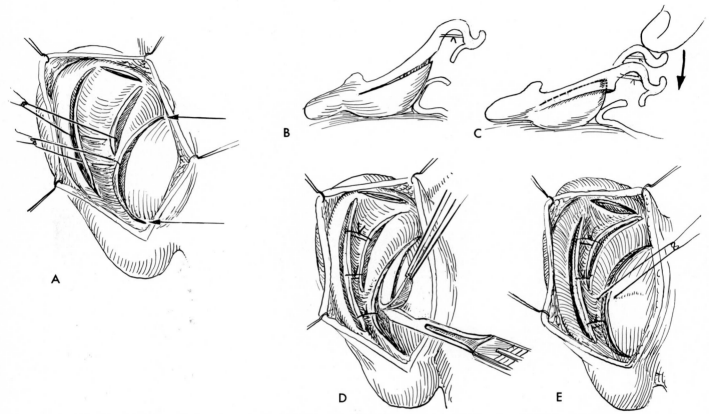

Figure 29–11.   Tubing of the cartilage is accomplished with clear nylon or Mersilene sutures (4–0). The first of these mattress sutures is placed immediately below the junction of the crura of the antihelix where it joins the body of the antihelix. The second is placed in the superior crus of the antihelix immediately above the crural junction. These sutures are tied with sufficient tension to produce the desired contour of the antihelix (*A*).

The contour of the tube may be maintained by passing straight needles through the tubed cartilage and at the proposed sites of the sutures before the sutures are positioned. By this means the contour of the tube is accurately gauged prior to insertion of the sutures. Once the sutures are in place, the needles are removed.

At this stage, correction of the protruding auricle has been achieved, and with pressure exerted on the scaphal region, the amount of conchal rim resection required to set the auricle back in a satisfactory position can be determined (*B* and *C*). An ellipse of conchal cartilage of required size is removed from the medial edge of the rim. Skin lying on the anterolateral aspect of the concha is undermined for a distance of 3 or 4 mm from the edges of the new conchal rim (*D*). The edges of the conchal and antihelix cartilages are approximated with a single interrupted 4–0 nylon suture (*E*).

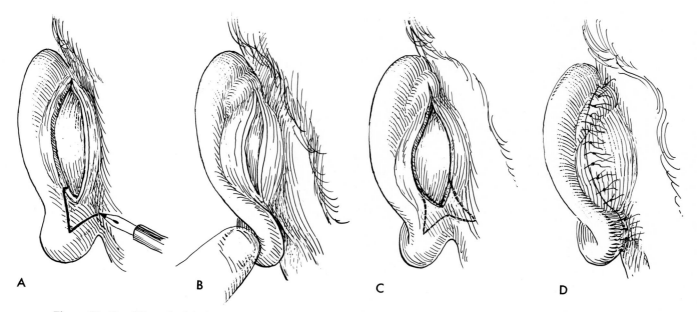

A   B   C   D

Figure 29–12. When the lobule of the ear protrudes, the skin incision is continued downward to the lobule in the shape of a "V" (*A*). Pressure of the freshly marked lobe skin against the mastoid skin makes an imprint outlining the mirror image of the skin to be resected (*B to D*). This W-shaped segment of skin is removed, hemostasis is secured, and the postauricular incision is closed with interrupted 5–0 nylon or 4–0 plain catgut sutures, fitting the small V-shaped incisions together.

A pressure dressing is applied; small pledgets of Acrilan wool (Chemstrand Corp.) or cotton wool soaked in sterile mineral oil are carefully packed within the convolutions of the corrected ear and covered with fluffed-out gauze. More Acrilan wool and a tube gauze head cap are applied, and mild pressure is maintained with a stretchable wrap bandage. The pressure dressing remains undisturbed for a period of five days.

A small fold of excess skin in the conchal fossa usually disappears within two or three months. It can be directly excised if in marked excess, although we have rarely had to do this.

This technique avoids sharp ridges resulting from folding of the cartilage and produces a natural-appearing concha, antihelix, and lobule.

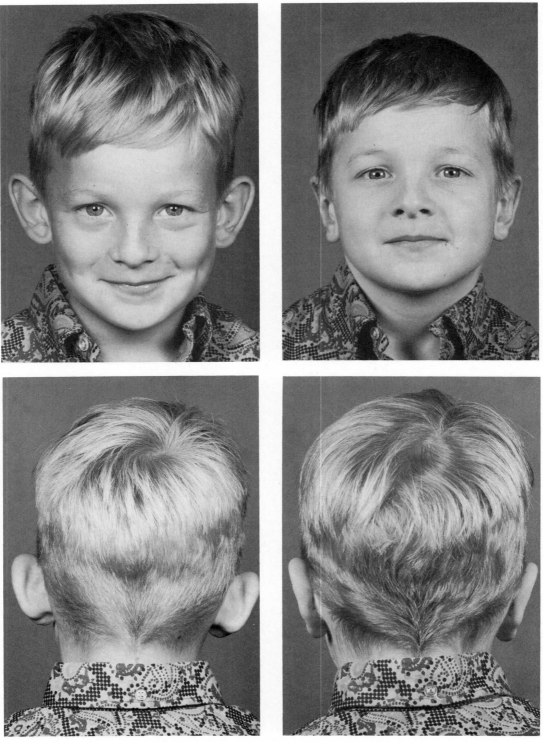

Figure 29–13. *See legend and illustration on the opposite page.*

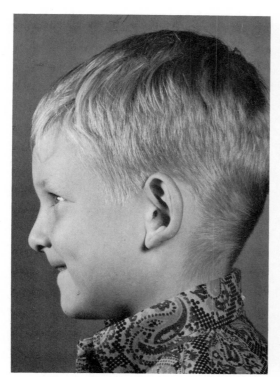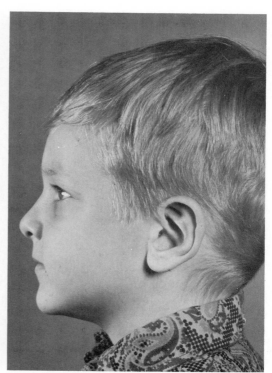

Figure 29–13.   A five-year-old boy with a typical lop ear deformity. Postoperative views were taken 15 months after correction by the Converse–Wood-Smith technique.

See illustration on the opposite page.

Figure 29–14.   The Mustardé Technique.

A method of correcting prominent ears by using buried mattress sutures was described by Mustardé in 1963. It is particularly applicable when the ear cartilage is thin and the ear deformity is not severe. When those conditions are not present, however, we prefer to use the Converse–Wood-Smith technique because more precise correction can be achieved.

It is essential that the perichondrium and adjacent soft tissue be stripped completely from the scalp aspect of the auricle from the point of junction of the concha with the mastoid to the helix rim, so that a smooth correction of the auricle can be made. The line of skin closure should be planned so as not to be in immediate juxtaposition with the buried mattress sutures.

In an ear formed of thin, easily correctable cartilage (A), a new antihelix fold is formed by finger pressure on the auricle, and the center line of the antihelix and the crura of the antihelix are outlined with ink (B). In the small ear, three sutures usually suffice; in the large ear, four or five buried mattress sutures may be necessary to achieve a smooth contour.

The position of these sutures is marked on the anterior aspect of the ear by ink dots so placed that a portion of cartilage 5 to 10 mm on either side of the midline is encompassed by the sutures. The points of suture entry are transferred from the auricular skin to the underlying cartilage by passing a 24- or 25-gauge hypodermic needle dipped in marking ink, so that on withdrawal of the needle, the marks of perforation are stained by the dye (C).

An ellipse of skin whose center line lies along the center line of the body of the antihelix and its posterior superior crus is excised down to and including perichondrium. After hemostasis is obtained, the perichondrium is raised from the scalp aspect of the auricle to the helix border and anteriorly to the point of junction of the concha with the underlying mastoid periosteum. This step is important to permit the smooth recontouring of the ear cartilage following insertion of the buried mattress sutures and to prevent the close apposition of the buried sutures to the skin wound.

The mattress sutures are inserted into the marks previously made on the cartilage (D), taking care to encompass the full thickness of the auricular cartilage—including, if possible, the perichondrium on its anterior aspect. We prefer to use 4–0 clear nylon sutures for this purpose, touching the end of the completed knot with the cautery to weld the nylon and insure that it will not unravel; 4–0 white Mersilene is also suitable for this purpose (E and F).

While looking at the anterior aspect of the auricle, the surgeon tightens the knots to produce a satisfactory antihelix contour; we prefer to begin with knots in the region of the body and cauda helicus and proceed superiorly. The sutures should be removed and replaced if a satisfactory contour does not result.

The skin is closed by intradermal 4–0 plain catgut sutures or by a continuous over-and-over 4–0 nylon suture. Protruding lobules can be corrected by the use of the fishtail excision already described (page 847). We do not favor the wedge excision of lobules advocated by Mustardé, for a lobular deformity can result from inadequate correction of the protrusion. Excision of excess conchal cartilage can be easily accomplished in the Mustardé operation, if this is required, and can produce a satisfactory result.

A pressure dressing, using accurately molded pledgets of Acrilan wool or cotton wool soaked in sterile mineral oil, is placed over the ear for seven to 10 days. A slightly elastic sleeping cap, which may be readily made from the upper elasticized end of a woman's stocking, is worn at night to splint the ears for four to six weeks.

See illustration on the opposite page.

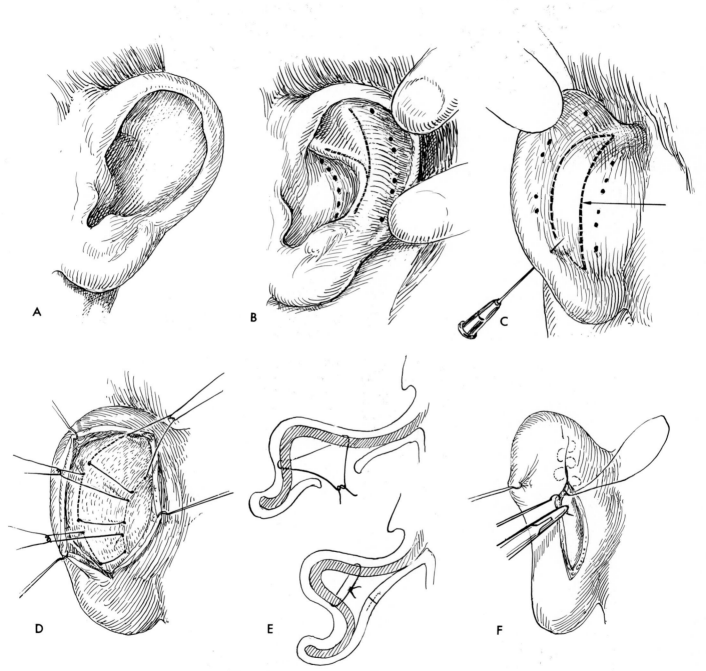

Figure 29–14. *See legend on the opposite page.*

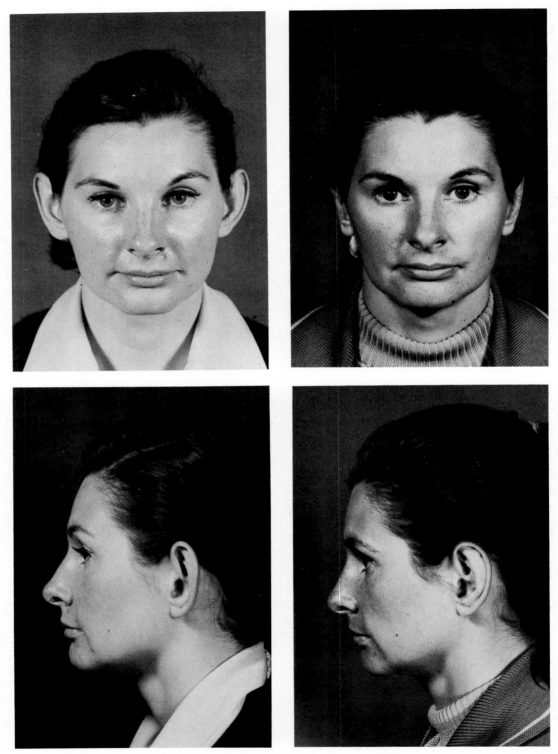

Figure 29–15. *See illustration and legend on the opposite page.*

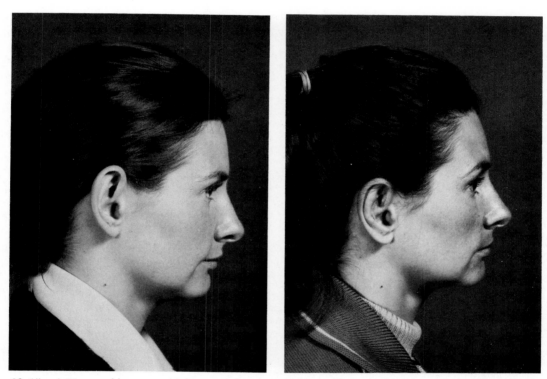

Figure 29–15.   A 25-year-old woman with lop ear deformity and thin, easily correctable ear cartilages. The postoperative views were taken two months after correction by the Owens-Mustardé technique.

See illustration on the opposite page.

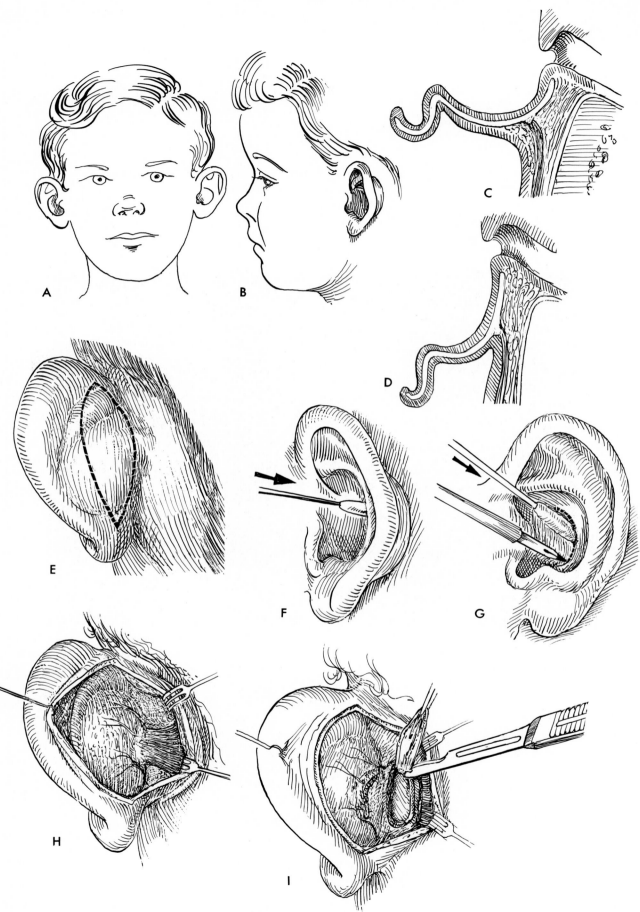

Figure 29–16. *See legend on the opposite page.*

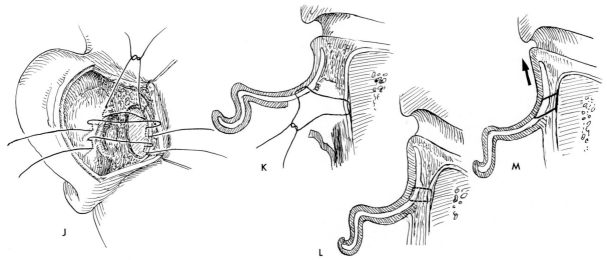

Figure 29–16. The Furnas Technique.

The principal indication for the use of this means of correction of the prominent ear deformity (Furnas, 1968) is the presence of a deeply cupped concha, whose posterior wall is high and detached from the underlying mastoid region, and a relatively well formed antihelix (*A* and *B*). In some instances this technique can eliminate the need for excision of a conchal cartilage strip.

A cross-sectional view of the detached concha is shown in *C* and may be compared with normally attached conchal cartilage (*D*).

The operative technique involves, first, estimation of the degree of detachment of the conchal cartilage and the amount of correction that may be achieved by pressure on the posterior wall of the conchal cavity with a cotton-tipped applicator (*F*). A line of junction between the posterior concha and the mastoid process, estimated from the point of pressure of the applicator, is marked in the depths of the conchal cavity to serve as an approximate guide to the points of insertion of the concha-mastoid sutures (*G*).

A posterior auricular segment of skin is excised (*E* and *H*). The concha is dissected anteriorly, and the fibers of the vestigial posterior auricular muscle and its ligament are divided, with care being taken to preserve the branches of the greater auricular nerve. A segment of the soft tissue overlying the mastoid fascia in this region is removed (*I*), and the deep fascia over the mastoid process is exposed. The area exposed should be about 1 × 2 cm, and its position is determined by trial and error placement of the conchal cartilage.

Sutures of 4–0 clear nylon are used to approximate and attach the cartilage to the fascia, using the previously placed marks in the depths of the conchal cavity as a rough guide to suture placement. Two or three sutures are generally required, and the thick mastoid periosteum and the full thickness of the conchal cartilage are picked up (*J*, *K*, and *L*). Sutures that are incorrectly placed or that distort the concha are removed and replaced. Care is exerted not to shift the conchal cartilage anteriorly, which will produce a narrowing of the external auditory meatus (*M*). The sutures are tightened and the final knots are welded by a quick application of the cautery to their ends.

If required, a fold is made in the antihelix, using the Converse–Wood-Smith or Mustardé technique.

The skin is closed as previously described, and a mild pressure dressing applied for seven to 10 days. The patient should wear a light elastic cap as a splint during sleep for four to six weeks.

See illustration on the opposite page.

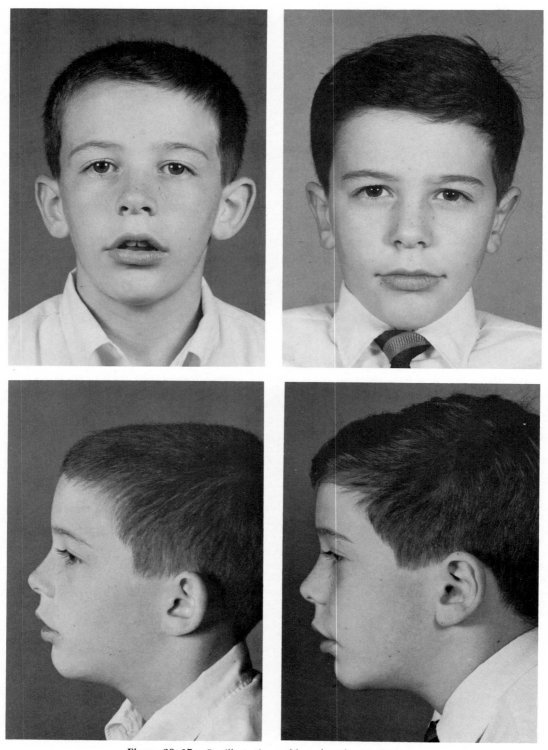

Figure 29–17. *See illustration and legend on the opposite page.*

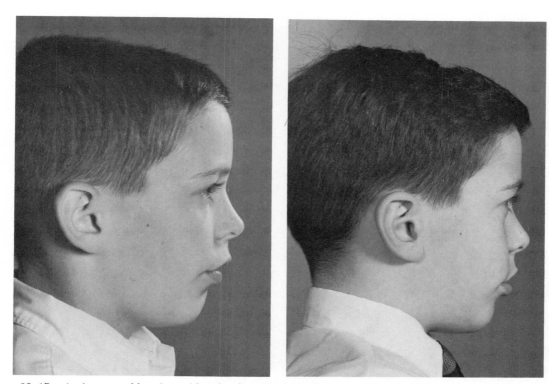

Figure 29–17.   A nine-year-old patient with a deeply cupped concha and a reasonably well-formed antihelix, whose appearance was improved by the Furnas technique. The postoperative photographs were taken six months after the operation.

See illustration on the opposite page.

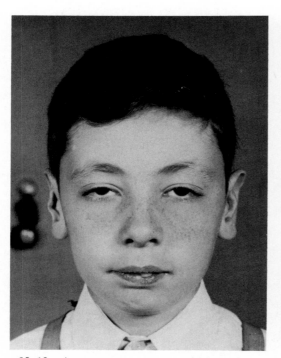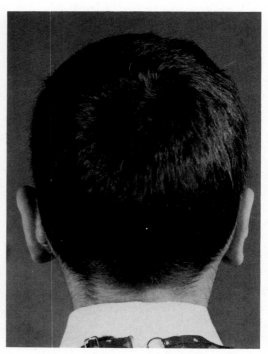

Figure 29–18.   An attempt to correct a "telephone deformity" created this excessive "plastered to head" appearance. Note the postauricular hypertrophic scar on the left.

reduced to two to three weeks, with further injections given as indicated by the resolution of the lesion.

Keloids

Keloid of the postauricular incision is one of the most frustrating of all postoperative complications and may require further operative procedures before a solution to the problem is reached. In the early stages of keloid formation, the use of intralesional steroid injections of triamcinolone acetonide has proved to be effective in a large percentage of patients. The drug is injected intralesionally on a weekly basis, and if early regression of the keloid has occurred, its use may be extended to every two weeks for some months, tapering off to once a month for a further two to three months before terminating the treatment.

The use of radiation in this area is fraught with danger, but on occasion has proved to be the only effective means of control of the keloids. When more advanced keloids occur in this region, surgical excision may need to be combined with radiation and delayed skin grafting of the radiated area, with final aid from the use of intralesional triamcinolone acetonide. Problems such as these have proved to be some of the most difficult keloid problems encountered in our practice and ones in which the results of therapy have left much to be desired.

(For references, see page 861.)

REFERENCES

Forehead and Brow

Baker, T. J.: The forehead lift. In Goulian, D., and Courtiss, G., (eds.): *Surgery of the Aging Face.* St. Louis, C. V. Mosby Co., 1978.

Bames, H. O.: Frown disfigurement and ptosis. Plast. Reconstr. Surg. 19:337, 1957.

Castanares, S.: Forehead wrinkles, glabellar frown and ptosis of the eyebrows. Plast. Reconstr. Surg. 34:406, 1964.

Connell, B. F.: Eyebrow, face, and neck lifts for males. Clin. Plast. Surg. 5:15, 1978.

Correia, P. de C., and Zani, R.: Surgical anatomy of the facial nerve, as related to ancillary operations in rhytidoplasty. Plast. Reconstr. Surg. 52:549, 1973.

Courtiss, E. H., Webster, R. C., and White, M. F.: Use of double w-plasty in upper blepharoplasty. Plast. Reconstr. Surg. 53:25, 1974.

D'Assumpçao, E. A.: A new instrument for rhytidoplasty. Brit. J. Plast. Surg. 23:301, 1970.

Edgerton, M. T., Webb, W. L., Slaughter, R., and Meyer, E.: Surgical results and psychosocial changes following rhytidectomy. Plast. Reconstr. Surg. 33:503, 1964.

Edwards, B. F.: Bilateral temporal neurotomy for frontalis hypermotility. Plast. Reconstr. Surg. 11:341, 1957.

Eitner, E.: Weitermitteilungen über Kosmetische Faltenoperationen in Gesicht. Wein. Med. Wchnschr. 85:244, 1935.

Fomon, S.: *The Surgery of Injury and Plastic Repair.* Chicago, The Williams & Wilkins Company, 1939.

Fomon, S.: *Cosmetic Surgery: Principles and Practice.* Philadelphia, J. B. Lippincott Co., 1960.

Fredricks, S.: The Lower Rhytidectomy. Plast. Reconstr. Surg. 54:537, 1976.

Furnas, D. W.: Landmarks for the trunk and the temporofacial division of the facial nerve. Brit. J. Surg. 52:694, 1965.

Gleason, M. C.: Brow lifting through a temporal scalp approach. Plast. Reconstr. Surg. 52:141, 1973.

González-Ulloa, M.: A trend of new operations to improve the results of rhytidectomy. Internat. Micr. J. Aesth. Plast. Surg. (Facial Plasty, 1974-A).

González-Ulloa, M.: Facial wrinkles, integral elimination. Plast. Reconstr. Surg. 29:658, 1962.

González-Ulloa, M., and Flores, E. S.: Rhytidectomy in the male — a new approach. Trans. Fifth Internat. Congress. Plast. Reconstr. Surg. London, Butterworth & Co., Ltd., 1970.

Griffiths, C. O.: A new approach to the operative management of forehead, brow, and frown rhytidectomies. Internat. Micr. J. Aesth. Plast. Surg. (Facial Plasty, 1974-B).

Hinderer, U.: Treatment of the aging face. Internat. Micr. J. Aesth. Plast. Surg. (Facial Plasty, 1974-B).

Hunt, H. L.: *Plastic Surgery of the Head, Face, and Neck.* Philadelphia and New York, Lea & Febiger, 1926.

Johnson, J. P.: The problem of the aging face. Plast. Reconstr. Surg. 15:117, 1955.

Joseph, J.: Nasenplastik und Sonstige Gesichtsplastik: nebst Einen Anhang über Mammaplastik. Curt Kabitzsch. Leipzig, 1931, p. 507–509.

Kaye, B. L.: The forehead lift: a useful adjunct to face lift and blepharoplasty. Plast. Reconstr. Surg. 60:161, 1977.

LeRoux, P., and Jones, J. H.: Total permanent removal of wrinkles from the forehead. Aesth. & Plast. Surg. 27:359, 1974.

Lewis, G. K.: Surgical treatment of wrinkles. Arch. Otolaryngology. 60:334, 1954.

Lexer, E.: Zur Gesichtsplastik. Arch. Klin. Chir. 92:749, 1910.

Litton, C.: Forehead lift: Coronal scalp approach. Presented at the annual meeting of the American Society for Aesthetic Plastic Surgery, Atlanta, April 15, 1976.

Loeb, R.: Technique for preservation of the temporal branches of the facial nerve during face lift operations. Brit. J. Plast. Surg. 23:380, 1970.

Marino, H.: Treatment of wrinkles of forehead. Prensa Med. Argent. 51:1368, 1964.

Marino, H.: The surgery of facial expression. Trans. Fifth Internat. Congr. Plast. and Reconstr. Surg. Butterworths, Melbourne, 1971, p. 1102.

Marino, H.: The forehead lift. Some hints to secure better results. Aesth. Plast. Surg. 1:251, 1977.

Mayer, P. M., and Swanker, W. A.: Rhytidoplasty. Plast. Reconstr. Surg. 6:255, 1950.

McDowell, F.: Editorial note in Regnault, P.: Complete face and forehead lifting, with double traction on "crow's-feet". Plast. Reconstr. Surg. 49:127, 1972.

Mitz, V., and Peyronie, M.: The superficial musculoaponeurotic system (SMAS) in the parotid and cheek area. Plast. Reconstr. Surg. 58:80, 1976.

Morel-Fatio, O.: Cosmetic surgery of the aging face. In Gibson, T. (ed.): *Modern Trends in Plastic Surgery.* Washington, Butterworths, Inc., 1964.

Noel, A.: La Chirurgie esthétique et sa rôle sociale. Paris, Masson et Cie, 1926.

Ortiz-Montasterio, F., Barrera, G., and Olmedo, A.: The coronal incision in rhytidectomy—the brow lift. Clin. Plast. Surg. 5(1):167, 1978.

Owsley, J. Q.: Platysma-fascial rhytidectomy; a preliminary report. Plast. & Reconst. Surg. 60:843, 1977.

Pangman, J. W., and Wallace, R. M.: Cosmetic surgery of the face and neck. Plast. Reconstr. Surg. 27:544, 1961.

Passot, R.: La Chirurgie esthétique des rides du visage. Presse Med. 27:P. 258, 1919.

Passot, R.: Chirurgie esthétique pure (technique et résultats). Paris, Doin et Cie, 1931.

Passot, R.: Quelques generalités sur l'operation correctif des rides du visage. Rev. Chir. Plast. 3:23, 1933.

Peterson, R. A.: Rhytidoplasty with emphasis on buccal, cervical, and submental regions. Video Tape 7601. Educational Foundation of the American Society of Plastic and Reconstructive Surgeons, Chicago, 1977.

Picaud, A. J.: Different forms of incisions and techniques in face-lifting. Trans Fourth Internat. Congr. Plast. and Reconstr. Surg. Amsterdam, Excerpta Medica, 1967, p. 1108.

Pitanguy, I., and Silveira Ramos, A.: The frontal branch of the facial nerve. The importance of its variations in face lifting. Plast. Reconstr. Surg. 38:352, 1966.

Pitanguy, I.: Ancillary procedures in face lifting. Clin. Plast. Surg. 5:51, 1978.

Rees, T. D., and Guy, C. L.: Patient selection and technique in blepharoplasty and rhytidoplasty. Surg. Clin. N. Amer. 87:(2), 353, April, 1971.

Rees, T. D., and Wood-Smith, D.: Cosmetic Facial Surgery. Philadelphia, W. B. Saunders Company, 1973.

Regnault, P.: Complete face and forehead lifting with double traction on "crows-feet". Plast. Reconstr. Surg. 49:123, 1972.

Skoog, T.: Plastic Surgery: New Methods and Refinements. Philadelphia, W. B. Saunders, 1974, 328.

Stephenson, K. L.: The History of Face, Neck, and Eyelid Surgery. In Masters, F. W., and Lewis, J. P. (eds.): Symposium on Aesthetic Surgery of the Face, Eyelid and Breast. St. Louis, The C. V. Mosby Company, 1972.

Tessier, P.: Ridectomie frontale—lifting frontale. Gazette Médicale de France 75:5565, 1968.

Uchida, J. I.: "A Method of Frontal Rhytidectomy". Plast. Reconstr. Surg. 35:218, 1965.

Viñas, J. C., Caviglia, C., Cortinas, J. L.: Forehead rhytidoplasty and brow lifting. Plast. Reconstr. Surg. 57:445, 1976.

Vinnick, C. A.: Personal communication, 1977.

Washio, H.: Rhytidoplasty of the forehead — an anatomical approach. Trans. Sixth Internat. Congr. Plast. and Reconstr. Surg. Paris, Masson et Cie, 1976, p. 430.

Chemabrasion

Ayres, S., III: Superficial chemosurgery in treating aging skin. Arch. Dermatol. 85:385, 1962.

Ayres, S., III: Superficial chemosurgery, its current status and relationship to dermabrasion. Arch. Dermatol. 89:395, 1964.

Baker, T. J.: Ablation of rhytides by chemical means. J. Fl. Med. Assoc. 47:451–454, 1961.

Baker, T. J.: Chemical face peeling and rhytidectomy, a combined approach for facial rejuvenation. Plast. Reconstr. Surg. 29:199, 1962.

Baker, T. J.: Chemical face peeling: An adjunct to surgical face lifting. South. Med. J. 56:412, 1963.

Baker, T. J., and Gordon, H. L.: Chemical face peeling. In Goldwyn, R. M. (ed.): The Unfavorable Result in Plastic Surgery. Boston, Little, Brown and Co., 1972, pp. 345–352.

Baker, T. J., Gordon, H. L., Mosienko, P., and Seckinger, D. L.: Long-term histological study of skin after chemical face peeling. Plast. Reconstr. Surg. 53:522, 1974.

Baker, T. J., Gordon, H. L., and Seckinger, D. L.: A second look at chemical face peeling. Plast. Reconstr. Surg. 37:487, 1966.

Batstone, J. H. F., and Millard, D. R., Jr.: An endorsement of facial chemosurgery. Br. J. Plast. Surg. 21:193, 1968.

Brown, A. M., Kaplan, L. M., and Brown, M. E.: Phenol-induced histological skin changes: Hazards, technique, and uses. Br. J. Plast. Surg. 13:158, 1960.

Combes, F. C., Sperber, P. A., and Reich, M.: Dermal defects treated by chemical agents. N.Y. Phys. & Amer. Med. 56:36, 1960.

Gillies, H., and Millard, D. R.: The Principles and Art of Plastic Surgery. Boston and Toronto, Little, Brown and Co., 1957.

Litton, C.: Chemical face lifting. Plast. Reconstr. Surg. 29:371, 1962.

Litton, C.: Followup study of chemosurgery. South Med. J. 50:1007, 1966.

Litton, C., Fournier, P., and Capinpin, A.: A survey of chemical peeling of the face. Plast. Reconstr. Surg. 51:645, 1973.

MacKee, G. M., and Karp, E. L.: Treatment of acne scars with phenol. Br. J. Dermatol. 64:456, 1952.

Rees, T. D.: Rehabilitation of the aging face. Geriatrics 20:1039, 1965.

Sperber, P. A.: Chemexfoliation— a new term in cosmetic therapy. J. Am. Geriatr. Surg. 11:58, 1963.

Sperber, P. A.: Treatment of aging skin and dermal defects. Springfield, Ill., Charles C Thomas, Publisher, 1965 a, Ch. 1, p. 3.

Sperber, P. A.: Chemexfoliation for aging skin and acne scarring. Arch. Otolaryngol. 81:278, 1965.

Spira, M., Dahl, G., Freeman, R., Gerow, F. J., and Hardy, S. B.: Chemosurgery — A histological study. Plast. Reconstr. Surg. 45:247, 1970.

Spira, M., Gerow, F. J., and Hardy, S. B.: Complications of chemical face peeling. Plast. Reconstr. Surg. 54:397, 1974.

Spira, M.: Treatment of acne pitting and scarring. Plast. Reconstr. Surg. 60:38, 1977.

Truppman, E. S., and Ellenby, J. D.: Major electrocardiographic changes during chemical face peeling. Plast. Reconstr. Surg. 63:44, 1979.

Dermabrasion

Converse, J. M., and Robb-Smith, A. H. T.: The healing of surface cutaneous wounds: Its analogy with the healing of superficial burns. Ann. Surg. 120:873, 1944.

DaSilva, N.: Dermabrasion with miniature electric suction dermatome. Plast. Reconstr. Surg. 30:690, 1962.

Eisen, A. Z., Holyoke, J. B., and Lobitz, W. C.: Responses of superficial portion of human pilosebaceous apparatus to controlled injury. J. Invest. Dermatol. 25:145, 1955.

Hynes, W.: The treatment of scars by shaving and skin graft. Br. J. Plast. Surg. 10:1–10, 1957.

Iverson, P. C.: Surgical removal of traumatic tattoos. Plast. Reconstr. Surg. 2:427, 1947.

Janson, P.: Eine einfache Methode der Entfernung von Tatauierungen. Dermat. Wschr. 101:894, 1935.

Kromayer, E.: Rotationinstrumente: Ein neues technisches Verfahren in der dermatologischen Kleinchirurgie. Chir. Dermat. Z. (Berlin) 12:26, 1905.

Kurtin, A.: Corrective surgical planing of skin; New technique for treatment of acne scars and other skin defects. A.M.A. Arch. Dermatol. 68:389, 1953.

Luikart, R., Ayres, S., and Wilson, J. W.: Surgical skin planing. N.Y. J. Med. 59:413, 1959.

Malherbe, W. D. F., and Davies, D. S.: Surgical treatment by dermatome for acne scarring. Plast. Reconstr. Surg. 47:122, 1971.

McEvitt, W. G.: Treatment of acne pits by abrasion with sandpaper. J.A.M.A. 142:647, 1950.

Spira, M.: Treatment of acne pitting and scarring. Plast. Reconstr. Surg. 60:38, 1977.

Rees, T. D., and Casson, P.: Indications for cutaneous dermal overgrafting. Plast. Reconstr. Surg. 38:522, 1966.

Webster, G. V.: Report at the Annual Convention of the American Society of Plastic and Reconstructive Surgeons, Hollywood, Florida, October, 1954.

Mentoplasty

Ballard, C. F.: The morphological bases of prognosis determination and treatment planning. Dent. Pract. 18:62, 1967.

Bell, W. H.: Surgical correction of mandibular retrognathism. Am. J. Orthod. 52:518, 1966.

Case, C.: A Practical Treatise on the Technics and Principles of Dental Orthopedia. Chicago, C. S. Case Co., 1921.

Converse, J. M.: Restoration of facial contour by bone grafts introduced through the oral cavity. Plast. Reconstr. Surg. 6:295, 1950.

Converse, J. M.: Degloving technique. In Kanzanjian, V. H., and Converse, J. M. (ed.): The Surgical Treatment of Facial Injuries. Baltimore, Williams and Wilkins Company, 1974, p. 1022.

Converse, J. M., Kawamoto, H. K., Jr., Wood-Smith, D., Coccaro, P. J., and McCarthy, J. G.: Deformities of the jaws. In Converse, J. M. (ed): Reconstructive Plastic Surgery. Philadelphia, W. B. Saunders Company, 1977, Chapter 30.

Converse, J. M., and Wood-Smith, D.: Horizontal osteotomy of the mandible. Plast. Reconstr. Surg. 34:464, 1964.

Friedland, J. A., Coccaro, P. J., and Converse, J. M.: Retrospective cephalometric analysis of mandibular bone absorption under silicone rubber chin implants. Plast. Reconstr. Surg. 57:144, 1976.

González-Ulloa, M., and Stevens, E.: Role of chin correction in profileplasty. Plast. Reconstr. Surg. 41:477, 1968.

Grabb, W. C.: The Hapsburg jaw. Plast. Reconstr. Surg. 42:442, 1968.

Hinds, E. C., and Kent, J. N.: Genioplasty: The versatility of the horizontal osteotomy. Oral Surg. 27:690, 1969.

Horowitz, S. L.: The challenge of facial deformity. Dent. Pract. 22:191, 1972.

Horowitz, S. L., Gerstman, L. J., and Converse, J. M.: Craniofacial relationships in mandibular prognathism. Arch. Oral Biol. 14:121, 1969.

Horowitz, S. L., and Hixon, E. H.: The Nature of Orthodontic Diagnosis. St. Louis, The C. V. Mosby Co., 1966, Chapters 15 and 17.

Jackson, I. T.: Use of tongue flaps to resurface lip defects and close palatal fistulae in children. Plast. Reconstr. Surg. 49:537, 1972.

Jobe, R., Iverson, R., and Vistnes, L.: Bone deformation beneath alloplastic implants. Plast. Reconstr. Surg. 51:169, 1973. (Discussions by Rees, T. D., and Spira, M.: Plast. Reconstr. Surg. 51:174, 1973.)

Junghans, J. A.: Profile reconstruction with Silastic chin implants. Am. J. Orthod. 53:217, 1967.

Lassus, C.: The horizontal osteotomy of the chin: Its indications. Rev. Stomatol. (Paris) 69:642, 1968.

Millard, R.: Adjuncts in augmentation mentoplasty and corrective rhinoplasty. Plast. Reconstr. Surg. 3:48, 1965.

Millard, R.: Augmentation mentoplasty. Surg. Clin. North Am. 51:333, 1971.

Obwegeser, H. L.: In Trauner, R., and Obwegeser, H. L.: The surgical correction of mandibular prognathism and retrognathia with consideration of genioplasty. 1. Surgical procedures to correct mandibular prognathism and reshaping of the chin. Oral Surg. 10:677, 1957.

Peck, H., and Peck, S.: A concept of facial esthetics. Angle Orthod. 40:284, 1970.

Pitanguy, I.: Augmentation mentoplasty. Plast. Reconstr. Surg. 42:460, 1968.

Rees, T. D.: Cosmetic Facial Surgery. Philadelphia, W. B. Saunders Company, 1973.

Riedel, R. A.: An analysis of dentofacial relationships. Am. J. Orthod. 43:103, 1957.

Rish, B. B.: Profile-plasty. Report on plastic chin implants. Laryngoscope 74:144, 1964.

Robertson, J. G.: Chin augmentation means of rotation of double chin fat flap. Plast. Reconstr. Surg. 3:471, 1965.

Robinson, M., and Shuken, R.: Bone resorption under plastic implants. J. Oral Surg. 27:116, 1969.

Robinson, M.: Bone resorption under plastic chin implants.

Follow-up of a preliminary report. Arch. Otolaryngol. 95:30, 1972.

Rubin, L. R., Robertson, G. W., and Shapiro, R. N.: Polyethylene in reconstructive surgery. Plast. Reconstr. Surg. 3:586, 1948.

Otoplasty

Barsky, A. J.: Plastic Surgery. Philadelphia, W. B. Saunders Company, 1938, pp. 199–221.

Becker, O. J.: Correction of protruding deformed ear. Br. J. Plast. Surg. 5:187, 1952.

Cocheril, R.: Essai sur la Restauration du Pavillon de l'Oreille. Paris Thèses. Lille. 1894.

Converse, J. M., Nigro, A., Wilson, F. A., and Johnson, N.: A technique for surgical correction of lop ears. Trans. Am. Acad. Ophthalmol. Otolaryngol. 59:551, 1956.

Converse, J. M., and Wood-Smith, D.: Technical details in the surgical correction of the lop ear deformity. Plast. Reconstr. Surg. 31:118, 1963.

Dieffenbach, J. E.: Die operative Chirurgie. Leipzig, F. A. Brockhaus, 1845.

Dufourmentel, C.: La greffe cutanée libre tubulée. Ann. Chir. Plast. (Paris) 3:311, 1958.

Ely, E. T.: An operation for prominence of the auricles. Arch. Otolaryngol. 10:97, 1881.

Furnas, D. W.: Correction of prominent ears by conchal mastoid sutures. Plast. Reconstr. Surg. 24:189, 1968.

Holmes, F. M.: A new procedure for correcting outstanding ears. Arch. Otolaryngol. 69:409, 1959.

Ju, D. M. C., Li, C., and Crikelair, G. F.: The surgical correction of protruding ears. Plast. Reconstr. Surg. 32:283, 1963.

Keen, W. W.: New method of operating for relief of deformity of prominent ears. Ann. Surg. 11:49, 1890.

Luckett, W. H.: A new operation for prominent ears based on the anatomy of the deformity. Surg. Gynecol. Obstet. 10:635, 1910.

MacCollum, D. W.: The lop ear. J.A.M.A. 110:1427, 1938.

McEvitt, W. G.: The problem of the protruding ear. Plast. Reconstr. Surg. 2:481, 1947.

Monks, G. H.: Operation for correcting the deformity due to prominent ears. Boston Med. Surg. J. 124:84, 1891.

Morestin, M. H.: De la réposition et du plissement cosmétiques du pavillion de l'oreille. Rev. Orthrop. 4:289, 1903.

Mustardé, J. C.: The correction of prominent ears using simple mattress sutures. Br. J. Plast. Surg. 16:170, 1963.

Mustardé, J. C.: The treatment of prominent ears by buried mattress sutures: A ten-year survey. Plast. Reconstr. Surg. 39:382, 1967.

Mustardé, J. C.: Plastic Surgery in Infancy and Childhood. Edinburgh, Churchill-Livingstone, 1971.

Pierce, G. W., Klabunde, E. H., and Bergeron, V. L.: Useful procedures in plastic surgery. Plast. Reconstr. Surg., 2:358, 1947.

Stark, R. B., and Saunders, D. E.: Natural appearance restored to the unduly prominent ear. Br. J. Plast. Surg. 15:385, 1962.

Stenstrom, S. J.: A "natural" technique for correction of congenitally prominent ears. Plast. Reconstr. Surg. 32:509, 1963.

Tanzer, R. C.: The correction of prominent ears. Plast. Reconstr. Surg. 30:236, 1962.

Wood-Smith, D., and Converse, J. M.: The lop ear deformity. Surg. Clin. North Am. 51:417, 1971.

Young, F.: The correction of abnormally prominent ears. Surg. Gynecol. Obstet. 78:541, 1944.

Part 6

TREATMENT OF BALDNESS

Chapter 30

Punch Grafts

NORMAN ORENTREICH, M.D.

For many years, it was known that autografts of black haircoat skin transplanted to white haircoat areas of spotted guinea pigs continued to grow black hair. In 1959, findings on skin autografts in man were presented at the New York Academy of Sciences (Orentreich, 1959). The transposition of autografts was studied in various diseases as well as in common baldness. In the case of baldness, it was found that autografts from the posterior fringe of the scalp (that long maintains hair growth while the rest of the scalp balds), when transplanted to the frontal scalp, continued to grow as though in their original sites. The basic technique of employing cylindrical punches to make practical use of this finding was published in the Annals of the New York Academy of Sciences, and subsequent refinements have been detailed in recent articles and books. As a testimonial to effectiveness, the procedure has become widely employed, especially in recent years. Persistent autograft hair growth in early transplanted patients has been observed for approximately 25 years.

However, since all hair loss is not common baldness or another type suitable for autograft correction, it is worthwhile to review the various alopecias and their treatments before discussing in detail the technique of hair transplantation.

Hair loss can be caused by injury to the living hair root or the keratinized hair shaft. If only the dead hair shaft is damaged, alopecia will be temporary because the underlying follicular apparatus continues to function adequately and will grow new hair. However, an inherently diseased root or toxic factors influencing a functioning follicle can stop hair growth and cause hair loss followed by: (1) immediate regrowth of new hair; (2) temporary failure to regrow hair; or (3) the persistent inability to regrow hair (Orentreich, 1960). If the follicle is completely destroyed, there is permanent loss of hair (Billingham, 1958; Miller, 1971).

CLASSIFICATION OF THE ALOPECIAS

Congenital alopecia may take the form of complete or partial (diffuse or patchy) absence of hair from birth (Cockayne, 1933). This may be associated with other cutaneous adnexal disorders. Rarely does normal hair develop.

Androgenetic alopecia is induced by androgens but only in persons genetically predisposed. Male pattern alopecia is the outstanding example of this type. Most hair loss in women (diffuse and/or patterned) is androgenetic. It results from endogenous or exogenous androgens triggering a hereditary predisposition to hair loss (Orentreich, 1966). Each individual hair follicle is genetically predisposed to respond or remain insensitive to androgenic (and other) influences that inhibit its growth.

Ninety-five percent of normal adult men have some androgenetic hair loss. It is usually patterned, but it frequently can be both diffuse and patterned. Seventy-five percent of adult women have some hair loss. It is usually of the so-called diffuse type; only occasionally is it of the male pattern type. The onset of androgenetic alopecia occurs earlier and the severity is greater in men than in women (Orentreich, 1964).

Alopecia Associated with Neoplastic Disorders

Space-occupying masses in the scalp can cause loss of hair by the pressure effects of displacement, dysplasia, and atrophy of the hair follicles, or by invasion and replacement of the follicular apparatus. Common cysts of the scalp, which often grow in clusters, frequently pose a pressure problem. Also to be considered are benign neoplasms such as cylindromas (turban tumors) and malignant lesions like leukemic nodular infiltrates (Leider, 1961). When surgical extirpation is indicated, the overlying alopecic skin should simply be observed for the next several months to determine if alopecia is only temporary.

Acquired Alopecias

Acquired alopecias are of several types: traumatic, hormonal, infectious, neurologic, psychiatric, nutritional, toxic (from poisons or drugs), and strictly dermatologic (Orentreich, 1960).

Traumatic Alopecias. Externally applied traction or pressure (as opposed to internal pressure owing to cysts and neoplasms) may be acute or chronic trauma. In acute trauma, with or without laceration, the hair loss that may occur at the site of injury is likely to be permanent if there is scarring. Chronic pressure may also produce localized alopecia. This type of hair loss may be seen after prolonged general anesthesia, especially if the patient is kept in the Trendelenburg position. Scalp edema may be the first symptom noticed in the area in which temporary hair loss later develops. Pressure and friction on the scalp of infants while lying will also cause a temporary hair loss. Physical trauma from acute traction (plucking, combing, or brushing) can cause breakage of the hair shaft or evulsion from the follicle. Breaking of the shaft does not interfere with continuity of growth, but evulsion usually produces a temporary cessation of hair growth. Chronic traction (tight pony-tails, braids, curlers, barrettes, headbands, or rubberbands) can cause hair loss at the site of tension. If the traction is removed early enough, no follicular damage occurs and permanent alopecia is avoided. However, prolonged traction can produce permanent hair loss. Avulsion, which is the tearing away of scalp tissue, can cause not only loss of the hair-bearing follicles and thus permanent alopecia but also injury to the skull. Burns from either extreme heat or cold can be sufficiently severe to destroy the hair follicle. Hair loss is permanent if there is necrosis of the follicle-bearing tissue (Stough et al., 1968).

Chemicals may come in contact with the hair and scalp through industry or cosmetics (Harry, 1955). Industrial exposure to sodium and/or calcium sulfide or dimethylamine can cause hair shaft breakage resulting in temporary hair loss without interfering with growth. A severe acute chemical dermatitis may also cause temporary hair loss. Only the severest primary irritant reaction or secondary bacterial infection with cicatrization can explain the permanent hair loss that is seen on rare occasions.

Exposure to x-rays, radium, radioisotopes, atomic bomb fallout or inadvertent short-wavelength radiation can produce temporary or permanent alopecia (Van Scott and Reinerston, 1957). In temporary alopecia, only the epithelial components are affected. In three to five weeks, the hair loss is almost complete, and within ten weeks, hair regrowth may be seen. Ionizing radiation involvement of the more resistant dermal papillae usually causes permanent hair loss and invariably produces radiodermatitis.

Hormonal Alopecia. The following clinical entities can produce this type of alopecia: hyperpituitarism, hypopituitarism, hyperthyroidism, hypothyroidism, hypoparathyroidism, hypocorticoidism, diffuse adrenocortical hyperplasia, androgen-secreting adrenocortical tumors, adrenogenital syndrome, androgen-secreting ovarian tumors, puberty, adrenarche, pregnancy, post partum, menopause, and diabetes mellitus.

Infectious Alopecia. Localized superficial infections seldom cause permanent hair loss (Leider, 1961). Deeper infection can cause temporary hair loss owing to breakage of the hair shaft or direct involvement of the follicle. If the follicle is destroyed, scarring is produced and the alopecia is permanent. The following organisms may affect the follicle and cause alopecia: viruses (e.g., herpes simplex, varicella, zoster, and variola) and bacteria (e.g., *Mycobacterium tuberculosis*, *M. leprae*, and pyogenic organisms). The follicles are also destroyed in folliculitis decalvans and acne varioliformis. Fungi usually cause temporary hair loss by breakage of the hair shaft; certain fungal infections, such as favus, may destroy the follicles. Kerion may also produce permanent hair loss. Temporary alopecia secondary to systemic illnesses, particularly those that cause high fevers, may begin to appear about ten weeks after the onset of the systemic disease. The following systemic infections are frequently associated with hair loss: bacterial, such as typhoid fever, scarlet fever, erysipelas, and pneumonia; viral, such as influenza; treponemal, such as syphilis; yeast, such as moniliasis; and protozoal, such as malaria.

Neurogenic and Psychiatric Alopecia. There is insufficient evidence to establish that neurogenic factors influence the follicle directly. Trichotillomania is the subconscious or conscious pulling out of the hair by the patient (Graham, 1966; Greenberg and Sarner, 1965). Scalp hair, eyebrows, and occasionally eyelashes are most frequently attacked (Orentreich, 1969a). This is often associated with trichorrhexis, the breaking off of the hair. Lichen chronicus circumscriptus (neurodermatitis), chronic scratching or rubbing can cause hair breakage and produce temporary localized friction hair loss. (Orentreich and Selmanowitz, 1970). On the other hand, repeated rubbing or biting of an area can occasionally produce a localized hypertrichosis.

Toxic (Pharmacologic or Occupational) Alopecia. Many organic and inorganic chemicals entering the system by inhalation, injection, ingestion, or topical application may affect hair growth and produce a toxic alopecia. Such alopecias may be divided into two groups: (1) non-specific chemical alopecias and (2) follicle-specific chemical alopecias. The non-specific types may be caused by heavy metals, whereas the follicle-specific types can be caused by antineoplastic compounds. Alopecia produced by these compounds is not likely to be permanent.

Nutritional Alopecia. Nutritional deprivation and metabolic disorder must be severe to produce hair loss; this may occur in kwashiorkor, sprue, and celiac disease. The common alopecias are not associated with nutritional deficiencies, but anemia, diabetes, hypervitaminosis A, and hypovitaminosis A may produce alopecia.

Dermatologic Alopecia. Alopecia areata with its forms are examples of the many types of bizarre-pattern alopecia of unknown etiology (Kopf and Orentreich, 1957; Orentreich, 1970 and 1966; Van Scott, 1958). A common alopecia of unknown etiology is alopecia areata. It has many variants — e.g., concentric, guttate, diffuse localized, diffuse generalized, ophiastic, totalis, and universalis. Hair loss usually occurs fairly suddenly and is seldom accompanied by other symptoms, though premonitory paresthesia sometimes occurs and mild erythema may be detected. The pathognomonic "exclamation point" hairs are present during the early active phase of the disorder (Van Scott, 1958). The course of the disease is unpredictable. Single patches frequently regrow spontaneously in a few months, yet recurrences are common. Extension to alopecia totalis or universalis, which occurs rarely, cannot be prognosticated.

Cicatricial alopecias, other than those already mentioned, include a number of cutaneous diseases with atrophy. They are pseudopelade of Brocq, lupus erythematosus, lichen planus (lichen planopilaris), and scleroderma.

TREATMENT OF THE ALOPECIAS

Before considering a surgical ameliorative approach for some of the alopecias, other treatments will be discussed.

Endocrine Therapy. With reference to scalp hair, estrogens generally stimulate and androgens inhibit growth of the genetically predisposed follicles (Orentreich, 1966). The previously mentioned endocrinopathies associated with hair loss can be helped by internal surgical correction and/or administration of hormones. Hair regrowth may

not occur until many months after surgery or the institution of appropriate drug therapy. In some cases, the correction of a hormonal imbalance, as in the adrenogenital syndrome, will merely prevent further hair loss; further, very intensive therapy is needed to produce regrowth of hair already lost.

Treatment of Infections. The best treatment for fungal infections of the scalp is the administration of adequate oral doses of griseofulvin until fungal cultures, Wood's light fluorescence, and the microscopic examination of hairs are negative. Bacterial folliculitis of the scalp is treated with appropriate antibiotics and monitored by culture and sensitivity studies. Abscesses, furuncles, and carbuncles should be incised and drained.

The systemic infections that influence the hair cycle phases and cause diffuse hair loss are likewise treated with the indicated antimicrobials. Since the telogen phase, to which many of the hair follicles may have been reverted, lasts 100 days, it may take three or four months or more before hair regrowth is observed.

Trichotillomania. The "trichotillo test" was devised to differentiate between self-inflicted alopecia (often denied by the patient) and alopecia areata. An alopecic area, roughly 5 cm square, is coated with four layers of collodion in ether or spray-on plastic surgical adhesive, with adequate drying time between layers (Orentreich, 1971; Orentreich and Selmanowitz, 1970). The patient is advised not to touch the patch and usually manages to comply, at least partially because of the substance's adherence. By three weeks, the site will appear darker; removal of the film will reveal early regrowth of hair. The test demonstrates the diagnosis clearly to the patient as well as the doctor. The test procedure may then be repeated as a treatment to achieve longer hair at the same site or growth elsewhere. Detailed psychiatric evaluations of patients with trichotillomania from the author's practice may be found in articles by Graham (1966) and Greenberg and Sarner (1965). Occasionally, an especially neurotic patient will pull off the occlusive patch, in which case suturing a patch in place (Pearlstein and Orentreich, 1968) will permit completion of the "trichotillo test."

Intralesional Corticosteroid Injections. Response to corticosteroid therapy is both diagnostic of and therapeutic for alopecia areata. Intralesional injections of relatively insoluble, aqueous suspensions of anti-inflammatory corticosteroids are the treatment of choice for alopecia areata and its variants alopecia totalis (whole scalp) and alopecia universalis (whole body) (Dillaha and Rothman, 1952; Dougherty and Schneebeli, 1955; Rony and

Cohen, 1955; Orentreich, 1958; Berger and Orentreich, 1960; Orentreich et al., 1960; Orentreich, 1971). Although most corticosteroids are effective, triamcinolone acetonide suspension (0.05 to 0.1 ml at 1 to 2 cm intervals of 5 mg/ml) is the most efficient for acute cases. For chronic, diffuse, or indolent forms, the longer-acting triamcinolone hexacetonide suspension (also 0.05 to 0.1 ml at 1 to 2 cm intervals of 5 mg/ml) is more beneficial. Mixtures of both suspensions totaling no more than 5 mg/ml may be used for cases of intermediate severity or persistence. Hair regrowth at the sites of injection should be evident within four to six weeks, at which time fill-in injections may be given as needed. To avoid local atrophy and/or delay of hair growth, previously injected sites should not be reinjected for three months. Prolonged therapy is usually not necessary to maintain continued hair growth.

The discomfort caused by the injections (needle stick and burning sensation) is minimized by preparatory freezing with Freon® or ethyl chloride. Alternatively, if a large area is to be injected, a few injections of lidocaine at the rim of the scalp effectively anesthetizes a large scalp area. Jet injection method is not preferable to 30-gauge needle injections; jet injection may produce severe bruising, discomfort, and tattooing with metal filings.

The regrown hair usually has the same texture and pigment as the patient's unaffected hair. Occasionally, and especially with alopecia totalis, the new hair is temporarily white or darker and curlier than normal.

The application of high potency topical steroids (e.g., 0.25 percent fluocinolone acetonide cream or 0.5 percent triamcinolone acetonide cream) under impervious occlusion can help, especially in children unwilling to have injections. Topical therapy is not a substitute for the subdermal injections (Orentreich, 1958). Oral administration of corticosteroids can regrow hair, but it should be avoided because the dosage required (minimum prednisone 15 to 20 mg/day) suppresses the adrenopituitary axis.

Cicatricial alopecias such as pseudopelade, discoid lupus erythematosus, and lichen planus can also be benefited by intralesional corticosteroid injections during the early inflammatory stage; topical and oral corticosteroids can also help.

HAIR TRANSPLANTATION: AUTOGRAFT AND HOMOGRAFT TECHNIQUES

In male pattern baldness, hair loss is greatest in the frontal scalp marked by hairline recession. Recent research has demonstrated that the hair follicles of this area tend to metabolize testosterone differently from the follicles of the occipital scalp fringe where hair growth persists (Takashima et al., 1970). As these differences are better understood, it is anticipated that ultimately, common balding will be preventable and possibly medically correctable by locally influencing the biochemical processes of the androgen-sensitive hair follicles (Orentreich, 1978). Until this goal is reached, surgical hair transplantation satisfactorily corrects the baldness of many patients with their own natural growing hairs rather than an artificial prosthesis. There will probably always be a place for hair transplantation in the management of traumatic and dermatologic cicatricial alopecias (Orentreich, 1959, 1970; Stough et al., 1968).

Certain forms of alopecia mentioned earlier should not be treated by the surgical transplant procedure. For example, surgery is contraindicated in alopecia areata. Surgically transplanted hairs in trichotillomania are likely to fall prey to the same fate as did the original hairs. Most infections of the scalp are limited to the superficial parts of the hair follicle, sparing the critical deeper portions. After the infection is eradicated, if the papilla is viable, the follicle is again capable of growing hair. Following removal of the offending causes, hair may grow in sites of alopecia due to traction or resulting from internal pressure such as cysts of the scalp. A six month period of observation for signs of regrowth of hair is appropriate. Adversely affected follicles are often thrown into the telogen phase of the hair growth cycle, the resting phase when hair growth ceases. This telogen phase lasts about 100 days in the scalp. If hair starts to regrow, it will do so at the rate of 0.33 mm/day, requiring weeks before short hairs are visible on the surface of the scalp (Myers and Hamilton, 1951; Kligman, 1959; Saitoh et al., 1969; Orentreich, 1969b).

The transplant technique has been successful for the treatment of male pattern alopecia, androgenetic alopecia in women (diffuse and/or patterned), and cicatricial alopecia. It is successful when the alopecic recipient sites can sustain autografts from remaining hair-growing donor sites (Orentreich, 1960, 1966; Ayres, 1964; Stough et al., 1968). When small areas of the scalp are avulsed, immediate replantation of the avulsed tissue may prevent alopecia.

For androgenetic baldness, hair-bearing skin from the donor areas (occipital and temporal) is placed in the bald recipient areas (frontal and dome). In the hair transplant process, "donor dominance" is exhibited by both donor and recipient grafts; each tissue maintains its original genetic characteristics despite transplantation. The term

Dominance Determination

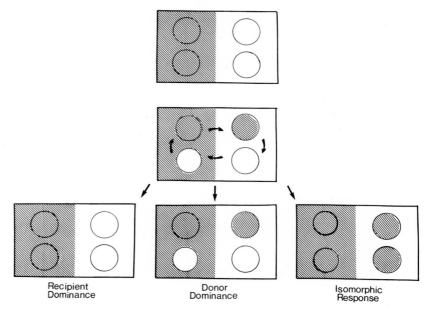

Figure 30–1. Examples of donor and recipient dominance as well as isomorphic response.

Recipient Dominance   Donor Dominance   Isomorphic Response

"recipient dominance" refers to autografts that take on the characteristics of the recipient site (Orentreich, 1959) (Figure 30–1).

Selection of patients and surgical planning should include the following: evaluation of donor area potential vis à vis the recipient area need; expectations of the patient; satisfactory hair styling; number of grafts required; cost of the procedure; cosmetic morbidity during the healing stages; wound-healing ability; and general health. Appropriate blood tests should be obtained before transplants are performed. Since black patients have a higher risk of keloid formation, a small number of trial plugs can be done. It is prudent to inform the patient with a written statement of the principles and details of the procedure, the sequence of events to expect in wound-healing and hair growth, medications and activities to avoid, and untoward occurrences that may take place.

Steps in Technique

First, the donor and recipient sites are cleansed with 70 percent alcohol. The hair in the donor area is clipped to a length of about 2 mm. It is preferable to clip a relatively narrow, transverse donor band insuring that the donor area can be easily hidden during the healing period by overlapping hair. Clipping (as opposed to shaving) allows visualization of the hair direction (angle inserted into the scalp), a critical factor for proper angulation of the punch cutting of donor plugs and proper orientation in the recipient sites. The donor and recipient areas are sprayed with Freon®

or ethyl chloride and anesthetized by the injection of a 1 or 2 percent lidocaine hydrochloride solution. Occasionally, epinephrine 1:100,000 in 2 percent lidocaine hydrochloride is used to control excessive bleeding or to prolong anesthetic action. Metal dental syringes, with 1.8 cc ampules of 2 percent lidocaine, are used because their hydraulic characteristics facilitate injection of scalp tissue.

Punches of various diameters (2.0, 2.5, 3.0, 3.5, 3.75, and 4.0 mm) have been designed specifically for hair transplantation surgery. They differ from the classic skin biopsy punch in these respects: the diameter of the shaft is relatively small, permitting efficient twirling of the punch for rapid cutting; the shaft is knurled, providing good grip; the cutting head cylinder is long and straight, in contrast to the truncated arrowhead design of some traditional skin punches; and a small hole is cut at the base of the cylinder to facilitate cleansing of the cup. Motor driven punches of the same characteristics are useful when a large number of grafts are performed at one sitting. The punch sizes most commonly used for hair transplants are 3.5, 3.75, and 4.0 mm in diameter. The same size punch is often used for recipient and donor sites, although a punch 0.25 to 1.0 mm larger can be used to obtain the donor tissue. Smaller punch grafts used to fill spaces between 4 mm grafts create a more natural cosmetic appearance, especially at the frontal hairline. Grafts larger than 4 mm do not heal as well and result in reduced hair density (Figure 30–2).

The advantage of the small full-thickness graft is its tendency to be vascularized in 24 to 48 hours.

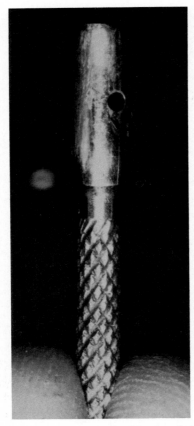

Figure 30–2. A 4-mm punch with a knurled shaft and a hole in the cylinder for easy cleaning and to vent air during the incision of the scalp. (Supplied by Robbins Instrument Company, Chatham, New Jersey.)

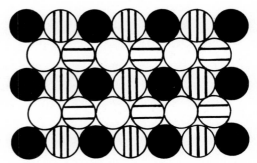

Figure 30–3. Grafts are separated by the width of the punch diameter. Four procedures are necessary to fill an area completely.

of 1 mm and then angled in the direction of hair growth. When working on the dome of the scalp, the punches are angled radially from the center of the calyx to coordinate with the usual pattern of hair on the dome. For the frontal scalp, the cuts are angled so the hair grows forward, as it naturally does (Figure 30–5).

The hair follicles should be cut parallel to the walls of the cylinder of the punch to prevent their being damaged. An examination of the hairs in the plugs can easily demonstrate whether the punch is being used at the correct angle (Figure 30–6).

The number of plugs cut at any one treatment depends on the degree of alopecia, the amount of cosmetic incapacitation the patient is prepared to accept, the frequency at which the treatments are given, and the maximal tolerance of the recipient site for grafts.

Ten to 60 plugs are usually transplanted at each visit. The recipient site should be allowed to heal for at least two weeks before additional grafting is performed in the same area. Other sites may be grafted the next day, taking care not to disturb previous grafts.

The bald grafts from the recipient site are discarded. Small tooth forceps are all that is usually needed to remove them. Small surgical scissors are used to cut any fibrotic anchoring band at its base to release the plug.

The donor site cuts can be much closer together than those of the recipient site but enough hair follicles must be left to cover the now semi-denuded donor area eventually (Figure 30–7).

The first nourishment of the graft is plasma, and the smaller the graft, the more adequate the nourishment. Recipient sites are usually separated by the width of the punch diameter to permit an adequate blood supply. After healing, additional plugs can be placed between the previously placed grafts. When doing only a single line of grafts (as at the hairline), it is feasible to place the grafts immediately next to each other. Later, smaller plugs can be used in the scalloped front line to create a more natural looking hairline (Figures 30–3, 30–4).

The bald site is punched using a twirling motion for increased cutting efficiency. The cut is first started at right angles to the scalp for a depth

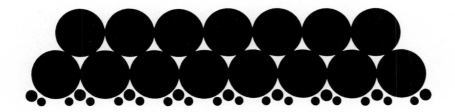

Figure 30–4. Small punches between 4-mm grafts to create a more natural hairline.

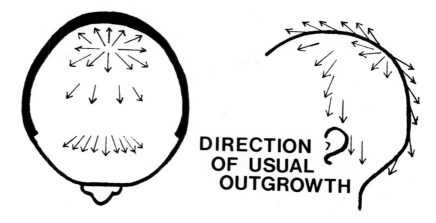

Figure 30–5. Usual pattern of scalp hair growth.

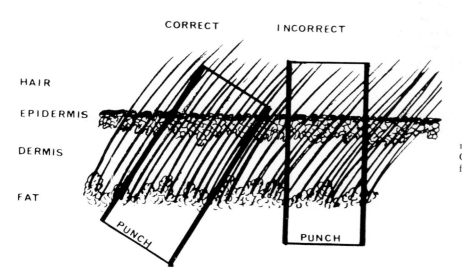

Figure 30–6. Correct and incorrect angle for cutting donor plugs. Correct method is parallel to hair follicle.

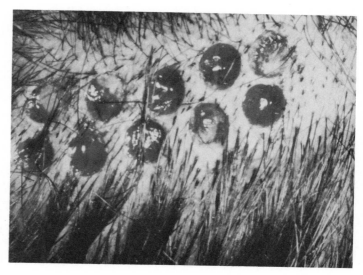

Figure 30–7. Donor sites prior to combing hair over defect.

The average 4 mm plug of hair-bearing scalp will contain from 12 to 15 hairs; the number will be less if the donor scalp hair is very sparse. The color of the donor hair may be dissimilar in shade or degree of graying. Donor graft selection should be designed to achieve the best cosmetic color result.

The donor plugs are also removed with a small tooth forceps. The skin plugs slip out of the scalp in the donor area with much greater ease than they do in the recipient site. If the plugs are attached to the underlying tissues by a fibrotic band, care must be taken to cut with the points of a small surgical scissors well below the level of the hair follicle. As each graft is removed, it is placed immediately on a 3 by 3 inch square of sterile gauze immersed in physiologic saline in a Petri dish. Grafts must never be permitted to dry.

After removal of the skin plugs, both donor and recipient areas are covered with wads of gauze that are held in place with an elastic cotton bandage. This encourages hemostasis while the donor grafts are prepared. Usually there is no bleeding after 10 or 15 minutes following removal of the plugs. Occasionally, if bleeding is excessive at a donor plug site, a 2–0 silk suture is placed, sometimes in a figure eight configuration, for hemostasis. These sutures can be removed within one to six days. If bleeding starts on planting of the donor plug, direct pressure is applied with gauze to produce hemostasis. Rarely does the recipient site require suture hemostasis; any such suture is removed the next day. In the presence of excessive recipient site bleeding, it is possible to suture the site without the graft and then to plant the graft the next day after suture removal. In this case, the donor plug is stored at 10° C, wrapped in sterile gauze and wet with sterile physiologic saline. Grafts will stay viable in this way up to three weeks, provided the gauze is kept moist with sterile physiologic saline.

Before the donor plugs are inserted into the recipient sites, they are gently cleansed of all spicules and loose hair while still immersed in saline. Excess fat and any attached galea aponeurotica are trimmed. Great care must be exercised not to damage the base of the hair follicles; if the dermal papilla of the follicle is removed, no hair can grow.

The donor grafts are placed in a manner oriented to conform to the angle cut in the scalp and to produce uniform angulation of the donor hairs in the recipient sites. Further hemostatic pressure may be required after placing the grafts. The fibrin clot that forms in minutes holds the plugs in place. The surgical areas are gently cleansed with 3 percent hydrogen peroxide and water. A thin layer of antibiotic ointment is spread over the implanted grafts, covered with gauze, and secured with an Ace bandage. The antibiotic ointment retains moisture, giving more rapid healing, better epithelialization, and minimal scarring of graft borders. Ointment dressing also reduces crusting on the surface of the grafts, which with dry dressings can be quite thick. A pressure dressing is applied to prevent disturbance of the grafts and to reduce postoperative bleeding or edema. This type of dressing is usually required when the number of grafts exceeds 20.

The hair immediately above is then combed over the donor site. The donor holes heal with a minimal cosmetic defect. At the recipient site, available hair may be gently combed over the grafts. If a hair prosthesis is worn, it may be carefully fitted into place over little or no dressing, taking care to make the wig attachments at untreated sites.

Postoperative Care

The patient is advised to take no alcoholic beverages or aspirin for the first 24 hours and to perform no strenuous physical activity for the first day and only limited physical activity for the next five days. The grafts should not be disturbed for 10 days. Great care is taken when combing or brushing near the graft sites; shampooing or showering of the head is avoided for five days. Thereafter, shampooing should be gentle until healing is complete. Picking at the graft crusts is forbidden; any crusts will eventually come off with shampooing or bathing. If bleeding occurs, the patient should apply pressure with gauze or a clean handkerchief directly to the site for 15 minutes; if bleeding persists, the physician should be called. The patient should expect mild discomfort, numbness, or altered local cutaneous sensations for weeks after the procedure. He should also be aware that although the hairs in the donor grafts appear to be growing the first month, they are really falling out. He should not expect hair regrowth for three months. There may be swelling from 24 to 48 hours after the procedure, which may spread to the forehead and eyelids. This can be helped by giving oral corticosteroids.

In the thousands of procedures performed, the complications encountered have been syncope during the procedure (1 out of 100), infection (1 out of 500), hypertrophic or keloidal healing (1 out of 1000 — including blacks), and venous aneurysm or arteriovenous shunt formation (1 out of 5000).

It is now over 25 years since the first hair

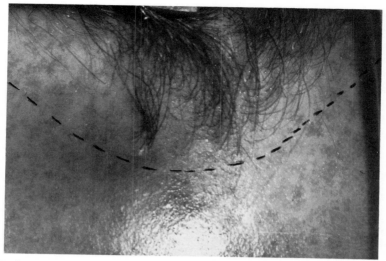

Figure 30–8.   Graft continues to grow while hairline is receding. Graft was initially placed at hairline margin.

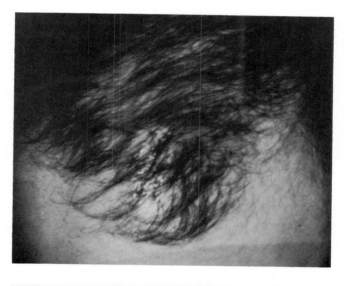

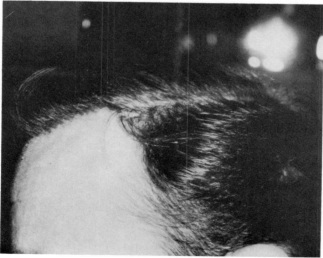

Figure 30–9.   Front of scalp showing multiple grafts several months after transplantation. Two years later frontal scalp grafting shows vigorous full growth of hair.

transplants were performed, and the transplanted donor hair is still growing in the recipient sites. In the hundreds of thousands of transplanted grafts, there has been no instance of failure to continue to grow hair, as long as the donor site has been in an area that continued to grow hair. Great care must be taken to select the donor area with an eye toward the future pattern of balding (Figures 30–8 and 30–9).

PRELIMINARY HOMOTRANSPLANTATION TRIALS

The technique of skin punch autotransplantation, used to redistribute hair on the scalp, is very suitable for homograft studies. The growth of hair in the donor graft is irrefutable evidence of a successful take and of continued integrity of the donor tissue; it dispels any argument that the transplanted skin has been replaced by the host's bald integument.

The approximate 21-day period usually encountered in skin homograft rejection is considerably shorter than the 90-day period required for hair growth in the donor graft. With intralesional triamcinolone acetonide administered at the rate of 1 mg per 4 mm graft every 30 days, the rejection phenomenon was suppressed and the hair growing potential was not inhibited. Reducing the dose of triamcinolone acetonide led to inflammation and rejection. Increasing the dose produced atrophy and suppression of hair growth.

The knowledge gained by dermatologists on the intralesional administration of steroids (Orentreich et al., 1960), combined with the technique of the scalp hair punch grafting, enabled sustained growth of homotransplanted hair for a year. Stopping the injections led to a rejection of the homograft.

(For references, see page 898.)

Chapter 31

Lateral Scalp Flaps

Ray A. Elliott, Jr., M.D., F.A.C.S.

*"Our future lot we can't behold,
but all that glits cannot be gold.
The surgeon's knife may be quite bold,
So all our options must be told."*

Patients' Plea, 1979

HISTORY

The use of lateral scalp flaps for the reconstruction of the anterior hairline for patients with male pattern baldness was proposed nearly 20 years ago by authors in the United States (Lamont, 1957) and in Europe (Correa-Iturraspe and Arufe, 1957; Limberger, 1959). These isolated reports of flap reconstruction were all but lost in the surgical literature after the introduction of a simple method of autogenous plug graft hair transplantation by Orentreich in 1959.

The popularity of the plug graft technique was almost instantaneous, and surgery for the treatment of baldness gained wide acceptance. Although the results with this method have often been dramatic, the appearance of the small clusters of hair was less than ideal in most cases. It was a search for a more normal density of hair, particularly for the anterior hairline, that prompted Vallis to develop the strip graft technique that he reported in 1964. Both of these pioneers have contributed a number of papers that relate their technique and experience (see Chapters 30 and 32).

There has been a cautious, renewed interest in flap reconstruction since Juri presented his clinical experience at the first International Congress of Aesthetic Plastic Surgery in Rio de Janeiro (1972). He proposed the use of large parietooccipital flaps to redistribute the existing hair. He used a single delayed flap for reconstruction of the anterior hairline and a second or even a third flap to span the residual parietal defects. Although the procedure was formidable, his results were truly dramatic. Since the publication of this technique (Juri, 1975), others have reported their experience with

his method (Medical News, 1977; Kabaker, 1978). Because of the dimensions of these large flaps, delay procedures have been recommended, and the difficult closure of the donor sites has required extensive undermining of the scalp and neck. A subsequent procedure for correction of the dogear of rotation is also described. In 1978, Juri published his technique for transposing a delayed occipital flap for the coverage of posterior defects, thus avoiding the need for plug grafts entirely.

AUTHOR'S METHOD

Early in my experience with plug grafts, I became disenchanted with the unnatural appearance of the result. My interest in the surgical treatment of baldness was renewed after seeing the beautiful results presented by Juri at the Congress in 1972. While awaiting the publication of his technique, and still unaware of the case report by Lamont, I developed a lateral scalp flap procedure that resembled that of Lamont, avoiding, however, the flap delays and graft in the donor area.

The technique varies from that described by Juri in that bilateral flaps are used for reconstruction of the anterior hairline. The narrower, shorter flap design does not require delay procedures; the dogear of rotation is distributed during the inset; and closure of the donor site requires no undermining. A method of flap rotation from the recipient site has been developed to facilitate the closure of the anterior portion of the donor defect. Plug grafts and an occasional supplemental flap have been used to provide hair for residual posterior defects. A preliminary paper (Elliott, 1977) and a detailed description of the method (Elliott, 1979) have been published. Others (Heimberger, 1977; Kabaker, 1978) have reported their experience with this method since my initial presentation to the American Society of Aesthetic Plastic Surgeons (1976).

Patient Selection

An analysis of the deformity and an assessment of the donor sites available for reconstruction are primary considerations. Equally important, however, is a careful evaluation of the patient. General health, motivation, and personal expectations must be considered. The age of the patient and the family history of baldness may also influence patient selection. Careful screening is essential if complications and untoward results are to be minimized. A significant number of patients seeking consultation will not be candidates for flap reconstruction.

Indications. The best candidates for flap reconstruction are those with a stable pattern of baldness in whom significant recession of the anterior hairline is a major complaint and luxurious lateral donor sites are preserved. Males between the ages of 26 and 55 have been treated with this method. Patients over the age of 50 should be screened with special attention to general health and motivation. As with other hair transplant procedures, patients with dense, dark hair will often have a better result than those with a low density of fine, blond hair, but good results have been observed in selected patients in the latter group.

Contraindications. Young men in their teens or early twenties are not good candidates for flap reconstruction. Progressive balding in the temple regions is likely to denude the base of the flap, and severe parietal recession might even affect the new anterior hairline of the central forehead. Patients with a generalized thinning and those with a strong family history of eventual balding in the lateral donor areas should be rejected. Traumatic scars that compromise the blood supply or diminish the hair in the donor site are obvious deterrents and may contraindicate flap reconstruction.

This procedure is not as simple as plug or strip grafting. Although it is readily accomplished with local anesthesia on an ambulatory basis, a longer operating time and greater patient stress can be anticipated. If the patient's general health suggests the need for hospitalization or general anesthesia, the surgeon must question seriously the advisability of performing the operation.

Patients without self motivation and those with fixed expectations of regaining their youth will be difficult if not impossible to satisfy and should be turned away. Improvement of self-image and an earnest desire to be more competitive in social and economic pursuits may be compelling and reasonable motivations, but every potential candidate must be questioned carefully to determine whether his expectations are reasonable and attainable. Although the majority of patients seeking cosmetic surgery today are well informed and well motivated, some unstable individuals will be seen. Experience with the interview will decrease the need for psychiatric evaluation to weed out these problem cases.

Patient Counseling. The art of surgery includes patient counseling regarding any planned treatment. It is particularly important in the field of cosmetic surgery. The procedure should be described in understandable terms with an accurate portrayal of the potential complications, cost, and anticipated disability. The limited width of the flaps, the permanent scarring along the new anterior hairline, and the need for supplemental procedures to improve the quality of the posterior coverage must be understood. The need for additional surgery in the event of progressive hair loss should also be discussed.

Alternative methods of treatment should be presented, including the probable advantages and disadvantages of each. It is important for the patient to realize that there is no surgical procedure available to increase the number of hair follicles; only an advantageous redistribution of existing hair can be offered. The more natural density of the hair follicles in a flap and the fact that each average size flap is equivalent to 250 to 300 plug grafts (0.4 cm diameter) will be important considerations.

PREOPERATIVE PLANNING

The nature of the defect and the density and location of the residual hair will influence the timing and number of procedures and the design of the flap. Accurate planning is important to the success of every case.

Choice of Procedures

When the pattern of baldness includes a recession of the entire anterior hairline, bilateral flaps are used to reconstruct the new hairline. The flaps are transposed in separate operations with an arbitrary interval of approximately four months. They are designed with sufficient length to overlap a few centimeters to provide additional coverage in the midline.

If there is a residual midfrontal forelock of good quality and the pattern of baldness is stable, shorter bilateral flaps are bridged across the temple recession to join the preserved forelock. If the residual hair in the midline is sparse in density or potential length, it should be ignored and a complete anterior hairline should be planned.

When there is an ample forelock but the patient is under 40 years of age, it is best to consider a unilateral flap until the fate of this midfrontal residual is certain. If the forelock is ultimately lost, a longer flap from the opposite side can be extended across the midline to join the short flap. Family history may be helpful in this planning.

The choice of procedures for the bald areas posterior to the new hairline will include hair plugs, additional flaps, and, perhaps, fractional excision. I have used all these methods alone and in combination, but plug grafts have been used most often.

Locating the Hairline

A curved, anterior hairline with bilateral elevation in the widow peak areas gives a more natural appearance and will satisfy the majority of patients. There is some recession of the hairline in most aging males; hence, the lower hairline of youth does not need to be restored. A higher hairline will decrease the size of the posterior defect and conserve the potential donor sites for more efficient coverage. The author agrees with Kabaker's recommendation that the distance from the midpoint of the hairline to the root of the nose should not be less than the measured distance from the nasolabial junction to the lower border of the chin.

The new anterior hairline should be continuous with the existing temple hair in every case. The dogear of rotation, revision of which will break this continuity, can and should be avoided routinely (see section on technique).

Flap Design

When reconstruction of the entire anterior hairline is planned, flaps that measure 12.5 to 15.0 cm in length will be required. If the length:base width ratio does not exceed 5:1, these flaps can be transposed without delay. In choosing a flap length, allowance is made for the curvature of the hairline and for some overlap in the mid forehead.

The lateral flap is based in the temporal region above the sideburn, with the superior incision starting at the temple hairline and the inferior incision beginning more posteriorly and well within the hair-bearing scalp. The superficial temporal artery will enter the base of the flap, but its precise location is not significant as it quickly exits on its nearly vertical course and is transected by the

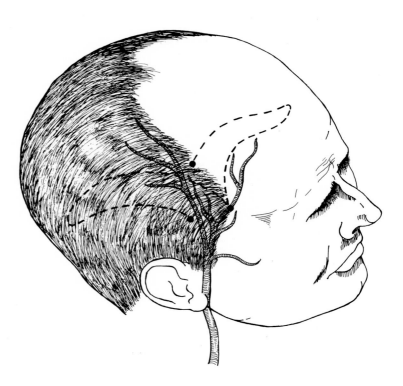

Figure 31–1. The design of the flap need not match the curvatures of the new hairline, nor must the flap be located in reference to the superficial temporal artery. Although this artery frequently enters the base of the flap, it quickly exits on the superior border.

superior incision. Palpation of the artery and the Doppler Flowmeter studies that have been recommended (Heimberg, 1977; Kabaker, 1978) are of no practical value, although they can be used to confirm the course of the artery. I have transposed bilateral scalp flaps successfully after ligation of both superficial temporal arteries when the procedure has been combined with a rhytidectomy.

Within a few centimeters of the base, the flap design narrows to a width of 2.5 cm. This width is maintained except for a slight terminal taper to provide a smooth posterior closure. Ideally, the flap will course posteriorly several centimeters above the ear and 2 to 3 cm below any area of parietal balding. The exact location of the flap depends upon the width of the donor site, but it is most important to avoid the balding areas. If the superior incision closely borders an area of hair loss and there is further balding, the new anterior hairline may become denuded. Supplemental flaps to the posterior scalp are less critical, and these can border on existing defects.

The flap design need not match the curvatures of the new anterior hairline, as the donor flap is flexible enough to follow any gentle undulations (Fig. 31–1). Some downward arching behind the ear is permissible but should be minimal. It is difficult to prejudge the exact location of the inset flap, so the author avoids the potential problems created by predetermined curves by using a gentle arc design in all cases.

When a shorter flap is planned to meet a residual forelock, I would recommend a minimum width of 2.0 cm. In practice, I seldom use a flap narrower than 2.5 cm, since the main objective is the transfer of hair follicles. It is well to remember as a rough guide that every 12.5 square cm of flap is equivalent to 100 plug grafts 0.4 cm in diameter.

TECHNIQUE

With the exception of an occasional case that has had an extensive concomitant procedure such as rhytidectomy, all the lateral scalp flap operations have been done on an ambulatory basis in the author's office operation suite. Light premedication, local anesthesia, and an occasional supplement with intravenous diazepam has been a satisfactory regimen.

Preparation

The hair is never clipped or shaved. In fact, patients are encouraged to let the hair in the donor sites grow during the interval between the consultation and operation to a length sufficient to give instant coverage of residual posterior defects. When additional procedures are planned, long hair in the transposed flaps can mask the operative sites until completion of the posterior coverage.

The entire head is cleansed and draped into the surgical field. Long hair is managed by wetting it and setting it aside with clips. This is a technique tested with rhytidectomy patients and no complications have resulted. The advantage of this excellent exposure of landmarks is obvious. Patient comfort is also enhanced. The patient is placed in the supine position with back elevation at 15 to 20 degrees.

Surgery

The flap design and anterior hairline are marked with a surgical pen, and all operative sites are infiltrated with 1 per cent Xylocaine containing 1:100,000 parts epinephrine. A spinal needle facilitates the injection of the anesthetic. An intravenous is started in all patients as a route for the administration of fluids or diazepam if required.

The markings are carefully checked and the flap is then elevated from posterior to anterior in the areolar plane, deep to the galea aponeurosis. The superior incision is beveled away from the flap to avoid damage to the hair follicles. The flap is tested for adequate length as the inferior incision is lengthened toward the base. Hemostasis is obtained with manual pressure until the entire flap is elevated, then clamps and suture ligatures are used. The cautery is used sparingly, if at all, in order to preserve the maximal number of follicles. The donor site is closed temporarily with towel clips and attention is turned to the anterior hairline.

The anterior hairline incision is carried to the plane of the frontal muscle with a bevel toward the forehead. The recipient site is undermined to a width of 2.5 cm to match the width of the flap. It is split in the midportion of its length and then backcut to within 1.5 cm of the donor flap. This portion of the recipient site is reserved as a sliding or rotation flap for closure of the anterior portion of the donor site, where tension is most pronounced (Figure 31–2).

Closure of the donor site is completed from posterior to anterior until excessive tension is encountered. If a rotation flap from the recipient flap is required, this flap is rotated 180 degrees. The dogear of rotation can be adjusted safely, preserving the part that contains the most hair follicles (Figure 31–3).

The transposed flap is inset along the new

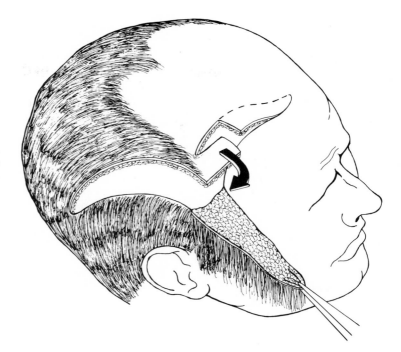

Figure 31–2. A rotation flap from the recipient site is used to avoid undue tension on the closure of the anterior portion of the donor site. The pedicle measures approximately 1.5 cm.

anterior hairline with interrupted or continuous fine, nonabsorbable sutures and a few half-buried, vertical mattress sutures. A single layer closure is sufficient and the maximal number of follicles are spared. The closure proceeds from lateral to medial, and the potential dogear is distributed with radially placed sutures as the flap is advanced toward the midline of the forehead. Undermining the forehead for one or two centimeters facilitates this distribution. There is always some resulting fullness laterally but this flattens in one or two weeks, obviating a revision. The overlapped tissue

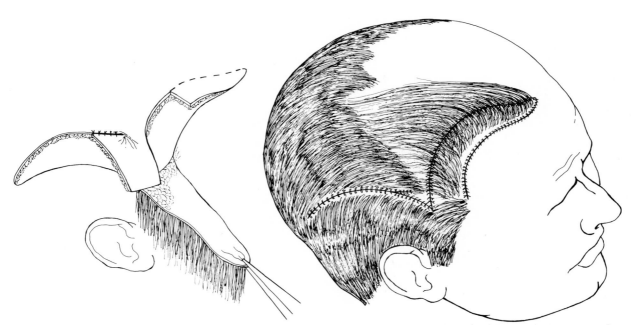

Figure 31–3. The flap is rotated 180° into the donor defect and supplies ample tissue for closure of the anterior portion of the defect. The dogear of rotation can be adjusted safely provided the base of the pedicle is not narrowed.

The donor site is closed with staples or sutures. No undermining is required. Overlapped and excess tissue in and from the recipient site is excised as the flap is inset and the donor site closed.

in the recipient site is excised and the inset of the posterior border of the flap is completed.

Skin staples facilitate the closure of most of the donor site and are used for inset of the upper border of the transposed flap from the recipient area. Skin staples are quite satisfactory for closure of the hair-bearing scalp; they save time and minimize tissue reaction.

A small Hemovac drain, fashioned from a number 22 pediatric scalp vein set and a blood vacuum tube, is inserted beneath the flap and a moderate compression dressing is applied. Demerol and codeine are prescribed, but pain medication is seldom required after the first 12 to 24 hours if the postoperative course is uncomplicated.

Postoperative Care

The drain is usually removed in 48 hours along with the dressing. Most of the sutures along the anterior hairline are removed at this time, except for the half-buried ones, and the remainder of the staples and sutures are removed within ten days. Cautious grooming is feasible as soon as the dressing is removed. A gentle shampoo is permitted on the sixth postoperative day, but dyes are avoided for at least two or three weeks after complete wound healing.

EXPERIENCE AND RESULTS

Since 1975, the author has performed the lateral scalp flap operation for a variety of candidates with male pattern baldness and to date, the patients have been pleased with their result. Figures 31–4 and 31–5 illustrate results achieved in two patients with male pattern baldness. Most of the early patients with bilateral flaps have returned for additional procedures to improve the quality of the posterior coverage; a few have been satisfied to groom the long anterior hair over the residual defects. A number of younger patients have had unilateral flaps and are awaiting progression or stabilization of their pattern of baldness before a second flap is designed.

The majority of patients who have returned for further surgery to improve the posterior coverage have been treated with plug grafts; fractional excision and z-plasty flaps have been used in a few cases with promising results. Where lateral scalp flaps have been used, the scalp has been too tight to permit large secondary excisions. The use of a z-plasty exchange of hair-bearing and non–hair-bearing flaps, on the other hand, has been helpful for breaking up large bald areas that are difficult to conceal. Fractional excision of smaller defects, although feasible in some cases, is not always necessary.

Bilateral flaps are seldom transposed in a single operation, but there have been exceptions. I prefer to stage bilateral flaps primarily because a unilateral procedure is less taxing on the patient, but also because it preserves the opportunity to use a longer flap from the second side in the event of a complication. Simultaneous closure of a second donor site may be more difficult because of increased tension. However, the technique for closure of the anterior portion of the donor site with a flap from the recipient site has helped to avoid undue tension in most cases. It should be noted that male face lift patients with pattern baldness are prime candidates for a one-stage operation that utilizes the redundant scalp in the flap design. The feasibility of combining these two procedures has already been discussed.

Pitfalls and Complications

The described technique has been remarkably free of problems. Careful patient selection, accurate planning, good surgical technique, and meticulous attention to detail are all essential. Wider experience with this method will help all of us to understand and to prevent potential complications even better.

Bleeding and Hematoma

Manual pressure by a well trained assistant and good hemostasis will control blood loss during the operation. No patient in the author's series has required a transfusion. Hematoma formation beneath the transposed flap may be heralded by persistent pain. This complaint should prompt an early inspection of the wound and gentle evacuation. Use of a small hemovac drain should be routine, but it is not a substitute for meticulous hemostasis.

Infection and Delayed Healing

Bacterial infection should be rare, as the blood supply in the scalp is excellent. However, secondary infection may result from delayed healing or wound separation if the donor site has been closed with undue tension. The anterior part of the donor site closure was troublesome until the rotation flap from the recipient was developed. This technique obviates the free graft suggested by Lamont (1957) and has virtually eliminated our problem with tension. Now that immediate adjustment of the dogear of rotation of this flap has proved to be safe, the author uses this method of closure in almost all cases.

Text continued on page 884.

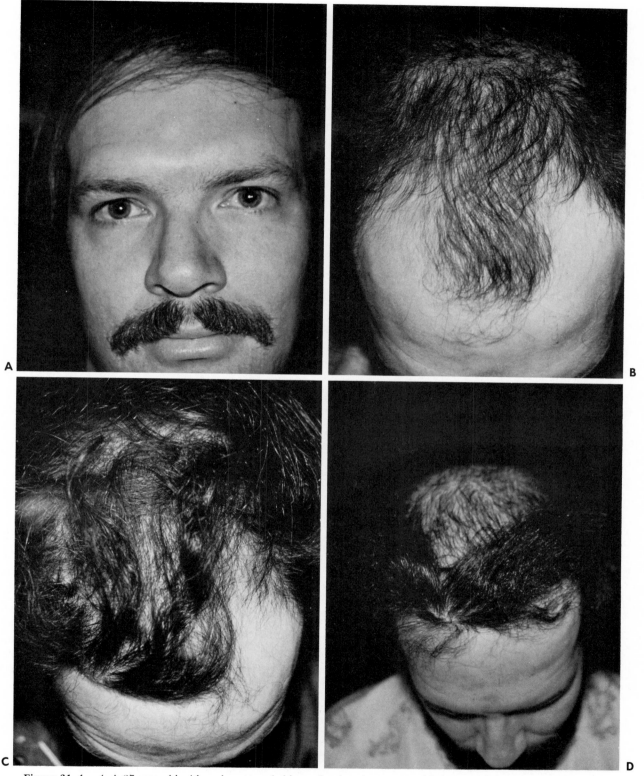

Figure 31–4. *A*, A 27-year-old with male pattern baldness that he tries to conceal by grooming lateral scalp over the defect.

B, The preoperative defect.

C, Right flap has been completed.

D, Both flaps have been completed and the hair has been separated to demonstrate the residual posterior defect.

Illustration continued on the following page.

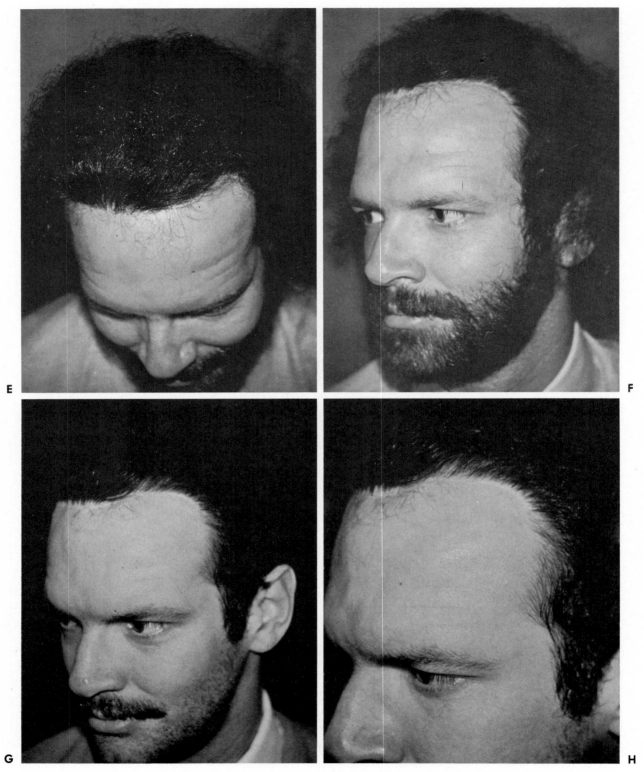

Figure 31–4 *Continued.   E* and *F*, The result at three months. There is good continuity of the new anterior hairline and the pre-existing temple hairline.

G and H, The result at one year. The hair is swept backward for maximum visualization of the scars.

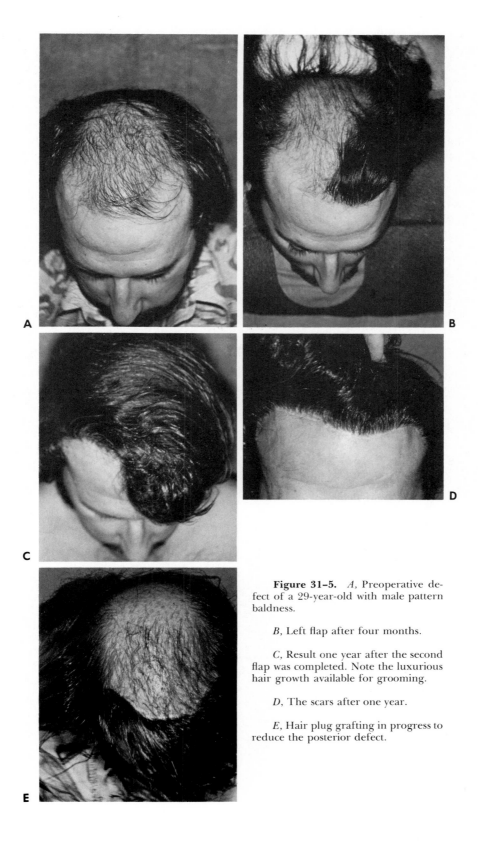

Figure 31–5. *A,* Preoperative defect of a 29-year-old with male pattern baldness.

B, Left flap after four months.

C, Result one year after the second flap was completed. Note the luxurious hair growth available for grooming.

D, The scars after one year.

E, Hair plug grafting in progress to reduce the posterior defect.

Necrosis and Alopecia

None of my patients have had a loss of flap tissue, although the distal few centimeters of the flap has developed an alopecia in several complicated cases. The subsequent regrowth of normal hair has been similar to the shock and recovery phenomenon seen routinely with plug and strip grafts. The potential for necrosis or permanent alopecia in the terminal portion of the flap presents an argument in favor of staging bilateral flaps, because a longer flap can be designed on the second side if necessary. It is well to discuss these potential complications during the consultation. Adjustment of the hairline, free grafts, and additional flaps may be used for salvage of selected cases if these problems are encountered.

CONCLUSION

Lateral scalp flap reconstruction of the anterior hairline has improved the quality of results in selected patients with male pattern baldness. At this point, scalp flaps should be considered as a valuable part of the armamentarium of techniques for the management of these patients. Undoubtedly, further refinements of technique will be suggested by interested and experienced surgeons. With a cautious, conservative accumulation of experience and accurate reporting of complications and long-term results, its rightful place will be defined.

I have had no experience with the proposed treatment of extensive baldness with flaps alone (Juri, 1975). The case histories have been dramatic with these larger flaps, but here again the technique must await a report on complications and long-term results.

The desire of surgeons and patients to obtain more instant and dramatic results than those seen with composite free grafts is understandable. The latter method has already withstood the test of time, and it continues to offer a good measure of patient satisfaction. However, I believe that the lateral flap technique will give a better quality result in selected cases.

(For references, see pages 898 and 899.)

Chapter 32

Strip Grafts

C. P. VALLIS, M.D.

Hair transplantation for male pattern baldness has become an increasingly popular operation during the past decade and a half. In carefully selected cases, modern techniques are quite successful in distributing a significant amount of hair from ageless hair-bearing areas of the scalp to the prematurely bald areas. Hair transplantation is now the most common cosmetic operative procedure in the male patient.

Several methods have been proposed for the replacement of hair in male pattern baldness. The most common is the punch graft operation. Free hair-bearing punch grafts were first described by a Japanese investigator, Okuda (1939). His work was not generally recognized, and it wasn't until 20 years later following the publication of Orentreich's classic paper (1959) that the age of hair transplantation began. The punch graft method consists of the transplantation of small cylinders of autologous full-thickness skin grafts from hair-bearing areas to bald areas by means of a skin biopsy punch. This has proved to be an ingenious and extremely appealing procedure to both surgeon and patient because of its utter simplicity.

The author (1964, 1967, 1969, 1971, 1972, 1976) originally described the use of a long strip of full-thickness hair-bearing skin graft from the scalp for the reconstruction of a new frontal hairline. When this procedure is used in conjunction with the punch graft method, very gratifying results can be achieved. The strip graft is essentially a composite segment of hair-bearing skin and subcutaneous tissue limited in width but unlimited in length. The strip graft operation, when properly executed by a qualified surgeon, can produce an acceptable hairline of good density (Figure 32–1).

Several other methods have been proposed for the replacement of hair in male pattern baldness. In an attempt to correct the condition, rotation flaps (Correa-Inturraspe and Arute, 1957), lateral pedical flaps (Elliot, 1977), parietal-occipital flaps (Lamont, 1957; Juri, 1975), and partial excision of full segments of hairless skin have been and are still being used. These methods have their proponents, and in carefully selected patients they have proved to be efficacious. However, because of their limited mobility, they are not as versatile as the punch graft or the strip graft, and they are rather complicated for such a benign condition as male pattern baldness.

SELECTION OF PATIENTS FOR HAIR TRANSPLANTATION

There are probably more deterrents to than indications for the hair transplant operation, but in carefully selected patients, a good growth of hair can be anticipated. Patients with adequate dense hair of good quality in the donor site may be candidates. Usually those with dark, coarse hair show a better and more dense growth of hair than those with fine, silky hair. Highly motivated patients who understand the limitations and discomfort of the operation are good candidates.

Criteria for Refusing a Patient

1. Severely bald patients with insufficient hair in the donor site — often just a narrow rim of hair around the parietal-occipital areas — should be refused.
2. Sparse or thin hair growth in all areas of the scalp is a contraindication.
3. Many patients with only minimal loss of hair complain that they are losing their hair rapidly, yet they have no real bald patches. They should be told to come back when there is actual recession or baldness.
4. The prolonged course of the multiple stage procedures may be a deterrent to many patients. It is essential not to hold anything back from the patient when discussing a proposed hair transplant procedure. It should be explained to him that this is a long series of tedious operative procedures, that consider-

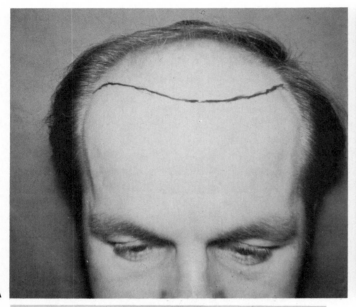

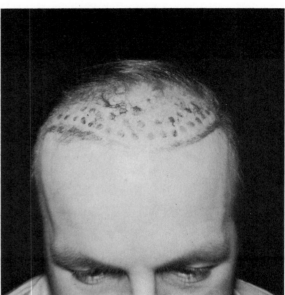

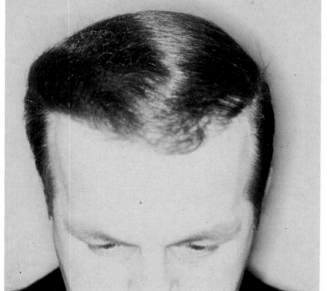

Figure 32–1. *A,* Proposed position of new frontal hairline in a 27-year-old man. *B,* Strip and punch grafts in position. *C,* Hair growth after six procedures.

able patience is required because the new growth is very slow, and that it will be several months before a full growth is obtained.

5. The limitations of the procedures should be carefully explained to every patient. They should be forewarned that regardless of the number of procedures performed, original growth of hair can never be regained. This information will also be a deterrent to some patients.

6. Emotionally unstable patients with a history of psychiatric disturbances should be refused.

7. Patients with any form of severe systemic disease, such as coronary insufficiency or uncontrolled high blood pressure, should not be accepted.

8. The creation of scars in the donor and recipient areas, although minimal, should be explained to all patients. This is a definite deterrent to some.

9. Patients with alopecia resulting from a diseased scalp should be referred to a dermatologist.

10. Patients with alopecia areata or any other type of alopecia not associated with typical pattern baldness or some form of trauma are usually not good candidates for transplant procedures.

TECHNIQUE

Strip grafts are not done in all patients undergoing hair transplants. In the author's practice, about one third of all patients receiving transplants will have strip grafts at some time during the course of their treatment. Several patients have no frontal recession but have baldness only on the crown of their scalp, and in these patients punch grafts alone are indicated. Most patients are not interested in having their original frontal hairline reconstructed. They simply wish to maintain their existing hairline. Many have marked thinning on top of the scalp and are simply interested in increasing the density of the hair in this area (Figure 32–2). There are also several patients who have only partial recession of the frontal hairline, and again, in these patients the punch graft method alone is utilized. In many cases, the punch graft procedure when done alone will add a significant amount of hair, and the use of any other method would be redundant. However, some individuals are anxious to recover as dense a growth of hair as possible in the frontal region. There are also those in whom the tufted effect caused by the punch grafts cannot be eliminated. In these patients the strip graft will greatly increase the amount of hair and enhance the natural appearance of the frontal hairline.

The strip graft procedure is usually done on patients who have obvious complete frontal recession requiring a totally new frontal hairline. In earlier operations, the frontal hairline was formed first with the strip grafts, and the punches were done subsequently as fill ins behind the strip. This often resulted in a rather obvious graft at a level some distance below the existing hairline. During the past several years, all new patients have been started with a series of punch graft procedures beginning at the existing hairline and gradually working faceward until a new frontal hairline is established. In most cases, the patient will be content with the result accomplished by the punch grafts. However, in patients who are anxious for more density, the strip graft should be suggested (Fig. 32–3).

Most of the problems that have been associated with hair transplant surgery are related to the reconstruction of a new frontal hairline. Regardless of which technique is used for the formation of this hairline, it is important that its position be carefully planned and designed preoperatively. Improperly placed punch or strip grafts create an undesirable aesthetic effect (Figure 32–4). It is essential that the proposed new hairline not run straight across the frontal region. There should be a widow's peak with some degree of posterior recession of the hairline on either side to give a more natural appearance. Transplants should not be placed in front of the temporal hair regardless of the degree of recession. Since the hair in the temporal region is clipped short in most individuals, it is very difficult to achieve a natural effect with transplants in this location. Two types of strip grafts are used in the author's practice: the linear strip and the running w strip. The operative techniques of both types will be described.

STRIP GRAFTS (Figures 32–5 through 32–9)

The strip graft operation is done as an office or outpatient procedure. A section of hair is shaved on the parietal-occipital area of the scalp. The patient is placed in a prone position on the operating room table, lying on his abdomen. The strip graft is roughly marked on the scalp with an applicator dipped in gentian violet solution. Although this patient may have had several previous punch graft procedures, care must be taken to preserve throughout the course of his treatment

Text continued on page 892.

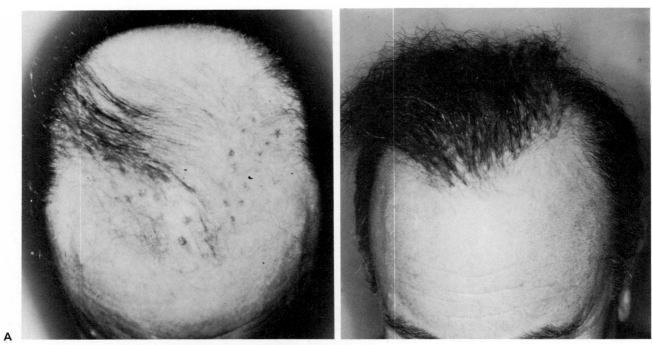

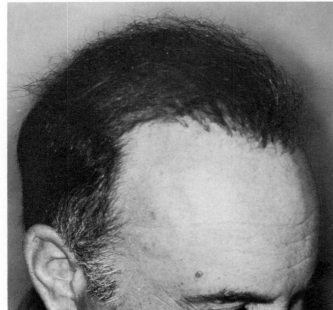

Figure 32–2. *A*, Marked thinning of hair is seen in this 56-year-old man. Note punch grafts. *B* and *C*, Hair growth after five punch-graft procedures. Note the tufted effect of the grafts.

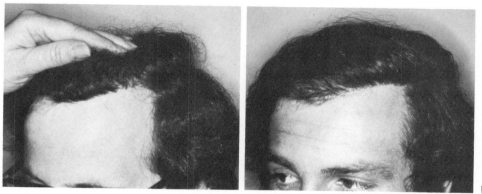

Figure 32–3. *A* and *B*, Two men, ages 22 and 25, one year after implantation of strips. Note density and naturalness of hairline.

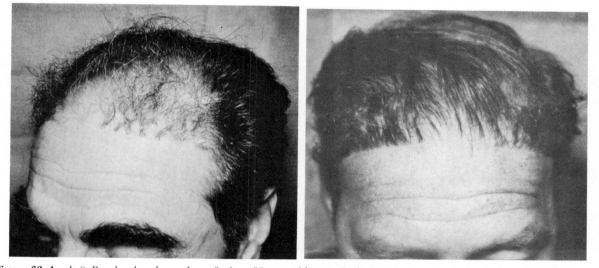

Figure 32–4. *Left,* Poorly placed punch grafts in a 52-year-old man. *Right,* Poorly placed strip grafts in a 40-year-old man.

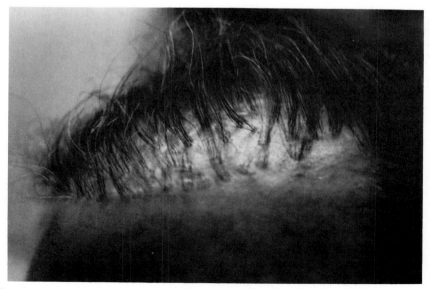

Figure 32–5. A 51-year-old man who has had 150 punch grafts. Note the tufted effect of the frontal hairline.

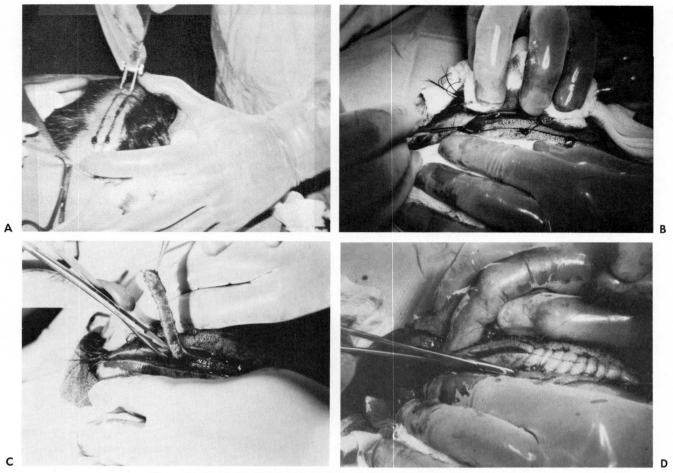

Figure 32–6. *A*, Parallel double-blade knife for taking strip graft.

B, Deeper incisions are made with single blade following angulation of hair follicles.

C, Resection of strip graft from fascial attachment.

D, Repair of donor wound with continuous suture.

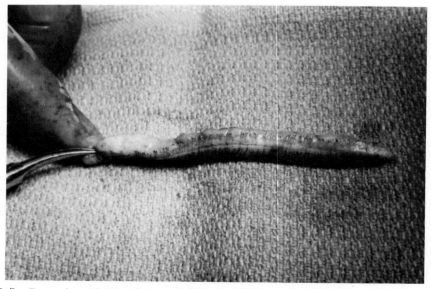

Figure 32–7. Free strip graft. Note the intact follicles and the layer of areolar tissue over the follicular bulbs.

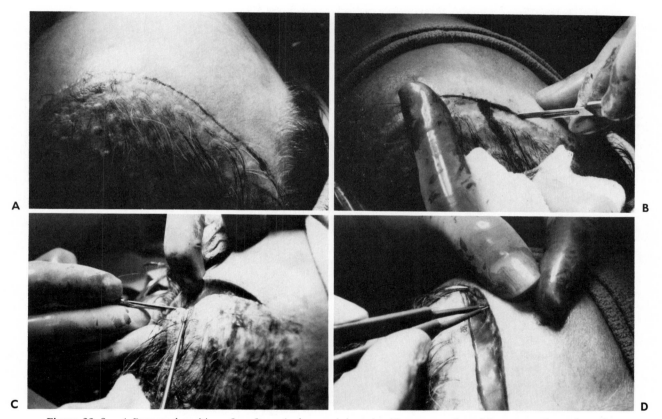

Figure 32–8. *A*, Proposed position of graft marked on recipient site. Note transection of front row of punch grafts.

B, Single linear skin incision.

C, Splitting of galea, causing wound to open wide.

D, Cauterization of bleeders with bipolar current.

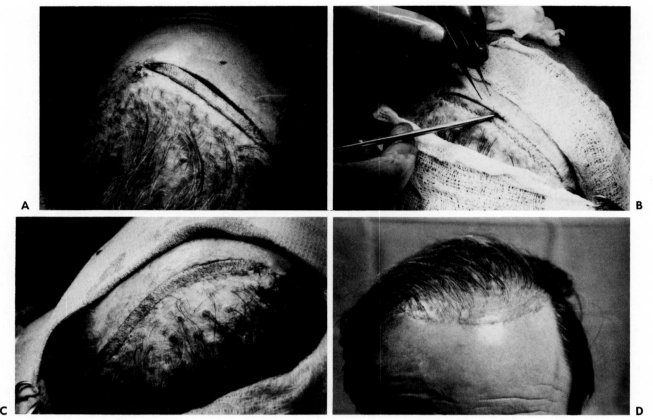

Figure 32–9. *A*, Placement of graft in recipient wound, with hair angulated inferiorly.

B, Suturing of graft with continuous 6-0 nylon.

C, Completed repair.

D, Appearance of graft one month after surgery.

an intact area of hair growth on the parietal-occipital areas of the scalp suitable for taking a strip graft of adequate length and width.

The length of the strip graft is limited only by the existing donor site and the length of the frontal area to be spanned. However, the width of the graft is strictly limited. Since the width determines the continued viability of the graft, a very wide graft would obviously fail to take. Formerly, it was believed that the graft should be cut no wider than 5 mm. Later, with experience, the author increased the width of the graft to as high as 9 mm. Although the 9 mm graft took very well in areas of the scalp untouched by previous surgery or trauma, it did not fare as well when placed close to previously applied punch grafts. A graft measuring 7 mm in width is used most frequently at present, since most patients have already had multiple punch grafts.

The width of the graft is also very important relative to the ultimate appearance of the hairline.

A very narrow strip less than 5 mm in width, although regaining circulation more readily, actually defeats the purpose of the strip graft operation. The resulting hairline is thin and sparse and does not have the density of hair that a wider strip would produce.

After the strip graft has been roughly marked, the local anesthetic is injected. A solution of 2 percent xylocaine without epinephrine is used. Pierce (1973) stressed the importance of not introducing a vasoconstrictor into the donor graft tissue. This insures quicker uptake of the circulation by the strip graft.

The strip grafts should be taken in a horizontal direction from the parietal-occipital areas of the scalp. The horizontal direction insures invisibility of the scar after healing. A simple instrument was designed to allow the surgeon to take a strip graft of a predetermined and uniform width. It is called the parallel double-bladed holder. It takes two number 15 scalpel blades and comes in varying widths from 5 to 10 mm. This instrument is used to make the initial incision in the donor site. This incision is carried through the epidermis no deeper than a millimeter or two, and then a single-bladed number 15 scalpel blade is used to make the deeper incisions on either side of the graft. When the deeper incision is made with the single blade, it is very important that it follows the slant and angulation of the hair follicles. Failure to do this will result in the destruction of several rows of the underlying follicular bulbs and will prevent a complete growth of hair in the graft. The incisions are carried down to the galea aponeurotica. The graft is lifted off its bed with a sharp pointed curved scissors or with a scalpel. Care should be taken to stay below the level of the hair follicles when the graft is being elevated.

After the strip graft has been removed from its bed, no attempt is made at hemostasis except for application of pressure on either side by the assistant. The wound is quickly closed with a continuous 3–0 polyethylene suture with a CE-10 needle. The graft that had been placed in a saline sponge is now carefully pared of excess fascia and fatty tissue. The paring of the fat should not be too excessive, and the hair follicles should not be exposed or damaged. The major circulation for the graft necessarily comes from the sides; consequently, an extra amount of fatty tissue under the follicles does not prevent the graft from taking.

After the donor site has been repaired, the patient, who has been lying on his abdomen during this portion of the procedure, is asked to turn over and lie on his back. The head of the table is elevated to a 30 degree angle, and the recipient area on the forehead is then prepared. The position of the graft has been previously designed and marked with gentian violet solution. (This is done with the patient in a sitting position before the operation is begun.) The frontal hairline is reconstructed in two stages: one strip is used to span half the frontal scalp on one side, and about two weeks to one month later, another strip is placed on the other side. It is essential that the strips form a complete hairline with no gaps. This is done by overlapping the grafts in the mid-forehead. It is possible to span the entire forehead with one long strip, although this increases the operative time considerably.

When the entire forehead is spanned in one operation, the graft is cut up into two segments and overlapped in the center of the forehead with a bridge of skin measuring approximately ⅛ inch between the ends of the graft. This is done to prevent indentation of the graft in the center of the forehead, often resulting from contraction of a long uninterrupted graft across the entire width of the forehead.

Local anesthesia using 2 per cent xylocaine solution with 1 to 100,000 epinephrine is injected subcutaneously along the line of incision. This effectively anesthetizes the ascending sensory fibers from the supraorbital nerve. The epinephrine helps greatly in reducing the amount of bleeding, but since the recipient area is not detached from the general circulation, any concentration of epinephrine will be eliminated in a few hours, thereby not hindering the reestablishment of circulation within the strip graft.

A simple linear incision is then made perpendicular to the skin extending through the skin and subcutaneous tissue and the underlying fascia or galea aponeurotica. Inadequate splitting of the underlying galea in the recipient area will not allow the wound to open widely enough to receive the graft, and in the end this will cause constriction of the graft with resulting barren growth of hair.

Bleeding in the recipient wound varies with different patients. In some, the bleeding is quite profuse with multiple pumping blood vessels, whereas in others, there may be only two or three actively bleeding blood vessels. Active bleeders are clamped with hemostats and ligated. The smaller bleeders are electrocoagulated with the bipolar cautery. Excessive electrocoagulation should be avoided to prevent undue injury to the recipient area. Complete hemostasis is important and further secured with weak epinephrine packs in the wound.

The carefully prepared strip graft is placed in the wound with the hair follicles pointed inferiorly. If the graft is thus placed, when the hair grows out there will be a full growth of hair right to the edge of the inferior margin. Also, when the patient combs his hair, the hairs will extend slightly downward before curving superiorly, thus camouflaging the linear edge of the graft. If the graft is not in this position, a pale white linear scar will result along the inferior margin of the graft. In many cases, the linear incision for the strip graft is placed through the front row of punch grafts. The incision actually transects the punch grafts, causing half of each graft to remain superior to the strip graft and the other half inferior to it. This maneuver creates enough irregularity in front of the strip graft to eliminate any sharp linear effect that a solitary strip graft may produce.

The graft is sutured to the skin superiorly and inferiorly with a continuous running 6–0 nylon stitch. Improper suturing of the graft in the recipient area very frequently results in poor take of the graft. A fine continuous suture used in the superficial layers of the skin without strangulation but with close coaptation of the skin margins without overlapping helps greatly in attaining a good take of the graft. When the suturing of the graft has been completed, a piece of gauze is gently but firmly rolled over the graft from one end to the other in order to eliminate any residual amount of blood that may be present under the graft.

A circular head bandage is used for pressure over the graft, although a small stent tied over the graft can be used. It is very important that the postoperative dressing is not placed too tightly. A tight dressing will result in embarrassment of the circulation at the site of the graft. An excessively tight dressing will also cause marked periorbital edema and ecchymosis, which may last for several days after the operation. A rayon dressing is initially placed over the strip graft to prevent adherence to the dressing material. The pressure dressing is kept on for two days, and then a small dressing is applied over the graft only. Dressings are not required after one week; the sutures are removed in nine days.

The patient is allowed to go home immediately after completion of the operation. He is advised to refrain from overactivity and he is also told to avoid excessive use of any alcoholic beverages and not to do anything that would tend to raise his blood pressure.

Two hundred and fifty milligrams of Ampicillin q.i.d. is prescribed for one week. Earlier, no prophylactic antibiotics were given, and in two cases, the strip grafts were lost because of a staphylococcal infection. Since oral penicillin has been given prophylactically, there has been no loss of grafts from infection.

THE RUNNING-W STRIP GRAFT
(Figures 32–10 and 32–11)

The one objection that has been raised against the strip graft procedure is that it forms an unnaturally straight hairline. In the author's cases, this complaint has been voiced only rarely. Actually, most patients state that the strip graft, because of the high density of hair that results, is preferred because it creates the desired fullness. Currently, the linear graft is used in most of the author's strip graft procedures.

In scar revisions, one of the common techniques employed to break up a straight line deformity is the running-W incision. It was thought that if a running-W incision were used to take the strip graft, any linear appearance of a new frontal hairline would be eliminated. A new instrument was designed whereby a strip graft with a running-W margin could be taken from the parietal occipital scalp and then placed in a running-W

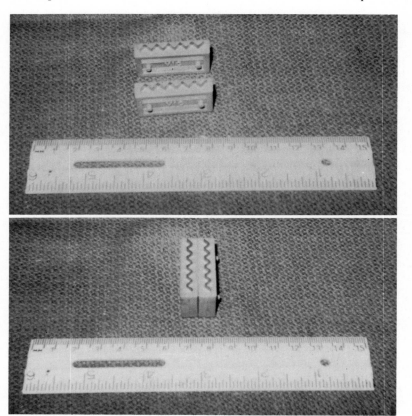

Figure 32–10. *Above,* Instrument for making running-W incision. *Below,* Two instruments joined for taking running-W strip graft.

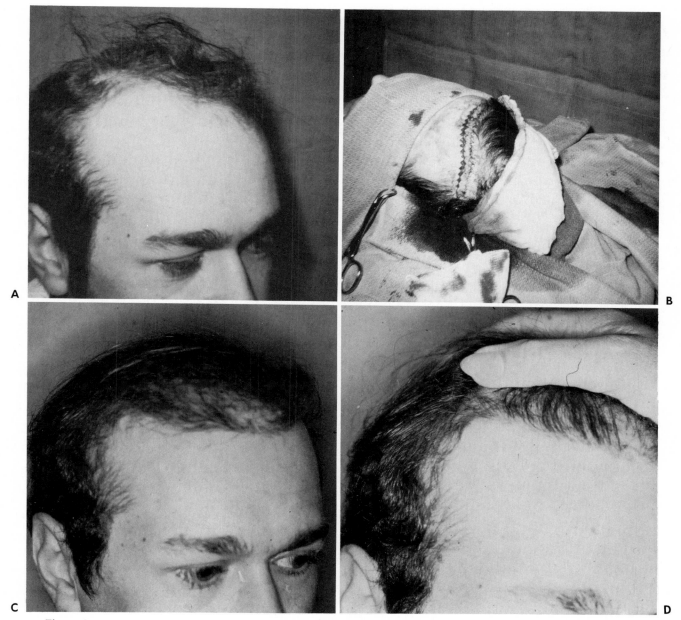

Figure 32–11.   *A*, Preoperative view of a 24-year-old man. *B*, Running-W strip graft in position. *C* and *D*, Results after six months.

incision made by the same instrument in the frontal scalp. The instrument is essentially a razor sharp running-W blade fused to a plastic holder. The blade measures 3 cm in length. The angle of each triangle is 90 degrees and each limb measures 4 mm in length. The strip graft in the parietal-occipital area is taken by placing two plastic holders together. This places the running-W blades 8 mm apart. The parallel blades are then pressed onto the scalp on previously marked lines in the parietal-occipital area. The blades are used simply as a "cookie cutter" to make a superficial skin incision. Any desired length of the graft can be

made by moving the parallel blades along the scalp. Once the superficial incision is made with this instrument, the remaining portion of the graft is taken with a number 15 scalpel blade. The graft is defatted and treated in a fashion similar to the usual linear strip grafts. When the author first began to use the running-W strip, the entire length of the graft on both sides had a running-W incision. However, it was found much simpler and more efficacious to make the running-W incision only in the central 3 cm or 6 cm of the graft and to construct either end of the graft with parallel linear incisions utilizing the parallel double-bladed holder. The incision in the donor site is repaired with a continuous 3–0 polyethylene suture.

A single running-W blade is used to make the incision in the recipient area. The knife is pressed along the previously designed line on the frontal area of the scalp. A superficial incision is made with the knife. The wound is further cut open with a number 15 scalpel blade, and the incision is carried down through the galea to allow the wound to open widely. The length of the recipient incision is similar to that of the strip graft. This graft fits perfectly into position and is sutured with continuous 6–0 nylon on both sides. Again, in placing the sutures, a superficial bite with the needle must be taken, and avoidance of strangulation of the graft is emphasized. A continuous suture is placed through the apex and valley of each triangle in order to insure close and smooth coaptation of the skin edges. All other details of the operative and postoperative course are exactly the same as for the linear strip graft. The running-w strip graft is more tedious and time consuming than the linear graft technique; however, results in 15 patients in whom this method was used have shown that the reconstructed frontal hairline has a satisfactory natural appearance, although the density of hair growth was not as great as that with the linear strip.

POSTOPERATIVE COURSE

The hair follicles in both the strip graft and the punch graft act alike. There is an initial false growth of hair for about three to four weeks. This hair is shed as the hair follicles go into a telogen phase, which lasts for two to three months after surgery. A new permanent growth then begins, and the new hair assumes the characteristics of the area from whence it came. Since hair growth proceeds at about 1 cm per month, a period of six months or more is required before a significant hair growth is noted.

At least two weeks or more should elapse before the second strip graft operation on the other side is performed. The operative and post-operative course for the second strip graft are exactly the same as for the first. Additional punch grafts can be done behind the graft as necessary, but these punch graft procedures should be delayed for at least three months after the second strip has been applied. There is one pitfall that a surgeon may discover if he becomes easily influenced by the patient's insistance to rush the final product by shortening the intervals between procedures. All the author's patients are advised that the

longer the interval between operations, especially with punch grafts, the better will be the ultimate result. With punch grafts, for instance, at least one month is allowed for procedures done in different areas of the scalp, and at least three to four months should elapse before additional punches are placed between previously implanted punch grafts.

Complications

If the patients are carefully selected and if the procedures are performed well technically, there should be few complications. In a small percentage of the strip grafts, there may not be a complete growth of hair in certain spots. This can be corrected easily by placing small punch grafts in the bald areas of the strip.

Occasionally, indentation of the strip graft may be noted postoperatively. This is usually due to the creation of a recipient wound deeper than the thickness of the strip graft, which causes the

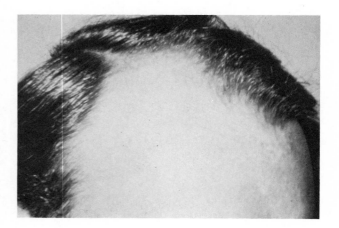

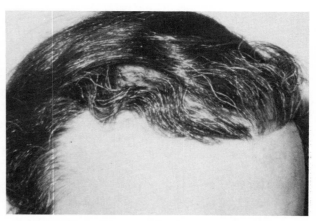

Figure 32–12. *Above,* Moderately severe recession in a 37-year-old man. *Below,* After six procedures.

strip graft to sit below the surface of the surrounding skin. In rare situations, the depth of the graft may be rather shallow owing to short hair follicles, and a different approach to the recipient site may be necessary. To provide for this, a strip of skin and subcutaneous tissue similar to the width of the strip graft can be excised. Incision is carried down to the galea, which is left undisturbed. This excised segment of skin could be just below a row of punch grafts or even between two rows of punch grafts.

The most unpleasant complication is the poorly positioned graft for the frontal hairline. Although it may show a profuse hair growth, it may present an appearance that is aesthetically worse than the preexisting condition. A poorly placed strip graft can usually be repositioned. Poorly placed punch grafts can be removed. This is usually done by removing the graft with a punch of similar size and suturing the wound transversely.

Another complication is numbness of the scalp behind the grafts. This numbness is more marked following the strip graft operation. The transverse incision transects the sensory fibers of the supraorbital nerve on both sides, and the numbness will last for several months after surgery. The numbness can be very desirable at first, since subsequent punch grafts can be done with very little additional local anesthesia. Normal sensation eventually returns after eight months to a year.

SUMMARY

Hair transplantation for male pattern baldness has been done on a large number of patients by dermatologists and plastic surgeons during the past 15 years. In selected cases, hair transplantation has been successful for adequate replacement of hair in bald areas of the scalp. In most cases, the punch graft technique alone is used. However, in selected cases, especially in younger individuals desiring a dense growth in the frontal area, the strip graft in conjunction with punch grafts can be used. The strip graft technique is more difficult to

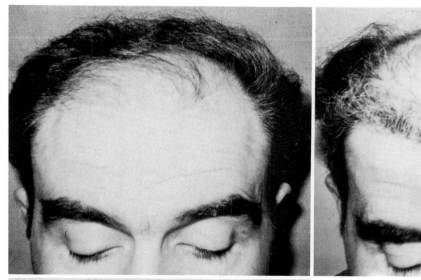

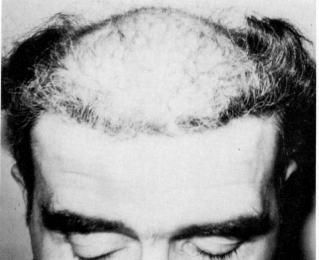

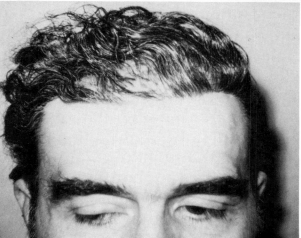

Figure 32–13. *A*, Severe recession in a 40-year-old man. *B*, Strip and punch grafts in position. *C*, Results after eight procedures.

perform, and it should only be done by a skilled surgeon. When the strip graft operation is properly executed, the results are very gratifying. Most impressive results have been with those who have had the strip graft operation combined with the punch graft method (Figures 32–12 and 32–13). The strip graft, like the punch graft, has proved to be extremely versatile. It can be transplanted in any conceivable direction and in any area of the scalp. It may be twisted into any desired shape so as to conform to any recipient site. It can also be made short or long and may be cut into smaller strips or even into small square grafts. If careful attention is paid to the simple steps of the operation discussed in this chapter, a surgeon will usually be rewarded with a complete take of the strip graft.

REFERENCES

Punch Grafts

Ayres, S., III: Conservative surgical management of male pattern baldness: An evaluation of current techniques. Arch. Dermatol. 90:493, 1964.

Berger, R. A., and Orentreich, N.: Abrupt changes in hair morphology following corticosteroid therapy in alopecia areata. Arch. Dermatol. 82:408, 1960.

Billingham, R. C.: A reconsideration of the phenomenon of hair neogenesis, with particular reference to the healing of cutaneous wounds in adult mammals. In Montagna, W., and Ellis, R. (eds.): The Biology of Hair Growth. New York, Academic Press, 1958, pp. 451–468.

Cockayne, E. A.: Inherited Abnormalities of the Skin and Its Appendages. London, Oxford University Press, 1933.

Dillaha, C. J., and Rothman, S.: Treatment of alopecia areata totalis and universalis with cortisone acetate. J. Invest. Dermatol. 18:5, 1952a.

Dougherty, T. F., and Schneebeli, G. L.: Use of steroids as anti-inflammatory agents. Ann. N.Y. Acad. Sci. 61:328, 1955.

Graham, F.: Trichotillomania, a symptom of adolescent identity crisis. Excerpta Med. Int. Congress Series. Psychosom. Med. 21:239, 1966.

Greenberg, H. R., and Sarner, C.: Trichotillomania. Arch. Gen. Psychiatry. 12:482, 1965.

Harry, R. G.: Modern Cosmeticology, Vol. 1. London, Leonard Hill, Ltd., 1955.

Kligman, A.: The human hair cycle. J. Invest. Dermatol. 33:307, 1959.

Kopf, A. W., and Orentreich, N.: Alkaline phosphatase in alopecia areata. A.M.A. Arch. Dermatol. 76:288, 1957.

Leider, M.: Practical Pediatric Dermatology. St. Louis, C. V. Mosby Co., 1961.

Miller, S. A.: Hair neogenesis. J. Invest. Dermatol. 56:1, 1971.

Myers, R. J., and Hamilton, J. B.: Regeneration and rate of growth of hairs in man. Ann. N.Y. Acad. Sci. 53:562, 1951.

Orentreich, N.: Clinical efficacy of triamcinolone acetonide and hydrocortisone acetate in dermatological patients. Monogr. Ther. 3:161, 1958.

Orentreich, N.: Autografts in alopecias and other selected dermatological conditions. Ann. N.Y. Acad. Sci. 83:463, 1959.

Orentreich, N.: Pathogenesis of alopecia. J. Soc. Cosm. Chemists 11:479, 1960.

Orentreich, N.: Alopecia. In Conn, H. F. (ed.): Current Therapy — 1964. Philadelphia, W. B. Saunders Company, 1964, pp. 427–430.

Orentreich, N.: Hair problems. J. Am. Med. Wom. Assoc. 21:481, 1966.

Orentreich, N.: Etiology of loss of eyelashes in a child. J.A.M.A. 207:961, 1969a.

Orentreich, N.: Scalp hair replacement in man. In Montagna, W., and Dobson, R. L. (ed.): Hair Growth. New York, Pergamon Press, 1969b, pp. 99–108.

Orentreich, N.: Hair transplants: Long-term results and new advances. Arch. Otolaryngol. 92:576, 1970.

Orentreich, N.: Disorders of the hair and scalp in childhood. Pediatr. Clin. North Am. 18:953, 1971.

Orentreich, N.: Medical treatment of baldness. Ann. Plast. Surg. 1:116, 1978.

Orentreich, N., and Selmanowitz, V. J.: Cosmetic improvement of factitial defects. Med. Trial Tech. Q. 1970, pp. 172–180.

Orentreich, N., Sturm, H., Weidman, A. L., and Pelzig, A.: Local injections of steroids and hair regrowth in alopecias. Arch. Dermatol. 82:894, 1960.

Pearlstein, H., and Orentreich, N.: Sutured dressing: An adjunct in the treatment of neurotic excoriations. Arch. Dermatol. 98:508, 1968.

Rony, H. R., and Cohen, D. M.: The effect of cortisone in alopecia areata. J. Invest. Dermatol. 25:285, 1955.

Saitoh, M., Uzuka, M., and Sakamoto, M.: Rate of hair growth. In Montagna, W., and Dobson, R. L. (eds.): Hair Growth. New York, Pergamon Press, 1969, pp. 183–201.

Stough, D. B., Berger, R. A., and Orentreich, N.: Surgical improvement of cicatricial alopecias of diverse etiology. Arch. Dermatol. 97:331, 1968.

Takashima, I., Adachi, K., and Montagna, W.: Studies of common baldness in the stumptailed macaque. IV. In vitro. Metabolism of testosterone in the hair follicles. J. Invest. Dermatol. 55:329, 1970.

Van Scott, E. J: Morphologic changes in pilosebaceous units and anagen hair in alopecia areata. J. Invest. Dermatol. 31:35, 1958.

Van Scott, E. J., and Reinerston, R. P.: Detection of radiation effects on hair roots of the human scalp. J. Invest. Dermatol. 29:205, 1957.

Lateral Scalp Flaps

Blanchard, G., and Blanchard, B.: Obliteration of alopecia by hair-lifting: A new concept and technique. J. Natl. Med. Assoc. (Canada) 69:639, 1977.

Correa-Inturraspe, M., and Arufe, H. N.: La cirugia plastica en las alopecias parciales definitivas del cuero cabelludo. La Semana Medica (Buenos Aires), 937, 1957.

Dingman, R. O.: Surgical treatment of defects of the scalp. J. Int. Coll. Surg. 30:148, 1958.

Elliott, R. A.: Lateral scalp flaps for instant results in male pattern baldness. Plast. Reconstr. Surg. 60:699, 1977.

Elliott, R. A.: Lateral scalp flaps. In Vallis, C. (ed.): The Treatment of Male Pattern Baldness. Springfield, Ill., Charles C Thomas, Publisher, 1979.

Gilles, H.: Note on scalp closure. Lancet 2:310, 1944.

Heimburger, R. A.: Single-stage rotation of arterialized scalp flaps for male pattern baldness. A case report. Plast. Reconstr. Surg. 60:789, 1977.

Juri, J.: Use of parieto-occipital flaps in the surgical treatment of baldness. Plast. Reconstr. Surg. 55:456, 1975.

Juri, J., Juri, C., and Arufe, H. N.: Use of rotation scalp flaps for treatment of occipital baldness. Plast. Reconstr. Surg. 61:23, 1978.

Kabaker, S.: Experiences with parieto-occipital flaps in hair transplantation. Laryngoscope 538:73, 1978.

Kazanjian, U. H., and Webster, R. C.: The treatment of extensive losses of the scalp. Plast. Reconstr. Surg. 2:360, 1946.

Lamont, E. S.: A plastic surgical transformation. Report of a case. West. J. Surg. *65*:164, 1957.

Limberger, S.: Die operative behandlung des haarverlustes. Medizinische (Stuttgart) *35*:1559, 1959.

Marcks, K. N., Travaskis, A. E., and Nauss, T. U.: Scalp defects and their repair. Plast. Reconstr. Surg. 7:237, 1951.

Medical News: The new wave in hair transplants. J.A.M.A. *237*:109, 1977.

Orentreich, N.: Autografts in alopecias and other selected dermatological conditions. Ann. N.Y. Acad. Sci. *83*:463, 1959.

Orentreich, N.: Hair transplants: Long-term results and new advances. Arch. Otolaryngol. *92*:576, 1970.

Orentreich, N.: Hair transplantation: The punch graft technique. Surg. Clin. North Am. *51*:511, 1971.

Vallis, C. P.: Surgical treatment of the receding hairline. Plast. Reconstr. Surg. *33*:247, 1964.

Vallis, C. P.: Surgical treatment of the receding hairline. Plast. Reconstr. Surg. *44*:271, 1969.

Vallis, C. P.: The strip graft method in hair transplantation. J. Am. Med. Wom. Assoc. *24*:890, 1969.

Vallis, C. P.: Hair transplantation for male pattern baldness. Surg. Clin. North Am. *51*:519, 1971.

Strip Grafts

Correa-Inturraspe, M., and Arute, H. D.: Plastic Surgery of partial alopecia. Semana Medica (Buenos Aires) *19*:937, 1957.

Elliott, R. A.: Lateral scalp flaps for instant results in male pattern baldness. Plast. Reconstr. Surg. *60*:699, 1977.

Juri, J.: Use of parieto-occipital flaps in surgical treatment of baldness. Plast. Reconstr. Surg. *55*:456, 1975.

Lamont, E. S.: A plastic surgery transformation. West. J. Surg. *65*:164, 1957.

Okuda, S.: Clinical and experimental studies on transplantation of living hairs. Jap. J. Dermatol. Urol. *46*:135, 1939.

Orentreich, N.: Autografts in alopecias and other selected dermatological conditions. Ann. N.Y. Acad. Sci. *83*:463, 1959.

Pierce, H. E.: Problems encountered with the strip graft transplant procedure. J. Natl. Med. Assoc. *65*:211, 1973.

Vallis, C. P.: Surgical treatment of the receding hairline: Report of a case. Plast. Reconstr. Surg. *33*:247, 1964.

Vallis, C. P.: Surgical treatment of the receding hairline. Plast. Reconstr. Surg. *40*:138, 1967.

Vallis, C. P.: Surgical treatment of the receding hairline. Plast. Reconstr. Surg. *44*:271, 1969.

Vallis, C. P.: The strip graft method in hair transplantation. J. Am. Med. Wom. Assoc. *24*:890, 1969.

Vallis, C. P.: Hair transplantation for male pattern baldness. Surg. Clin. North Am. *51*:519, 1971.

Vallis, C. P.: The strip graft method in hair transplantation. *In* Ervin E., and Ervin, E., Jr.: Skin Surgery. 4th Ed. 1976. Charles C Thomas, Springfield, Illinois.

Vallis, C. P.: Hair transplantation. *In* Goldwyn, R. M. (ed.): The Unfavorable Result in Plastic Surgery. Boston, Little, Brown and Co., 1972.

Part 7

BODY
CONTOURING

Chapter 33

Breast Reduction and Mastopexy

SHERRELL J. ASTON, M.D., F.A.C.S.,
AND THOMAS D. REES, M.D., F.A.C.S.

HISTORY

It is not known who performed the first reduction mammaplasty in a female. Paulas of Aegina (AD 625–690), a well known Byzantine surgeon, described a reduction mammaplasty in the sixth book of his *Epitome of Medicine Paulas*, but this procedure was designed for the correction of gynecomastia. There is no record suggesting the procedure was used to treat hypertrophy in females. Later writings by Haly ben Abbas (AD 732–1096) and Albucasis (1013–1106) redescribed Paulas of Aegina's gynecomastia operation, but they did not document that the procedure was performed in a female. Four hundred years later, Ambroise Paré (1510–1590) gave credit to Paulas of Aegina and Albucasis for the first reduction mammaplasty operations.

Several historical reviews have credited the first reduction mammaplasty for hypertrophy of the female breast to Will Durston in 1669. A review of the literature shows that Durston was not a surgeon by the standards of his time, and he did not perform a mammaplasty on the "big-breasted woman" about whom he wrote.

Dr. Gaillard Thomas (1882), described to the New York Obstetrical Society an inframammary incision for removing benign tumors from the breast without breast mutilation. Czerny (1895) was the first to "deal in the plastic manner with defects of the breast." He removed a fibroadenoma from the breast and substituted a lipoma from the same patient "with good results." Pousson (1897) reported, in the Bulletin et Memoire de la Société de Chirurgie de Paris, removing a crescent-shaped section from the upper anterior portion of the breasts in order to treat bilateral mammary hypertrophy in a young woman. Skin and subcuta-

neous tissue was excised down to the pectoralis muscle fascia, and the breast was elevated and suspended by suturing it to the pectoralis fascia. A month before Pousson published his technique, Michel (1897) had already presented Pousson's patient, completely healed, to the Société d'Anatomie de Bordeaux, thus documenting a favorable result with the technique.

Verchère (1898) described excision of a triangular segment of breast tissue from the upper outer quadrant of the breast and axilla and skin closure in the shape of a "Y." Hippolyte Morestin (1869–1919), an accomplished general surgeon with an interest in plastic surgery, described to the Société de Chirurgie de Paris in 1903 the removal of a benign tumor from the breast through a buttonhole incision in the hair-bearing portion of the axilla. The paper "De l'ablation esthétique des tumeurs du sein" was read for Morestin by Demoulin.

During the same meeting at which Morestin made his presentation, Guinard reported operating on a patient with macromastia using semicircular incisions in the submammary folds to remove a large amount of skin and breast tissue. Two years later, in 1905, Morestin reported an operation for mammary hypertrophy using a seven centimeter horizontal incision placed in the inframammary fold. Dissection was carried to the retromammary space, the breast was dissected off the pectoralis fascia, and a large discoid portion of the breast was excised. In 1907, Morestin presented his collective experience with treating mammary hypertrophy to the Société de Chirurgie de Paris, and in 1909, he described to the same Société the correction of a case of breast asymmetry with unilateral hypertrophy. The enlarged areola was reduced at a second operation. Joseph (1925) suggested that the technique of discoid breast reduction should be credited to Morestin and Guinard, and that the procedure should be known as the "Morestin-Guinard method."

Dehner (1908) described a mastopexy technique that involved excision of ellipses of skin and subcutaneous tissue from the superior portions of the breast down to the pectoralis muscle and suspension of the breast to the periostium of the third rib. This technique was a modification of that previously described by Pousson in 1897.

Girard (1910) performed a mastopexy through Thomas's submammary incision. The gland was separated from the pectoralis fascia and elevated. Its posterior surface was suspended from the pectoralis fascia and the second rib with a heavy catgut suture. Gobell (1914) suspended the breast from the third rib with fascia lata strips placed behind the breast tissue.

Kausch (1916) reported excision of skin, subcutaneous tissue, and gland circumferentially around the areolar, but nipple necrosis occurred. To prevent necrosis, he suggested a two stage procedure resecting hypertrophic breast tissue through concentric incisions first laterally and, at a second stage, medially. The result was marred by scarring.

These early breast operations did little to correct ptosis or reduce any but minimal hypertrophy. The procedures removed skin and subcutaneous tissue with elevation of the nipple; the glandular tissue was reduced very little. Support was insecure, as it depended on skin tightening over a large breast volume and/or suspension of the breast to the pectoralis fascia and/or ribs. With the development of the nipple transposition technique, an overall reduction of the breast mass became feasible.

Introduction of nipple transposition began the modern era of breast reduction. Nipple transposition through a buttonhole incision in the skin flap is generally credited to either Morestin in 1909 or Villandre in 1911. However, Auber (1923), of Marseilles, was the first to report the technique. A few months after Auber's paper (1923), Kraske (1923) described a technique used by Lexer in 1912 which combined transposition of the nipple and midline excision from the lower quadrants of the breasts. In 1923, Lotsch reported correction of ptosis using a periareolar and vertical midline incision to transpose the nipple and fashion a new skin brassiere. Lotsch described a second operation in 1928 that included skin excision vertically and horizontally and excision of glandular tissue.

Transposition of the nipple was performed by Dufourmentel in 1916, but it was not published by

him until 1925. During the discussion of Dufourmentel's presentation of nipple transposition to the Société Chiruguire Paris in 1925, Villandre noted that he had performed a similar procedure in 1911. He credited Morestin as previously performing a similar operation. Mornard (1926) stated that he had learned the procedure from Morestin in 1909. Axhausen (1926) was the first to report complete separation of the skin from the underlying breast tissue in order to resect the gland, transpose the nipple, and resect excess skin.

The main problems in design of the early transposition techniques were (1) extensive undermining between the skin and gland and (2) the necessity of maintaining a large glandular mass in order to provide adequate nipple blood supply.

Dartigues (1924, 1925, 1928) described separate procedures to correct varying degrees of ptosis. Severe ptosis required total mammectomy with free nipple and areolar grafts. Joseph (1925) described a two stage technique in order to transpose the nipple and areola on a pedicle under a narrow cutaneous bridge. Passot (1925) used the Thomas submammary incision to resect the gland from the inferior and posterior surface of the breast and transposed the nipple beneath a cutaneous bridge to its new position. Noël (1928) excised ellipses of skin above the areola in order to correct ptosis. Later the same year, she reported refinements of the technique that included transposition of the nipple under a subcutaneous bridge followed by resection of breast tissue two weeks later.

Biesenberger (1928) described elevation of the skin from the underlying breast, "S"-shaped excision of the lateral portion of the gland, rotation of the remaining glandular pedicle and attached nipple upward and counterclockwise, and creation of a new skin brassiere. Nipple slough and skin necrosis was slightly more common with this technique than with those developed subsequently.

The Biesenberger technique provided an adequate method of glandular resection and breast resculpturing. However, some believe that Biesenberger based this procedure on an inaccurate concept of the blood supply to the breast, which failed to account for the importance of the lateral thoracic artery. Most of the complications that occurred with the Biesenberger operation were due to the lack of blood supply to the nipple and skin.

Schwarzmann (1930) fashioned a periareolar "cutis bridge" for maintenance of the blood supply to the nipple. This technique provided a superiorly based dermoglandular pedicle to vascularize the nipple-areolar complex.

The surgical principles of Biesenberger's operation for nipple-areolar transposition, gland resection, skin resection, and breast resculpturing and Schwarzmann's vascularized nipple-areolar complex provided two major advances leading to modern reduction mammaplasty techniques. All currently popular breast reduction techniques, except free nipple transplantation procedures, are based on the principles of these two operations.

Gillies and McIndoe (1939), in an attempt to reduce the incidence of avascular necrosis of the nipple, resected a V-shaped wedge from the upper middle segment of the breast, followed by "mobilization of the inner and outer pedicles which were reduced in size to form a U-shaped tube of breast tissue carrying the nipple at the apex of the U."

McIndoe and Rees (1958) reported 347 patients operated by the McIndoe modification of the Biesenberger technique. They concluded that nipple necrosis following the McIndoe-Biesenberger operation was often the result of periareolar hematomas compressing the blood supply rather than of primary circulatory insufficiency.

The Biesenberger technique, or a modification thereof, was practiced throughout the world as the operation of choice for reduction mammaplasty with nipple transposition until Strömbeck introduced his technique in 1960. Some surgeons continue to use modifications of the Biesenberger technique (Carlsen and Tershakowec, 1975; Vilain, 1976).

Maliniac (1932) reported a two stage breast reduction procedure after a study of the blood supply of the breast that indicated to him that previous descriptions were inaccurate. Ragnell (1941) arrived at conclusions similar to Maliniac's regarding the relationship between blood supply and complications of reduction mammaplasty. He also adopted a two stage procedure in very large breasts, and in 1946, Ragnell reported his experience with 500 cases of reduction mammaplasty. Today, two staged operative techniques are rarely if ever indicated. An occasional patient may fail to have the sufficient reduction in breast size following surgery, thus requiring a second procedure.

Mammectomy with free nipple grafting is credited by Maliniac (1950) to Lexer in 1912. However, Thorek in 1922 was first to document the technique. Dartigues (1928) claimed originality for the procedure, but this claim was challenged by Thorek. Thorek's operation was a partial mastectomy using a Passot type incision and transplantation of the nipples as free composite grafts of areola, muscle, and ductile tissue. In 1946, Thorek reported 25 years' experience with free nipple transplantation reduction mammaplasty. The technique was widely adopted in America and was championed by Adams (1947, 1949), Conway (1952, 1958), Marino (1952), Longacre (1953), and May (1956).

Wise (1956) reported a method of breast reduction using fixed patterns. In 1963, 1972, and 1976, he reported free nipple grafting using fixed breast reduction patterns. Felix and associates (1970) reported their experience with the Strömbeck reduction technique and free nipple grafts. Free nipple transplantation is the procedure of choice in gigantomastia, where moving the nipple a long distance on a pedicle would jeopardize its survival.

MODERN REDUCTION TECHNIQUES

As noted, Biesenberger (1927) and Schwarzmann (1930) made two major contributions to the development of modern reduction mammaplasty. Another major influence came 30 years later when Strömbeck (1960) modified a keyhole pattern originally introduced by Nedkoff in 1938. He extended the concept of a dermal bridge technique, described by Schwarzmann in 1930, to reintroduce on a practical basis the dermal pedicle for nipple transposition. Strömbeck used a pattern similar to that described by Wise (1956) to predetermine the shape of skin flaps and a horizontal dermal-parenchymal bridge for preservation of the principal arteriovenous and cutaneous nerve system to insure nipple survival. Gland is resected from above and below the dermal pedicle. Subsequently, Strömbeck (1964) reported that the dermis can be incised through to the subcutaneous fat on one or both sides of the pedicle in patients with short glandular bridges where tension and retraction develops when the nipple is moved to its new position. In 1973, Strömbeck reported his experience with this technique in 570 patients.

The Strömbeck operation became the prototype for a number of operations using a dermal bridge for nipple-areolar survival and resection of gland without skin undermining. Independently, Pitanguy (1960) reported a horizontal dermal bridge and "keel" shaped resection of gland from the inferior and central portions of the breast. Pitanguy credited the 1923 Lexer-Kraske operation with influencing his procedure. Cordoso de Castro (1976) described a modification of the Pitanguy technique using curved incisions to define the medial and lateral breast flap borders and resection of the breast tissue on a horizontal plane. He believed this modification produced breasts that were less tense and more desirable in shape. Similarly, Pitanguy advocated varying the curve of the incisions according to the individual breast.

Skoog (1963) described a laterally based dermal flap separated from the gland at the subcutaneous level. In a later presentation (1974), he suggested that the flap be made thicker by including a layer of glandular tissue in order to prevent curling, folding, and venous obstruction of the flap.

In 1972, McKissock described his now popular bipedicle vertical dermal pedicle for nipple transposition. This technique of reduction mammaplasty has gained wide acceptance because of its simplicity of design and its safety. McKissock pointed out that the dermal bridge functions mainly as a structural support to hold the flap together. Nipple survival depends on an intact parenchymal blood supply in the base of the pedicle for nourishment and venous drainage.

Dufourmentel and Mouly (1961) described a lateral wedge excision of skin, fat, and gland with a resultant lateral oblique scar. In the opinion of these authors, the lack of a scar on the medial aspect of the breast outweighs the long lateral oblique scar that may extend beyond the inframammary crease or fall into the axilla. They subsequently described four variations of the oblique technique in order to manage the wide range of breast problems associated with hypertrophy and/or ptosis. Unlike most techniques, preoperative measurements and planning of resection are not made with the patient sitting; instead, markings and measurements are made with the patient in the supine position in the operating room.

Regnault (1974) reported on reduction mammaplasty with the B technique, which results in a lateral oblique scar without a medial extension. In design and resection it is similar to the Dufourmentel-Mouly technique, but it emphasizes a more medial resection of the inferior portion of the breast. The lateral extension of the scar is slightly shorter with this method than with the Dufourmentel-Mouly technique.

Shatten and associates (1971, 1975) wrote of wide experience with their lateral wedge resection technique. This procedure differs mainly from that of Dufourmentel and Mouly in the use of a laterally based dermis-fat breast flap that is rotated superiorly and medially and becomes the core around which the remaining skin and breast flaps are closed. The dermis-fat gland flap in the Dufourmentel-Mouly operation is based more medially. Shatten determines the position of the nipple at the end of the operation after the breast flaps have been closed. Variations in the lateral wedge excision have been reported by Elbaz and

Verheecke (1972) and Meyer and Kesselring (1975).

Weiner and associates (1973) reported on a technique of breast reduction using a superior dermal pedicle for nipple transposition. This technique should not be used if the new nipple site is to be more than 7.5 centimeters above its original location. A disadvantage of this operation is the necessity of complete separation of the nipple from the gland in cases of marked hypertrophy. Arufe, Erenfryd, and Saubidet (1977) wrote about a superior dermal pedicle similar to Weiner's technique but retained glandular tissue in order to preserve the important blood supply to the superior medial breast tissue. Gsell (1974) described a superior based vertical dermal flap similar to the McKissock pedicle but transected at the inframammary end. This is risky, since much of the blood supply to the parenchyma is transected. Nipple necrosis is apt to be high with this technique.

Aufricht (1949) introduced an inferior mammary pedicle technique. Robertson (1967) and Arons (1976) reported experience with the technique of inferior flap mammaplasty performed in conjunction with free nipple grafting. Courtiss and Goldwyn (1977) reported an inferior dermal pedicle technique as an alternative to free nipple-areolar grafting in patients with severe macromastia or ptosis. In their technique, the inferior dermal pedicle extends transversely across the full length of the inframammary fold incision. A keyhole pattern similar to that described by McKissock is also used. Advantages of their technique include (1) excellent vascularity of the pedicle, (2) reduction of pedicle length and subsequent reduction of the potential for kinking upon closure, and (3) good nipple-areolar sensation through preservation of the fourth and fifth intercostal nerves. Robbins (1977) reported an inferior dermal pedicle similar to that of Courtiss and Goldwyn but limited to the medial portion of the inframammary fold.

Ribeiro (1975) described an inferior pedicle technique. He avoided a vertical scar by bringing the nipple and areolar under and through the superior skin flap and into position. Breast sculpturing is done by tubing the inferior dermal pedicle and passing it beneath the superior skin flap.

Kaplan (1978) reported reduction mammaplasty with resection of three out of the four breast quadrants and transposition of the nipple without preservation of a dermal pedicle. The nipple survived on the parenchyma of the superior quadrant in 85 breasts and of the inferior quadrant in 80 breasts. There was no nipple necrosis in the 165 breasts reported. The technique is a variation of the Penn (1960) technique, with wide skin flap undermining and resection of the medial and lateral breast quadrants.

Significant contributions have been made by many surgeons not noted herein. In recent years, excellent textbooks of plastic and reconstructive breast surgery have been edited by Goldwyn (1976) and Georgiade (1976).

INDICATIONS FOR SURGERY

Most patients requesting breast reduction arrive at their decision after careful consideration. Patients vary in age from teen-agers to septuagenerians. Complaints are usually multiple and include physiologic and psychologic factors. The chief indication for breast reduction is discomfort owing to excessive weight of one or both breasts.

Heavy pendulous breasts are frequently painful. Chronic mastitis may be present. Premenstrual congestion often exacerbates symptoms. Pains in the shoulders, neck, and upper back are usual. Uncomfortable and unsightly grooves form in the shoulders from pressure exerted by brassiere straps supporting the heavy breasts. Intertrigo is often present in the submammary crease, which is constantly moist. Kyphosis and arthritis of the cervical spine may develop secondary to postural attitudes adopted to compensate for the weight of large breasts (Conway, 1952). A protuberant abdomen frequently accompanies the kyphosis.

In addition to the physical discomfort of large breasts, patients find their daily routine hampered by the mass of the breast tissue. Physical activities such as athletics are limited. Many patients are socially uncomfortable because of psychosocial and psychosexual attitudes and connotations related to the breasts. Friends and peers exacerbate the psychologic discomfort by remarks made in jest, and social adjustment may be seriously handicapped. This is especially true for teen-agers when self-image is of major importance and emotions are volatile. Large breasts may become the secondary sex characteristic that trouble patients most. Goin, Goin, and Gianini (1977) documented psychologic studies of a group of breast reduction patients and found that some adolescent patients with large breasts had not incorporated their breasts into their self-image. Instead, the breasts were viewed as obstacles and handicaps, external to the patients themselves.

It is also difficult and expensive to obtain properly fitting brassieres. Some patients find it necessary to have blouses, dresses, coats, and other clothing items custom made. This extra financial burden is significant for many patients.

Breast asymmetry with unilateral hyperplasia is another indication for reduction mammaplasty. Marked unilateral hyperplasia can result in scoliosis. Serious psychologic problems may result from the emotional stress associated with unilateral hyperplasia. Patients with chronic mastitis or severe fibrocystic disease combined with a strong family history of malignant breast disease, multiple biopsies and "cancer phobia" may be candidates for subcutaneous mastectomy (Malianic, 1950; Longacre, 1959; Freeman, 1962, 1969; Lewis, 1965; Bader, Pelletiere and Curtin, 1970; Goulian and McDivitt, 1972; Wiener et al., 1973). Breast reduction is not sufficient treatment for such patients.

Patient Evaluation

The ideal candidate for breast reduction is normal in weight, stature, and height. However, the majority of patients requesting surgery vary from slightly to significantly obese. Obese patients should be required to lose excess weight preoperatively. It is incongruous if a massively obese patient is concerned only with her breast size. Lack of dietary control in some patients is related to the large breasts and associated with distorted self-image. Some patients — usually teen-agers and young adults — diet religiously following breast reduction, lose weight, and adopt a new life style. However, preoperative weight reduction is clearly preferable.

A thorough medical history and physical examination, including the breast and axilla to test for intrinsic breast disease, are necessary to identify systemic diseases that may contraindicate major surgery. A history of easy bruisability, hemorrhage, or other signs suggesting blood dyscrasias must be investigated. No aspirin-containing compounds should be consumed for ten days prior to surgery, since aspirin decreases platelet cohesiveness resulting in an increase in bleeding. Patients taking birth control pills and other estrogen-containing hormones are alleged to have greater interoperative bleeding. Such medication should be discontinued ten days before surgery. The surgical procedure should not be scheduled during the three or four days prior to menses or during the first two or three days of the menstrual cycle. The glandular tissue bleeds profusely at such times.

A detailed history of the breasts is important. When did they become large? Was the growth related to taking hormones? Are the hormones still being taken? Are the breasts still increasing in size? Is pregnancy planned in the near future? Has there been pain and tenderness, nipple discharge, or signs of inflammation? Have masses or lumps been noted, and, if so, have they been investigated? Mammograms, thermograms, or xeroradiograms should be obtained when indicated.

Examination is made with the patient sitting or standing. The size of the breast relative to the body habitus is observed. The distance of the nipples from the suprasternal notch and the midline of the chest are measured individually. Differences in the two breasts as to size, level of the inframammary fold, or level of superior attachment of the breast to the chest wall are noted. This helps the surgeon in ascertaining asymmetry of which the patient may be unaware.

Striae in the upper quadrants of the breast skin will remain following surgery. Patients should be so informed, since they are often of the mistaken opinion that striae can be removed. Planned surgical incisions and postoperative scars should be described in detail.

Breast markings are best made on the evening prior to or morning of surgery before the patient receives premedication. Making markings in a busy operating room just prior to induction of anesthesia becomes hectic for a premedicated patient. All preoperative measurements and markings are made with the patient sitting or standing with the breasts dependent. Nipple position, inframammary crease location, and pattern design change when the patient is supine and the breasts fall laterally.

Informed Consent

The general details of the planned breast reduction procedure are explained in clear terms to the patient. Complications including hypertrophic scars, hematoma, and nipple necrosis are discussed with the patient. The location of the surgical scars is described. Many patients have been misinformed by well meaning friends regarding the nature of incisions for breast reduction. Incisions drawn on the skin with indelible ink clearly demonstrate their location.

The patient should be made aware that severe complications such as thrombophlebitis, pulmonary embolus, and even death can occur with any major operative procedure. The low incidence of such complications with reduction mammaplasty can also be pointed out.

Patients are advised that lactation and breast feeding may not be possible following reduction mammaplasty because of interference with the mammary ducts in all cases of free nipple grafts and in many transposition operations.

Patients should be questioned as to the level of sensuality and eroticism they experience associated with their nipples. There is often some loss or diminution of sensation following reduction mammaplasty, although it is usually transient in nature — particularly following nipple transposition procedures. Nipple erectility returns to normal in most patients.

Patients requiring free nipple areolar grafts should be informed that the areola may remain shiny and flat in appearance. Nipple projection will be slight or absent. The subject of nipple sensitivity is discussed in the section dealing with complications of breast reduction.

NEW NIPPLE SITE

Selecting a new nipple site is critical. A nipple placed in too high a location is difficult to correct. It is wise to locate the nipples slightly lower than the ideal position, since the nipples tend to migrate superiorly in the months following surgery. Such a cephalic migration occurs as the skin brassiere stretches and the breast mass "settles out" from under the nipple. For the Strömbeck and McKissock procedures, the new nipple site is predetermined and cut at the beginning of the procedure. The Pitanguy technique allows more flexibility, as the final location is determined after the new breast is reshaped. Location of the new nipple site depends on several factors including length of the torso, body habitus, dimensions of the thoracic cage, breast mass, and, most importantly, the position relative to the inframammary fold.

Determining the new nipple site is similar for reduction mammaplasty and mastopexy. Exceptions to this statement will be noted.

The suprasternal notch, midclavicular points, and midline of the sternum are marked. A vertical line is drawn from the midclavicular points through the nipples, down the inferior pole of the breast, across the inframammary crease, and onto the chest wall (Figure 33–1, A). If one nipple is situated significantly more laterally or medially than the other, the vertical line can be shifted in the direction necessary to give better symmetry. The vertical line from the midclavicular point is not parallel to the midaxis of the body but diverges in a lateral direction through the nipples.

The index finger of one hand is placed under and behind the breast up to the inframammary crease. The opposite index finger palpates through the breast to determine the level of the tip of the finger in the inframammary crease, and the surface of the breast is marked at this point (Fig. 33–1, B). This is approximately the new nipple site. The actual new nipple site should be placed 1.0 to

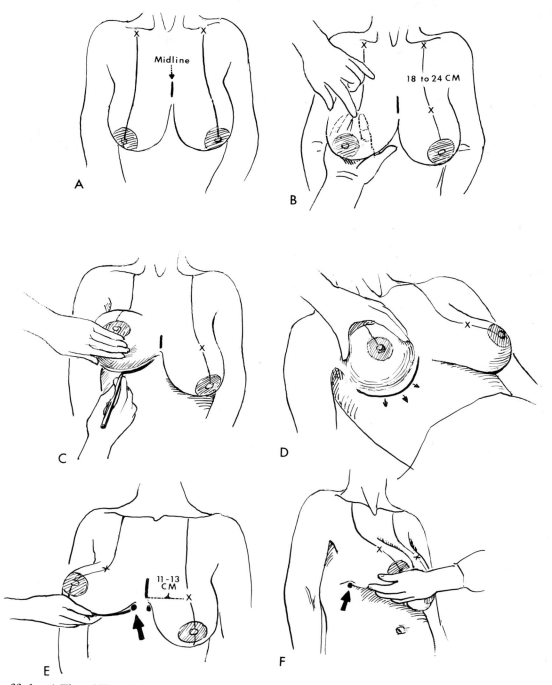

Figure 33–1. *A*, The midline of the breast and the midline of the anterior chest wall are marked.

B, The projection of the inframammary crease onto the anterior surface of the breast is determined.

C, The inframammary fold is marked with the patient standing.

D, In the supine position, the previously marked inframammary crease appears too low. This marking should not be changed when the patient is supine.

E and *F*, The medial and lateral limits of the inframammary fold are marked.

1.5 cm lower, to allow for upward migration. Depending upon the height of the patient, the size of the thorax, and the age of the patient, nipples are situated 18 to 24 cm from the sternal notch and 11 to 13 cm from the midsternum. When the breasts are very large and the skin is stretched, there is a greater tendency for the nipples to move up after the weight and stretch are reduced. Correction of mild ptosis may only require a small amount of upward nipple movement — as little as 1 or 2 cm. The final nipple position should be at the apex of the breast cone, pointing forward, slightly upward, and laterally.

The inframammary crease is marked by gently elevating the breast and sweeping the tip of the marking pencil in the inframammary crease (Fig. 33–1, C). The inframammary crease location, determined with the patient sitting or standing, must remain constant throughout the surgical procedure. When the patient is placed supine, the inframammary crease appears to be higher than when marked in the upright position, as the breast mass shifts cephalad and laterally (Fig. 33–1, D). The inframammary crease marking must not be redrawn when the patient is supine.

When possible (Fig. 33–1, E,F), the medial and lateral limits of the inframammary incision are marked at the points where the overhanging fold of breast tissue will hide the incision postoperatively. Otherwise, it will be difficult for the patient to wear certain kinds of clothing.

When the new nipple sites are determined and the inframammary crease is marked, pertinent drawings for the reduction mammaplasty technique selected for the individual patient are then completed.

SELECTION OF OPERATIVE TECHNIQUE

Any one of the several standard nipple transposition operative procedures can be adapted to correct mild to severe macromastia. Patients with extreme hypertrophy ("gigantomastia") are best treated by free nipple grafting, as are those with dense, sclerotic, and unyielding parenchyma. Two or three techniques well understood and used with flexibility will permit the surgeon to handle a full range of problems from slight ptosis to extreme hypertrophy. The techniques favored by the authors are McKissock, Pitanguy, and Strömbeck for moderate to marked hypertrophy and ptosis and the free nipple graft for gigantomastia and very thick breasts.

All transposition procedures involve resection of gland and tailoring a new skin brassiere. It makes no difference whether glandular resection is done superiorly and inferiorly or medially and laterally, as long as the residual breast tissue retains its vascularity and can be sculptured to the desired breast shape. The arterial supply of the mammary gland comes mainly from the lateral thoracic artery, the perforating branches of the internal mammary artery, and the branches of the intercostal arteries. There is considerable controversy as to which of these branches is of primary importance in maintaining the blood supply to the gland and nipple. An any rate, sufficient blood supply must be present in the glandular tissue that remains following reduction mammaplasty.

Mild hypertrophy can be corrected by the technique of Aries (described by Pitanguy). The advantages of this technique are minimal tissue disturbance and avoidance of a transverse scar in the inframammary crease. In the Aries-Pitanguy technique, a vertical ellipse of skin and gland is resected below the nipple. This procedure is most useful when very mild hypertrophy accompanies slight ptosis. It is especially useful in cases where a small reduction in volume of one breast is necessary to correct breast asymmetry.

ARIES-PITANGUY TECHNIQUE

The basic principles of the Aries-Pitanguy operation are resection of a small portion of the central lower portion of the breast and skin flap elevation to transpose the nipple to its new position.

The approximate level of the new nipple position is determined as previously described. The amount of breast tissue to be resected is determined and outlined as a lozenge-shaped resection lying immediately inferior to the areola. Skin incisions are made down through the dermis along the outlines of the breast tissue to be resected (Figure 33–2, A). The areola is dissected, leaving the dermal ring attached circumferentially (Fig. 33–2, B).

The skin is undermined in a subcutaneous plane only to the width necessary to permit upward shifting of the gland to the desired level (Fig. 33–2, C). Limited undermining also permits downward shift of the excess skin and a plumping out or filling of the superior portion of the breast by forcing the tissue cephalad. Excess gland is excised as a wedge below the nipple (Fig. 33–2, D). Manipulation of the breast and the skin flap at this point determines the approximate site of the new nipple.

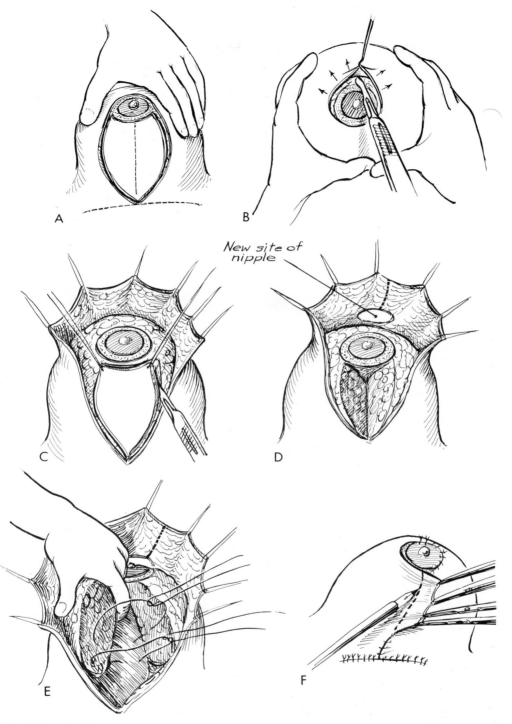

New site of nipple

Figure 33–2. *A,* A periareolar incision is made, and a lozenge shape of skin and breast tissue between the lower border of the areola and inframammary crease is outlined for excision.

B, Periareolar skin is undermined far enough to permit superior elevation of the nipple-areolar complex to its new position.

C, The planned lozenge-shaped resection is made. For the correction of ptosis without macromastia, the lozenge-shaped area is de-epithelialized maintaining all tissue bulk.

D, Excision completed.

E, Breast tissue is approximated with buried absorbable sutures, and the nipple-areolar complex is elevated to its new position.

F, Excision of excess skin.

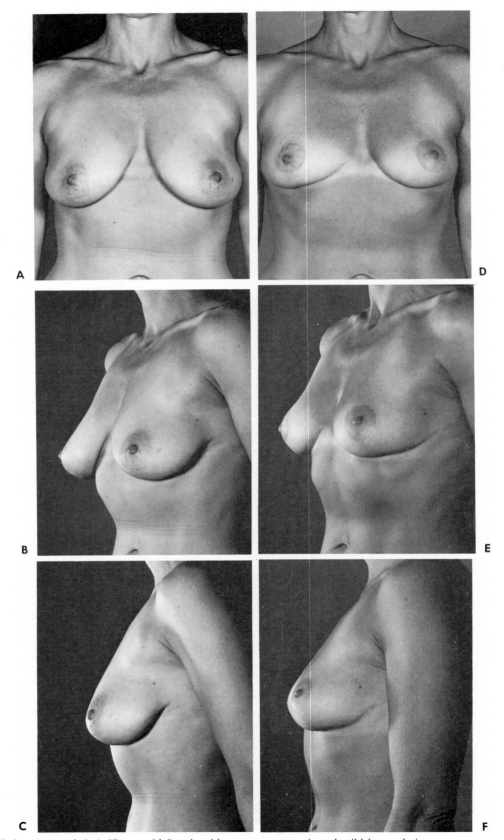

Figure 33–3. *A, B,* and *C,* A 37-year-old female with postpartum ptosis and mild hyperplasia.

D, E, and *F,* Two years following small amount of reduction and mastopexy by the Aries-Pitanguy technique there is no significant return of ptosis.

The cut breast tissue is approximated in the midline with absorbable sutures (Fig. 33–2, *E*). This helps force the nipple and areola in a cephalad direction.

The skin flaps are draped around the areola, excess skin is removed below the nipple, and the vertical incision is tailored and sutured in position (Fig. 33–2, *F*) (see Figure 33–3).

A disadvantage of the Aries-Pitanguy technique is that the vertical scar may extend below the inframammary crease as "dogears" are chased. A short horizontal incision in the inframammary crease is preferable to an incision extending below the inframammary crease, and this should be designed without hesitation.

The technique of Dufourmentel and Mouly (1965, 1968), which places the incision in a radial line extending obliquely and laterally towards the axilla, is also particularly well suited to correct mild or moderate hyperplasia. The B technique of Regnault and the lateral wedge excision of Shatten are of similar value. The lateral wedge excision techniques are difficult to master. Consistent good results, particularly in large breasts, are difficult to achieve. The nipples in such patients tend to have a "cross-eyed" appearance.

MCKISSOCK TECHNIQUE

The McKissock vertical pedicle technique is readily applicable to the reduction of mild, moderate, and severe degrees of breast hypertrophy (Figure 33–4). This technique should not be used in cases of gigantomastia, nor where nipple transposition of more than fifteen cm is necessary. The McKissock technique is applicable to the majority of breast reduction patients. Advantages of the McKissock technique include (1) well vascularized dermal-parenchymal pedicle for nipple-areolar nourishment, (2) easily mobilized pedicle for nipple transposition, (3) excellent exposure of medial,

Text continued on page 917.

Figure 33–4. *A,* A keyhole pattern is centered appropriately to the new nipple site.

B, The width of the keyhole and the width of the medial and lateral breast flaps are adjusted according to the individual breast.

C and *D,* The width of the keyhole determines the contour of the new breast. The "lazy S" configuration of the inferior margin of the medial lateral skin flaps provides breast volume centrally and relatively less volume medially and laterally to help obtain the desired conical breast shape.

Illustration continued on the following page.

Figure 33–4 *Continued.* *E* and *F*, The vertical dermal pedicle is outlined.

G, The vertical dermal pedicle is de-epithelialized.

H, Medial and lateral wedges of breast tissue are resected.

I, The upper half of the vertical dermal pedicle is freed from the pectoral fascia.

Illustration continued on the opposite page.

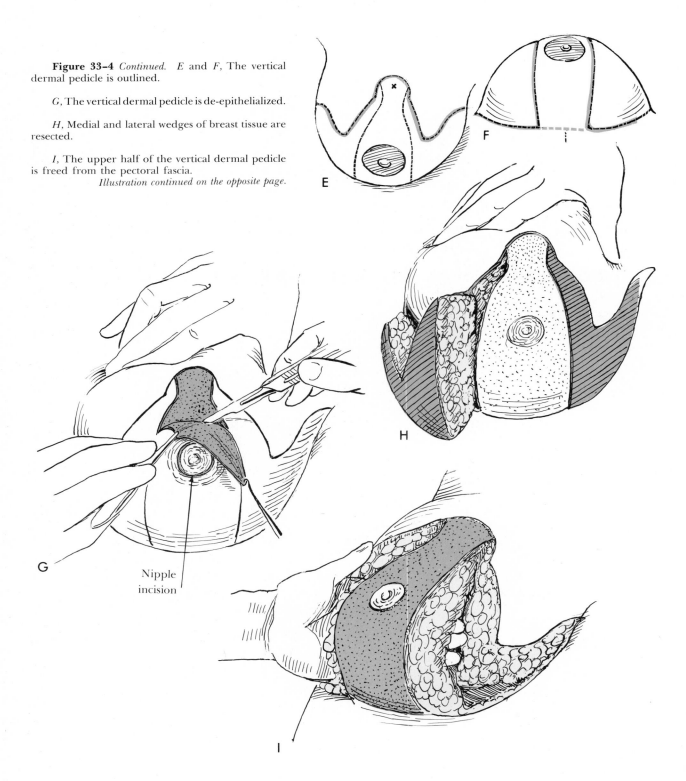

Nipple
incision

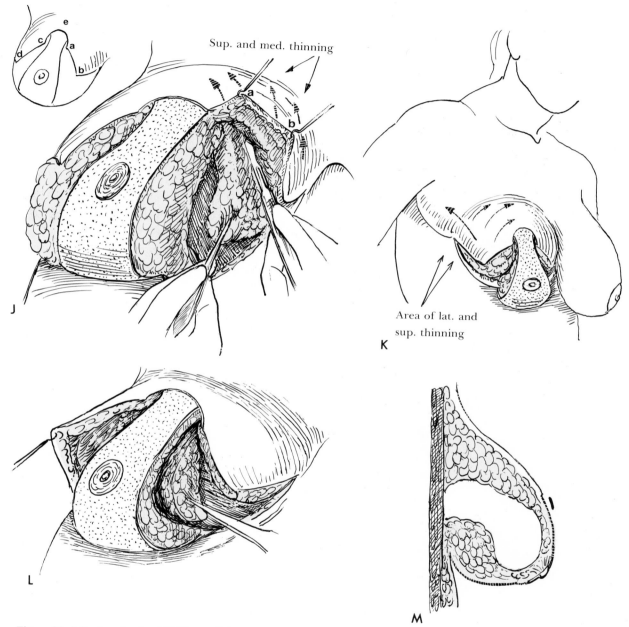

Figure 33–4 *Continued.*   *J* and *K,* The medial and lateral breast flaps and the breast superior to the dermal pedicle are thinned as indicated.

L and *M,* Parenchyma is resected from the upper half of the vertical dermal pedicle. Parenchyma approximately 1.0 to 2.0 cm thick is left on the superior portion of the pedicle. Parenchyma in the inferior half of the pedicle remains full thickness.

Illustration continued on the following page.

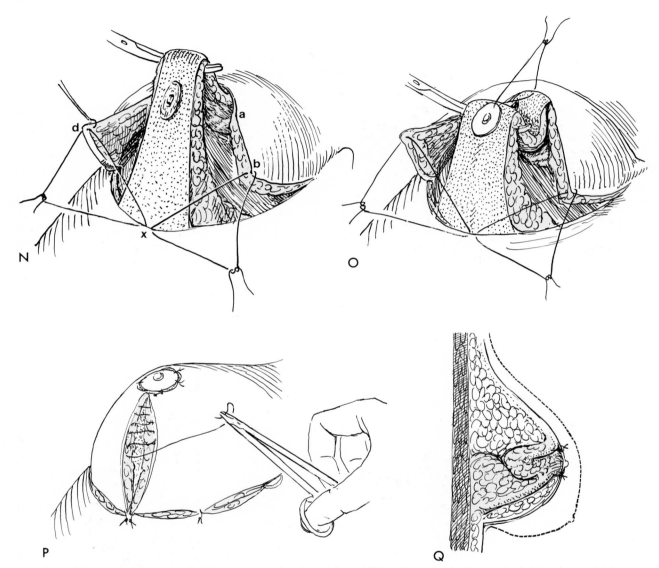

Figure 33–4 *Continued.   N*, A stitch begins approximation of the medial and lateral skin flaps to the inframammary fold.

O, The vertical dermal pedicle is folded superiorly to bring the nipple-areolar complex to its new site.

P and *Q*, The medial and lateral skin flaps are sutured. Any discrepancy in length of the medial and lateral skin flaps and inframammary fold can be adjusted as the flaps are sutured.

middle, and lateral gland for resection, and (4) flexibility in design of skin flaps for the individual breast. The McKissock technique is difficult to execute in the very large breast of the gigantomastia patient because of unwieldy length of the vertical pedicle.

The basic principles of the McKissock technique are (1) a modified keyhole pattern, (2) a bipedicle vertical dermal flap for architectual support of the nipple-areolar complex, and (3) vascularization of the flap from vessels passing through the parenchyma. McKissock believes most of the circulation enters the inferior pedicle. The new nipple sites and the inframammary creases are determined and marked as previously described. The keyhole and medial and lateral skin flaps are outlined using a celluloid pattern for marking the new areola window and keyhole. Celluloid patterns with areola windows of 3.5 cm, 4.2 cm, and 4.8 cm can be used for almost any breast size encountered. The pattern simplifies marking the areola window, keyhole widths, medial and lateral skin flap widths, and the vertical dermal pedicle. However, the pattern provides only the basic outline; the drawings must be modified so as to obtain the desired result in each patient.

The pattern is placed on the midclavicular line with the areola windows centered around the new nipple site, and indelible ink marks the pattern (Fig. 33–4, A, B). The pattern gives fixed reference points for exact measurements. This is extremely important in establishing breast symmetry. Adjustments are easily made to narrow the keyhole, shorten the length of the medial and lateral skin flaps, or vary the width of the vertical pedicle as necessary for the individual breast.

The width of the medial and lateral skin flaps (areola to inframammary crease distance) is determined 4.5 to 5.5 cm from the points where the diverging keyhole lines intersect the areolar circle (Fig. 33–4, B). Five cm is the average; however, the flap width varies with the planned new breast size. If the flaps are made too long, the breasts will "settle" from under the nipple, finally locating the nipples in a high position. The smallest width possible without excessive tension is used. The width of the flap can be narrowed during the final tailoring if it is considered excessive in length.

The width of the keyhole is of major importance (Fig. 33–4, C). If it is too wide, there will be excessive excision of skin from the medial portion of the breast. Flap closure will be tight and the breast will be flat on the bottom. If the keyhole is too narrow, there will be a horizontal skin excess and too great a discrepancy between the combined length of the medial and lateral skin flaps and the

inframammary fold to which they are sutured. Therefore, the central portion of the breast will bulge inferiorly postoperatively.

Lines are next drawn medially and laterally from the points determined as the inferior limits of the width of the medial and lateral skin flaps to meet the inframammary line at the points determined as its medial and lateral limits. These lines are made in a lazy S configuration to provide a generous breast volume centrally and relatively less volume medially and laterally (Fig. 33–4, C, D). This helps obtain the desired conical breast shape.

Vertical lines are marked from approximately the halfway points of the new areolar window inferiorly down the anterior surface of the breast to below the inframammary crease (Fig. 33–4, E, F). These lines determine the width of the vertical dermal pedicle and should be 5 to 7 cm apart at the inframammary fold. In some patients, the vertical lines will pass through a portion of the areolar pigmentation, and in others, the vertical lines may run tangential to the existing areolar pigmentation. The most important point is that the pedicle be slightly wider than the planned new areolar size.

An assistant grasps the breast with both hands at its base and applies gentle but firm pressure circumferentially, thereby stretching the areolar skin. An areolar "cookie-cutter" of the desired size (3.5 to 4.5 cm, depending on the breast size to be constructed) is centered around the nipple and pressure is applied. A ring impression made in the areolar skin is incised circumferentially. Quadrants of the new smaller areola are scored at the periphery with the scalpel to facilitate the areola positioning later. All ink markings on the breast are scored superficially with the knife; otherwise, they may become difficult to find as the surgical field becomes active.

The vertical pedicle as previously measured and outlined is deepithelialized (Fig. 33–4, G). Care is taken not to undermine the areola. Usually, deepithelialization is more easily performed above the areola. A buttonhole in the skin through the epidermis is more desirable than a buttonhole through the dermal bed into the subcutaneous tissue. However, intermittent interruption of the dermis does little harm to the areola blood supply, as the important vessels are located in the parenchyma. The breast is stabilized between the hands of the surgeon and the assistant to facilitate cutting. The triangle of breast tissue medial to the vertical pedicle is first resected (Fig. 33–4, H). Beginning adjacent to the deepithelialized vertical pedicle, the gland is incised perpendicular to the chest wall down to the prepectoral fascia. The outer skin incision is incised and the gland is again cut through down to the chest wall. The breast tissue is easily dissected from the pectoral fascia. The triangle of skin and breast lateral to the vertical pedicle is incised and removed in a similar fashion. The superior one half of the vertical pedicle is undermined at the level of the chest wall, producing a bucket handle effect (Fig. 33–4, *I*). This permits mobilization of the pedicle to allow easier access to the medial and lateral quadrants of the breast and to permit upward mobility of the nipple-areola.

After removal of the medial and lateral triangles of breast tissue, the remaining breast flaps are generally too thick to allow pliability and restructuring of the breast. Thinning of the flaps is necessary. Dissection at the level of the pectoral fascia separates the breast tissue from the chest wall medially. Skin hooks are placed along the margin of the medial breast flap and the gland is resected as indicated (Fig. 33–4, *J*). The maneuver is repeated laterally. In large, fat breasts, superior trimming is required (Fig. 33–3, *K*). Lateral resection often requires removing the tail of the breast from the axilla. Parenchyma is now resected from beneath the superior one half of the vertical pedicle, leaving 1 or 2 cm of parenchyma attached to the dermis (Fig. 33–4, *L, M*). Parenchyma in the inferior half of the pedicle remains full thickness, since according to McKissock the main vascular and neural supply to the nipple-areolar complex passes through the inferior pole.

After hemostasis is obtained with electrocautery, temporary approximating sutures are placed in the dermis of the skin flaps. The opposite breast is resected in a similar fashion. When resection of the second breast is complete, the temporary sutures are removed from the first breast and a comparison is made of the remaining volume of gland in the two breasts. In a systematic fashion, the medial and lateral flaps and the superior portion of the two breasts are compared. The dermal pedicles are compared for width and thickness of remaining gland. Necessary resections are made to produce symmetry. The resected tissue should be weighed separately on a scale.

Flap closure is begun by approximating the inferior borders of the medial and lateral skin flaps to their new position along the inframammary fold (Fig. 33–4, *N*). Most often, this is approximately the midpoint of the vertical dermal pedicle. The point of attachment of the medial and lateral skin flaps to the inframammary fold can be varied either in a medial or lateral direction several millimeters as necessary to line up the breast flaps in the best manner.

Careful folding of the superior portion of the vertical dermal pedicle positions the nipple and areola in the new position (Fig. 33–4,*O*). If the dermal parenchymal pedicle is quite long, it may sometimes be necessary to resect a small additional amount of breast tissue from the superior medial portion of the breast in order to allow room for the pedicle to fold superiorly. A 5–0 nylon suture is placed from 12 o'clock on the areola to the skin at the mid-superior portion of the areolar window. The areolar window flaps are closed (Fig. 33–4,*J*, inset *A* to *C*). Sutures are placed at 12, 3, and 9 o'clock between the areola and areolar window skin. Placement of these sutures is aided by scoring of the areolar quadrants at the onset of the operation. If the surgical field is not sufficiently dry at this point, flat suction drains can be placed from lateral to medial, passing beneath the bucket handle of the vertical pedicle. The drains exit through the lateral extent of the inframammary incision. A separate stab wound for a drain is not necessary and produces an extra scar.

The flaps are sutured in place from the lateral and medial ends toward the center of the breast (Fig. 33–4, *P, Q*). A great deal of discrepancy between the length of the flaps and the inframammary incision can be corrected as the closure is made. Small dog-ears can be excised at the ends of the inframammary incisions. The breast tissue is approximated with a few sutures of 4–0 absorbable suture, and the skin is approximated with intracuticular Prolene suture along the vertical and horizontal incisions. Final approximation of the areola is carried out with interrupted 5–0 nylon sutures. (See Figures 33–5 and 33–6.)

STRÖMBECK TECHNIQUE

The Strömbeck technique utilizes a horizontal dermal and parenchymal pedicle for transposition of the nipple-areolar complex. The horizontal pedicle is nourished by branches of the lateral thoracic and internal mammary arteries. The Strömbeck technique was originally designed to reduce very large breasts, but it is most useful to reduce breasts of moderate size requiring resection of 500 grams or less. Fatty or sclerotic tense breasts are the most difficult to reduce by any method. Infolding of the Strömbeck horizontal pedicle is particularly difficult in such breasts. Transecting dermis on one or both sides may be necessary in order to position the nipple in the desired location and can be done with impunity according to Strömbeck.

The advantages of the Strömbeck technique

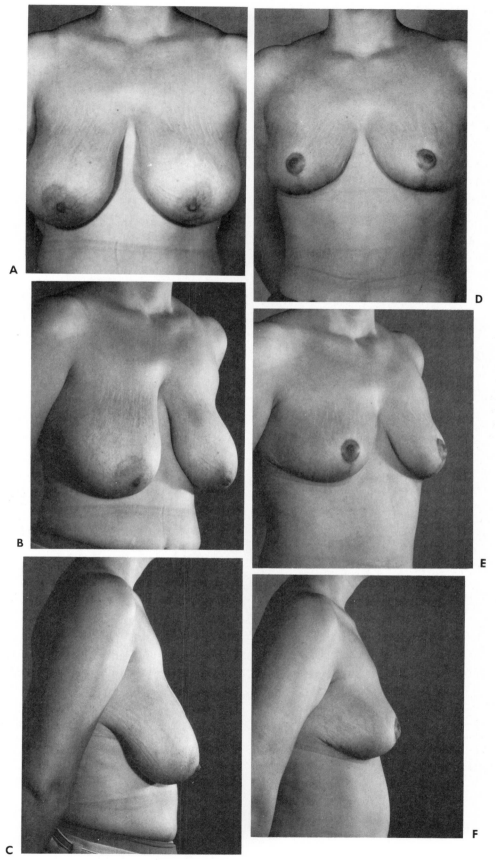

Figure 33–5.   *A, B,* and *C,* A 28-year-old female with large, pendulous breasts after two pregnancies. *D, E,* and *F,* The breasts were each reduced approximately 470 grams by the McKissock technique. The lateral extension of the inframammary incisions stops beneath the normal breast fold. Sleeveless blouses and similar revealing clothing can be worn without exposing incisions.

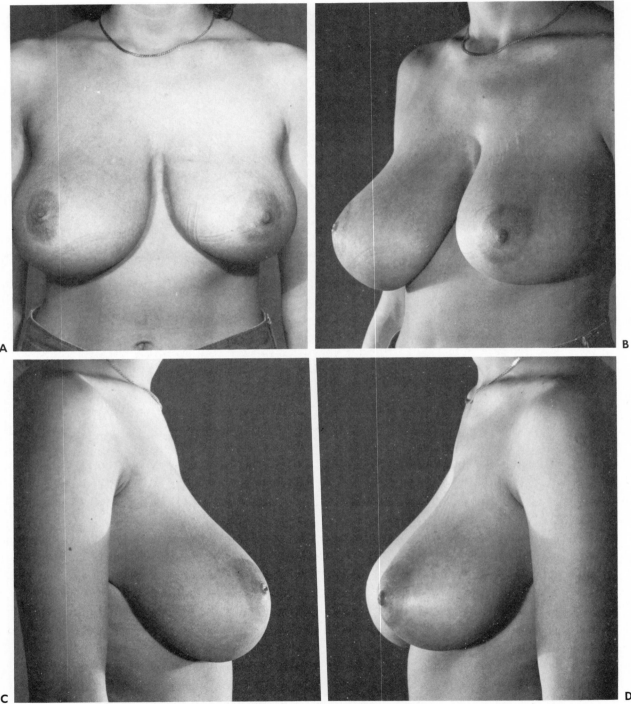

Figure 33–6. *A–D,* A 19-year-old female with large, ptotic breasts and asymmetry. Note nipple position is near level of inframammary folds.

E–H, Seventeen months following 799-gram reduction of the right breast and 484-gram reduction of the left breast by the McKissock technique. There is some flatness of the medial quadrants of the breast as a result of keeping the medial extension of the inframammary incision from the midline. The lateral extensions of the inframammary incisions are approximately the length of the original inframammary skin fold.

Illustation continued on the opposite page.

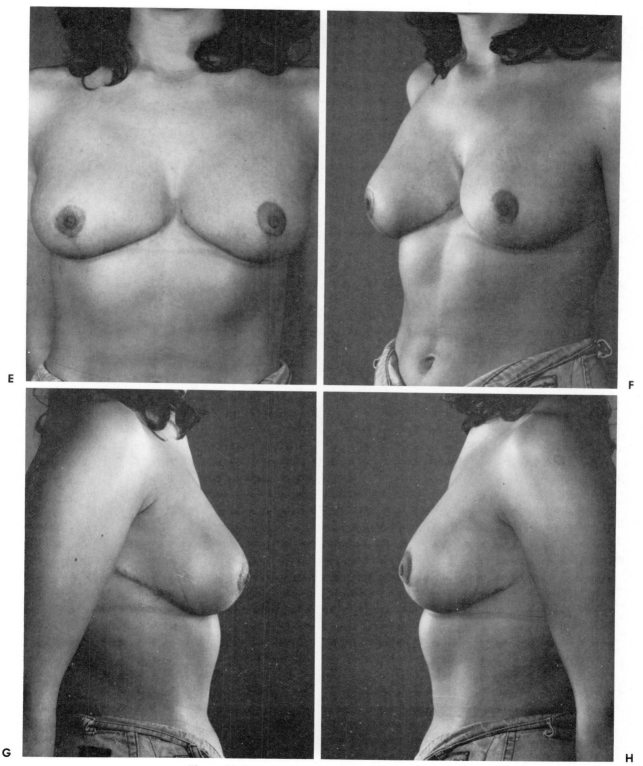

Figure 33–6 *Continued.   See legend on the opposite page.*

are (1) a relatively simple pattern to follow, (2) a good blood supply to the nipple-areolar complex, and (3) no skin flap undermining is required. Two disadvantages are (1) difficulty in transposing the nipple to its new site in very large or pendulous breasts and (2) flatness of the inferior breast post-operatively.

Selection of a new nipple site and marking the inframammary line have been previously discussed in this chapter. The transparent celluloid Ström-beck pattern (Fig. 33–7, *A*) is placed on the breast. The midline of the pattern corresponds to the vertical line from the midclavicle through the nipple (Fig. 33–7, *B*). The upper border of the areolar window of the pattern is centered 1.5 cm above the new nipple site. The areolar window and lower borders of the pattern are marked with indelible ink (Fig. 33–7, *B, C*).

The breast is gently supported and moved laterally (Fig. 33–7, *D*), and the lower medial breast is folded in so as to determine the point on the inframammary crease to which the lower corner of the future medial skin flap will approximate. This point is marked on the inframammary crease (Fig. 33–7, *E*). The lower edge of the medial skin flap is then easily determined, so that it will fit the in-framammary incision (Fig. 33–7, *F*). The breast is again gently supported and moved medially. The lower part of the breast is folded in so as to determine if the lower edge of the lateral flap will meet the point on the inframammary crease just marked as the point to which the medial flap would reach (Fig. 33–7, *G*). If the lower corner of the lateral flap does not reach this point on the in-framammary crease, the lateral flap must be lengthened by moving the lower lateral corner medially (line *B-C* versus *B-X*, Fig. 33–7, *G*), but the

upper corner (at the areolar window) is not changed. In effect, this narrows the keyhole. The lower edge of the lateral skin flap is now easily determined and marked to fit the inframammary incision. Every effort should be made to stop the inframammary fold incision both medially and laterally at the points where the overhanging breast will cover the incision. This is in part determined by the inferior margins of the medial and lateral skin flaps. However, it is usually possible to "cheat" a little bit medially on the lateral flap and laterally on the medial flap.

The opposite breast is marked in a similar fashion. The positions of the superior borders of the areolar windows must be identical and the medial borders of the medial and lateral skin flaps must be identical in measurement (4.5 to 5 cm) in order to assure breast symmetry (Fig. 33–7, *H*). If there is asymmetry in the size of the two breasts, the inferior borders of the medial and lateral skin flaps and the lengths of the inframammary inci-sions will not be the same on the two breasts.

The upper corners of the medial and lateral skin flaps are connected by a curved incision, *BC*, with the concave side directed upward and extend-ing to 2 cm above the areola (Fig. 33–7, *I*). The lower corners of the medial and lateral skin flaps are joined by a similar horizontal incision, *DE*, which passes approximately 1 cm below the areola (Fig. 33–7, *I*). The transverse pedicle is thus out-lined.

The breast is distended by circumferential pressure applied around its base in order to stretch the skin of the areola. The desired new areolar size is established with a cookie-cutter marker (3.5 to 4.5 cm, depending upon the new breast size), and a superficial incision is made to the dermis to outline

Text continued on page 927.

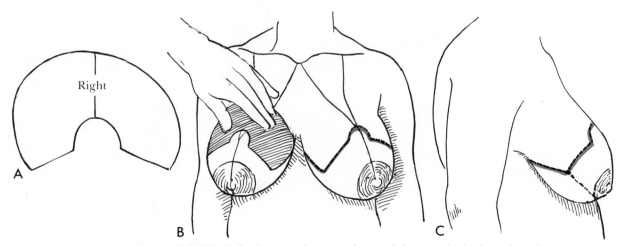

Figure 33–7.   *A, B,* and *C,* A celluloid Strömbeck pattern is centered around the new nipple site and marked.

Illustration continued on the following page.

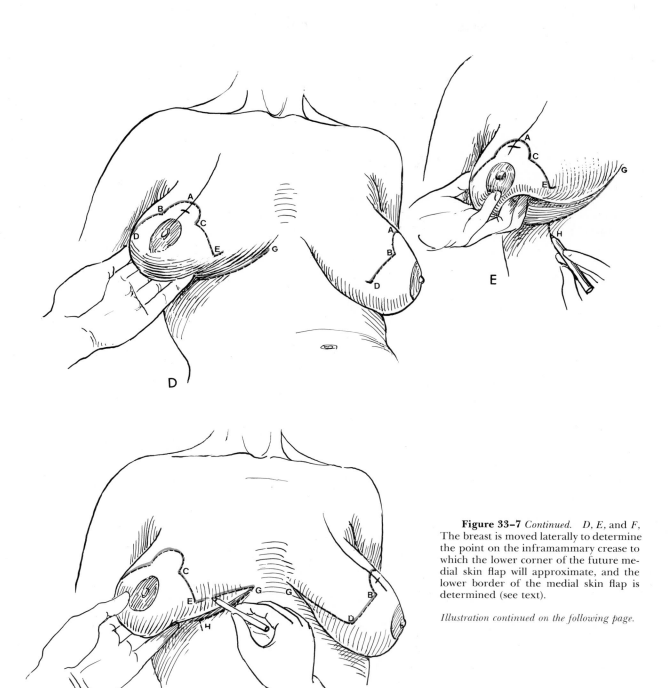

Figure 33–7 *Continued. D, E,* and *F,* The breast is moved laterally to determine the point on the inframammary crease to which the lower corner of the future medial skin flap will approximate, and the lower border of the medial skin flap is determined (see text).

Illustration continued on the following page.

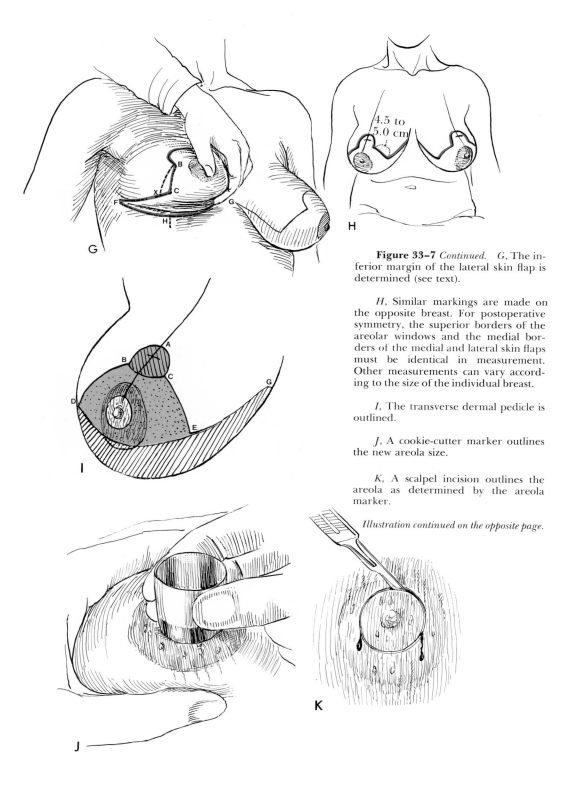

Figure 33–7 *Continued.   G*, The inferior margin of the lateral skin flap is determined (see text).

H, Similar markings are made on the opposite breast. For postoperative symmetry, the superior borders of the areolar windows and the medial borders of the medial and lateral skin flaps must be identical in measurement. Other measurements can vary according to the size of the individual breast.

I, The transverse dermal pedicle is outlined.

J, A cookie-cutter marker outlines the new areola size.

K, A scalpel incision outlines the areola as determined by the areola marker.

Illustration continued on the opposite page.

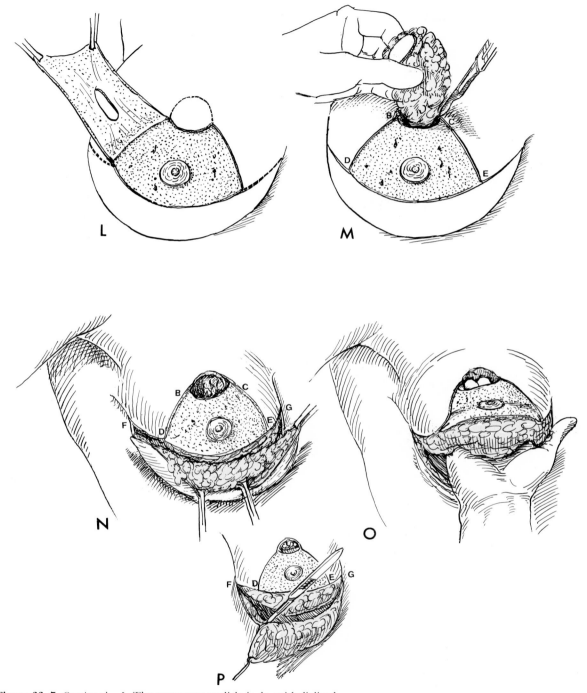

Figure 33–7. *Continued.* *L*, The transverse pedicle is de-epithelialized.

M, A core of skin, subcutaneous tissue, and gland is resected at the new areolar site down to the pectoral fascia.

N, The upper border of the breast segment to be resected is incised down to the fascia.

O, The transverse pedicle is freed from the chest wall.

P, Resection of the breast tissue is completed.

Illustration continued on the following page.

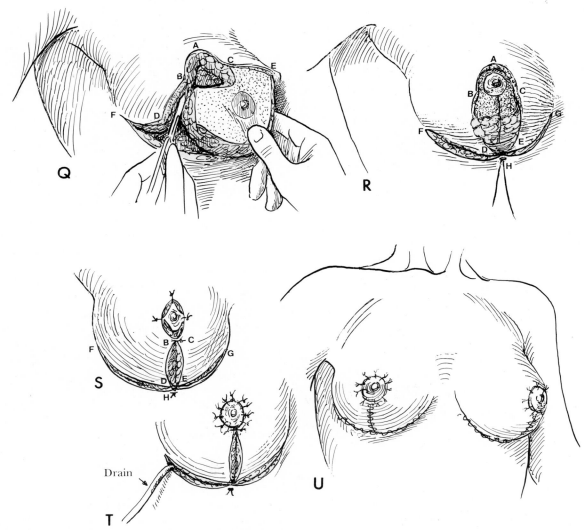

Figure 33–7 *Continued.*   *Q,* The dermis can be divided medially and laterally when necessary to move the nipple-areolar complex to its new position.

R, Recontouring of the breast is begun by suturing the medial skin flap (Point E) and the lateral skin flap (Point D) to Point H along the inframammary crease. The nipple-areolar complex is moved into its new position. The entire lateral pedicle can be cut if pedicle mobility is needed.

S, The areolar windows and areolar quadrants are sutured.

T, A drain is placed beneath the breast and brought through the lateral incision.

U, Breast flaps are closed from lateral to medial and from medial to middle of the breast to accommodate any discrepancy in flap lengths and to prevent dogears at medial and lateral corners of the inframammary incision.

the new areola (Fig. 33–7, J, K). Even though a cookie-cutter is used with a fixed diameter, the size of the areola will in part depend on the amount of stretching of the areolar skin at the time the marking is made. Equal amounts of pressure should be applied to both the right and left breast in order to create similar nipple areolar sizes. The transverse pedicle is deepithelialized (Fig. 33–7, L). Care must be taken not to undermine the areola as it is approached. Deepithelialization is aided if the circumferential pressure around the breast distends the surface. Skin, subcutaneous tissue, and gland are resected at the new areola site down to the pectoral fascia (Fig. 33–7, M). The core of resected tissue should be no greater in diameter than the new areolar window because excessive resection of tissue may contribute to a retracted nipple postoperatively. Further resection of breast tissue in this area can be carried out if indicated when the breast flaps and transverse pedicle are mobilized for closure.

Digital dissection inferiorly along the fascia beneath the breast lifts the inferior portion of the gland and undermines the transverse pedicle. The breast is cut down to the fascia along the upper border of the lower segment of breast tissue for resection (Fig. 33–7, N). Manual stabilization of the breast prevents beveling the incision and unplanned resection of a portion of the parenchyma from beneath the transverse pedicle. The thickness and mobility of the transverse pedicle can be examined as the inferior aspect of the transverse pedicle is completely freed (Fig. 33–7, O). Resection of the inferior breast tissue is completed by first cutting along the inferior mammary line and then dissecting the breast off the pectoral fascia (Fig. 33–7, P).

Reshaping of the breast is begun by suturing together the lower edges of the medial (Point E) and lateral (Point D) skin flaps to Point H (previously determined as the point at which the medial and lateral skin flaps would meet on the inframammary fold) along the inframammary crease (Fig. 33–7, Q, R). If the glandular pedicle is short and it is difficult to transpose the areola to its new position, the dermis can be cut through down to the subcutaneous fat on one side (Fig. 33–7, Q). The dermis can actually be cut on both sides if the pedicles are short and there has been no glandular resection off the areolar carrying pedicle. When necessary, the entire lateral pedicle can be cut to move the areola into its new position. It is thought to be safer to cut the lateral side of the pedicle than to cut the medial side, which carries a better blood supply coming from the internal mammary artery.

The upper corners of the medial and lateral skin flaps (Points B and C) are sutured together and the areolar quadrants are sutured (Fig. 33–7, S). If the surgical field is not sufficiently dry, a vacuum drain is placed beneath the breast flaps and brought out laterally through the inframammary incision (Fig. 33–7, T). The separate stab wound incision is not indicated for a drain. The breast parenchyma is approximated with 4–0 absorbable sutures and the skin is closed along the vertical and horizontal incisions with intracuticular Prolene. The areola is sutured in place with interrupted 5–0 nylons (Fig. 33–7, U). (See Figures 33–8 and 33–9.)

PITANGUY TECHNIQUE

The Pitanguy technique can be used to correct slight to marked hypertrophy. Pitanguy also used his technique for correcting gigantomastia, with or without free nipple grafting. The Pitanguy technique also facilitates free nipple grafting in very large or pendulous breasts. However, this requires a great deal of experience with the procedure and is not recommended for routine corrections of gigantomastia.

The advantages of the Pitanguy technique are (1) flexibility in nipple positioning intraoperatively, (2) preservation of lactation in many patients, and (3) excellent breast shape. The main disadvantages are the free-handed approaches to measurement and resection, which limit its use for inexperienced surgeons. This very flexibility is one of the most attractive features of the operation for the experienced surgeon.

Pitanguy Operative Procedure

The Pitanguy reduction mammaplasty involves a "keel" shaped segment of breast tissue resected from the inferior and middle of the gland and the nipple-areola transposed on a transverse dermal pedicle.

A vertical line is made from the midclavicular point through the nipple and inframammary crease. The inframammary crease is marked. The new nipple site (Point A, Fig. 33–10) is identified on the midclavicular line by placing the index finger in the submammary fold and marking the point on the skin surface just below the level of the submammary fold as originally described by Pitanguy and described previously in this section. Point A does not represent the exact center of the nipple, but it is the point very near where the nipple will be when the operation is complete. Precise nipple

Text continued on page 932.

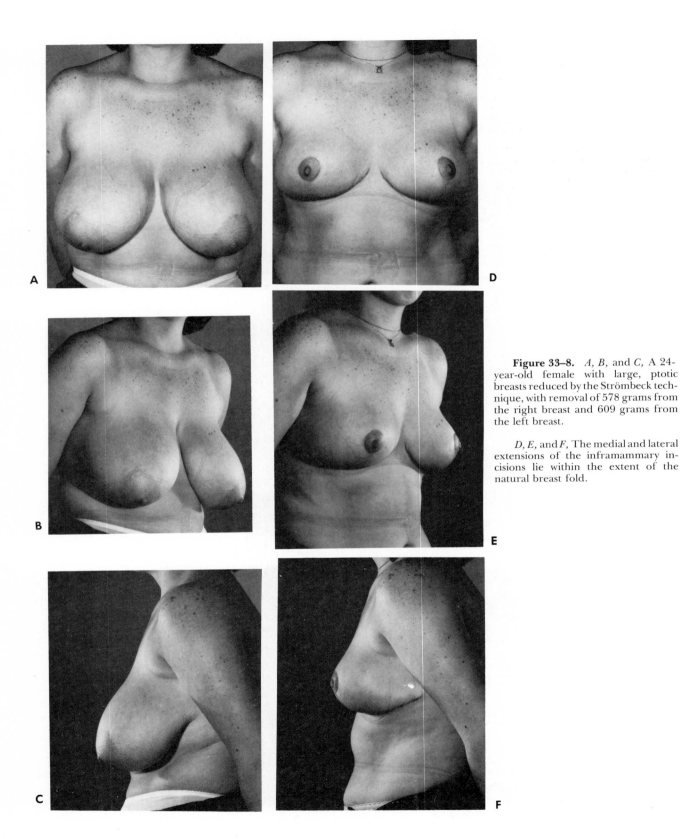

Figure 33–8. *A, B,* and *C,* A 24-year-old female with large, ptotic breasts reduced by the Strömbeck technique, with removal of 578 grams from the right breast and 609 grams from the left breast.

D, E, and *F,* The medial and lateral extensions of the inframammary incisions lie within the extent of the natural breast fold.

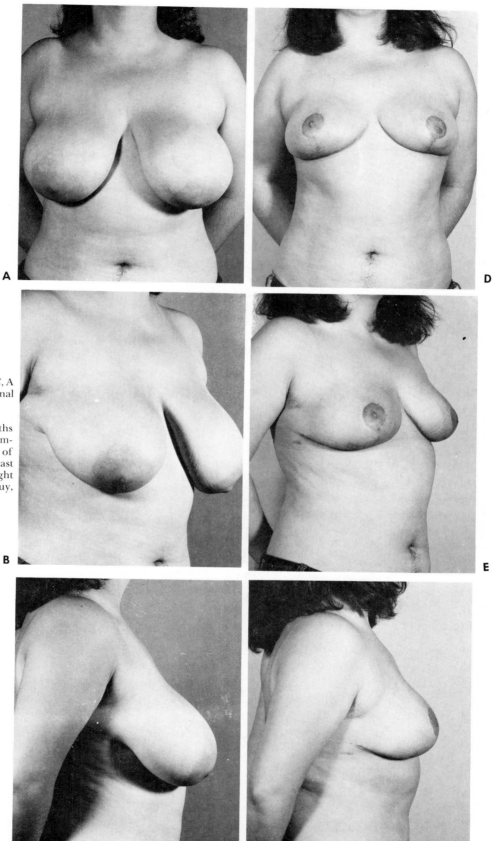

Figure 33–9. *A, B,* and *C,* A 21-year-old female with virginal hypertrophy.

D, E, and *F,* Seven months following reduction by the Ström-beck technique, with removal of 630 grams from the left breast and 470 grams from the right breast. (Courtesy of Cary L. Guy, M.D.)

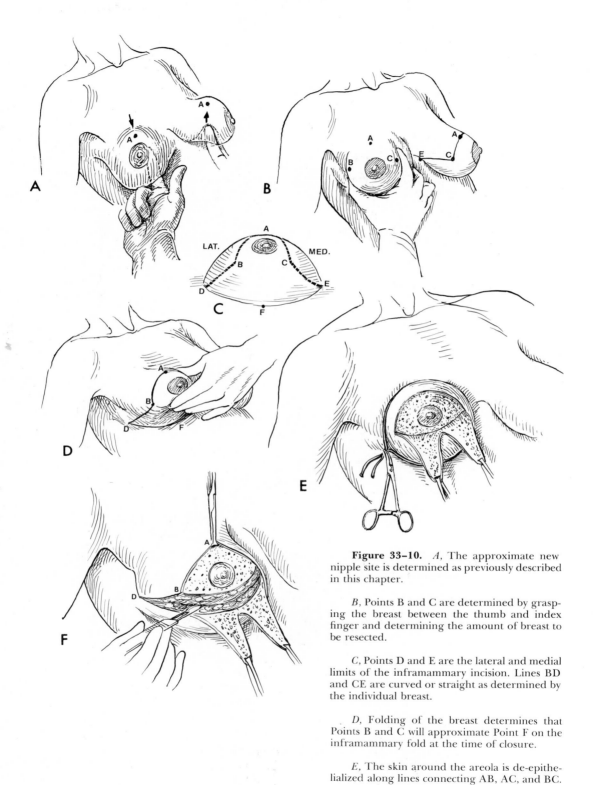

Figure 33–10. *A,* The approximate new nipple site is determined as previously described in this chapter.

B, Points B and C are determined by grasping the breast between the thumb and index finger and determining the amount of breast to be resected.

C, Points D and E are the lateral and medial limits of the inframammary incision. Lines BD and CE are curved or straight as determined by the individual breast.

D, Folding of the breast determines that Points B and C will approximate Point F on the inframammary fold at the time of closure.

E, The skin around the areola is de-epithelialized along lines connecting AB, AC, and BC.

F, Breast resection is begun.

Illustration continued on the opposite page.

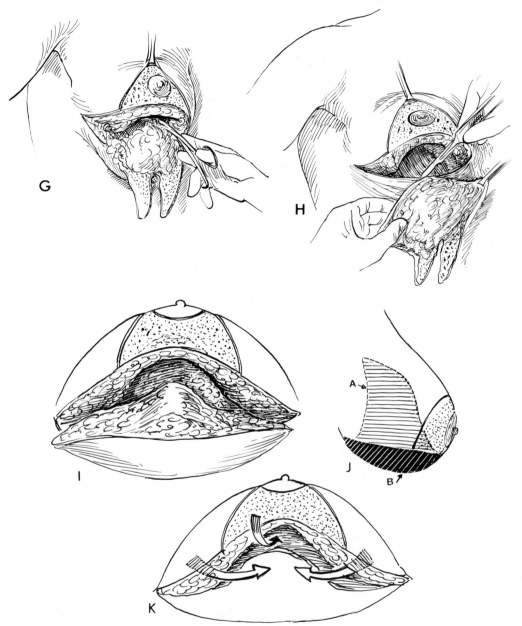

Figure 33–10 *Continued.*   *G*, A boat-keel–shaped resection is made in the mid-breast.

H, Breast resection is completed.

I, J, and *K*, Breast resection is visualized in two parts, keel (A) and base of keel (B).

Illustration continued on the following page.

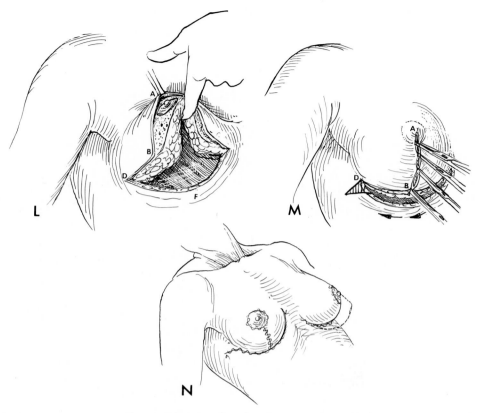

Figure 33–10 *Continued.*   *L,* Breast closure is begun by approximating Points B and C to Point F on the inframammary crease. The nipple-areolar complex is pushed cephalad. Full-thickness skin excision is made at the new areolar site.

M and *N,* Closure is completed.

placement is made at the end of the operation. The amount of breast tissue to be resected is determined by establishing fixed reference points. Points *B* and *C* (Fig. 33–10) are determined by grasping the breast with the thumb and index finger. Points *B* and *C* should not be placed higher than a transverse line passing through the nipple. Distances *AB* and *AC* (Fig. 33–10) are approximately 6 to 7 cm in length unless the breasts are asymmetrical or unusual in shape, thus requiring asymmetrical markings.

Points *D* and *E* represent the lateral and medial extremes respectively of the lines of resection that are marked at the ends of the inframammary incision (Fig. 33–10, *C*). Lines *CE* and *BD* can be straight or curved as determined for the individual breast. Points *B* and *C* are in part determined by estimating the amount of breast tissue to be removed and by folding the breast in such a fashion as to determine at which 'Points *B* and *C* will approximate to Point *F* (Fig. 33–10, *D*).

With all points established, the areolar diameter of the desired size is marked around the nipple. An incision is then made circumscribing the areola.

Skin around the areola is deepithelialized at least 4 to 5 cm in all directions (Fig. 33–10 *E*). Deepithelializing extends inferiorly from point *A* and between Points *B* and *C* and to below the areola similar to the Strömbeck operation.

Resection of breast tissue is begun by cutting through the skin and subcutaneous tissue down to the parenchyma along lines *CE*, *BC*, and *BD* (Fig. 33–10, *F*). The incision is beveled so that the glandular resection in the shape of a boat keel is made according to the volume determined to be removed (Fig. 33–10, *G*). A superior medial portion of the keel is first dissected, and the breast tissue is then removed by cutting along the inframammary fold (Fig. 33–10, *H*). The resected portion of breast tissue can be visualized in two parts (Fig. 33–10, *I, J, K*): part *A,* the superior medial portion of glandular resection, and part *B,* the base of the keel, which extends transversely across the breast the full length of the inframammary fold incision (Fig. 33–10, *J*).

The breast flaps are brought together in the midline with catgut sutures in glandular tissue to help approximate Points *B* and *C* (Fig. 33–10, *L*).

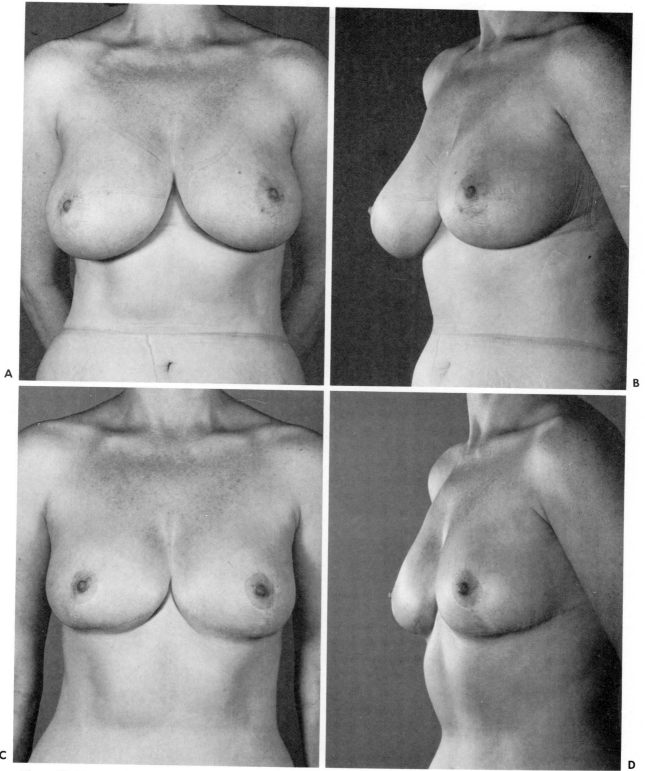

Figure 33–11. *A* and *B*, Moderate mammary hyperplasia corrected by the Pitanguy technique of reduction mammaplasty. *C* and *D*, Postoperative photographs one year following 400-gram reduction of the right breast and 280-gram reduction of the left breast.

The nipple is pushed upward toward the apex by the breast tissue remaining medially and laterally. Skin flap revisions can be made by trimming *AB, AC, BD,* or *CE* as indicated.

The skin is approximated in the midline of the breast in such a fashion that lines *AB* and *AC* are sutured together (Fig. 33–10, *M*). The patient is placed in a semi-sitting position and the apex of the breast cone is marked bilaterally. A suture fixed at the sternal notch aids measurement for symmetry of the two breasts. The cookie-cutter or napkin ring used originally to outline the areolar size is centered about the determined new nipple site and pressed into the skin. Full thickness skin excision allows the nipple-areolar complex to be brought into its new position (Fig. 33–10, *M*).

The breast tissue along the inframammary fold is approximated with 4–0 absorbable sutures. The horizontal and vertical incisions are sutured with intracuticular Prolene sutures, and steristrips are applied. The areola is sutured in place with multiple interrupted 5–0 nylon sutures (Fig. 33–10, *N*). (See Figure 33–11.)

FREE NIPPLE-AREOLAR TRANSPLANTATION

Free nipple transplantation is the procedure of choice in extreme hypertrophy, pendulousness, or gigantomastia for several reasons: (1) the vascular supply of the nipple can be jeopardized by nipple transposition techniques because of the great distance necessary to elevate the nipple. The free nipple graft is a composite graft of skin, smooth muscle, and remnants of ductile elements. Properly handled, defatted, and applied to a healthy dermal bed, graft viability approaches 100 percent. (2) The loss of lactating function is readily accepted by such patients; reduction of breast volume is the prime concern. Gigantic breasts usually have poor lactating function in any event. In the past, some of the controversy between surgeons favoring nipple transposition and those favoring nipple transplantation revolved around the question of functional lactation. It was the opinion of those favoring nipple transposition that to destroy lactation, particularly in the young woman, is physiologically and psychologically unsound. Those favoring nipple transplantation argued that most patients seeking reduction mammaplasty are little concerned about maintaining functional lactation. (3) Erotic sensitivity and erectile function is usually less than normal in very large breasts before surgery. The varying loss or diminution in sensitivity is therefore less critical.

Some sensation and erectile function returns to some free nipple grafts over varying months postoperatively. (4) There is no limit to the breast volume that can be removed. (5) Operating time and blood loss are kept to a minimum. (6) The cosmetic result of breast shape and contour following free nipple graft technique equals that of nipple transposition in gigantic breasts.

Maliniac (1950, 1959) cited opinions by Warren, Geschiskter, Huggins, and Treves to support his belief that free nipple transplantation produced a potential carcinogenic hazard by interfering with ductile egress. There is no hard scientific evidence to support the thesis that breast tissue without ductile egress has a higher chance of becoming malignant as suggested by Maliniac. In fact, there is no evidence to suggest any relationship between plastic surgical operations and breast malignancy (Rees, 1977). Instances when malignancies have been reported following breast plastic surgery appear to be coincidental when examined by statistical analysis.

FREE-NIPPLE GRAFT TECHNIQUE

Free nipple-areolar grafting can be adapted to most breast reduction techniques. It is particularly adaptable to the Pitanguy reduction technique. The technique favored by the authors is as follows:

With the patient in a standing or sitting position, a vertical line is drawn from the midclavicle through the nipple (Fig. 33–12, *A*). The inframammary crease is marked and the planned new nipple site is determined as previously described (Fig. 33–12, *B*). In large hypertrophies and gigantomastia, the skin is excessively stretched above the areola and therefore the new nipple site should be slightly lower than would be selected for a breast of a lesser size. A Strömbeck type pattern with a 5 cm areolar window is centered over the midclavicular line approximately 1.5 cm above the new nipple site. The areolar recipient site and the medial and lateral skin flaps are marked according to the pattern. The keyhole width can be adjusted as needed (Fig. 33–12, *C*). Manipulation and folding of the inferior medial and lateral quadrants of the breast as described for the Strömbeck operation accurately determines the inferior edges of the medial and lateral skin flaps. The open areolar window is made a complete circle by an incision connecting the two diverging borders of the breast flaps on an appropriate arc (Fig. 33–12, *C*).

The areolar recipient site is deepithelialized (Fig. 33–12, *D*). A 4.5 cm cookie-cutter areolar

Text continued on page 938.

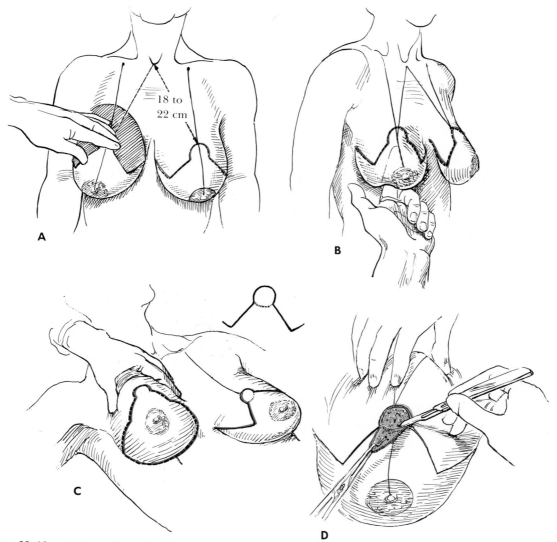

Figure 33–12. *A*, *B*, and *C*, A celluloid keyhole pattern is centered around the new nipple site, which is determined as described early in the chapter. The areolar recipient site is outlined.

D, The areolar recipient site is de-epithelialized.

Illustration continued on the following page.

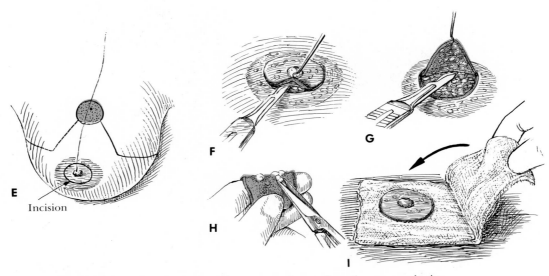

Figure 33–12 *Continued.   E,* A cookie-cutter marker outlines the new areola size.

F and *G,* The new nipple-areolar complex is excised as a full-thickness skin graft.

H and *I,* The nipple-areolar complex is defatted and preserved in a saline-soaked gauze.

Illustration continued on the opposite page.

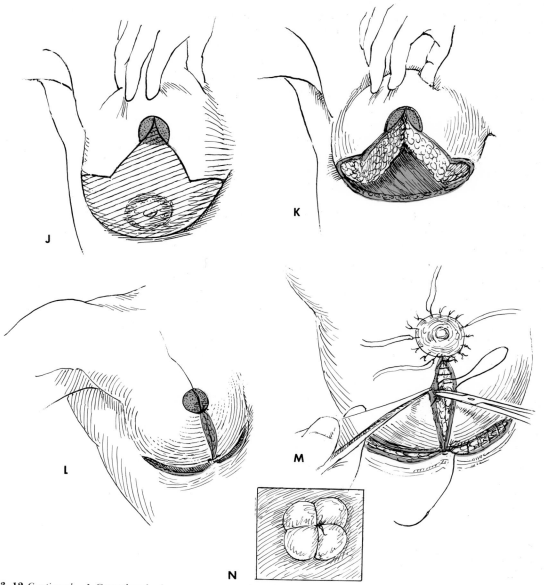

Figure 33–12 *Continued.* *J*, Cross-hatched area represents the portion of the breasts to be resected.

K, Breast tissue is resected.

L, Recontouring of the breast by flap approximation.

M and *N*, The nipple-areolar complex full-thickness graft is sutured into the new site and secured with a bolus tie-over dressing.

marker outlines the new areolar boundaries (Figure 33–12, E). The nipple-areolar complex is dissected beneath the dermis as a full-thickness graft containing epidermis, dermis, muscle, and some ductile elements (Fig. 33–12, F, G). The graft is defatted and thinned down to the dermis, although a few residual muscle fibers will do no harm (Fig. 33–12, H). The prepared graft is placed in a saline soaked gauze and placed in a safe position until it is needed later in the operating procedure (Fig. 33–12, I).

The diverging borders of the medial and lateral skin flaps are extended into the areolar recipient site in such a way as to remove a small triangle of dermis from the middle of the recipient site (Fig. 33–12, J). This triangle is kept small by arcing the flap extremes of the areolar circle. By removing the small central triangle, the recipient site will not have folds in it when the breast flaps are approximated.

All breast tissue lying within the keyhole pattern on the breast is then resected down to the pectoral fascia. The medial and lateral skin flaps can be thinned as indicated if excess bulk remains (Fig. 33–12, K). The medial and lateral skin flaps are rotated to the middle of the breast, adjusted as necessary, and sutured in place appropriately (Fig. 33–12, L). Deep sutures of absorbable material are used to approximate the glandular tissue.

The vertical and horizontal skin incisions are approximated with an intracuticular Prolene suture. The full thickness nipple-areolar graft is placed on the recipient site and carefully sutured in place (Fig. 33–12, M). Placement of the graft is facilitated by having designated the quadrants with a scalpel prior to removing the full-thickness skin graft. A tie-over bolus dressing stabilizes the graft (Fig. 33–12, N). The tie-over dressing is removed on the fifth or sixth postoperative day. (See Figures 33–13, 33–14, and 33–15.)

CORRECTION OF PTOSIS WITHOUT HYPERPLASIA

Some descent of the breast tissue is the normal response to gravity and is part of the normal aging process. In many women, the relationship of the nipple to the submammary crease remains fairly constant as aging occurs — the gland, nipple, and skin descend together. Ptosis is present when the skin, gland, and nipple descend in such a way that the nipple is at or below the inframammary crease. The position of the nipple relative to the inframammary crease is the most important anatomic consideration in diagnosing breast ptosis. Ptosis almost always accompanies hypertrophy. Ptosis

also frequently occurs in breasts that are small or average in glandular volume. Ptotic breasts function normally but are aesthetically unsatisfactory.

Some of the contributing causes of ptosis are postpartum or menopausal atrophy, dermochalasis, and weight loss. The anatomic makeup of some breasts makes them ptotic from the very onset of glandular response to hormones in the teen-age years.

If the nipple lies above the inframammary crease, the breast is not ptotic. Laxity of the breast skin envelope following weight loss or postpartum atrophy may, however, suggest "sagging breasts." The real problem in such patients is hypoplasia of the superior breast quadrants and settling of existing breast tissue inferiorly in a loose skin envelope. Simple augmentation mammaplasty is the treatment of choice in these patients.

The degree of breast ptosis varies according to certain anatomic factors. Regnault's (1976) classification of ptosis is used here. (1) First degree or minor ptosis — the nipple position is at the level of the inframammary fold, above the lower contour of the gland and skin envelope. First degree ptosis can be corrected by a periareolar and small vertical skin excision and/or augmentation mammaplasty. If the breast volume is at all adequate, the skin operation alone is the procedure of choice because of the high incidence of fibrous capsule contracture associated with augmentation mammaplasty.

(2) Second degree or moderate ptosis — the nipple position is below the level of the inframammary fold but remains above the lower contour of the breast and skin envelope. Second degree ptosis should always be corrected by making a new skin brassiere. Some patients can be improved with simple augmentation, but this does not correct the ptosis. If hypoplasia accompanies the ptosis, a small prosthesis for augmentation can accentuate the improvement obtained by the mastopexy.

(3) Third degree or major ptosis — the nipple position is below the inframammary fold and at the lower contour of the breast and skin envelope. Third degree ptosis must be corrected by fashioning a new skin brassiere. Augmentation without skin reduction will resemble a "ball in a sock" effect. Augmentation can accompany the mastopexy if hypoplasia is present.

Most of the currently accepted breast reduction techniques can be modified and used to perform a mastopexy. The area of skin that would be excised in a breast reduction operation is deepithelialized to maintain maximal bulk or excised without gland excision if breast volume is adequate. The skin flaps overlying the gland are not undermined.

Regnault (1974) used the B technique with its

Text continued on page 942.

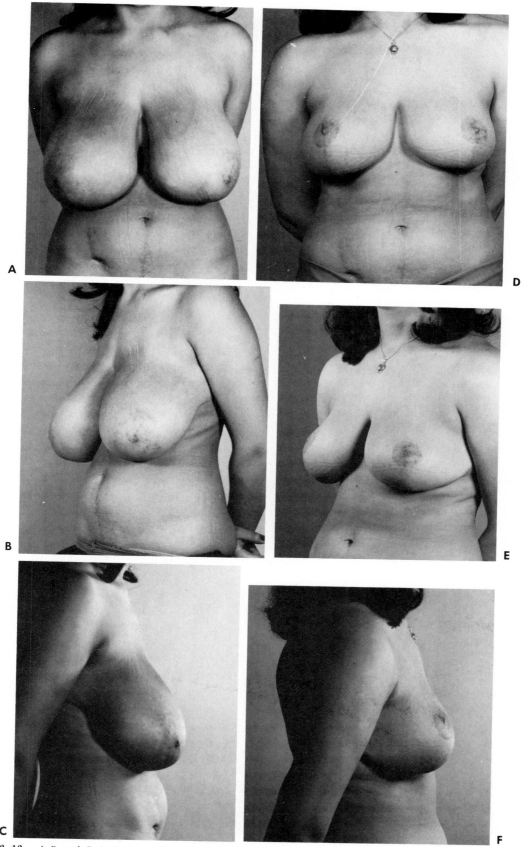

Figure 33–13. *A, B,* and *C,* A 14-year-old female with virginal hypertrophy of the breasts. *D, E,* and *F,* One year following reduction mammaplasty with free nipple grafts and removal of 1125 grams from the right breast and 1050 grams from the left breast. The areola and nipple texture is similar to the preoperative texture. (Courtesy of Cary L. Guy, M.D.)

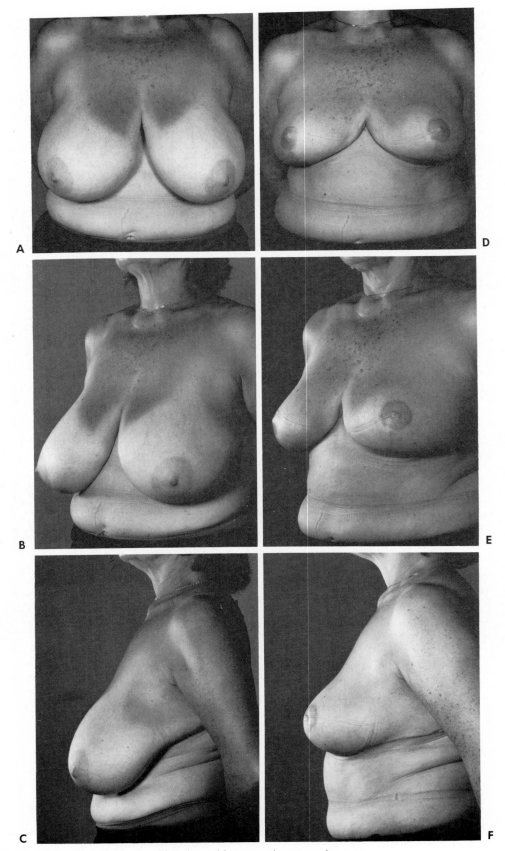

Figure 33–14.   *A, B,* and *C,* A 58-year-old patient with severe gigantomastia.

D, E, and *F,* Twelve months following reduction mammaplasty with free nipple graft technique. More than 1250 grams of tissue were resected from each breast.

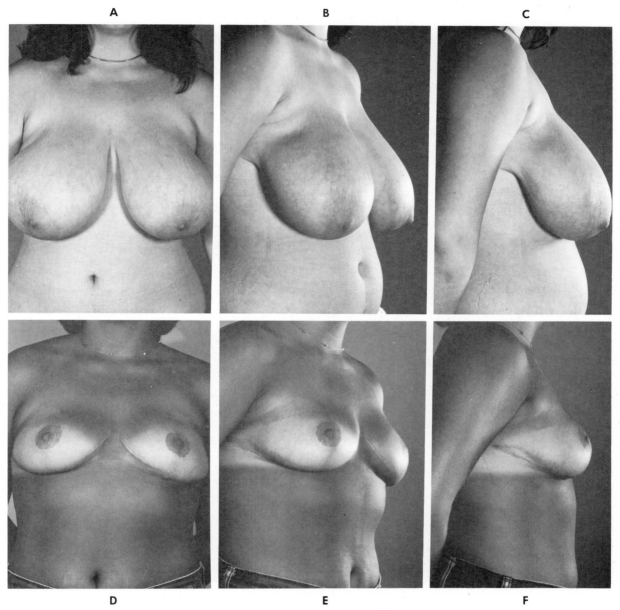

Figure 33–15. *A, B,* and *C,* A 15-year-old patient with severe gigantomastia with tense, firm, heavy breast tissue.

D, E, and *F,* One year following breast reduction by free nipple graft with removal of 1194 grams from the right breast and 1100 grams from the left breast and elevation of the nipple position approximately 12 centimeters.

inferior lateral oblique scar for mastopexy. Many surgeons have found the Strömbeck technique or a variation of it to be readily adaptable for correction of ptosis. Kahn, Hoffman, and Simon (1968) reported their experience with this method. The technique of Dufourmentel and Mouly (1965, 1968) is well suited for the correction of the small ptotic breast. The incision is placed in a radial line extending laterally towards the axilla, and the incision is hidden by most clothing styles. The vertical dermal pedicle technique of McKissock (1972) can be used for mastopexy, but there is no advantage in making a bipedicle flap when the medial and lateral glandular tissue is not isolated. Goulian (1969, 1971, 1972, 1976) has geometrically designed precise equilateral triangles, which are deepithelialized to perform a "dermal mastopexy." The Aries-Pitanguy procedure is also readily used for correcting ptosis. However, a horizontal incision is preferable to extension of the vertical incision below the inframammary crease as suggested in early descriptions of the technique. Biggs, Brauer, and Wolf (1978) reported excellent results with mastopexy in conjunction with subcutaneous mastectomy in patients with (1) ptosis and downward pointed nipples, (2) large skin envelopes, and (3) a high breast on the contralateral side, as may occur following a breast reconstruction.

Regardless of the surgical technique selected, the major points in planning a mastopexy are (1) determining the new nipple site, as described in the discussion of breast reduction, (2) designing the new skin brassiere by determining horizontal and vertical skin redundancy (mastopexy is the creation of a new skin brassiere), (3) preservation of all possible tissue in small breasts to retain volume, (4) reshaping of the breasts when volume is sufficient, and (5) augmentation of volume with implants when required.

The midclavicular to nipple line, a new nipple site, and the inframammary line are determined with the patient sitting or standing as previously described for breast reduction techniques. Measurements from the suprasternal notch to the new nipple positions may help establish symmetry, but fixed numerical measurements are of little meaning. The design of a new skin brassiere varies according to the degree of ptosis and the amount of skin excess (Fig. 33–16, A). A keyhole pattern is centered about the new nipple site and an open areolar window is marked. Pinching together the redundant skin midway between the areola and the inframammary crease helps determine the necessary keyhole width and establishes the middle markings of the medial and lateral skin flaps.

Larger, more ptotic breasts will require a wider keyhole. Cases of mild ptosis may not require a keyhole type pattern. Instead, skin excision or deepithelialization below the nipple is elliptical in shape and stops at the inframammary crease.

The length of the limbs of the medial and lateral skin flaps is important (Fig. 33–16, B, C). For small to moderate breasts, the skin flaps should be 4.5 cm in length, and for larger breasts, 5 cm in length. More than 5 cm will make the areola to inframammary crease distance too long, so that the nipple will eventually rest in a high position. The inferior borders of the medial and lateral skin flaps (Points b and b'. Fig. 33–16, C) should be sutured to their new position (Point C) along the inframammary fold before the inferior margins of the skin flaps are marked and excised. Such a technique insures that the horizontal incisions will be kept to the minimal length (Fig. 33–16, D). In patients with mild ptosis, the upward movement of the nipple may be only 1 or 2 cm (Fig. 33–16, E). This may be only the amount by which the areola is reduced in circumference. The new nipple site in mild ptosis is selected by determining the apex of the breast cone that will be present when the redundant skin is removed. In moderate or severe ptosis, the new nipple site is determined by locating on the anterior surface of the breast the inframammary fold and placing the nipple one centimeter lower. Postoperative breast sagging is not as significant a problem as it is in reduction mammaplasty; however, a certain amount of skin stretch occurs with time. When there is a difference in the degree of ptosis on the two breasts, it is important to plan the final position of the nipples so that they are equal (Fig. 33–16, F). In some patients with first degree ptosis, the medial extension of the horizontal scar can be kept to a minimum while the lateral extension is somewhat longer (Fig. 33–16, G). The dog-ears of skin that result from approximating the medial and lateral skin flaps should be trimmed to equalize the incision lengths. Patients with breast asymmetry or hyperplasia of one breast and ptosis of the other require a mastopexy on the ptotic side and a breast reduction on the contralateral side (Fig. 33–16, H). Asymmetry may result from ptosis of one breast and hypoplasia of the opposite. The appropriate treatment of these patients is therefore a mastopexy in combination with breast augmentation. In all cases of asymmetry, symmetrical locations of the new nipple site are important in the final appearance of the breasts. Symmetrical locations of nipple position can be difficult when the skin of one breast has been subjected to a much greater skin stretch than the opposite side.

Text continued on page 950.

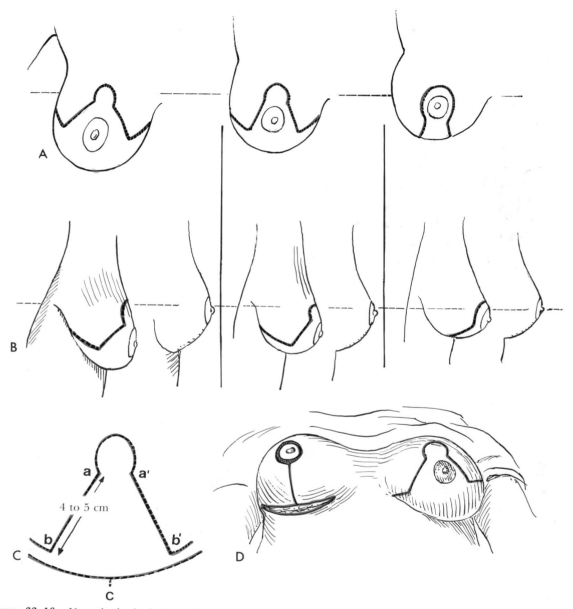

Figure 33–16. New nipple site is determined as previously described in this chapter.

A and *B*, The width of the keyhole is determined by the degree of ptosis and the amount of skin excess.

C, Lines ab and a′b′ are most often 4.5 to 5 centimeters in length.

D, The horizontal incision is kept to minimum lengths if Points b and b′ (33–16 *C*) are sutured to Point C on the inframammary crease before inferior margins of skin flaps are excised.

Illustration continued on the following page.

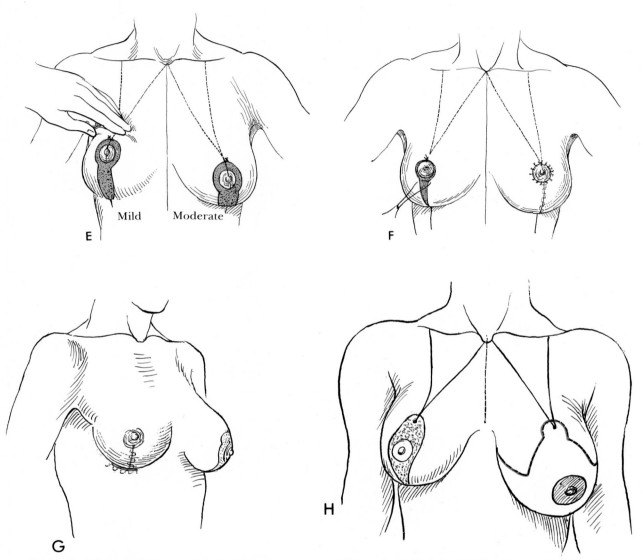

Figure 33–16 *Continued.* *E* and *F,* Ptosis asymmetry is corrected by symmetrical new nipple positions and appropriate mastopexies.

G, The horizontal incision is kept short for correction of first-degree ptosis.

H, Right breast ptosis is corrected by mastopexy and the left breast is reduced. New nipple sites are symmetrically placed.

Illustration continued on the opposite page.

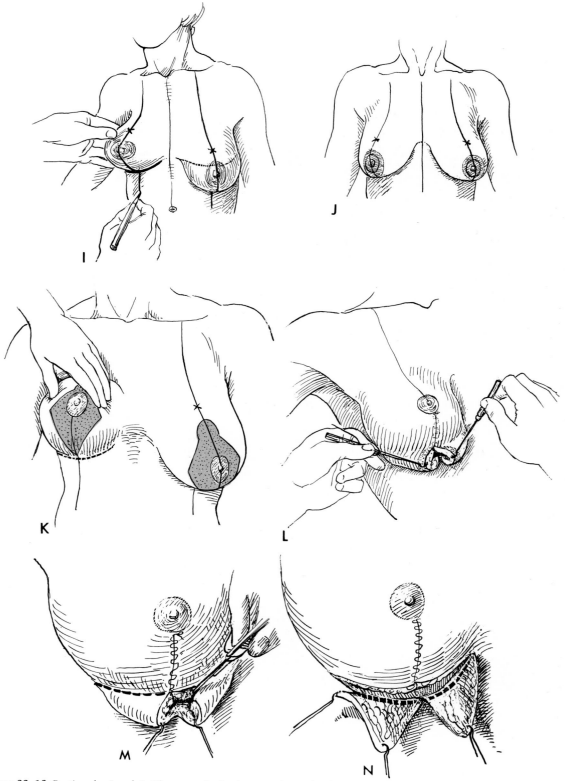

Figure 33–16 *Continued.   I* and *J,* The new nipple sites are determined, and the breasts are marked for correction of third-degree ptosis.

K, Keyhole patterns are de-epithelialized.

L, Skin flaps are approximated to the midpoint on the inframammary line.

M and *N,* Excess skin along the inferior borders of the medial and lateral skin flaps is marked with ink and excised. The inframammary incision is maintained at minimum length.

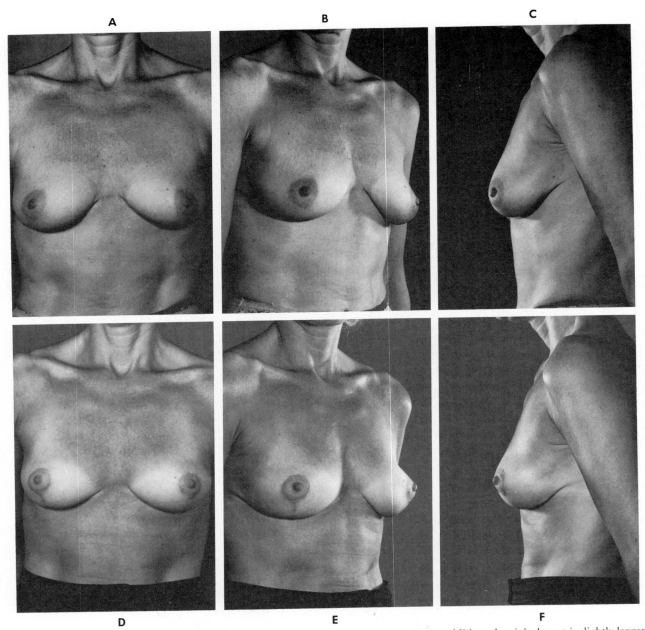

A   **B**   **C**

D   **E**   **F**

Figure 33–17.   *A, B* and *C,* A 45-year-old female with first-degree breast ptosis. In addition, the right breast is slightly larger than the left breast.

D, E, and *F,* One year following Aries-Pitanguy mastopexy and slight reduction of the right breast.

Illustration continued on the opposite page.

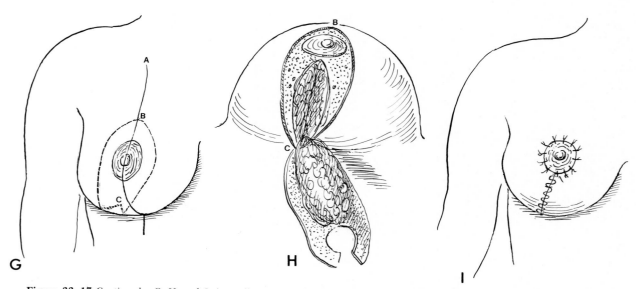

Figure 33–17 *Continued.*   *G, H,* and *I,* A small amount of breast tissue was resected from the mid-de-epithelialized area.

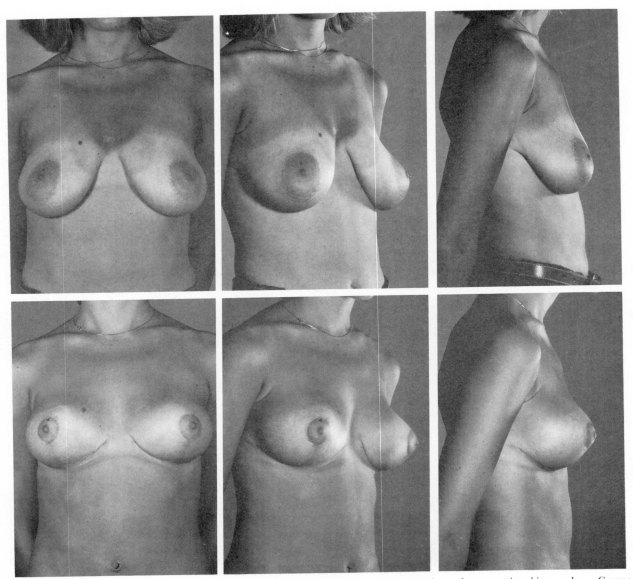

Figure 33–18.   A 20-year-old patient with second-degree ptosis, adequate breast volume, but excessive skin envelope. Correction was made by the mastopexy technique shown in Figure 33–16.

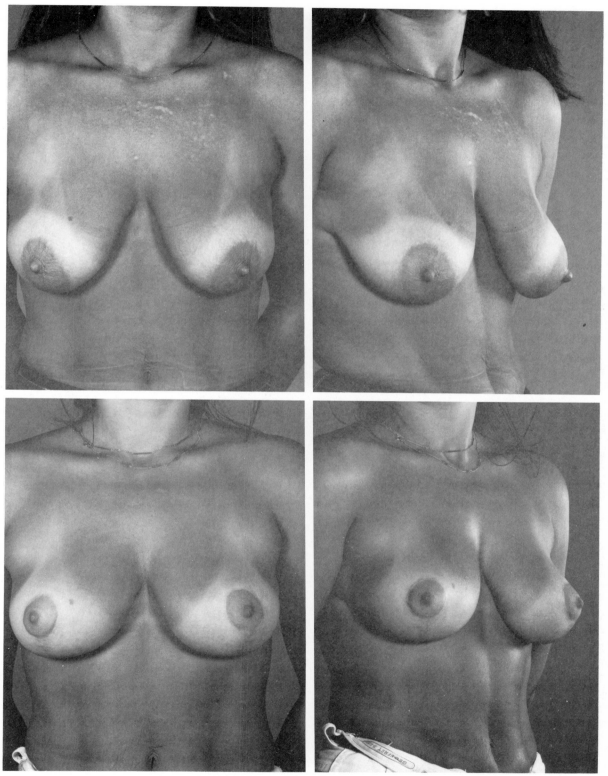

Figure 33–19.   A 22-year-old patient with third-degree ptosis. Correction was made by the mastopexy technique described in Figure 33–16.

Figure 33–16, I through O shows the steps in performing a mastopexy for third degree ptosis (nipples below the level of the inframammary fold).

The midclavicular line with extension through the nipples and onto the chest wall is outlined, and the new nipple sites are determined with the patient sitting (Fig. 33–16, I). The new areola size is established with an areolar cookie-cutter marker (Fig. 33–16, J). An appropriate keyhole pattern is drawn and the redundant skin is deepithelialized (Fig. 33–16, K). The medial and lateral skin flaps are approximated to the appropriate point on the inframammary fold. The nipple-areolar complex is sutured in its new location (Fig. 33–16, L).

The redundant inferior margins of the medial and lateral skin flaps are marked with ink and excised on the superior edge (Fig. 33–16, M). The redundant skin triangles are then excised along the inframammary crease. Thus the horizontal inframammary fold incisions are kept to a minimal length (Fig. 33–16, N). When a small amount of reduction is indicated to establish breast symmetry, a lozonge-shaped resection of breast tissue can be removed from the midportion of the deepithelialized area (Fig. 33–17). (See Figures 33–18 and 33–19.)

POSTOPERATIVE CARE FOLLOWING REDUCTION MAMMAPLASTY OR MASTOPEXY

Telfa strips are placed over the horizontal and vertical incision lines and Telfa "doughnuts" are placed over the nipple. This allows postoperative visualization of the nipple-areolar color. Bulky dressings are not required. When the patient has sufficiently recovered from anesthesia, bathroom privileges with assistance are permitted. A regular diet is given as soon as requested by the patient.

Postoperative pain is usually mild to moderate. Severe pain requires evaluation of the patient for possible hematoma. Narcotic analgesics should be given as necessary to make the patient comfortable. Most patients will not require a narcotic after the first 24 to 36 hours postoperatively. Anxious and apprehensive patients may require Valium or some other tranquilizer to help maintain a calm, peaceful postoperative course, but this is not common in breast reduction patients. An antiemetic should be given to relieve postoperative nausea.

A previously selected comfortable brassiere is put on when the patient is fully awake and can sit up. This provides support to the breast, minimizes discomfort, and provides a sense of security to the patient. Severe midback pain can occur if the patient is abruptly or roughly elevated off the operating table while still under anesthesia in order to apply a brassiere or dressing. Brassieres with small chest bands may put pressure on the inframammary portion of the incision. This pressure can be relieved by placing a small gauze bandage under the chest band or by removing the brassiere for 12 to 18 hours when the incisions will be much less sensitive. The brassiere can be removed when necessary for comfort during the first few days postoperatively without untoward effect. The brassiere is worn day and night for the first 14 days, except for intermittent periods to relieve the sensation of constant pressure. After this time, the brassiere is not necessary when the patient is in bed. After the sixth postoperative week, continuous brassiere support is no longer required.

Drains are removed from the breast on the second morning postoperatively and the patient is discharged.

All periareolar and any other interrupted sutures are removed on the sixth postoperative day. Steristrips are applied to support the incisions. Showering and bathing are permitted after this time. Intracuticular sutures are removed on the 12th to 14th day postoperatively. Normal activities are resumed on a graduated schedule. Many patients are anxious to return to their jobs as soon as possible. Sedatory workers can return to work after 10 days. Vigorous activities such as golf, running, and tennis are restricted until the sixth postoperative week.

Complications of Breast Reduction

Breast reduction by any technique is a major surgical procedure and therefore is associated with complications. Rees and Flagg (1972) described the complications of breast reduction and mastopexy. There are relatively few complications following a simple mastopexy operation.

The overall complication rate of breast reduction varies from 10 to 25 percent in a large number of patients operated on by various techniques (Ragnell, 1946, 1957; Conway, 1952; Conway and Smith, 1958; McIndoe and Rees, 1958; Strömbeck, 1964, 1968, 1973; Skoog, 1963, 1974). The published mortality rate for reduction mammaplasty is zero.

Strömbeck (1971) noted a definite correlation between the volume of breast tissue resected and the incidence of complications. In his series of 1106 breasts, 15 percent of 74 breasts, each of which had 1000 grams of tissue resected, had complications, as compared with 0.5 percent of 399 breasts from which 250 grams were resected.

Hematoma. Hematoma is the most frequent and troublesome complication of breast reduction; even so, it is uncommon. The generous vascular supply to the breast comes from the internal mammary artery perforators, the intercostals, and the long thoracic artery. Meticulous hemostasis during the surgical procedure is the best prophylaxis. Most major hematomas occur from a large single vessel that has lost its tie or sloughed a cauterized end. Jackson-Pratt drains can be placed beneath the breast flap to remove serosanguineous drainage but will not prevent a hematoma from a significantly bleeding vessel. Large hematomas should be evacuated immediately on discovery under general anesthesia. Failure to reduce the internal pressure on the skin may result in skin and nipple slough.

Nipple Slough. Nipple slough is a dreaded complication of reduction mammaplasty, since the aesthetic result is permanently marred. Reports indicate that partial or total nipple necrosis occurs in approximately 1 percent of all cases. The cause of nipple slough depends in part on the surgical technique used. In all transposition techniques, care must be aimed at protecting the vascular pedicle. In the McKissock type of operation, the parenchyma should not be violated beneath the lower half of the pedicle, according to McKissock.

Cyanosis of the nipple and areola indicates venous congestion and marginal vascularity. Such congestion may herald the onset of circulatory stasis and eventual partial or total nipple slough. A bluish congested areola lasting 24 to 48 hours is uncommon but does occur. Ice compresses may help during this period. Persistent engorgement and cyanosis herald a significant problem. The breast should always be dressed in a fashion so the nipple and areola are visible. If cyanosis is noted, the dressing should be removed and the breast should be examined for hematoma. Localized hematomas can cause or contribute to congestion.

In nipple transposition procedures, the most common causes of nipple and areola slough are: (1) excessive resection of parenchyma leaving an inadequate blood supply, (2) congestion secondary to a small localized hematoma, (3) stretching the dermal pedicle too tight, (4) torsion of the dermal or breast pedicle, and (5) excessive tightness of the skin brassiere causing compression of the pedicle.

Nipple sloughs are best treated conservatively until complete demarcation and eschar separation occurs. The exact loss can then be ascertained. The same principle applies regardless of whether one is dealing with a nipple transposition or full-thickness graft. If the loss area is not over 25 percent of the areolar surface area, a small scar revision several months later will probably suffice. Larger areas of loss will require a reconstructive procedure. A full-thickness graft of labia majora will probably give the best color and texture match for "filling in" a defect. If the defect is small enough, a small graft from the opposite nipple may be possible. Total areola reconstruction is best performed with a full-thickness labia majora graft or a split-thickness skin graft from the upper medial thigh near the groin crease where the pigmentation in the graft is excellent.

Skin Slough. Small areas of skin slough occur most commonly in the tips of flaps at the junction of the vertical and horizontal incision related to tension on the tip of the flaps by the sutures and the weight of the breasts. The area involved is usually 1 cm or less. Small sloughs are treated conservatively. A dry eschar is encouraged. Minimal débridement should be done when the eschar separates.

Major skin slough is rare following the nipple transposition and partial amputation techniques where skin undermining is minimal or not done at all. Wide skin undermining as in the Biesenberger operation was associated with more skin survival problems. Skin slough is related to trauma, tension, or compression from an underlying hematoma. The underlying fat and breast tissue may also be necrotic.

Large skin sloughs are treated aggressively. As soon as the margin of necrosis is demarcated, the area should be excised and sutured closed if possible. This aggressive approach will save weeks of healing time. Débridement and later a split-thickness skin graft is another alternative, but granulation tissue does not grow readily on fat or breast tissue. Many weeks may pass before the wound is ready for grafting.

Fat Necrosis. Fat necrosis is usually associated with interference of the tenuous blood supply to the fat such as localized hematoma, abscess formation, congestion, or excessive pressure. Drainage from liquified fat can be prolonged and progressive. If the fat necrosis is extensive, it will involve the overlying skin, and the skin may become necrotic. In general, the incidence of fat necrosis increases as the size of the breast increases. However, it is uncommon with the nipple transposition procedures currently in use.

Diagnosis of fat necrosis is not difficult. There is a palpable hardness of the breast initially, followed in a few days by redness, fluctuation, skin necrosis, or sinus tracts. A temperature of 38° or 39° C for the first three to four days postoperatively is suggestive of fat necrosis, if no other cause for the temperature is obvious.

Small areas of necrosis should be treated conservatively with irrigation and cleansing of any sinus tract. Liquified fat can be expressed at intervals. Healing may take many weeks. Extensive area of fat necrosis should be treated more aggressively with surgical débridement and wound closure.

Infection. Massive infections following reduction mammaplasty are rare since the advent of antibiotic therapy. When infection does occur, sound surgical procedures of drainage, culture, and appropriate antibiotic therapy are indicated.

Nipple Retraction. Nipple retraction following reduction mammaplasty is chiefly caused by two factors: (1) excessive tension on the areola-bearing pedicle, and (2) excessive resection of breast tissue just beneath the nipple.

Retraction is more frequent with the Strömbeck technique. Nipple retraction is less apt to occur following the McKissock, Skoog, or Pitanguy technique. Minimal retraction resulting from the force of gravity and the pressure of the glandular mass pushing forward almost always subsides in a few days. When tension exists on the horizontal pedicle, Strombeck advises cutting the dermal pedicle (where the tension is greatest) through to the subcutaneous tissue close to the vertical borders of the flap during primary surgery. Cutting the dermis is sometimes successful in giving a permanent eversion; however, the nipple may retract again as postoperative edema subsides. The tendency for retraction can be minimized if a small plug of tissue is removed from the new nipple site. Pitanguy does not remove a core of tissue from the upper breast for this reason.

If nipple retraction persists after four to six months, surgical correction is required. The periareola scar is excised along its inferior half and the offending band is sectioned. Sometimes, undercutting the nipple is required. This has the disadvantage of severing the ducts. If these techniques free the nipple but the inversion tendency remains, a buried purse-string suture around the base of the areolar may be necessary. It is rarely impossible to correct a retracted nipple.

Malposition of the Nipple-Areolar Complex. The most common error in judgment made by surgeons performing reduction mammaplasty is to locate the new nipple site at a position that is too high. The skin of the inferior quadrant of the breast loosens and stretches with gravity and time, and the breast mass "falls out" from beneath the nipple. The new nipple site should always be positioned at least 0.5 cm lower than the measure-ment that seems to be correct. The distance from the submammary fold to the nipple should be no more than 4.5 to 5 cm. This lessens the degree of breast sag from beneath the nipple.

Correcting a highly located nipple requires actual downward repositioning of the nipple-areolar complex and, in most instances, shortening the distance from the inframammary fold to the areola. Both maneuvers may be required in some patients. In addition, a prosthesis placed behind the breast to make the main projection of the breast directly behind the nipple (Millard, Mullin, and Lesavoy, 1976) may be required in selected patients. Moving the nipple and areola to a lower position on the breast always leaves undesirable scars on the upper breast. Misplacement of the nipple off the vertical dimension of the breast axis is an error in judgment and is best avoided.

Scars. Scars are subject to hypertrophy, spreading, and, rarely, to keloid formation. Vertical breast scars frequently widen to some degree but rarely hypertrophy. Periareolar scars occasionally thicken but usually soften and flatten with time.

The inframammary incisions have a distinct tendency to hypertrophy. These incisions should be placed exactly in the submammary fold, where they are under minimal tension and are well camouflaged. The submammary incisions should not join across the midline of the chest unless there is a "web" of breast tissue across the midline requiring excision.

Hypertrophic scars are best treated in time with small doses of interlesional steroids. An occasional patient will benefit from scar excision and meticulous closure many months after the original surgery.

Cysts. Small inclusion cysts sometimes develop in the area of buried dermis from epithelial elements or appendage remnants. Most undergo spontaneous resolution if left alone, but excision may occasionally be necessary.

Sensory Changes. Courtiss and Goldwyn (1976) studied 625 breasts preoperatively and found that the areola is the most sensitive part of the breast, with the skin adjacent to the areola being less sensitive and the nipple itself the least sensitive of the breast skin. Almost all breasts demonstrated uneven sensory patterns. Patients studied by these authors included those having augmentation mammaplasty, reduction mammaplasty by transposition techniques, reduction mammaplasty by free nipple-areolar grafts, gynecomastia correction, and mastopexy. Patients with large breasts requesting reduction mammaplasty had less sensation than did patients with small breasts who were evaluated prior to augmentation mammaplasty. Women with small or moderate breasts who had never been pregnant had greater sensation in their nipples and areola. The principal finding in this study was that patients having plastic surgery of the breast for reduction, augmentation, or subcutaneous mastectomy had at least transient loss of pain, crude touch, and light pressure sensation. There was frequently permanent loss of pain recognition in the areola and nipple. A large number of patients reported that erectility was normal even though pain sensation was markedly diminished or absent. Some patients reported that they could not tell when their nipples were erect because they had reduced feeling in that area. Erectility and crude touch returned faster than did pain sensation in patients having

augmentation mammaplasty. As one would anticipate, thin nipple and areolar grafts from which the muscle had been removed failed to become erect. Patients who had reduction mammaplasty by transposition techniques most often had erectile function of the nipple.

An unexpected finding in this study was that the patients having augmentation mammaplasty by either inframammary or periareolar incisions showed a decrease in sensation of the nipple and areola. Two years postoperatively 15 percent of the patients still had impaired sensory perception, although crude touch and light pressure appreciation had returned. Many of these patients had normal erectile function and many had enhanced sensuality.

(For list of references, see pages 1066 to 1071.)

Chapter 34

Mammary Augmentation, Correction of Asymmetry, and Gynecomastia

SHERRELL J. ASTON, M.D., F.A.C.S., AND
THOMAS D. REES, M.D., F.A.C.S.

Augmentation mammaplasty is a common operation. Available data suggest that approximately 30,000 women undergo this procedure each year in the United States. Augmentation mammaplasty is a relatively simple operation to correct a specific and easily diagnosed problem with good results. The principal problem of breast augmentation is the periprosthetic fibrous capsular contracture that develops in approximately 40 per cent of patients a few weeks to many months following the operation. However, patient satisfaction and acceptance is very highly reflected in the exceedingly low incidence of implant removal.

WHY AUGMENTATION?

Modern society has established the well developed female breast as an important characteristic of femininity. Emphasis on youth and vigor, increased social consciousness of physical acceptability, more liberal and open attitude toward sexual relationships, revealing clothing fashions, and more time spent in leisure and social activities, where all of these factors interact, have taken a toll on the female who is deficient in breast development. A lack of self confidence and feeling of inadequacy can result from small breasts.

All aspects of a patient's life often become influenced. The patient may be shy and withdrawn. Some women become so emotionally concerned with their small breasts that it is impossible for them to assume a normal role in courtship and marriage. Sexual frigidity related to feelings of inadequacy can occur. A salutory personality change following augmentation mammaplasty is not uncommon.

The majority of patients requesting augmentation mammaplasty are not emotional cripples. The primary goal—to enhance self image by increasing the breast size and improving the shape—can be most helpful both for patients with primary hypoplasia and those with postlactation or postmenopausal atrophy. However, patients requesting breast reconstruction following mastectomy are severely handicapped and often are emotionally crippled. The need for reconstruction is amplified in such patients.

There is rarely need for psychiatric evaluation as a prerequisite for the procedure unless the complaints are bizarre. There is a sparsity of psychiatric data of patients having breast augmentation. Edgerton and McCleary (1958) and Edgerton, Meyer, and Jacobson (1961) studied 65 patients and found that the majority were married, approximately 30 years of age, and often involved in a major marital conflict. In general, the patients studied were "active, competitive, 'on the go', people who were physically graceful, often pretty and socially at ease." A history of major unhappiness in childhood was elicited in most. Gifford (1976) documented a history of major childhood unhappiness in patients seeking breast augmentation. During preoperative and postoperative psychiatric evaluation of these patients, Gifford found the following characteristics: "(1) the search for something more than increased sexual attractiveness for some kind of total personality change; (2) the insistance that any physical change be 'part of me', 'not artificial', 'real' in the sense of congruent with the ideal self which has been impaired, even if 'ideal' existed only in the patient's imagination or at some specific earlier period in life; (3) self-esteem following operation that cannot be fully accounted for by realistic satisfaction with a good aesthetic result."

Shipley, O'Donnell, and Bader (1977) challenged previous psychologic studies of patients seeking augmentation both in data interpretation and lack of control group studies. These investigators studied women seeking breast augmentation and compared them to two control groups (small breasted women and average breasted women). They found no support for "the conclusions of early investigators that women seeking breast augmentation suffer from low self esteem or poor general body image. There was also no evidence of depression, social malfunctioning, or a high instance of either major gynecological surgery or psychiatric counseling."

The female seeking augmentation differed from other women primarily in her negative evaluation of her breasts, her greater emphasis on dress and physical attractiveness, and a desire to dress in a more daring or sexually revealing fashion. In a follow-up study three months after augmentation, Shipley, O'Donnell, and Bader (1978) found that the patients remained well adjusted, were much happier with their breasts, dressed as they desired, and had an enhanced body image.

HISTORY

The modern era of breast augmentation began approximately 25 years ago. Berson (1945), Bames (1950, 1953), Conway and Smith (1958), and Watson (1959) reported their experience with transplantation of free dermis-fat or fat-fascia grafts to increase breast size. These techniques had the disadvantages of unsightly donor site scars, absorption of the grafts (up to 50 percent or more), and a high incidence of fat necrosis and chronic drainage. This method of breast augmentation has been abondoned in favor of using alloplastic prostheses now available.

Breast augmentation and reconstruction with local flaps of deepithelialized tissue was reported by Maliniac (1950), Marino (1952), O'Conor (1964), and Goulian and McDivitt (1972). Longacre (1953, 1956, 1959) reported in detail his technique of pedicle flap augmentation of the hypoplastic gland, either congenital or acquired. Dermis-fat pedicle flap reconstruction is of value following total or subtotal subcutaneous removal of mammary tissue for benign or premalignant conditions. However, postoperative scars and lack of adequate volume limit such procedures for the majority of patients.

Injection of the breast with Paraffin to increase breast volume was introduced by Gersy in 1889, and it subsequently led to many complications (Fig. 34–1). Breasts injected with foreign substances are prone to the development of firm nodules months to years following injections. The injection of liquid silicone into the breast for augmentation was first reported by Uchida in 1961. Unfortunately, this practice was taken over by some unscrupulous practitioners in the early 1960's and led to multiple complications including nodules, cyst formation, chronic edema, skin breakdown, and occasionally death (Nosanchuk, 1968; Boo-Chai, 1969; Chaplin, 1969). Responsible researchers studying liquid silicone injections have consistently condemned the use of liquid silicone for breast augmentation, since the results are unpredictable, can mask true breast pathology, and are inferior to breast augmentation with modern prostheses.

Boo-Chai (1969), Kopf and associates (1976), and Ortiz-Monasterio and Trigos (1972) have reported on large series of patients with complications following injections of foreign materials into the breasts. It is impossible to identify the exact mixtures or compounds that have been injected into many of the patients. Silicone alone or adulterated with additives is present in most. Pathologic specimens indicate nonspecific inflammatory reactions often associated with substances other than silicone. The treatment of patients with complications following injections of any substance into the breast is difficult and frustrating. Nodules, masses, and cysts are frequently present (Figure 34–2). Some patients have localized inflammation of an intermittent nature which may or may not involve the skin. When the dermis has been injected, skin necrosis is a real possibility. Excision of localized nodules may be of benefit to some patients, but most patients have generalized involvement of the breast tissue requiring a subcutaneous mastectomy as a minimal procedure. Parsons and Thering (1977) suggested routine subcutaneous mastectomy in such patients because of the difficulty in performing breast examinations and the

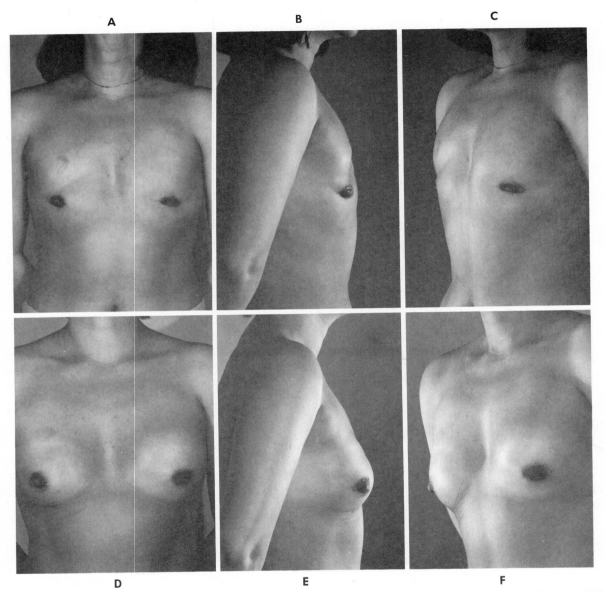

Figure 34–1. A young Taiwanese woman seven years following injection of paraffin or liquid silicone into the breasts in Taiwan and subsequent attempted removal of granulomas and immediate insertion of prostheses by another physician. Bilateral infections and partial slough of the left areola occurred.

A, B, and *C,* When the patient was first seen, there were persistent granulomas bilaterally and significant distortion of the left nipple and areola. First-stage reconstruction one year later consisted of removal of persistent granulomas and insertion of small prostheses for skin expansion.

D, E, and *F,* Second-stage reconstruction six months later by iasertion of a 210-cc gel prosthesis on the right and a 240-cc gel prosthesis on the left. Fourteen months following the last surgical procedure, the patient had developed very slight fibrous capsular contractures.

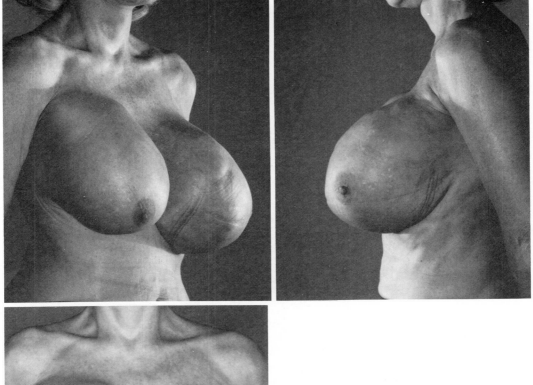

Figure 34–2. A 68-year-old patient three years following augmentation mammaplasty by gel prostheses *and* large volumes of liquid silicone by an unscrupulous practitioner. Nodules, masses, and cysts were numerous. The left breast was chronically infected.

inconclusive nature of mammograms; however, to date there is no evidence to support an increased incidence of malignancy associated with liquid silicone injection. Mastectomy should be reserved for patients with a significant involvement of the breast tissue and overlying skin. The results of mastectomy and prosthetic reconstruction for silicone injected breasts has been cosmetically limited and often unacceptable.

Early experience with prosthetic implants for breast augmentation was stimulated by the work of polyvinyl sponge implants in dogs (Grindlay and Clagett, 1949; Grindlay and Waugh, 1951; Moore and Brown, 1952). These reports indicated that implants of Ivalon (polyvinyl) were inert and nontoxic and produced minimal inflammatory re-

sponse and thin fibrous capsules around the implants. Polyvinyl sponge was found to break down after implantation for a long period. Openheimer, Openheimer, and Staut (1952) produced sarcomatous tumors in rats by implantation of many different types of plastic materials, and Dukes and Mitchley (1962) produced similar tumors in rats by implanting Ivalon sponge. Edgerton and McCleary (1958) expressed doubt that these atypical "sarcomas" were comparable to human malignancies. After more than 25 years, accumulated evidence does not indicate a causal relationship between breast augmentation and malignancy.

Ivalon sponge for breast augmentation was first reported by Pangman in 1951. Etheron, or polyvinylether, quickly became the most widely used sponge implant. Experience with Ivalon and Etheron implants were reported by Pangman (1953), Pangman and Wallace (1954), Edgerton and McCleary (1958), Edgerton, Meyer, and Jacobson (1961), Conway and Dietz (1962), and Pickrell (1962). Ingrowth of fibrous tissue into all open cell sponge implants with subsequent hardness, shrinkage irregularities, and asymmetries gave extremely unfavorable results. The incidence of infection and drainage was much higher with the porous sponges than with new prostheses.

Cronin and Gerow (1963) first described a prosthesis of dimethylpolysiloxane (silicone) gel contained in a silastic envelope. The prosthesis was the first so called "natural-feel" silicone gel prosthesis. This prosthesis or a variation of it has gained ubiquitous approval by plastic surgeons the world over as the material of choice for breast augmentation. The original implants were teardrop in shape and backed with a Dacron mesh "fixation patch" to allow ingrowth of fibrous tissue to secure them in position to the chest wall. Fibrous capsular contracture often produced firmness and wrinkling of the prosthesis. Erosion and extrusion of the implants were rare. In recent years, significant refinements have been made in the design of gel-filled prostheses. Elimination of Dacron patches has been accompanied by a decrease in the incidence of fibrous capsules (Williams, 1972). The silastic envelope has been thinned and made in various shapes (teardrop, round, and low profile), and the viscosity of the silicone gel has been decreased. Currently popular low-profile, round, thin-wall silastic envelopes containing "soft" gel are favored by most surgeons. These are far superior to the prototypes.

The Ashley prosthesis (1970, 1972), a "Y"-chambered silicone envelope filled with silicone gel, has an outer layer of fine-celled polyvinyl sponge. According to Ashley, collagen growth into the outer shell produces fixation, reduces shearing motion, and thereby reduces overall collagen formation and breast firmness. These findings are not shared by other surgeons, although the Y prosthesis has been used in breast reconstruction after mastectomy by many.

Histologic studies of tissue reaction to polyurethane have shown an intense foreign body reaction and breakdown of the polyurethane over time (Hollenberg, 1963; Ridgon, 1973; Imber et al., 1974; Lilla and Vistnes, 1976). Cocke, Leathers, and Lynch (1975) placed polyurethane-covered prostheses in five patients following subcutaneous mastectomy and subsequently removed the prostheses from three patients three weeks to twenty months later because of fluid collection, cellulitis, and skin nodules. Retained fragments of polyurethane bound into the tissues of two of the patients induced foreign body reaction for several months after the prostheses were removed. Smahel (1978) did histologic studies of fibrous capsules of four patients during removal of polyurethane prostheses. He concluded that during the early stages after implantation, the structure of the capsule was determined by the spatial arrangement of the foam (polyurethane) and its connection to the silicone shell. Later, fibrotic tissues subjected the foam to pressure and tension causing mechanical destruction of its adhesion to the silicone prostheses. After separation from the prosthesis, the polyurethane particles became incorporated deep in the fibrous capsule. The capsule showed a definite centrifugal tendency forcing the foreign body (polyurethane) outward from the capsule into the surrounding tissue. Foreign body reaction to the polyurethane was intense. Smahel believed that capsulectomy at the time of prostheses removal is indicated if there is an unfavorable reaction after polyurethane implantation.

Inflatable silicone balloon prostheses were championed by Arion (1965), Tabari (1969), Jenny (1969), Rees, Guy, and Coburn (1973) and others. Initially filled with Dextran and later normal saline, the inflatable implants were credited with a high degree of normal breast consistency and 'flow' characteristics. The early inflatable implants were associated with a troublesome incidence of leak and deflation, thought to be the result of fatigue in the capsule where small wrinkles occurred, producing constant shearing force.

The quality of inflatable implants has been improved in recent years, but, like the gel-filled implants, the problem of spherical fibrous capsular contracture occurs frequently enough to be troublesome.

The "double lumen prosthesis" was introduced in 1974. These prostheses are synthesized with two lumens; one is filled with silicone gel and the other with saline, which is inflated to the desired volume at the time of implantation. Double lumen prostheses are of two types. In the first, the saline bladder is deep to the gel lumen. The volume of saline can be reduced by percutaneous needle puncture after healing, and fibrous contracture produces a stable capsule. The fibrous capsule can, of course, contract around the saline-emptied smaller prosthesis, similar to the contracture that occurs when a large prosthesis is replaced with a smaller one at open capsulotomy. The second type is a gel-filled lumen located deep to the saline-filled bladder. Implants with large and small volumes of each lumen have been made so that the volume of saline can be reduced as desired. This is thought to act as a filter to absorb the "silicone molecular bleed" from the gel. Such a filter action could be important if 'silicone bleed' proves to be a major cause of spherical fibrous contracture. Hartley (1976) has reported a large experience with this prosthesis.

CHOICE OF PROSTHESIS

The choice of prosthesis rests with the individual preference of the surgeon. There is no proven significant functional difference in host response to gel-filled, saline inflatable, or double lumen prostheses. Each type can be inserted through any of the standard incisions. Gel-filled implants are preferred by most following subcutaneous mastectomy or as a replacement for other implants at secondary surgery where the breast tissue has become attenuated. When marked hypoplasia is present, inflatable implants may be too soft. The saline can shift against the breast wall on ballotment. Generally, the consistency and flow characteristics of inflatable implants more nearly simulate breast tissue than the other types of prostheses. Inflatable implants are particularly helpful in correcting breast asymmetry, since the volume can be adjusted with the prosthesis in place. Inflatable implants have a reported deflation rate of 2 to 8 percent. Palpable folds in the prosthetic capsule can occur when the surrounding fibrous tissue contracts.

Silicone gel-filled implants are fabricated in various shapes: teardrop (as were the original Cronin implants), oval, or round. Inflatable implants with center-fill or side-fill valves are usually round in shape. Teardrop or oval implants are more difficult to position, and they must be secured in position by a suture through a "suture loop" attached to the implant. With contraction of a spherical fibrous capsule, teardrop or oval implants most often assume a round shape.

Proponents of saline-filled prostheses believe that there is a lower incidence of fibrous capsular contracture with this implant (Rees, Guy and Coburn, 1973; Reiffel, Rees, Guy, and Aston, 1978).

INDICATIONS FOR BREAST AUGMENTATION

The primary indication for augmentation mammaplasty is an inadequate volume of breast tissue. Hypomastia may be developmental in nature or the result of postmenopausal involution.

Small breasts can also result from massive weight reduction. In hypomastia there is a deficiency of skin and underlying gland, whereas patients with breast tissue involution usually demonstrate some skin redundancy. Insertion of an appropriately selected prosthesis can give an excellent correction to either problem; however, the latter often requires concomitant mastopexy.

If breast ptosis accompanies small breast volume, a mastopexy is indicated. Augmentation and mastopexy can be performed together or separately according to the decision of the patient and surgeon.

The correction of developmental breast asymmetry is particularly rewarding and will be discussed subsequently.

Resection of a portion of the breast for a large benign tumor or cystic breast disease may reduce the breast mass sufficiently to produce noticeable asymmetry. A small breast prosthesis can remedy the problem, provided the pathologic diagnosis does not contraindicate the use of a prosthesis.

Patient Evaluation for Augmentation

Complete medical history and physical examination are important to rule out any systemic disease that may contraindicate major surgery. Gross evidence of breast pathology should be investigated by examination, mammography or xeroradiography. A history suggestive of problem bleeding or any other signs suggesting blood dyscrasias should be investigated. No aspirin-containing compounds should be taken for ten days prior to surgery. Aspirin decreases platelet cohesiveness. Patients taking birth control pills and other estrogen-containing hormones seem to have greater intraoperative bleeding than do others. When feasible, the medication should be discontinued ten days before surgery. The surgical procedure should not be scheduled during the three or four days prior to menses or during the first two or three days of the menstrual cycle, when the glandular tissue bleeds profusely.

The patient is examined while sitting or standing. The breast history and examination will determine if the small breasts are due to congenital hypoplasia, postpartum or postmenopausal involution, or a combination of factors. Breast asymmetry is pointed out to the patient. Mild to moderate breast asymmetry frequently has not been noticed by the patient. The size of the breasts and their relationship to the thoracic cage are noted. Chest wall asymmetry, which will influence the postoperative result, is likewise pointed out to the patient. The amount of skin and glandular tissue is evaluated to determine the appropriate amount of augmentation. When ptosis is present, its degree and its influence on augmentation are discussed with the patient (see Chapter 33 for section on breast ptosis).

PROSTHESIS LOCATION

Breast prostheses are most commonly placed between the posterior breast capsule and the underlying pectoral fascia. Dissection in this tissue plane is facilitated by its relative avascularity. Inframammary, periareolar, transareolar, or axillary skin incisions may be used for exposure. Some surgeons advocate placing prostheses behind the pectoral muscle. The submuscular plane is easily reached through a standard mammary crease incision or via an axillary approach. Dempsey and Latham (1968) and Griffith (1968) reported submuscular augmentation. Proponents of submuscular implantation believe the implants are more normal to palpation and the effects of capsular contraction are less obvious (if present). The chief disadvantage is that the prostheses can move up and laterally on contraction of the pectoralis muscle. The implants so placed can be located too high and excessively separated from the midline. Regnault (1977) reported transecting the pectoralis major muscle at its inferior and medial insertion, allowing the muscle to contract superiorly over the lower quarter or third of the breast prosthesis, leaving this portion covered only by mammary and superficial soft tissue. Regnault reported that almost all breasts in her series were without spherical fibrous capsular contractures. Papillon (1976) suggested only partial muscle division. Complications associated with submuscular prostheses implantation without muscle transection were minimized by this technique. Pickrell and associates (1977) reported favorable results with submuscular prostheses without transecting the pectoralis muscle. They reported no capsular contractures in their series.

Robles, Zimman, and Lee (1978) described undermining the deep surface of the pectoralis muscle inferiorly and medially to its costal insertions, detaching the pectoralis from the costal insertion, and continuing the dissection inferiorly in the subcutaneous tissue to the level of the seventh or eighth rib, some 4 or 5 cm below the level of the sulcus produced by the normal attachment of the pectoralis muscle to ribs. This large subpectoral pocket, used primarily by these surgeons for reconstruction of subcutaneous mastectomy patients, prevented upward displacement of the prosthesis owing to the pectoralis muscle activity in their opinion.

INFORMED CONSENT

The general details of breast augmentation should be explained in simple terms to the patient. The most common complications, including spherical fibrous capsular contracture, infection, and hematoma are discussed with the patient. Forty to 50 per cent of patients having mammary augmentation develop some degree of capsular contracture around the breast prosthesis from a few weeks to many months following surgery. This fact should be emphasized.

Patients should be informed that hypesthesia, anesthesia, and loss of erectility and erotic sensation can all occur; however, they are uncommon. There is temporary loss of sensation in the nipples in 7 to 15 percent of patients undergoing augmentation mammaplasty owing to injury to the fourth, fifth, or sixth intercostal nerves.

The planned incision and postoperative scars are described, and the fact that surgical scars are always visible on close inspection is explained. The possibility of keloids is noted.

ANESTHESIA

General or local anesthesia as preferred can be used for routine augmentation mammaplasty. Local anesthesia using 0.5 percent xylocaine with 1:200,000 epinephrine is the preference for ambulatory surgery.

Adequate premedication (according to the surgeon) should be given prior to local anesthesia to provide sedation and analgesia. The type and variety of drugs utilized vary widely from surgeon to surgeon. Combinations of barbiturates, narcotics, and diazepam are favored by most in dosages that can be reversed should overnarcosis result.

The cutaneous sensory innervation to the breast comes from the supraclavicular branches of the cervical plexus and also from the anterior and lateral perforating branches of the second, third, fourth, and fifth intercostal nerves. The deep nerve supply to the gland proper is derived almost entirely from the fourth, fifth, and sixth intercostal nerves.

Excellent anesthesia of the entire breast area is obtained by local infiltrating of the incision site with a small gauge needle and then raising three small wheals on the chest wall with the same needle in the lower medial quadrant, the lower lateral quadrant, and the upper midportion of the breast. A small gauge, three inch spinal needle is then inserted through the wheals and passed in a radial fashion in the plane between the subcutaneous tissue and pectoral fascia medially and laterally and between the posterior breast capsule and the muscular fascia beneath the breast.

AUGMENTATION TECHNIQUES

Several incisions have been described for breast augmentation including the inframammary, periareolar, transareolar, and axillary incisions. The choice of incision for an individual patient should be based on anatomy, the preference of the patient, and the preference of the surgeon. The authors prefer the periareolar and inframammary incisions. Excellent exposure is gained through such incisions, and they heal with relatively inconspicuous scars. Axillary incisions avoid incisions on the breast but provide limited exposure to the wound. This can be of significance in obtaining adequate hemostasis. Transareolar incisions can distort the nipple and interfere with the ducts and nipple sensation.

An incision in the inframammary fold is ideal for ptotic breasts and those with sufficient fullness of the inferior quadrants to hide the inframammary fold when the patient is in an upright position. Periareolar incisions are ideal for small breasts with good skin tone where there is minimal ptosis. The areola must be of sufficient diameter to support this incision. A very small areola contraindicates this approach. In general, periareolar incisions heal with minimal scars. However, patients with deeply pigmented areolae frequently have a small white scar that is obvious on inspection.

INFRAMAMMARY FOLD INCISION

With the patient sitting or standing, a 3 to 4 cm incision is marked in the inframammary crease in the midline of the breast directly centered under the nipple and areola (Figure 34–3). This places the incision in the position where it is under the least amount of constant stress. Incisions that are placed above the inframammary crease or those that extend laterally or medially are constantly under more stretch and are frequently larger and thicker than incisions placed in the midline of the breast. If the incision is outlined in the inframammary crease with the patient sitting or standing, the postoperative incision will lie in the inframammary crease. When the patient is placed in the supine position, the drawn incision will appear to be 1.0 to 1.5 cm below the crease, as the breast moves superiorly (Fig. 34–3B). This incision should not be redrawn, as the incision outlined with the patient in the upright position is the desired location.

An incision is made through the skin, subcutaneous tissue, and breast tissue down to the muscle fascia (Fig. 34–3C). Careful dissection with scissor tips permits delineation between the posterior capsule of the breasts and the pectoral fascia (Fig. 34–3D). Once the desired plane has been visualized, blunt finger dissection is facilitated. The index finger is used to sweep the posterior capsule of the breast from the muscle fascia by a gentle rotating motion of the finger (Fig. 34–3E). The opposite hand is used to support the breast tissue and to manipulate the breast onto the surface of the dissecting finger.

The dissection extends to the sternal border medially, over the second and third ribs superiorly, to the midaxillary line laterally, and to the inferior attachment of the breast tissue at the level of the inframammary crease (Fig. 34–3F). The size of the pocket dissected must be generous relative to the size of the breast prosthesis selected. Although the size of the planned prosthesis can be roughly determined preoperatively in most patients, an occasional retromammary pocket will not be as large as anticipated. If the pocket is not dissected to sufficient size, the skin overlying the prosthesis appears tense and the edges of the implant can be apparent through the skin. The breast appears to "stand off" the chest wall. If the size of the retromammary pocket is adequate for the implant size, the edges will not be seen through the breast tissue and the breast will have a normal pleasing contour and feel (Fig. 34–3G). Very large pockets that permit prosthesis mobility and possible false bursa formation may reduce the incidence of fibrous capsules.

Meticulous hemostasis is important. The fiberoptic light retractor (Fig. 34–3H) provides excellent exposure and the electrocautery provides a source of coagulation. The prosthesis can be placed through the inframammary incision (Fig. 34–3I,J). The insertion of a silicone gel prosthesis is aided by wetting the prosthesis and the surgeon's gloves with saline to reduce friction between the surface of the prosthesis and the gloves. A gentle squeezing and "milking" of the prosthesis between the fingertips will slide the prosthesis into place. A relatively large prosthesis can be inserted through an incision of 3 to 4 cm.

When the prosthesis is in position, the index finger is placed into the pocket and the prosthesis

Text continued on page 965.

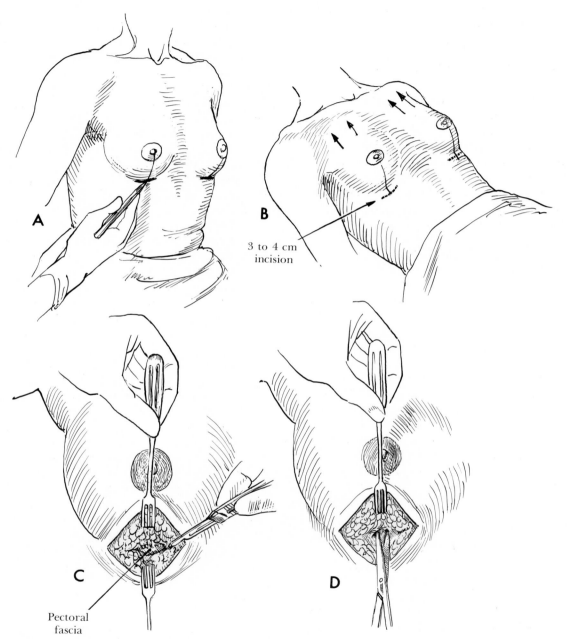

3 to 4 cm
incision

Pectoral
fascia

Figure 34–3. Augmentation mammaplasty, inframammary incision.

A and *B*, Incision outlined with patient sitting. In supine position, the incision appears too low, but the position should not be altered.

C and *D*, Incision to muscle fascia and scissor dissection begun on surface of muscle fascia.

Illustration continued on the opposite page.

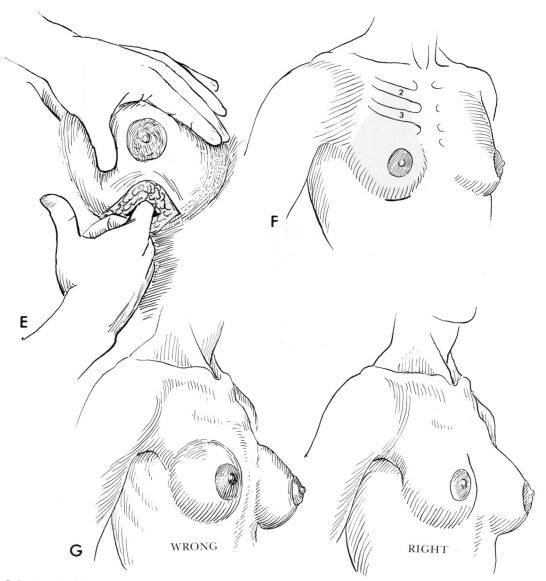

Figure 34–3 *Continued.* *E*, Retromammary pocket dissected on surface of pectoral fascia.

F, Extent of pocket as discussed in text.

G, The size of the pocket must be adequate to accommodate the prosthesis without its margins being obvious through the skin.

Illustration continued on the following page.

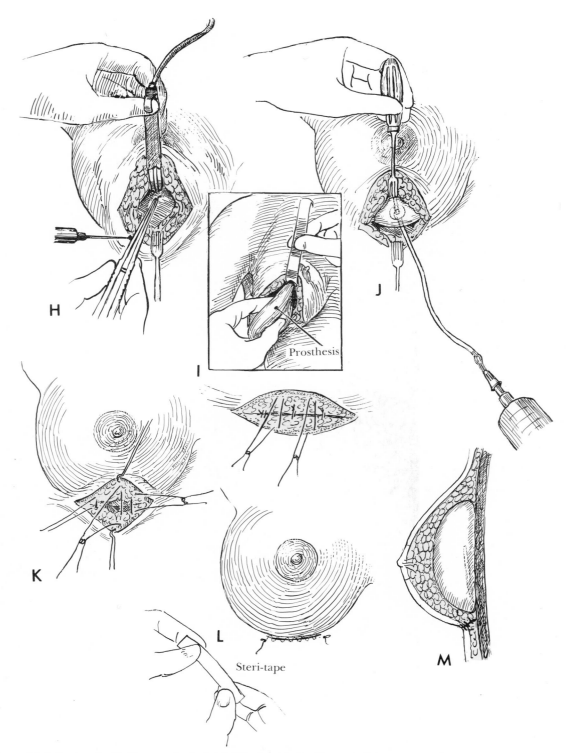

Figure 34–3 *Continued.*   *H*, Hemostasis obtained with the aid of a fiberoptic light source and electrocautery.

I and *J*, A silicone-gel or inflatable prosthesis placed in the retromammary pocket.

K, L, and *M,* The incision in the breast tissue is closed with absorbable suture material, and the skin is approximated with intra-cuticular Prolene. Steristrip tapes are applied to support epithelial approximation.

is gently moved about to insure that it is unfolded and filling the pocket. If the pocket is tight, further peripheral dissection is performed. Patients with apparently symmetrical breasts may appear to have one breast slightly larger than the other when the prostheses are initially placed into the pockets. Such asymmetry is usually the result of unequal dissection of the pockets.

The breast tissue is approximated with three to four sutures of 4–0 absorbable suture material such as Vicryl, and the skin is closed with an intracuticular 4–0 Prolene suture, which is removed seven days postoperatively. Steristrip tapes are applied to support epithelial approximation (Fig. 34–3K,L,M). (See Figures 34–4 through 34–7.)

PERIAREOLAR AUGMENTATION

An incision at the junction of the hyperpigmented skin of the areola and surrounding breast skin is well camouflaged. Such incisions are possible when the diameter of the areola permits. It is preferable in very small breasts where the inframammary incision is difficult to position and is

Text continued on page 969.

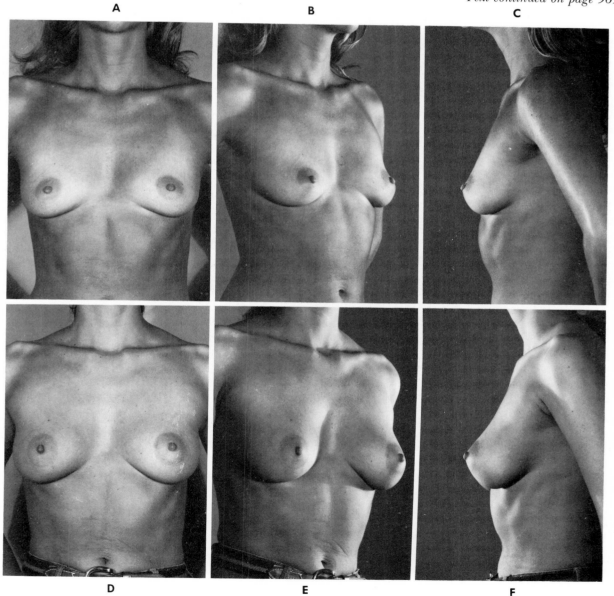

A   B   C

D   E   F

Figure 34–4.   *A, B,* and *C,* Superior quadrant atrophy following lactation and a short period of breast-feeding.

D, E, and *F,* An overall increase in breast volume was obtained with 145-cc gel prostheses placed through inframammary incisions. Larger prostheses may have distorted the natural breast shape. This patient has remained without fibrous capsule contracture for three years following augmentation.

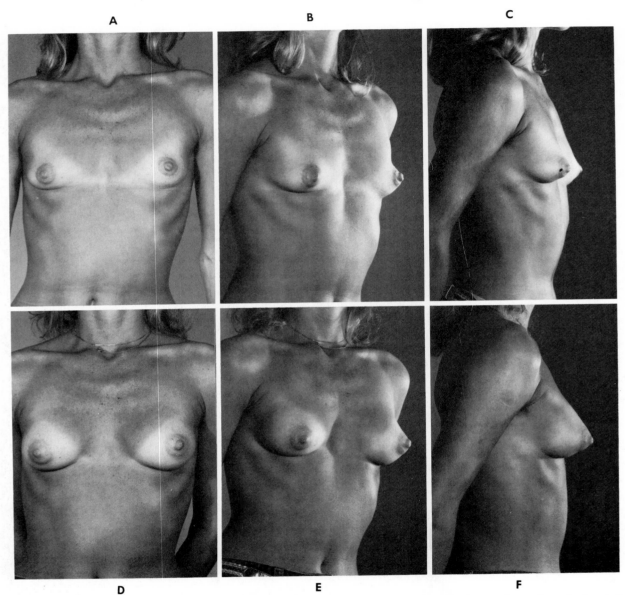

A   B   C

D   E   F

Figure 34–5. *A, B,* and *C,* Small breasts with a minimal amount of superior quadrant breast tissue and a tendency for herniation of breast tissue into the areolar area.

D, E, and *F,* Following augmentation with 120-cc saline inflatable prostheses, a natural breast contour is present. Large-volume prostheses would produce an unnatural appearance of the breasts in this kind of patient owing to the thin overlying tissues, wide rib cage, and small diameter of the base of the breast.

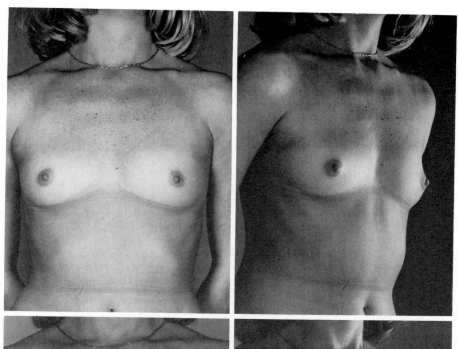

Figure 34–6. *A* and *B,* A 26-year-old patient with a small amount of breast tissue.

C and *D,* One year following augmentation through inframammary incisions with 180-cc gel implants. The breasts are round in appearance owing to the tightness of the overlying chest wall tissues and a moderate fibrous capsule.

E and *F,* One year following removal of 180-cc gel implants and replacement with 240-cc gel implants because of patient's persistent request for increased volume. Wide undermining in all directions was made at the time of the surgical procedure. The persistent roundness and suggestion of a prosthesis is seen through the skin.

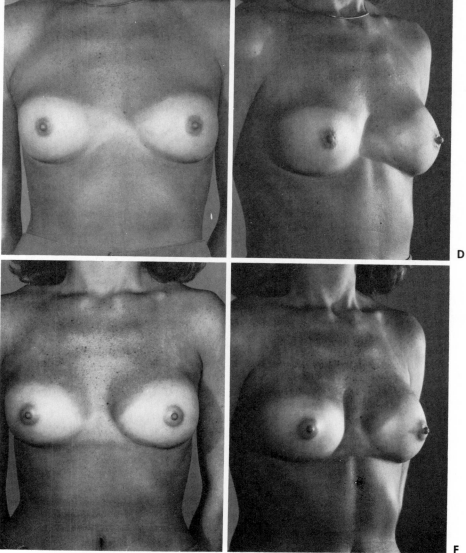

A   B   C

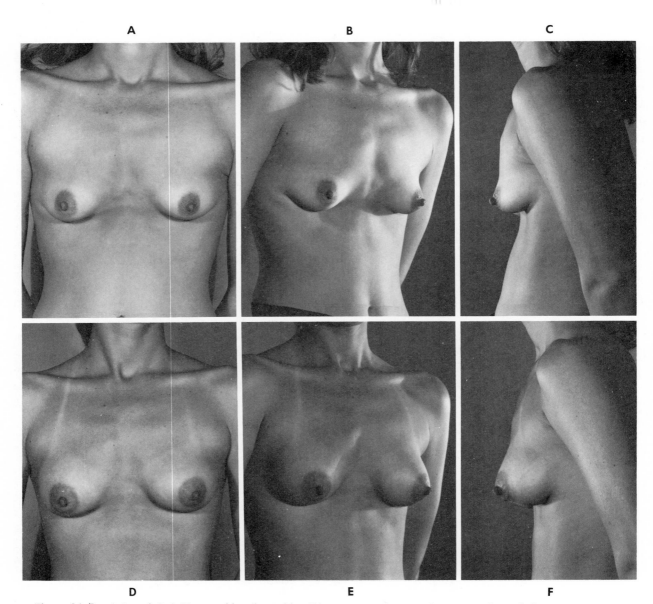

D   E   F

Figure 34–7.   *A, B,* and *C,* A 22-year-old patient with mild pectus excavatum and mammary hypoplasia.

D, E, and *F,* The anterior chest wall deformity is in part camouflaged with 130-cc gel prostheses inserted through inframammary incisions.

apt to be visible. Hypertrophic or prominent periareolar scars can develop but are uncommon.

The planned incision is drawn from three o'clock to nine o'clock at the junction of the hyperpigmented skin of the areola with the surrounding breast skin (Figure 34–8A). An incision is made through the skin and subcutaneous tissue down to the breast (Fig. 34–8B). The cut edge of the areolar skin has a tendency to retract superiorly 3 or 4 mm, exposing the anterior surface of the breast. There are two approaches to the pectoral fascia: (1) a small horizontal incision (3 cm) through the breast tissue, (Fig. 34–8C) and (2) subcutaneous dissection down to the inferior pole of the breast and then retrograde dissection beneath the breast tissue (Fig. 34–8D). The approach shown in Figure 34–8C is most commonly used. The breast is incised straight down to the prepectoral fascia (Fig. 34–8E, F). A 3 cm incision along the horizontal dimension usually suffices. Small retractors are

placed in succession to the depth of the transected breast tissue to permit a single cut through the breast parenchyma to the pectoral fascia. When the posterior breast capsule has been reached, the pectoral fascia is seen as a pale blue layer. The plane of dissection between the posterior breast capsule and the pectoral fascia is confirmed by gently sliding the breast back and forth, noting the gliding motion of the posterior breast capsule over the pectoral fascia.

Scissors are used to incise the posterior breast capsule and establish the dissection plane (Fig. 34–8G).

Blunt finger dissection separates the posterior breast capsule from the pectoral fascia (Fig. 34–8H). Retraction with the opposite hand manipulates the breast over the dissecting finger. This maneuver aids in delineating the retromammary pocket.

The retromammary pocket is dissected me-

Text continued on page 973.

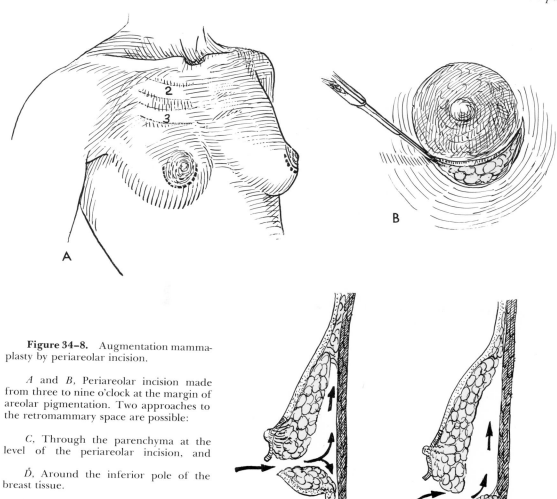

Figure 34–8. Augmentation mammaplasty by periareolar incision.

A and *B*, Periareolar incision made from three to nine o'clock at the margin of areolar pigmentation. Two approaches to the retromammary space are possible:

C, Through the parenchyma at the level of the periareolar incision, and

D, Around the inferior pole of the breast tissue.

Illustration continued on the following page.

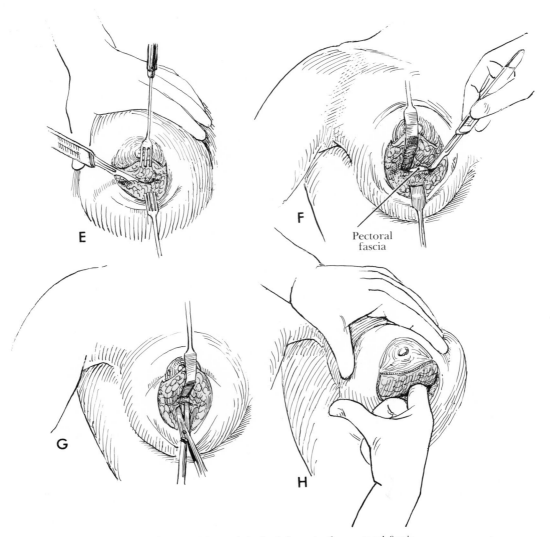

Pectoral
fascia

Figure 34–8 *Continued.*   *E* and *F*, The parenchyma is incised down to the pectoral fascia.

G, Scissor dissection begins developing pocket anterior to the pectoral fascia.

H, Finger dissection creates retromammary pocket.

Illustration continued on the opposite page.

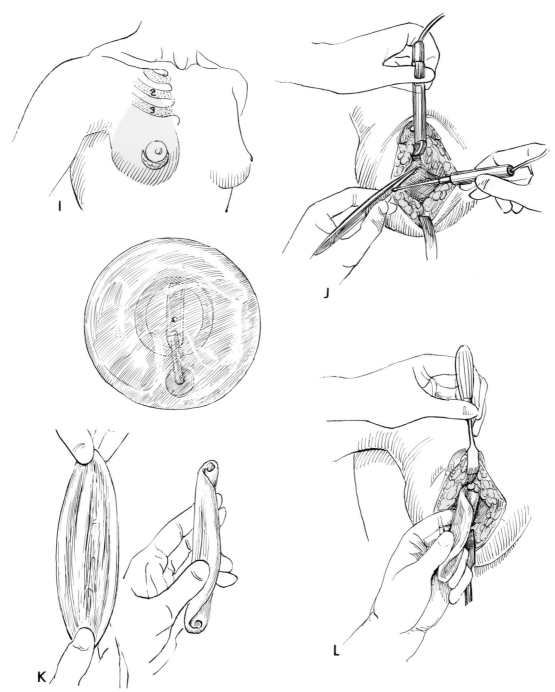

Figure 34–8 *Continued.*   *I*, Extent of retromammary pocket discussed in text.

J, Hemostasis obtained with the aid of a fiberoptic light source and electrocautery.

K and *L*, Inflatable prosthesis tubed and inserted through a small hole in the parenchyma.

Illustration continued on the following page.

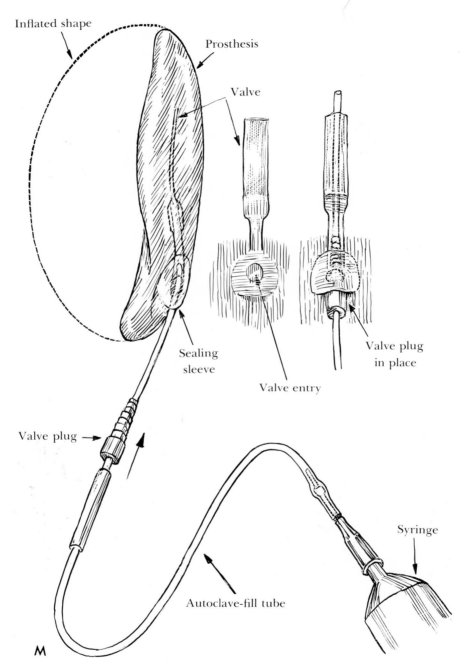

Inflated shape

Prosthesis

Valve

Sealing
sleeve

Valve entry

Valve plug
in place

Valve plug

Autoclave-fill tube

Syringe

M

Figure 34–8 *Continued.   M,* Diagram of inflatable prosthesis and its filling system.

Illustration continued on the opposite page.

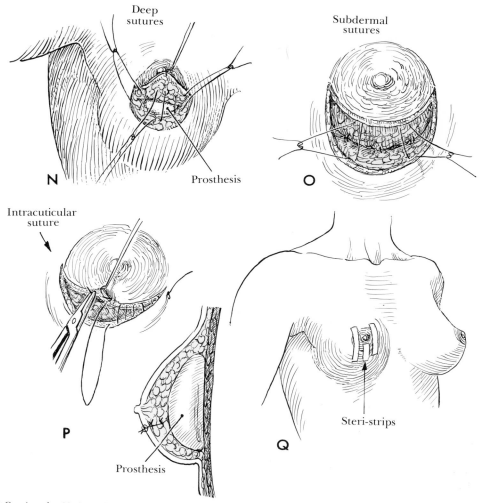

Figure 34–8 *Continued.* *N, O,* and *P,* Prosthesis inflated, parenchyma incision closed with absorbable sutures, and skin approximated with intracuticular suture.

Q, Epithelial approximation is assured with Steristrip tapes.

dially to the lateral border of the sternum, superiorly to the level of the second or third rib, laterally to the midaxillary line and inferiorly to the attachments of the breast at the inframammary fold (Fig. 34–8*I*).

Meticulous hemostasis is obtained with the aid of a fiberoptic retractor. Electrocautery is used to coagulate vessels (Fig. 34–8, *J*).

A silicone prosthesis is placed in the dissected pocket. An empty balloon prosthesis is most easily inserted. The empty balloon is rolled up into a tubular shape, inserted into the pocket, and unrolled (Fig. 34–8, *K, L*). A gel prosthesis should be moistened with saline to facilitate its insertion.

The inflatable prosthesis is filled with saline after insertion and the valve is closed or plugged. Air is aspirated from the prosthesis. The filling and aspiration can be performed before or after

the prosthesis is placed in the retromammary pocket.

Several balloon prostheses are available. The surgeon should be familiar with the component parts of the particular prosthesis used including the valve, valve entry, sealing sleeve, valve plug, and autoclave-fill tube prior to putting the prosthesis in the retromammary pocket (Fig. 34–8, *M*).

When the desired volume is injected, a finger is placed inside the pocket to determine that the prosthesis lies in the desired position and the balloon is not folded or wrinkled. Further blunt finger dissection can release residual tightness of the breast tissue over the implant.

The breast tissue is approximated with a single layer of 4-0 absorbable suture. Care is taken to not puncture the prosthesis as the incision is closed (Fig. 34–8, *N*).

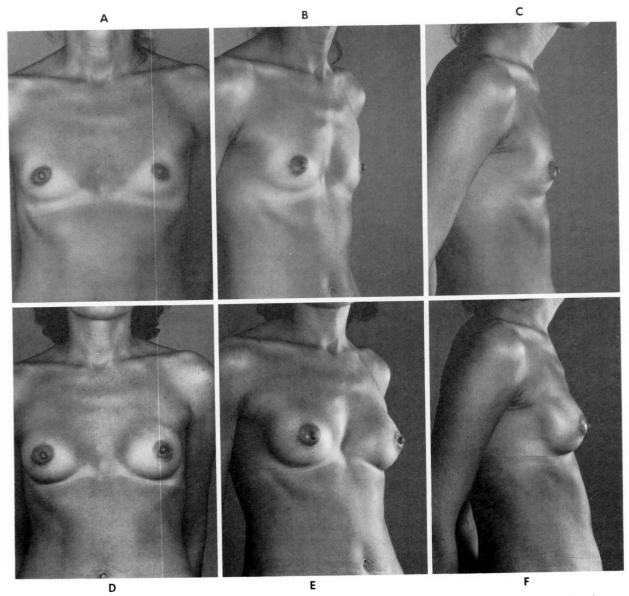

Figure 34–9. *A, B,* and *C,* A 34-year-old woman with a minimal amount of breast tissue and tight anterior chest wall skin following one full-term pregnancy. The left breast is situated somewhat higher on the anterior chest wall and is slightly smaller than the right breast.

D, E, and *F,* The patient following 120-cc augmentation of the right breast and the 140-cc augmentation of the left breast using saline inflatable prostheses through periareolar incisions.

Two or three 4–0 absorbable subdermal sutures line up the areolar incision, which is then closed with an intracuticular 4–0 Prolene (Fig. 34–8, *O, P*).

Epithelial approximation is assured with Steristrip tapes (Fig. 34–8, *Q*). (See Figure 34–9.)

POSTOPERATIVE CARE

A comfortable stretch brassiere is worn as soon as the patient can cooperate. Care should be exercised in sitting up a sleeping patient to avoid painful back sprain. The bra is worn day and night for two weeks, except for bathing. This provides comfort and a source of security for most patients. When the prostheses are placed under the pectoralis muscle, no brassiere is worn for four to six weeks to allow the dependent weight of the implants to "stretch out" the lower portion of the pectoralis muscle. This appears to help prevent cephalic displacement of the submuscular implants.

Patients operated on an outpatient basis are discharged to their home or to a recovery facility two or three hours following surgery. For the protection of the patient, an adult should accompany the patient home.

Pain after augmentation mammaplasty is variable but usually minimal to moderate in degree. Tylenol with Codeine (30 mg) usually suffices for analgesia. Severe pain is an indication for examination of the wound to rule out hematoma.

If given, prophylactic antibiotics should be started to obtain high blood levels during the intraoperative period. Activities are limited to necessary traveling. Bed rest, with kitchen and bathroom privileges, is ordered on the day of surgery. Vigorous physical activities requiring pectoral muscle activities (tennis, swimming, etc.) are restricted for three weeks. Normal daily functions are not limited. Many patients return to work three or four days after surgery.

Intracuticular skin sutures are removed on the seventh postoperative day. Breast massage by the patient to maintain the full size of the pockets is advised by some surgeons. Such manipulation is thought to mitigate against spherical contraction. The implanted prosthesis is pushed medially, laterally, inferiorly, and superiorly one dozen times in each direction three times per day for six months and then continued once or twice per day.

The goal of breast massage is to produce a large pseudobursa around the prosthesis rather than a constricting fibrous capsule. The patient is instructed to move the implant actively. Some patients are afraid they will "damage" their new breasts and thus their exercise will be limited. Surgeons who advocate massage must thoroughly educate their patients. Few patients will exercise as often or for as long as they are instructed.

COMPLICATIONS OF AUGMENTATION

Complications of breast augmentation with a dermis-fat graft, a dermis-fat flap, injection of foreign materials, and polyvinyl implants have been discussed. The following discussion of complications and sequelae applies to the silicone bag type of prosthesis now in wide use.

Firmness

Breast firmness of varying degrees secondary to spherical fibrous capsular contracture (SFCC) occurs in one or both breasts in 40 percent or more of patients following augmentation mammaplasty. The incidence of SFCC is sufficiently high to consider it an untoward sequelae of the surgery rather than a complication. It is the result of the natural healing process and is not pathologic. Massage, pressure bandages, lack of pressure bandages,

steroids, replacement of prostheses with smaller prostheses, long immobilization, and early mobilization have all been advocated to reduce the incidence of contracture. The authors have no conclusive data to suggest that any of these modalities is significantly effective.

It is not known why some patients develop only slight firmness and others develop hard breasts that may be uncomfortable and painful. Calcification of fibrous capsules and extremely hard breasts have been reported (Redfern, Ryan, and Su, 1977; Benjamin and Guy, 1977). Severe capsular contractures often produce visible and palpable asymmetries. One or both breasts may be rounded, tense, and unnatural. The edge of the breast prosthesis may become palpable and occasionally visible when there is only a small amount of overlying breast tissue. Saline-filled implants, more frequently than gel-filled ones, develop a palpable "buckle" as the inflatable balloon is squeezed by the contracting scar tissue capsule. Breast firmness may develop a few weeks postoperatively or not until after many months or several years (Williams, Aston, Rees, 1975). Often, patients report an acute episode of breast discomfort or tenderness just prior to noting breast firmness. This may represent hematogenous bacterial seeding of the fibrous capsule. The degree of firmness is in part related to the thickness and the contracture of the fibrous pseudosheath that develops around the prosthesis. Williams (1972) documented firmness in 65 percent of a series of patients augmented with Cronin gel prostheses with Dacron patches on the back but had an incidence of firmness of only 1 percent when similar implants without Dacron patches were used. Whether or not there is a greater incidence of fibrous capsular contracture associated with saline or gel-filled implants is still under investigation. Statistical data is inconclusive at this time. The microscopic appearance of the fibrous capsules has been studied by several investigators in recent years (Imber et al., 1974; Thomson, 1973). In baboons, Williams, Aston, and Rees (1975) showed that a hematoma in the subpanniculus caronsus pocket, after the implantation of silicone discs, was associated with the formation of a surrounding fibrous capsule thicker than that developing around similar implants in a pocket emptied by constant suction drainage for one week.

The etiology of SFCC is speculative and, no doubt, multifactorial. Suggested causes include, among others, mechanical irritative effects of the prosthesis, subclinical infection, motion of the pectoralis muscles, organized seromata, delayed rupture of small vascular channels, residual hematoma in the submammary pockets that organize, and tissue response to silicone molecules. "Silicone bleed" from the surface of the silicone prosthesis has been suggested as a possible etiology of SFCC. Silicone elastomer membrane is a semipermeable membrane through which many substances pass including drugs, gases, liquids, and certain size polymer chains of silicone gel. It is well known that a gel prosthesis left in contact with an absorbent material, such as tissue paper, will leave a "greasy stain" after a few hours. The "stain" is much heavier from a gel prosthesis, but it is also obvious with saline-filled prostheses. Clinically, foreign-body reaction to silicone gel in axillary lymph nodes has been documented 10 years after subpectoral augmentation mammaplasty (Hausner, Schoen, Pierson, 1978). There was no evidence of prosthesis rupture when removed en bloc with a radical mastectomy specimen for carcinoma. The exact role of silicone bleed and its relationship to fibrous capsular contracture is not known at present. If silicone bleed were a major factor in capsule formation, a higher incidence of contracture would be anticipated around silicone gel-filled implants than around inflatable implants. One theory suggests that silicone particles are phagocytized by cells surrounding the prosthesis and contribute to the SFCC.

Investigators have documented the presence of silicone particles within fibrous capsules (Wilflingseder, Propst, and Mikus, 1974). Domanskis and Owsley (1976) studied specimens of fibrous breast capsules under an electron microscope and a light microscope. Multiple areas of particulate foreign material, consistent with the appearance of droplets of dimethylopolysiloxane, were found in the specimens. An active foreign body reaction was observed at the interface between the capsule and the implant as well as throughout the tissue subjacent to the deposits of foreign material. These authors postulated the presence of transmembrane extravasation of silicone as being a theoretical explanation of the etiology of capsular contracture of the breast after augmentation mammaplasty. However, similar studies documenting the presence of silicone particles have not been able to correlate silicone particles with clinical hardness (Rudolph et al., 1978). Electron microscopic studies have positively documented myofibroblasts within the fibrous capsule wall (Rudolph, 1978). However, the relationship of silicone to the myofibroblast and clinical firmness is uncertain.

At present, closed compression capsulotomy as described by Baker, Bartels, and Douglas (1976) is in vogue as the primary treatment of fibrous capsules. Manual pressure applied to the breast by the heels of the hands ruptures the capsule. Considerable hydraulic pressure is exerted on the capsule through the prosthesis by this technique. With the patient supine and under mild sedation, pressure is applied in succession horizontally, vertically, and obliquely, obtaining further tearing of the capsule in each direction in an attempt to gain circumferential release. A quite noticeable "pop" is palpable and frequently audible as the initial capsule rupture occurs. The breast becomes instantaneously soft if the maneuver is successful.

The advantages of the procedure are its simplicity and its noninvasive nature. It can be performed on an outpatient basis. Although some patients will reform capsules in three or four months after this procedure, others have maintained soft breasts for more than one year. The procedure can be repeated up to several times as necessary, as long as it is effective.

Complications of closed compression capsulotomy are few but may be significant. Bizarre shaped breasts occur with incomplete capsule rupture (Baker, Bartels, Douglas, 1976; Vinnick, 1976). Hematoma following capsular tear that ruptures a blood vessel may require surgical evacuation. Implant rupture with extravasation and silicone gel into the surrounding tissues — even into the axilla and upper extremity — has been reported (Huang, Blackwell, and Lewis, 1978). Goin (1978) reported a large axillary mass and severe axillary pain simultaneous with a closed capsulotomy, suggesting high pressure injection of silicone gel through the tissues and into the axilla. Subsequent histologic studies confirmed silicone in axillary lymph nodes. Leaked silicone gel can produce granulomatous reactions presenting as breast nodules or masses on the trunk distant from the breasts (Eisenberg and Bartels, 1977; Capozzi, DuBou, and Pennisi, 1978). Experimental studies of tissue response to ruptured gel-filled mammary prostheses in rats have shown a significant increase in capsule thickness as compared with the capsule around intact prostheses. The gel was also noted to migrate through the fibrous capsule and into surrounding tissue (Vistnes, Bentley, and Fogarty, 1977). Inflatable implants may rupture and deflate during compression closed capsulotomy (Feliberti, Arrillaga, Colon, 1977).

A "gamekeeper's thumb" has been reported by surgeons performing this procedure (Tolhurst, 1978). Pressure should be applied to the base of the breast with the heels of the hands and not by squeezing between the fingers and thumbs. Capsules not responding to closed capsulotomy can be treated by open capsulotomy.

Open capsulotomy releases and excises the contracting capsule. The breasts are soft in the early postoperative period. Silver (1972) left the capsule intact and reinserted the prosthesis deep to the capsule. Dempsey and Latham (1968) suggested placing the prosthesis behind the pectoralis muscle to buttress the implant. Williams (1972) resects a strip of capsule 1 to 2 cm wide around the periphery of the fibrous capsule, and if the capsule is thicker than 2 to 3 mm, he suggests a total capsulectomy. Mladick (1978) suggested stripping the capsule from the posterior breast prior to removing the prosthesis and then resecting any remnant of capsule with breast attached. Many surgeons widely incise the contracted capsule based on the theory that the major contracture phase has occurred.

The use of steroids to limit capillary proliferation and fibroplasia has been reported as helpful in preventing capsular contracture in augmentation mammaplasty. Williams (1972) and Peterson and Burt (1974) instilled triamcinolone solution into the retromammary implant pocket. Postoperatively, steroids administered in this way can gravitate to the inferior gutter of the implant pocket. It is questionable if a single dose is effective over several weeks.

Perrin (1976) attempted sustained release of steroids across the implant-wound interface. He instilled methylprednisolone Na hemisuccinate (125 mg) in inflatable implants in solution with saline. He reported an incidence of "significant" capsule formation in less than 5 per cent of 100 patients.

Marked atrophy of breast parenchyma and skin flaps has been reported following instillation of local doses of steroids in the retromammary pocket or within the prostheses (Fredricks, 1976; Cohen, 1978; Persoff, 1978). The effects of smaller doses of intraluminal steroids (Solumedrol 20 mg) are being evaluated. It is hoped that smaller doses will obviate some of the local side effects.

The effects of triamcinolone acetonide on the architecture and composition of the fibrous capsules developing around gel-filled prostheses in rats was evaluated by Vistnes, Ksander, and Kosek, (1978). No difference in capsule thickness, total protein count, or collagen content was noted in the steroid-treated animals when compared with implanted control animals.

When triamcinolone acetonide was delivered over a long period by continuous diffusion from within a gel-filled prosthesis, the thickness of the capsule around the prosthesis was decreased and the protein and collagen composition of the remaining capsule was modified (Ksander, Vistnes, and Fogarty, 1978). Modification in the capsule did not, however, significantly alter the firmness of the capsule.

The therapeutic efficacy of steroids in preventing a spherical fibrous capsular contracture around breast prostheses has not as yet been established.

Hematoma

The incidence of hematoma following augmentation mammaplasty is less than 1 percent. Careful hemostasis with the aid of a fiberoptic light source is mandatory. Hematoma formation is easily recognized; a painful swollen breast that is excessively firm to palpation is highly suggestive. Hematomas should be promptly evacuated. The prosthesis is removed, hemostasis is obtained, and the breast pocket is irrigated with saline to remove small clots from the tissue. A prosthesis is reinserted and the wound is closed in the conventional fashion with suction drainage. Failure to evacuate a hematoma is associated with a very firm breast immediately following surgery that is likely to result in fibrous capsule. Hematomas provide an excellent culture medium for bacteria.

Infection

Infection is rare following breast augmentation with silicone prostheses. In the authors' series, its incidence is less than 1 percent. Prophylactic broad spectrum antibiotics may be given orally for 24 hours preoperatively and for four days following surgery. The breast and chest walls are washed with pHisoHex soap beginning two days before surgery (Betadyne is preferred as a skin prep). Infection is indicated by a warm, tender, swollen breast. Infection usually occurs within the first few postoperative days, but it can occur as late as five to ten years after surgery (Hayes, 1977; Williams, Aston, and Rees, 1975). Infection is treated by solid surgical principles. The prosthesis is best removed, and the pockets should be evacuated and drained. Appropriate full spectrum antibiotics are administered. Prostheses should not be replaced for at least three months following clinical evidence of infection.

A subclinical infection by *Staphylococcus epidermidis*, which is frequently present in breast ducts, may be significant in the etiology of fibrous capsules.

Wound Dehiscence

Wound dehiscence is associated with infection, hematoma, serous fluid collection, and improper wound closure. Some serous fluid forms around most prostheses early after surgery; it is generally absorbed into the tissues. Significant collection of serous fluid is uncommon with modern prostheses. Inflammation or infection can result in excessive fluid collection. Pressure on the area of least resistance in an improperly closed wound will cause dehiscence at the point of least resistance in the absence of infection. The wound should be promptly resutured. Atrophy secondary to local steroid therapy instilled in an inflatable prosthesis can result in extrusion. Ellenberg and Bartels (1977) suggested that the incidence of breast atrophy would be lessened by methylprednisolone sodium succinate as the steroid of choice. Wound breakdown from any cause (including skin slough) clearly results in implant extrusion.

Pain

Breast pain after the initial postoperative period is uncommon following augmentation mammaplasty. Prolonged and persistent pain is usually associated with SFCC. Hard breasts are uncomfortable and occasionally associated with intermittent pain. Breasts may also be tender on palpation when SFCC is present.

Sensory Changes

Injury to the nerves during surgery or pressure from the implants may be associated with postoperative hypesthesia of the periareolar area. The incidence of sensibility loss to the nipple is reported to be 7 to 15 percent (Courtiss and Goldwyn, 1976; Papillon, 1976). Papillon (1976) reported full return of sensibility to the nipples following implant removal more than five years after augmentation. Hypesthesia is as common with periareolar incisions as with inframammary incisions.

Scars

Periareolar or inframammary incisions generally heal well. Hypertrophy or keloid formation can occur in any breast scar, and patients should be so forewarned. Appropriate therapy includes excision and intralesional steroids.

Prosthesis Malposition

Prosthesis displacement of the implants is less apt to occur if accurate dissection of the retromammary pocket is carried out. Disruption of the fibrous attachments of the breast at the inframammary crease may result in inferior displacement of the prosthesis. The inframammary crease can be reestablished with permanent sutures and adequate support of the breast for five to six weeks.

Excessive dissection medially and superiorly is unusual because of the natural barrier of the sternum, and the effect of gravity on the prosthesis mitigates displacement of the prosthesis superiorly or medially. Such displacement is usually associated with SFCC. Dissection of the pocket too far laterally will result in lateral displacement of the prostheses.

Prostheses placed behind the pectoral muscles are subject to superior and lateral displacement from the forces of contracture of the pectoral muscles. Detachment of the medial insertions of the pectoralis muscle to the fourth and fifth ribs and costal margins aids in establishing the prosthesis in a more favorable position to overcome the effects of muscle contraction.

Implant Deflation and Rupture

Inflatable balloon implants have a deflation rate of 1 to 2 percent. Shearing forces from breast movement between the walls of the implant at the site of a "wrinkle" with eventual fatigue of the silicone capsule and eventual rupture is a common cause. A faulty valve can also result in deflation. A less common cause is traumatic rupture, which can occur in gel prostheses.

MAMMARY ASYMMETRY AND DEVELOPMENTAL ABNORMALITIES

Mammary asymmetry varies from slight difference in the size and shape of the breast to unilateral hypomastia or amastia with or without a nipple (athelia). Some breast asymmetry is present in most women. This is consistent with the normal variations that exist in the two sides of the body. Frequently, the difference in size of the two breasts is not of sufficient magnitude that it is detected by the patient.

The incidence of significant mammary asymmetry is not known. Many women with the problem probably never seek surgical correction because of the embarrassment and psychologic stress of exposing their deformity. Pitanguy (1974) found noticeable asymmetry in 4 per cent of 1273 patients undergoing mammaplasties. The incidence in the general population is probably higher.

The etiology of significant breast asymmetry is variable. Bilateral micromastia is usually a developmental deficiency. Unilateral micromastia associated with contralateral macromastia is also a congen-

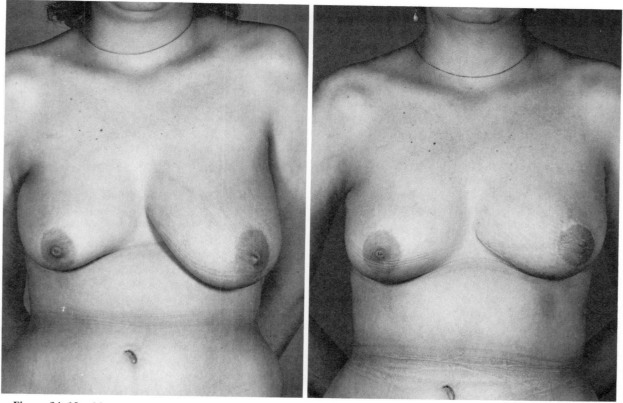

Figure 34–10.   Mammary asymmetry corrected by augmentation of the right breast with 175-cc saline-filled prosthesis and Pitanguy technique mastopexy of the left breast.

ital anomaly. Virginal hypertrophy is an end organ response to hormonal stimulation. Surgical procedures, lacerations, crush injuries, radiation therapy, burns, and any other trauma to the breast bud during infancy and childhood may destroy or restrict normal breast growth and development.

Breast asymmetry may be unilateral or bilateral. Hypoplasia or hyperplasia with associated ptosis can occur on either side. The hypoplastic or hyperplastic breast may be associated with a normal breast on the contralateral side. All possible combinations of large and small breasts on the two sides can occur. Deformities of the thorax such as pectus excavatum, pectus carinatum, and scoliosis may be associated with a congenital breast deformity.

Slight to moderate asymmetry of the anterior thorax is frequently seen in patients requesting augmentation mammaplasty. The height of the rib cage at its junction with the sternum can differ from side to side so that one side protrudes more than the other.

When one breast is small and the other is normal in size, augmentation of the small breast is indicated. When one breast is large and the opposite is small, a reduction mammaplasty may suffice or be combined with augmentation of the small breast (Figure 34–10). Both breasts may be small

and require asymmetrical augmentation. Inflatable implants are particularly useful in correcting asymmetry.

INDICATIONS FOR SURGERY

Alleviation of psychologic distress is the primary indication for correction of breast asymmetry. Inappropriate development of sex characteristics can result in severe emotional distress in teenagers (Schoenfeld, 1964). Body image is extremely important during adolescence. Rees (1968), Corso (1972), Simon, Hoffman, and Kahn (1975), and Hueston (1976) reported psychologic disturbances associated with breast asymmetry. Social maladjustments and behavioral problems requiring psychiatric care are not uncommon in patients with significant breast asymmetry.

Fitting of brassieres and other clothing can be difficult and expensive. Some patients eliminate certain revealing clothing such as sporting attire and bathing suits because of fear of revealing their asymmetry.

Treatment of breast asymmetry requires accurate evaluation and diagnosis of the existing deformity. Appropriate application of the principles of breast reduction, mastopexy, and breast augmentation as presented in this chapter will significantly improve the anatomic problems for most patients. Custom made prostheses or inflatables may be necessary for patients with chest wall deformities or pectoral muscle absence. Areola and nipple reconstruction is occasionally necessary.

Psychologic support should begin at the first consultation. Most patients find some comfort in learning that the incidence of breast asymmetry is relatively high. Necessary surgical procedures including limitations and possible complications should be discussed with the patient and the relatives. Some deformities, such as unilateral micromastia and contralateral hypertrophy and ptosis, will always cause asymmetry. However, the appropriate correction of shape and volume can make the residual asymmetry easy to camouflage by clothing.

Patients who have had surgical correction of breast asymmetry are some of the happiest patients seen in the practice of plastic surgery. Few have complaints about persistent minor asymmetry, postoperative scars, and so forth. Frequently, patients who are shy and withdrawn preoperatively literally "blossom" postoperatively. Improvement in self confidence and self image is often evident after surgery.

Amastia

Amastia — total absence of the mammary gland, nipple, and occasionally the pectoralis major muscle — is rare. Trier (1965) reviewed the subject in detail.

Polymastia

Polymastia — supernumerary mammary glands — is most often seen as bilateral axillary breasts (Rees, 1964, 1967; Kaye, 1974, 1975). Such deformities represent prolonged or separated tails of the normal breast buds, which developed along the embryologic mammary ridges. Aberrant glandular tissue may occur at sites other than the axilla but is almost always situated laterally. Etiologic theories of supernumerary breasts differ. The embryologic theory (DeCholnoky, 1939; Haagensen, 1971; Hamblen, 1945; Hamilton, Boyd, and Mossman, 1945) holds that supernumerary breasts occur because of the persistence and later development of the primordial breast tissue along the milk lines, where regression ordinarily occurs.

Another theory (Hughes, 1950) proposes that supernumerary breasts are caused by independently migrating nests of primordial breast cells that locate and develop in a random fashion. Such a theory would explain the unusual occurrence of a fully developed dorsal supernumerary breast as reported by Hanson and Segovia (1978).

Aberrant glands without an associated nipple may first become obvious during pregnancy when hyperplasia of the glandular tissue occurs. Polythelia may or may not be associated with aberrant glands. Normal lactation may occur in ectropic glands. It has been suggested that aberrant mammary glands may represent a reversion of ancestral characteristics, since, in general, they follow the form of lower animals.

Aberrant breast tissue can develop along with any breast diseases, either benign or malignant, that occur in normal breast tissue (DeCholnoky, 1939, 1951; Copeland and Geschickter, 1950; Cutler, 1961; Cogswell and Czerny, 1961; Hiraide and Akai, 1968; Brightmore, 1971; Haagensen, 1971; Smith and Greening, 1972). There is controversy as to whether there is a greater incidence of malignancy in ectropic breast tissue than in normally situated breasts. The aesthetic deformity of axillary breast tissue, and the possibility of breast pathology (Copeland and Geschickter, 1950), are strong indications for surgical removal. The surgical technique described by Kaye (1974, 1975) permits removal of breast tissue and excess skin, leaving a horizontal scar hidden high up on the inner surface of the arm and axilla.

Polythelia (accessory or supernumerary nipples) usually occurs 5 to 6 cm below the usual nipples and is located slightly more medially toward the midline. Supernumerary nipples can occur anywhere along the embryonic mammary ridge. In the adult, the milk line begins laterally in the axilla and crosses medially as it approaches the groin.

Mammary tissue is usually absent in significant amounts in supernumerary nipples. Accessory nipples alone are rarely of consequence. However, excision is indicated, particularly when there is associated glandular tissue, because of the possibility of malignant change.

The Tuberous Breast

The tuberous breast is an unusual breast deformity so named because of its resemblance in shape to a tuberous plant root (Rees and Aston, 1976; Williams, 1976). It is difficult to treat. The base of the tuberous breast is deficient in both its horizontal and vertical dimensions, and with development, the breast projects forward but lacks characteristic fullness. The nipple and areola are usually overly developed.

"The tuberous breast" is a generic term that

includes two breast deformities of similar appearance but significant anatomic difference. Both are characterized by small truncated glands with apparently normal function. In one type, there is a vertical and horizontal deficiency that is proportional. The deficiency results in a concentric small base, a small tuberous shaped breast, and a large nipple-areolar complex with apparent herniation of the breast tissue into the areola (Figure 34–11A).

In the second type, the breast is more deficient in the vertical than in the horizontal dimension

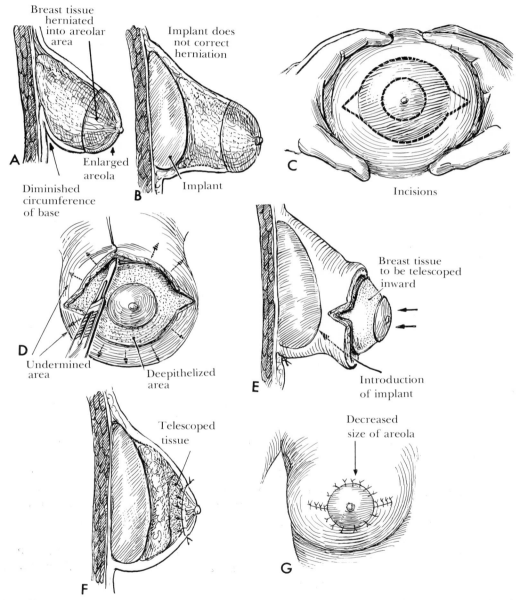

Figure 34–11. *A*, Tuberous breast deformity.

B, Anticipated result following standard augmentation mammaplasty.

C, Correction of herniated nipple deformity by telescoping technique. New areolar size and skin incisions outlined.

D, Excess areola deepithelized. Skin and subcutaneous tissue dissected off breast capsule.

E, Prosthesis placed in retromammary pocket on pectoral fascia.

F and *G*, Breast tissue telescoped into new skin brassiere and incision sutured.

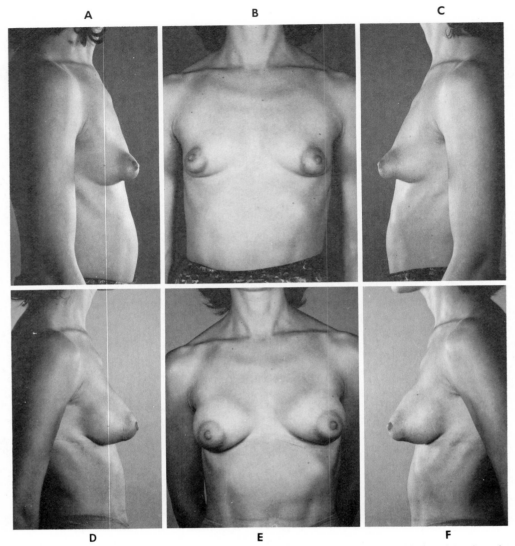

Figure 34–12.   *A, B,* and *C,* Mammary hypoplasia and tuberous breast with herniation of breast tissue into the nipple-areola complex.

D, E, and *F,* Six months following periareolar incisions for augmentation mammaplasty with 165-cc silicone-gel prostheses. The nipple-areolar complex "hangs off" the prostheses.

and the base of the breast is small. In this, the breast is ptotic with the nipple pointing downward but without apparent herniation of parenchyma into the nipple-areolar complex. The circumference of the areola, too, is smaller and more normal in size. The first type may be considered the true tuberous breast.

Routine augmentation mammaplasty of the true tuberous breast with herniation of the parenchyma accentuates the deformity (Figure 34–12). The nipple and areola are literally pushed to protrude even further (Fig. 34–11*B*). The entire breast then droops over the implant. Williams (1976) has termed this type the "snoopy breast." Correction requires reduction of the circumference of the areola sufficient to confine the underlying breast tissue by telescoping it posteriorly towards the chest wall. In effect, the skin brassiere is recon-

structed and the areola is reduced over existing breast parenchyma. Augmentation mammaplasty then increases the breast to the desired volume.

Surgical Technique for Correction of the Tuberous Breast

Projected incisions are drawn that describe a new areolar diameter (4.5 to 5 cm) and that allow for tailoring of lateral "dogears." Lateral triangular skin excisions may or may not be required (Fig. 34–11*C*). When there is only moderate enlargement of the areola, triangular excisions of the dogears may not be necessary. The initial incisions are made on the new areolar boundary and beveled outward so as to split the dermis to preserve the subdermal plexus of vessels and nerves. The lateral skin wedges are excised and the dissection is carried to the subcutaneous plane. The breast parenchyma is then denuded of skin flaps, and

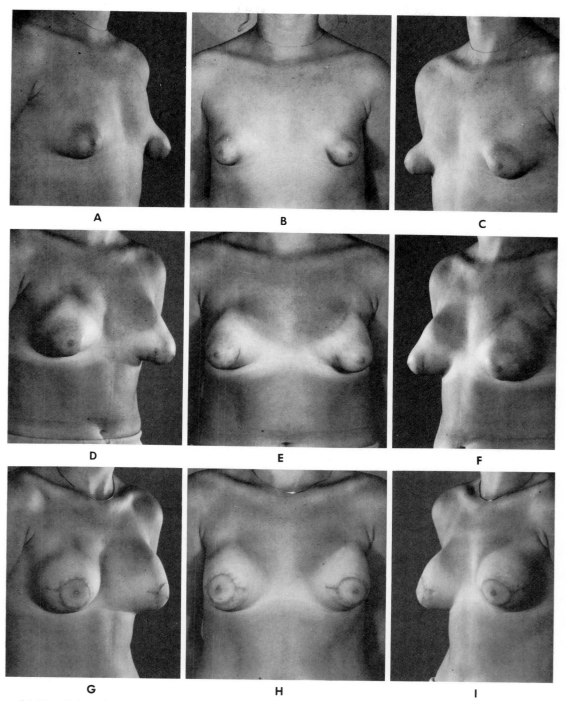

Figure 34–13. *A, B,* and *C,* Pure tuberous breast deformity.

D, E, and *F,* Breast tissue protrudes from anterior surface of prostheses four months following augmentation mammaplasty with 130-cc silicone-gel prostheses.

G, H, and *I,* Breasts have more "normal" shape three years following telescoping procedure described in text.

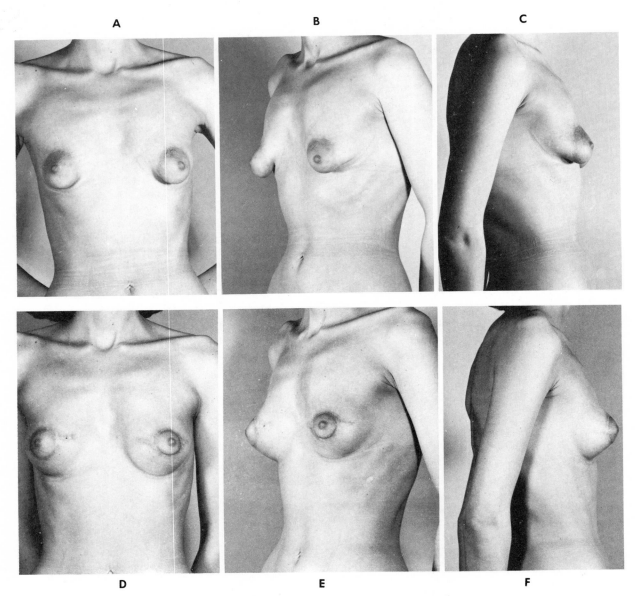

Figure 34–14. *See legend on the opposite page.*

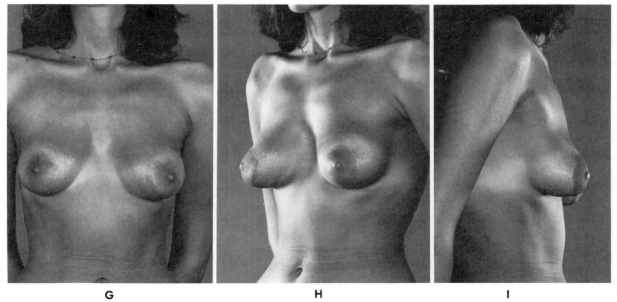

Figure 34–14.   *A, B,* and *C,* True tuberous breast deformity.

D, E, and *F,* Three months and (*G, H,* and *I*) two years following correction by technique described in text. (Courtesy of Cary L. Guy, M.D.)

skin flaps are elevated off the breast parenchyma circumferentially (Fig. 34–11*D*).

A prosthesis is inserted through an incision at the inferior aspect of the gland and placed in the usual retromammary pocket posterior to the breast capsule on the pectoralis fascia. Frequently, there is significant asymmetry in breast size, making inflatable prostheses the best choice (Fig. 34–11*E*).

The herniated nipple and areola are telescoped posteriorly, and the skin brassiere is closed with deep absorbable sutures and intracuticular sutures supported by interrupted sutures in the skin (Figures 34–11*F,G,* 34–13, and 34–14).

In the second type of tuberous breast deformity in which the areolar herniation is not a feature, retromammary augmentation with a prosthesis of the surgeon's choice may suffice. This simple step, however, may not correct the entire problem, since the breast parenchyma is foreshortened, particularly in the vertical dimensions (Figure 34–15) of its base, so that augmentation alone may result in a breast resembling a "whipped cream topping" on a dessert (Figure 34–16*A,B*). The total diameter of the breast parenchyma can be increased by incising the posterior capsule of the breast in a radial fashion from the center extending to the margins of the breast tissue. The radiating incisions help

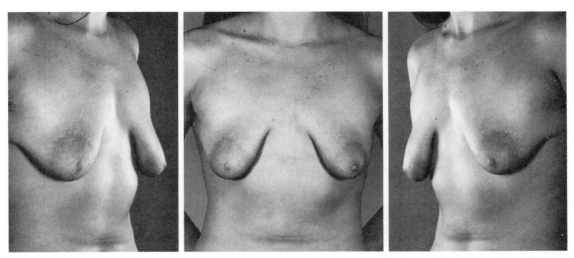

Figure 34–15.   The base of the breast is more deficient in the vertical dimension. The breasts literally hang from the chest wall.

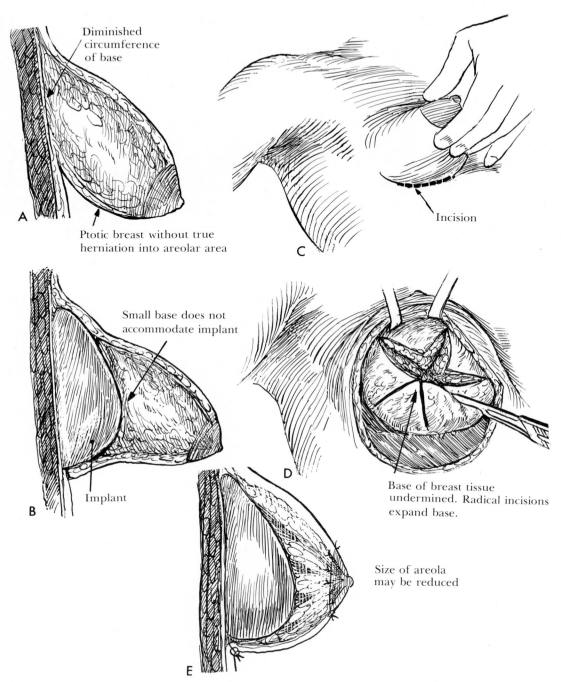

Figure 34–16. *A,* Diagrammatic representation of ptotic tuberous breast deformity (Type II).

B, Anticipated result with standard augmentation mammaplasty.

C–E, Technique for correction of breast deficient in vertical dimension.

C, Inframammary incision.

D, Breast dissected off the prepectoral fascia. Radial incisions into breast parenchyma permit breast to unfold.

E, Expanded breast tissue redraped over prosthesis.

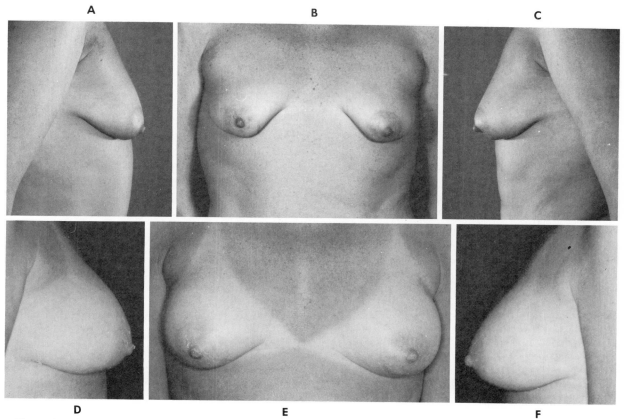

Figure 34–17.   *A, B,* and *C,* Tuberous breast, Type II, with short vertical dimension of base of breast.

D, E, and *F,* Result following technique described in text and augmentation with 165-cc, low-profile, silicone-gel prostheses.

the breast to unfold and become less tuberous in shape by expanding its base. The technique for correcting this type of deformity is as follows.

With the patient in a sitting position, an inframammary incision is outlined in the fold (Fig. 34–16*C*). The length of this incision must depend on the breast size and the necessary amount of unfolding of the breast. After the patient is surgically prepared, the skin incision is made and dissection is carried down to the pectoral fascia. Blunt and sharp dissection separates the posterior breast capsule from the pectoral fascia. Radial incisions are made at approximately every 60 degrees around the circumference of the base of the breast, beginning at the midportion of the dome of the posterior surface of the breast capsule and extending medially, laterally, superiorly, and inferiorly (Fig. 34–16*D*). The incision is made through approximately three fourths of the thickness of the breast tissue. The breast now unfolds much like parallel incisions in the galea aponeurotica, that permit further advancement of a scalp flap. Hemostasis is obtained and a breast prosthesis of the desired size is placed in the retromammary pocket

(Fig. 34–16*E*). Skin closure is carried out in two layers (Figure 34–17).

SUBCUTANEOUS MASTECTOMY AND AUGMENTATION

The use of breast prostheses to fill out the skin envelope following subcutaneous mastectomy has stimulated a great deal of interest in recent years. Rees (1977) reviewed this problem in detail and his findings are summarized here.

Indications for subcutaneous mastectomy according to some surgeons concerned with the problem of premalignant breast disease are (1) severe or progressive fibrocystic disease (usually accompanied by frequent biopsies), (2) intractable mastodynia, (3) extensive intraductal papillomatosis, (4) a high incidence of familial breast cancer, (5) unilateral breast malignancy in a young woman, (6) a suspicious or positive mammogram without gross clinical findings, (7) lobular carcinoma in situ (bilateral in 35 per cent), (8) multiple fibroadenomas, (9) giant duct ectasia, and (10) parenchymatous irregularities resulting from infection, surgical trauma, or previous biopsies. Authorities in breast disease disagree as to which pathologic conditions of the breast are to be considered premalignant, and the methods of exact diagnosis in patients with such problems as progressive fibrocystic disease are inexact.

Analysis of patients with breast pathology has shown that patients with multiple intraductal papillomas and/or ductal hyperplasia with atypia are in a "high risk" group for developing mammary carcinoma (Bader, Pelletiere, Curtin, 1970). Patients with multiple papillomas have an incidence of carcinoma 12 to 13 times greater than the normal for their prospective age group. Significant intraductal hyperplasia with microscopic atypia is associated with a higher potential for malignancy than are well differentiated papillomas. Indication for subcutaneous mastectomy in this group of patients is suggested by the occult carcinomas found in subcutaneous mastectomy and breast reduction specimens (Pennisi and associates, 1971). Pennisi, Capozzi, and Terez (1977) reported these findings on 419 subcutaneous mastectomies to the subcutaneous mastectomy data evaluation center established at the Saint Francis Memorial Hospital in San Francisco: lobular neoplasia, 65 patients; adenocarcinoma, 12 patients; infiltrating carcinoma, 11 patients; papillary carcinoma, 1 patient; medullary carcinoma, 1 patient. There was thus a 6.1 percent incidence of unsuspected carcinoma.

The adequacy of glandular resection by subcutaneous mastectomy is questioned by many. It is generally agreed that the usual techniques of subcutaneous mastectomy do not remove all glandular tissue (Freeman, 1969; Goldman and Goldwyn, 1973). Extensive procedures including removal of pectoral fascia and as much as possible of the subcutaneous tissue containing the lymphatics in the skin flaps have been advocated (Bader, Pelletiere, and Curtin, 1970). Removal of the nipples and areolae and replacement as free grafts have been suggested to reduce the amount of residual breast tissue (Horton and associates, 1974; Rubin, 1976). The potential for malignancy is considered to be reduced in direct proportion to the amount of tissue removed.

Modern breast prostheses have made subcutaneous mastectomy an acceptable alternative to simple mastectomy in properly selected patients. However, Peacock (1975) believed that the biologic principles of breast pathology are too little understood to make subcutaneous mastectomy an acceptable prophylactic procedure. Many surgeons with experience in performing subcutaneous mas-

tectomy and reconstruction with prostheses prefer a two stage procedure. The first stage consists of gland resection and skin tailoring. The second stage consists of mammary reconstruction with a prosthesis placed either subpectorally or beneath the skin flaps as the situation dictates. One stage procedures (resection of gland and immediate placement of a prosthesis) have been associated with a higher incidence of skin flap breakdown and implant extrusion (Kelly, Jacobson, Fox, and Jenny, 1966; Freeman, 1967; Grossman, 1973). Subpectoral implants have been advocated as a way of reducing skin flap problems for one stage procedures (Jarrett, Cutler, and Teal, 1978). Mladick (1978) warns against opening up a new tissue plane for immediate subpectoral breast reconstruction because of the relatively high incidence (6.1 percent) of carcinoma found in subcutaneous mastectomy specimens. When all histologic studies are complete, subpectoral reconstruction may proceed on safer grounds. All the usual problems of implant surgery may be encountered following this procedure.

Subcutaneous mastectomy and implant reconstruction is an acceptable and reasonable approach for the patient at high risk of developing breast carcinoma. However, few patients who have undergone this procedure are entirely pleased with their postoperative results. The breasts are often firm or hard from spherical fibrous capsule contracture and are frequently distorted in shape. Breasts may be uncomfortable or painful. Consolation lies in the belief that the likelihood of developing breast cancer has been reduced, yet the breast mound has been maintained.

BREAST CANCER AND PLASTIC SURGERY OF THE BREAST

Based on currently available statistics, it is not possible to establish a relationship between plastic surgical procedures on the breast and the development of malignant breast tumors. Data obtained by groups of independent investigators have indicated a lower incidence of breast carcinoma following augmentation mammaplasty than that in the general female population. Although it may be fallacious to assume the incidence of breast carcinoma is decreased following augmentation mammaplasty, reasonable interpretation of the available data indicates that there is no increased incidence of malignancy following plastic surgical procedures on the breast.

Maliniac (1959) reported breast carcinoma that developed in a breast following reduction mammaplasty using a free nipple graft technique. It was his opinion that the malignant potential in the breast had been accentuated by the obstruction of ductile egress. There are few hard data to support this opinion.

Snyderman and Lizardo (1960) obtained data on 5008 reduction mammaplasties operated by various techniques. Four cases of carcinoma were found upon preoperative examination. A frozen section diagnosis of carcinoma during the operation was made in five patients, and nine other malignancies were found upon permanent pathologic sections. In 2516 augmentation mammaplasty patients, three carcinomas were found at long-term followup. Two malignancies were found preoperatively, one was found intraoperatively, and one was found on follow-up examination in 1648 cases of gynecomastia. The overall incidence of carcinoma in the 9172 breast plastic surgery operations was 0.3 percent. Hoopes, Edgerton, and Shelly (1967) estimated that at the time of their review, over 40,000 breast augmentations had been performed. However, they were able to identify only six patients in whom carcinoma had developed following augmentation. The prosthetic materials used in these six patients were polyvinyl sponge, silicone sponge, RTV silastic, Cronin implants, Pangman implants, and silicone fluid injections. Hoopes and associates noted that approximately 2000 cases of breast cancer would be expected in the 40,000 females during their lifetimes. It was surprising that only six malignancies could be found.

DeCholnoky (1970) estimated that 50,000 patients had undergone augmentation mammaplasty by 1969. In a worldwide questionnaire study, he obtained reports on 10,941 augmentations performed by 265 qualified plastic surgeons. Eighty of the patients were in their second or third decade of life. Only one additional case of carcinoma was found to add to the six reported by Hoopes and associates (1967). At that time, polling of general surgeons with a great deal of breast surgery experience failed to produce other cases of malignancy following augmentation. Despite more recent reports of carcinomas occurring in breasts containing prosthetic implants (Perras and Papillon, 1973; Johnson and Lloyd, 1974; Franz and Herbst, 1975; Aston, 1978), there is no evidence that the incidence of breast cancer is increased in patients with breast prostheses. It is most likely that enough implants have been put in enough breasts in the appropriate age group over a sufficient number of years that the true incidence of breast carcinoma in all women will begin to appear in augmented women in the next few years.

Patients undergoing plastic breast operations should be carefully evaluated and examined preoperatively, interoperatively, and postoperatively. Mammograms should be obtained when indicated, as they may be of help in patient evaluation. Robertson (1977) demonstrated changes in postoperative mammograms following reduction mammaplasty with the McKissock technique. No doubt changes can occur on mammograms with any technique owing to the changes in the anatomy with pedicle folding and mobilization of breast flaps. However, none of the findings reported on the mammograms suggested carcinoma.

MAMMAPLASTY AND MAMMOGRAMS

There is considerable controversy regarding the indications or contraindications for mammograms in mammaplasty patients. Mendes, Filho, and Ludovici (1968) advocated preoperative mammography before all types of mammaplasties in order to have a record for later comparison. Perras and Papillon (1973) required mammography for any patient more than 35 years old before any cosmetic breast surgery and yearly postoperative mammograms for patients having subcutaneous mastectomy as a prophylactic procedure for premalignant disease. Rintala and Svinhufvud (1974) clinically evaluated the effect of augmentation mammaplasty by comparing preoperative and postoperative mammography and thermography results. They interpreted their findings as indicating that a correctly performed augmentation does not interfere with interpretation of postoperative mammograms or thermograms, and augmentation may even facilitate the interpretation of the films in cases of severe hypoplasia.

Cohen, Goodman, and Theogaraj (1977) used xeromammography to study five patients with saline-filled implants and five with silicone gel-filled implants. Their data "suggests that all breast prostheses interfere somewhat with the interpretation of mammograms, but that saline-filled implants allow a much better determination than do gel implants." They further concluded that xeromammography is a better diagnostic procedure than film mammography. The conclusions are controversial both in regard to the benefits of saline-filled implants and xeromammography. Either saline-filled or gel-filled implants can interfere with film mammography or xeromammography (Snyder, 1978; Wolfe, 1978). Pennisi (1978) and Wolfe (1978), in discussing the Cohen et al. article, emphasized the recently advised moratorium on widespread use of mammography in the belief that the radiation delivered by mammography may increase the number of breast cancers in years to come.

GYNECOMASTIA

The term "gynecomastia" was introduced by Galen in the second century AD. He defined gynecomastia as an unnatural increase in the fat of the breast in males. Although Galen was aware of glandular enlargement of the male breast occurring as a separate entity, he did not consider this gynecomastia. The first recorded description of a reduction mammaplasty was the technique of Paulas and Aegina in the seventh century AD. This procedure was designed for the correction of large breasts in males. There is no documentation that it was used in females. Letterman and Schurter (1976) and Simon and Hoffman (1976) have written extensive reviews of gynecomastia.

Gynecomastia may be defined as enlargement of the male breast owing to an increase in the glandular tissue. Collections of fat tissue in the breast area are considered "pseudogynecomastia."

During adolescence, it is normal for the male breast to undergo a small amount of hypertrophy. Usually, involution occurs before the age of 21 years. Nydick and associates (1961) studied the breasts of 1890 normal boys in a summer camp and found an incidence of gynecomastia of 38.7 percent in caucasians and 28.9 percent in blacks. Most gynecomastia occurred in the 14 to 14½ year age group. Gynecomastia persisted through two seasons in 27.1 percent of the cases and through three seasons in 7.7 percent.

Gynecomastia developing in a prepubertal patient must be evaluated for its etiology. A testicular tumor is a strong possibility (August, Chandra, Hung, 1972; Johnstone, 1967).

Breast enlargement in the adult male may be due to excess adipose tissue or a combination of adipose tissue and mammary tissue. A small discrete mass composed of periductal connective tissue surrounding mammary ducts and containing hypoplastic epithelium is found frequently in the adult male. It must also be kept in mind that breast carcinoma does develop in the adult male.

Gynecomastia in the late adolescent and adult male may be associated with various endocrine disorders including hyperthyroidism and hypothyroidism, pituitary chromophobe adenoma, acromegaly, and benign and malignant adrenal tumors. Testicular tumors, particularly chorionepithelioma, are found in association with gynecomastia. Teratomas and other interstitial cell tumors may also be associated with gynecomastia. The exact hormonal influence on the breast is not known. Gynecomastia also occurs with diseases of the liver and is frequently seen associated with cirrhosis. The administration of hormone is often associated with gynecomastia. This is frequently seen in patients receiving estrogen for attempted control of prostatic carcinoma.

Harmon and Aliapoulious (1972) reported gynecomastia following heavy use of marijuana in three young men. The major active component in marijuana, cannabinol, was noted to be chemically similar to Estradiol.

Klinefelter's syndrome includes gynecomastia and is associated with testicular atrophy with hyalinization of the testicular tubules. Absent spermatogenesis, markedly diminished or absent cells of Leydig, and increased urinary levels of follicle-stimulating hormones are also characteristic of this syndrome. The majority of these patients are chromatin positive and/or have a significant clone of cells with an XXY karyotype. A few have XXY/XY mosaicism. A relationship between breast cancer and Klinefelter's syndrome has been noted (Cuenca and Becker, 1968). Prophylactic mastectomy in all patients with Klinefelter's syndrome has been suggested by Becker (1972).

Treatment

The initial approach to gynecomastia in adolescents should be conservative. Increased breast size is normal and usually transient, lasting no more than two years. If gynecomastia is excessive or lasts more than two years, a full evaluation of the patient for possible etiology is indicated, to be followed by appropriate treatment of the gynecomastia. Gynecomastia in the young male is analogous to a breast deformity in the teenage female. The occurrence of an abnormality in a secondary sex characteristic at this critical emotional period in life, when the self image plays a major role, may produce significant psychologic problems if not corrected.

Numerous surgical incisions have been described for the correction of gynecomastia, including those of Campos (1942), Malbeck (1945), Maliniac (1950), Barsky, Kahn, and Simon (1960, 1964), Pitanguy (1966), Simon, Hoffman, and Kahn (1973), and others.

The majority of cases of gynecomastia consist of breast enlargement without excessive overlying skin. The authors prefer to use an inferior periareolar incision (Webster, 1946) from three o'clock to nine o'clock just inside the pigmented

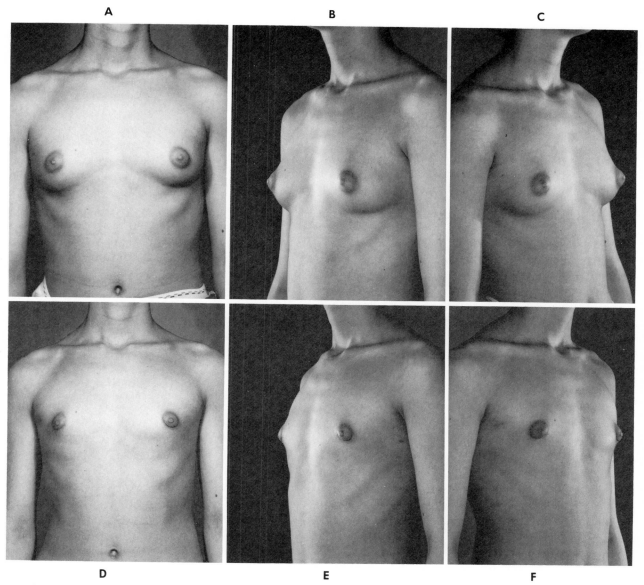

Figure 34–18.   *A, B,* and *C,* A 19-year-old male with gynecomastia and negative endocrine evaluation.

D, E, and *F,* Correction by technique described in text.

area of the areola. Large amounts of breast tissue can be removed by this approach, and the incision heals remarkably well (Figure 34–18). The two major technical points of this technique are (1) a thick nipple-areolar flap to prevent adherence of the nipple and areola to the chest wall and (2) beveling of the resection at the periphery in order to prevent an unsightly depression of the chest wall.

A perioareolar incision extending from three o'clock to nine o'clock at the junction between the hyperpigmented areolar skin and the surrounding skin of the breast is outlined (Figure 34–19*A*). A large volume of breast tissue can be removed through this semicircular incision without radial extensions. A radial extension at either three

o'clock or nine o'clock or both can be made if the volume of breast tissue is so large as to make removal through the semicircular incision impossible. The planned skin incision is incised from three o'clock to nine o'clock and taken down through the subcutaneous tissue into the breast tissue. A skin hook is placed on the cut edge of the areola, and dissection is deepened into the breast tissue for approximately 1 cm in depth (Fig. 34–19*B*). The breast tissue is then cut across beneath the nipple-areolar complex in order to fashion a button of breast tissue that will later be important to prevent a sunken flat nipple and areola on the anterior chest wall (Fig. 34–19*C, D*).

A plane is established between the subcutaneous tissue and the underlying breast tissue, and

Text continued on page 995.

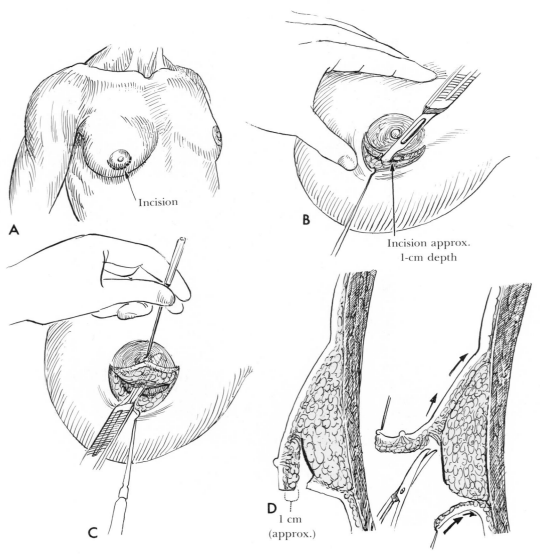

Figure 34–19.   *A* and *B*, Periareolar skin incisions from three to nine o'clock extended approximately one centimeter deep into breast substance.

C and *D*, Undercutting of nipple-areolar complex to leave button of tissue beneath areolar to prevent flat nipple and areola after resection of gynecomastia.

Illustration continued on the opposite page.

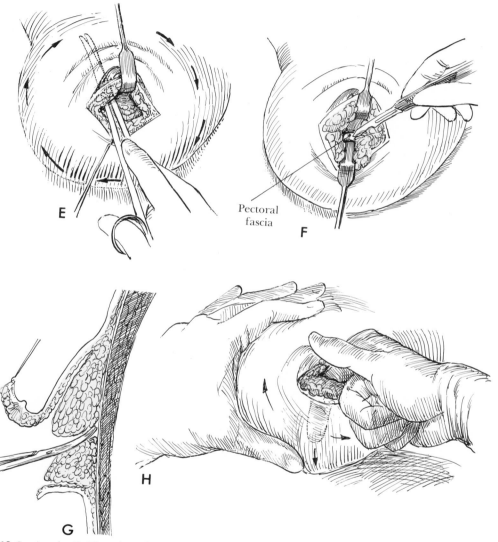

Figure 34–19 *Continued.   E,* Dissection of skin from underlying breast tissue in the subcutaneous plane.

F, G, and *H,* Parenchyma is divided down to the pectoral fascia. Finger dissection separates parenchyma from pectoral fascia.

Illustration continued on the following page.

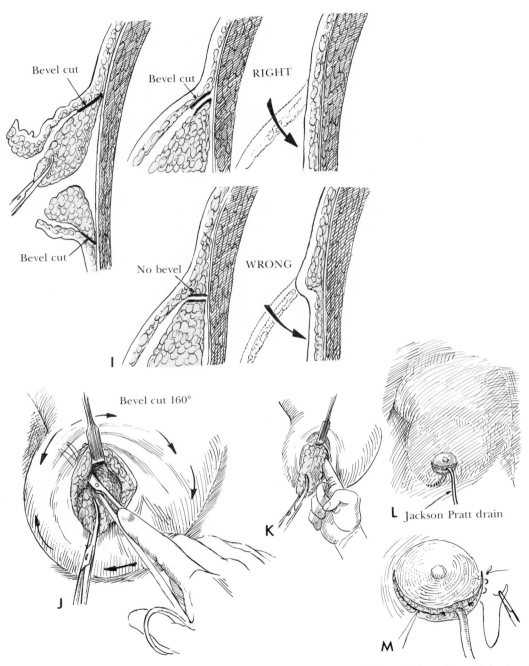

Figure 34–19 *Continued.* *I* and *J,* Subcutaneous plane of dissection and prepectoral plane of dissection are joined at the margins of parenchyma by bevel cut so as to not leave a step deformity at the limits of the parenchymal excision.

K, Parenchyma is delivered through skin incision.

L and *M,* A flat, vacuum suction drain is placed in the residual cavity, and the incision is closed in two layers.

dissection is made 360 degrees (Fig. 34–19*E*). The dissection plane is easily developed between subcutaneous tissue and the breast tissue in most patients. When the breast volume is large, it can be divided down to the middle of the breast to the pectoral fascia, establishing two separate masses of breast tissue to be removed. Small gynecomastia masses can be removed by beginning the dissection at the inferior pole of breast mass and then separating the breast tissue from the pectoral fascia (Fig. 34–19*F*,*G*).

Complete separation of the breast tissue from the overlying skin is the first step. Exposure of the pectoral fascia is obtained by dissecting around the inferior pole of the breast or incising straight down through breast tissue. Blunt dissection is used to separate the posterior breast tissue capsule from the underlying pectoral fascia (Fig. 34–19*H*).

At the margins of the gynecomastia, scissors are used to bevel the cut at the junction of the subcutaneous tissue and the anterior chest wall (Figure 34–19*I*). Failure to bevel the peripheral extension of the gynecomastia will result in a "scooped out" depression on the anterior chest wall. This deformity is unsightly and quite difficult to correct.

The breast tissue is delivered through the periareolar incision (Fig. 34–19*K*). When all the redundant tissue has been removed, hemostasis is obtained with the aid of electrocautery. Hematoma and seroma formation are the most common complications following gynecomastia resection. A small Jackson-Pratt drain is placed in the dependent portion of the subcutaneous pocket, and the wound is approximated with absorbable sutures placed between the subcutaneous tissue beneath the nipple and the inferior skin flap (Fig. 34–19*L*). The skin is approximated with intracuticular prolene sutures (Fig. 34–19*M*). The thickness of the button-of-breast tissue between the nipple-areolar complex can be decreased prior to wound closure if it is determined to be too thick. Failure to retain a button of adequate thickness will result in a flat depressed nipple on the anterior chest wall.

When the gynecomastia is feminine in appearance and redundant skin will surely be present following resection of breast tissue, the lateral oblique technique described by Dufourmentel and Mouly will provide an acceptable postoperative scar. Letterman and Schurter (1972) combined the Dufourmentel-Mouly lateral oblique technique with the Skoog superior medial dermal pedicle to support the nipple-areolar complex on large breasts. Patients with considerable skin redundancy are best treated with a transverse simple mastectomy and free nipple grafting. Most often, patients requiring this approach are seen after a massive weight loss.

(For list of references, see pages 1066 to 1071.)

Chapter 35

Breast Reconstruction After Mastectomy

JOHN BOSTWICK, III, M.D.

Female breasts are certainly a primary symbol of femininity. This focus is intensified by Western culture and fashion, which stress pleasing breasts as a basic aspect of a woman's attractiveness. The increasing number of patients requesting aesthetic change of their breasts has encouraged plastic surgeons to develop and refine techniques to modify breast size, shape, and contour. As the experienced plastic surgeon learns, the patient who requests breast surgery often has motivations that are more complex and involved than a simple increase in sexual attractiveness. There is usually a more deep-seated desire to improve general self-esteem, self-confidence, and self-assertiveness.

The woman who develops a cancer of the breast must face simultaneously the significant threat of death and the psychic devastation accompanying complete loss of the breast. This loss frequently evokes a decrease in self-esteem and concept of self and a general feeling of unattractiveness. Breast cancer is the most common cancer in women, and it usually occurs at a time of life marked by situational disappointments. This can add up to a very depressing outlook for the patient.

General surgical tradition has dismissed breast reconstruction following mastectomy as frivolous, unnecessary, and not in the patient's best interest. Women requesting reconstruction were often led to feel "ungrateful" for the surgical procedure that saved their life. The development of successful and reliable techniques of breast reconstruction in a carefully selected group of these patients has resulted in some of the most positive, rewarding, and dramatic improvements in self-esteem and

self-confidence that are seen in the field of plastic surgery.

HISTORY OF BREAST RECONSTRUCTION

Radical mastectomy for the local treatment of breast cancer was developed at the turn of the 20th century, and its primary proponent, W. S. Halsted, advised against the "plastic" repair of the defect (Halsted, 1907). Local treatment remained, and surgeons traditionally advised their patients against any form of reconstruction. The techniques of breast reconstruction during the first three fourths of this century did little to encourage the general surgeon to change this position. Breast sharing (Reinhard, 1932) and local and distant staged pedicle flaps (Gillies and Millard, 1957) required multiple procedures and usually fell short of a pleasing and satisfying reconstruction.

Many advances in techniques of aesthetic breast surgery such as reduction mammoplasty and mastopexy have been developed during the past 20 years. Scientific advances of silicone chemistry and the subsequent large experience with breast augmentation have given us useful material for simulation of a breast mound (Cronin and Gerow, 1964). Subcutaneous mastectomy (Freeman, 1962) and total prophylactic mastectomy with reconstruction (Horton et al., 1974) and the pectoral muscle and serratus anterior muscle flaps have advanced the techniques necessary for breast reconstruction.

Recent strides in reconstructive surgery, particularly the application of the latissimus dorsi musculocutaneous flap, allow a group of techniques necessary for breast reconstruction following radical mastectomy to be performed in one stage (Bostwick et al., 1978, 1979).

SELECTION OF PATIENTS

Selection of patients who are breast reconstruction candidates following mastectomy for cancer involves the same myriad of social and psychologic considerations used for any aesthetic surgery candidate. Basic criteria that must be evaluated are previous psychiatric treatments and the patient's and surgeon's concept of a successful result. As in all aesthetic surgery, the desired end result is a happy patient. Current techniques make successful breast reconstruction a possibility in virtually all women regardless of the extent of surgical or radiation treatment. It must also be understood and constantly remembered that local recurrence or appearance of distance metastases is a natural part of female breast cancer following radical mastectomy. Cooperation and communication with the patient's oncologic breast surgeon is essential in selection of the proper patient for reconstruction. A recent prospective study to identify breast cancer patients with high risk of early recurrence after initial mastectomy reveals several important clinical factors. In addition to patient age, menopause status, tumor size, and positive axillary lymph nodes, the degree of tumor differentiation and blood vessel invasion are important predictors of recurrence in premenopausal patients (Cancer Journal, 1978). A suitable candidate for breast reconstruction following radical mastectomy has a realistic understanding of the possibilities and limitations of reconstruction. The patient with a primary tumor with minimal risk of local recurrence is a good candidate for reconstruction.

Patients with a tumor less than 2 cm in diameter and with no involved axillary nodes or one should have the lowest risk of developing recurrence based on available statistics (Haagensen, 1971). Patients with more advanced disease have a higher risk of recurrence both locally and systemically, and these factors must necessarily be considered when the surgeons and the patient decide to attempt reconstruction following radical mastectomy. Most local recurrences manifest during the first two years following the mastectomy.

Many patients have indicated that they would certainly rather spend their last days or years with two breasts than without them, and it is difficult to deny these patients with a risk of dying of metastatic disease a chance to feel "whole" again. This is certainly an area that requires extensive communication and understanding among all involved, and each decision must be made on an individual basis. Assessment of possible distant metastatic disease is necessary prior to any breast reconstruction. This is best done in cooperation with the patient's oncologist or oncologic surgeon. There is no evidence that breast reconstruction affects the natural course of breast cancer. We do know its universally positive effect on the patient's self-esteem and general outlook on life.

TIMING OF BREAST RECONSTRUCTION

The woman with a carcinoma of the breast faces both the threat of the cancer and the loss of a primary female symbol. There is often a feeling of "panic" and severe situational depression. She is often relieved simply with the knowledge that breast reconstruction is a possibility after mastectomy. While most women would like to have their breast restored to its initial appearance at the time of mastectomy, primary reconstruction is probably not in the patient's long-term best interests. Radical mastectomy is accompanied by a number of complications such as skin loss, hematoma, and infection. Any of these would result in considerable difficulty if simultaneous breast reconstruction is undertaken. It is also advisable to define the stage of the tumor prior to reconstruction. This is possible only with assessment of the final permanent pathologic specimen.

Reconstruction at some time following mastectomy allows evaluation of the patient's reaction to the deformity and communication among the patient, her general surgeon, and the plastic surgeon. In patients with favorable tumors and minimal likelihood of local recurrence, the breast is usually reconstructed as soon as the mastectomy wound has healed and any local wound complications such as skin loss or seroma have subsided. This usually takes a minimum of six weeks. If the patient requires chemotherapy or radiation therapy or has a poor prognosis, it is advisable to wait one to two years. The author prefers that chemotherapy be completed prior to reconstruction.

Preoperative communication between the oncologic surgeon and the plastic surgeon can be very helpful and perhaps can lead to an earlier and less involved reconstruction. Position of the incision, preservation of the pectoralis major muscle, and uninvolved skin can certainly make the difference between the insertion of a breast implant and the necessity for major flap transposition.

TECHNIQUE OF RECONSTRUCTION

When breast reconstruction is being planned, the surgeon must evaluate the adequacy of the skin cover and the presence of the pectoralis major muscle and the anterior axillary fold. He must also determine the proposed size, shape, and contour of the breast mound. The proposed nipple areola reconstruction, symmetry, and potential malignancy of the opposite breast must be considered. A plan must then be determined based on these variables.

Breast Reconstruction with Adequate Skin Cover and Pectoralis Major Present

Patients with adequate skin cover and a pectoralis major muscle can obtain a pleasing breast contour with insertion of a silicone breast prosthesis beneath the skin and pectoralis major and serratus anterior muscle. The implant is inserted through the mastectomy incision. Usually, a 200 to 300 cc implant can be easily inserted. If a larger breast is desired, a larger prosthesis can be placed during a second procedure a few months later. Experience with the placement of the silicone breast prosthesis in the subcutaneous position under the thin skin flaps following radical mastectomy has shown eventual fibrous capsulation, intense firmness, and discomfort and distortion of the reconstructed breast. The subpectoral placement usually gives a softer breast and does not carry the risk of implant exposure and subsequent necessity of removal. In placing the implant in the subpectoral position, the most common problem is a high position of the implant. The initial dissection must extend well beneath the rectus fascia just below the pectoralis major origin on the sixth rib for 2 to 3 cm *below* the proposed inframammary crease. A serratus anterior muscle flap is used for lateral coverage of the implant.

The incision is usually made by excising a portion of the mastectomy scar but not in the area of the proposed nipple-areola site. An incision is then made between the serratus anterior muscle and the pectoralis major muscle, and the muscle flap is dissected from the deep surface of these muscles. The lower medial fibers of the pectoralis major are detached from the lateral sternal border. The implant is placed beneath the muscles and pre-

placed sutures between the pectoralis major and serratus anterior are secured.

With preoperative planning, most women who have a modified radical mastectomy can undergo reconstruction without a major flap transfer. This should make the procedure more attractive, and more readily available to the largest group of patients.

Reconstruction with Addition of Skin and Muscle

Patients who have tight, thin, or irradiated skin require the addition of distant pedicled tissue. Patients without the pectoralis major muscle have a hollowness of the infraclavicular area and anterior axilla, which generally limits their choice of clothing and which can be a more significant aesthetic defect than the missing breast. The development of the latissimus dorsi musculocutaneous island flap has provided a reliable one stage procedure for simultaneously replacing missing skin and pectoralis major muscle, filling the axillary hollowness, and re-creating the anterior axillary fold (Fig. 35–1).

The skin over the latissimus dorsi muscle is nourished by perforating muscular vessels from the underlying muscle. The entire muscle and its overlying skin will survive as an island based on its thoracodorsal pedicle. An ellipse of skin (usually situated beneath the brassiere in back) along with the entire muscle can be transposed anteriorly based on the preserved thoracodorsal pedicle and can restore the skin and muscle defect following a radical mastectomy (Figs. 35–2 and 35–3). For patients undergoing radical mastectomy, the flap is transferred as an island, after determining that the thoracodorsal pedicle is intact (Fig. 35–4).

The muscle is sutured to the divided insertion, the sternal and clavicular origin of the pectoralis major, and to just below the proposed inframammary crease. This ameliorates the infraclavicular and axillary defect and allows the implant to be placed entirely beneath skin and muscle. The skin island is sutured into the defect following excision of the mastectomy scars. A silicone breast implant is then placed beneath the latissimus dorsi musculocutaneous flap (Fig. 35–5). The author usually places the new nipple-areola and modifies the opposite breast at the same procedure. The flap donor site on the back is closed primarily. For patients who underwent a modified radical mastectomy, a skin island and enough muscle to cover the implant is transferred. This type of reconstruction has been predictable and reliable. The breasts have usually maintained their pleasing contour and soft-

Text continued on page 1005.

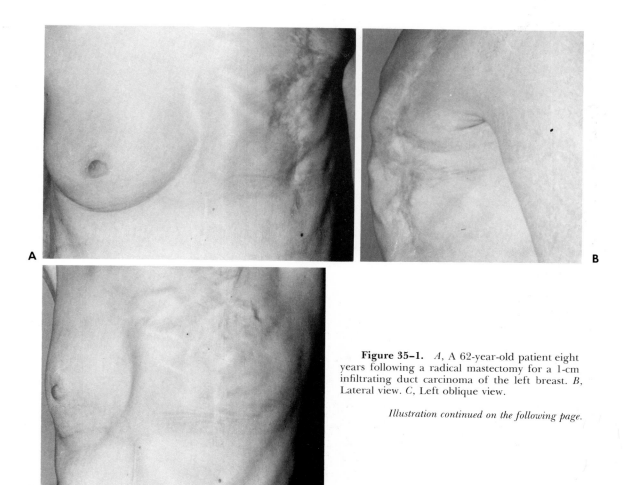

Figure 35–1. *A*, A 62-year-old patient eight years following a radical mastectomy for a 1-cm infiltrating duct carcinoma of the left breast. *B*, Lateral view. *C*, Left oblique view.

Illustration continued on the following page.

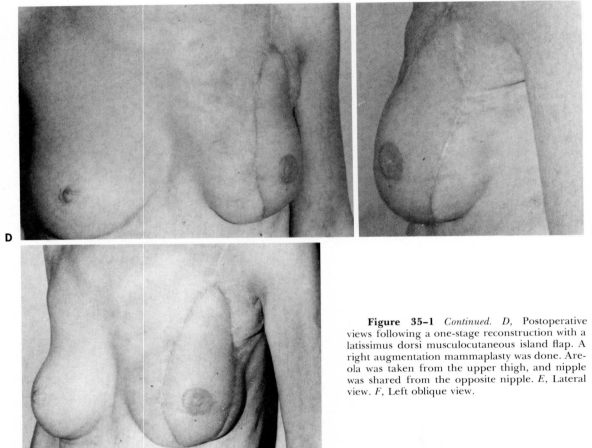

Figure 35–1 *Continued. D,* Postoperative views following a one-stage reconstruction with a latissimus dorsi musculocutaneous island flap. A right augmentation mammaplasty was done. Areola was taken from the upper thigh, and nipple was shared from the opposite nipple. *E,* Lateral view. *F,* Left oblique view.

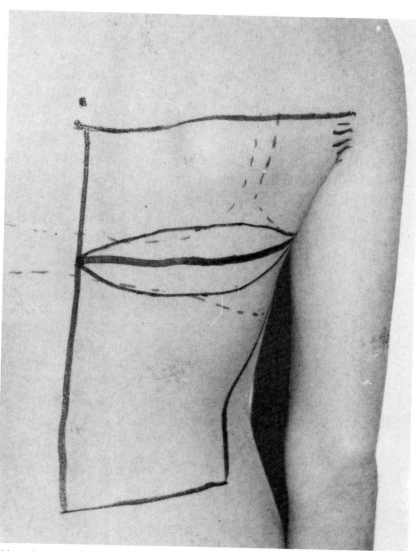

Figure 35–2.   Markings for the latissimus dorsi musculocutaneous island flap. The skin island is taken so that final closure is covered by the brassiere.

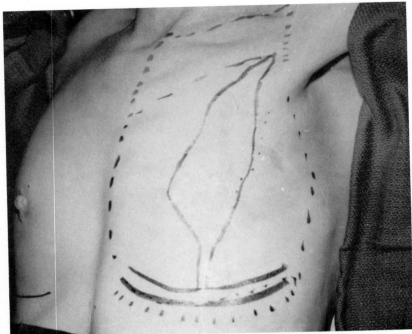

Figure 35–3.   Preoperative markings. The mastectomy scar to be excised. The mastectomy defect is recreated up to the clavicle, to the sternum and 2 cm below the proposed inframammary crease.

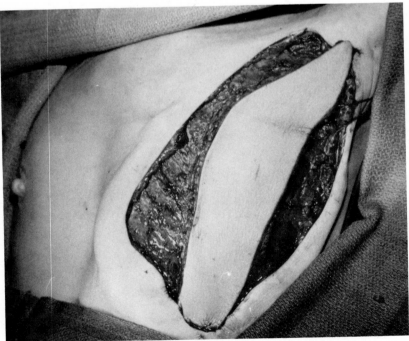

Figure 35–4.   The flap of skin and muscle is transferred. The muscle is sutured to the divided margins of the pectoralis major — the clavicle and sternum. It is also sutured to the rectus fascia below to recreate an inframammary crease.

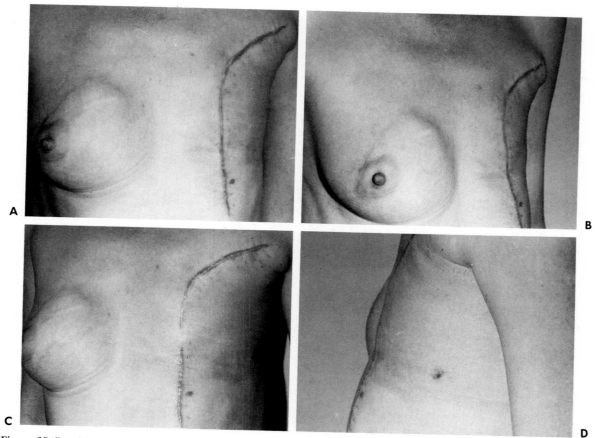

Figure 35–5. *A*, A 44-year-old patient two months following a left modified radical mastectomy for a 1-cm infiltrating ductal carcinoma with no axillary metastases. *B*, Right oblique view. *C*, Left oblique view. *D*, Lateral view.

Illustration continued on the following page.

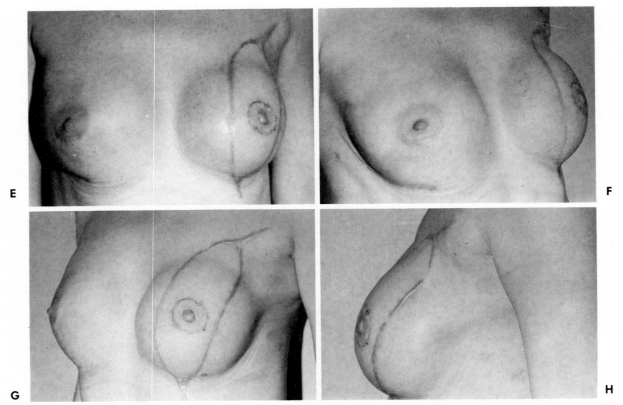

Figure 35–5 *Continued.*   *E*, Postoperative. The skin was replaced with a latissimus dorsi musculocutaneous island flap. A silicone implant was placed completely beneath the latissimus dorsi muscle. A right subcutaneous mastectomy with immediate submuscular reconstruction was done. *F*, Right oblique view. *G*, Left oblique view. *H*, Lateral view.

ness, and there has been no functional loss from transposition of the latissimus dorsi anteriorly.

In patients in whom the pectoralis major muscle has been removed but sufficient skin has been preserved, the latissimus dorsi muscle may be transferred without an overlying skin island. An incision in the brassiere line is necessary to dissect the muscle, and a second incision in the axilla is necessary to divide the insertion. The muscle is then transferred anteriorly and sutured to the divided ends of the pectoralis major insertion and origin.

The latissimus dorsi is now the first choice when a major tissue transfer is necessary. If the latissimus dorsi is not available because of previous pedicle division or the patient's decision not to have a back incision, the upper transverse abdominal flap is the next choice. This axial pattern flap based on perforators over the rectus fascia may be elevated primarily to the posterior axillary line and transposed to replace skin — particularly when there is a vertical or oblique incision.

Nipple-Areola Reconstruction

A mound on the chest does not look like a breast without a nipple-areola. The first choice of tissue for nipple-areola reconstruction is the opposite nipple-areola. If other tissue is used, the upper inner thigh is preferred (Fig. 35–6) rather than the labium, which usually is too dark. If a pink areola is desired, retroauricular skin is the choice. Tissue for nipple reconstruction from the earlobe and toe has been satisfactory. Augmentation of nipple projection has been obtained with auricular cartilage.

The nipple-areola is usually placed at the time of initial reconstruction, particularly if a surgical procedure is being performed on the opposite nipple-areola. Subcutaneously placed implants usually undergo fibrous capsulation, and it is advisable to delay nipple-areola reconstruction in these patients.

MANAGEMENT OF THE OPPOSITE BREAST

For breast reconstruction to be satisfactory, there should be symmetry. The current techniques of augmentation mammoplasty, reduction mammoplasty, and mastopexy are all necessary, at times, to obtain this symmetry. As a general rule, bilateral silicone implants behave more symmetrically than does reconstruction on one side when the opposite breast is shaped by mastopexy or reduction mammoplasty.

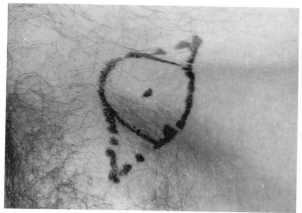

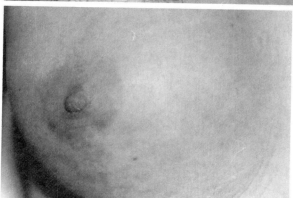

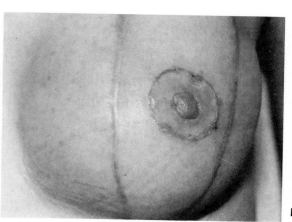

Figure 35–6. *A,* Areolar donor site—upper inner thigh (same patient as in Figure 35–5).

B, Nipple reconstruction from lower half of opposite nipple and areola from upper inner thigh.

C, Donor site from opposite nipple.

The risks of development of a second primary cancer in the opposite breast must be considered. Factors contributing to a second cancer are age, family history, the type of initial primary cancer (particularly lobular carcinoma), and pathologic changes. Communication with the general surgeon is helpful in planning treatment of the opposite breast.

Often, a prophylactic total mastectomy with immediate reconstruction is recommended. This is usually combined with reconstruction of the opposite breast, as it provides the best opportunity to obtain a symmetrical result. It is the one procedure that is attractive to most patients.

COMPLICATIONS

Local or systemic recurrence of the breast cancer is a part of the natural history of the disease following initial local treatment. Careful selection of patients based on the criteria of tumor type, size, and involved nodes reduces the number of patients who develop recurrence. A requisite of breast reconstruction is that the patient and a significant other person in her life understand the possibility and risks of local recurrence.

Capsular contracture about the implant and subsequent asymmetry is often seen following reconstructions. This is particularly common when the implant is placed subcutaneously. This complication has a much lower incidence when the silicone implant is placed beneath adequate skin and a functioning muscle. This muscle may be either the preserved pectoralis major and serratus anterior or the transposed latissimus dorsi. If the thoracodorsal pedicle has been divided, the skin island may still transpose over the atrophic latissimus dorsi muscle, supplied by collaterals into the latissimus dorsi. There is insufficient muscle to fill the postmastectomy defect completely. Division of the insertion of the latissimus dorsi must be avoided under this situation. These patients may benefit by a dermis-fat graft to the infraclavicular area to fill the defect. This may be obtained from the lower abdomen at the time of an abdominoplasty. It has been the author's experience that custom designed implants in the infraclavicular area usually develop capsular contractures and often require removal because of discomfort.

(For list of references, see page 1071.)

Chapter 36

Abdominoplasty

SHERRELL J. ASTON, M.D., F.A.C.S.

HISTORY

During the past eight decades, many operations have been described to correct abdominal wall deformities that resulted from laxity of abdominal wall structures, herniation of intraabdominal contents, adipose accumulation, weight loss, or a combination of these factors (Aston and Pickrell, 1977). Operative procedures in use around the turn of the 20th century were primarily concerned with hernia repair and resection of excess abdominal panniculus. They were accomplished by large full-thickness wedge excisions of skin and adipose tissue down to the muscle fascia, herniorrhaphy, and closure without undermining.

In France, Demars and Marx performed an extensive fat resection from the abdominal wall in 1890. Gaudet and Morestin (1905) reported transverse closure of large umbilical hernias, resection of excess skin and fat, and preservation of the umbilicus to the French Congress of Surgery. Desjardin (1911) used a vertical incision to resect 22.4 kg of skin and adipose tissue. Morestin (1911) reported a series of five patients undergoing massive dermolipectomy utilizing transverse incisions.

In Germany, Weinhold (1909) reported his experience with a combination of vertical and transverse cloverleaf shaped incisions, and two years later Jolly (1911) reported a low transverse incision. Shepelmann (1918) described a vertical spade shaped resection of skin and adipose tissue extending from the xiphoid to the pubis.

In the United States, Kelly (1899) used the term "abdominal lipectomy" to describe transverse resection of a large pendulous abdominal wall, and in 1910 he reported his experience with this technique used on eight patients at the Johns Hopkins Hospital. The incision extended across the midabdomen into the flanks, permitting removal of a wedge of panniculus adiposus, hernia repair, and wound closure without undermining. Thorek

(1939) described a technique, which he called "plastic adipectomy," for resecting "fat aprons" using oblique transverse incisions directed so as to meet at an apex on the fascia, thus eliminating a dead space when the edges were approximated. He removed the umbilicus en masse with the fat apron, and at the end of the surgical procedure, transplanted the umbilicus as a composite graft to the desired location. The success rate of umbilical grafting was not reported, but Thorek suggested the alternative of circumscribing the umbilicus, leaving it attached to the abdominal wall, and bringing the umbilicus out through the skin at the end of the operation.

The operations above were primarily aimed at relief of the functional problems associated with hernias and large pendulous abdomens. However, the cosmetic benefits were obvious. Kelly stated that "quite apart, however, from the tremendous physical and, in some cases psychical benefit, I personally recommend and would do the operation in extreme cases for the cosmetic benefit" (1910).

The early abdominal wall operations were the forerunners of procedures that have subsequently been described as "abdominoplasty" techniques and are mainly performed for cosmetic benefit. The vast majority of patients requesting abdominoplasty have much less deformity than the abdomens on which the early procedures were performed.

Numerous and variable abdominoplasty techniques have been described. The primary difference in all the currently popular techniques is the shape of the skin incision. The goals of all techniques are (1) to permit resection of excess skin, (2) to close muscular diastasis if present, (3) to tighten the aponeurotic laxity, and (4) to leave a scar that can be hidden under the smallest possible article of clothing such as bikini panties or a bikini bathing suit. Important factors in selecting a technique for an individual patient include the shape of the abdominal wall, the aesthetic and functional deformity, and the preference of the surgeon. Although skin incisions vary in design, they can be classified according to their positions on the trunk as (1) transverse, (2) vertical, or (3) a combination of transverse and vertical.

TRANSVERSE INCISIONS

Low transverse incisions of various designs are most frequently used. The necessary operation can be adequately performed, and the resultant scar can be hidden under minimal clothing. Demars and Marx (1890), Kelly (1899), Gaudet and Morestin (1905), Morestin (1911), Jolly (1911), Thorek (1939), Flesch-Thebesius and Weinhelmer (1931), Somalo (1940), and others helped establish the principles for more recently described transverse incisions. The early operations primarily involved skin and fat resection with minimal or no undermining of the abdominal wall.

Vernon (1957) combined a low transverse incision with two of the major contributions to modern abdominoplasty techniques: (1) undermining of the abdominal flap and (2) transposition of the umbilicus. Kelly (1910) suggested umbilical transposition but did not report having performed it.

Spadafora (1962) excised the lower abdominal panniculus using a transverse sinusoidal incision that curved downward from the level of the pubic hairline in the midline to below the inguinal fold and then extended above the anterior superior iliac spine laterally. The upper abdominal wall was undermined and the umbilicus was transposed to a new site. There is no significant advantage to this difficult to cover incision.

Pitanguy (1967) reported 300 consecutive abdominal lipectomies utilizing a low horizontal incision following the limit of the pubic hair growth, crossing the inguinal fold, and continuing horizontally to a point corresponding to a vertical projection of the anterior superior iliac spine, and then curving downward on the lateral sides of the hips in order to conceal the scars in the area normally covered by a bikini swimsuit (Figure 36–1). Curving the incision downward laterally helps compensate for the excessive length of the superior skin flap. In 1975, Pitanguy presented a series of 539 patients operated by this technique, and he reemphasized the necessity of either upward or downward extension of the incision laterally to compensate for the difference in the length between the upper and lower cutaneous borders. It is

significant that this report presents the largest series of abdominoplasties found in the surgical literature. Few would argue that Pitanguy has had the greatest influence of any single surgeon on the development of body sculpturing surgery throughout the world.

Callia (1967) described a low curved transverse incision that extended from the level of the pubic hairline medially to 2 to 3 cm below the inguinal crease laterally (See Figure 36–1) This incision is very similar in shape to that later described by Regnault. However, Regnault's incision is not placed below the inguinal crease. The advantages of the Callia incision are (1) the residual scar rides up into the groin crease postoperatively and (2) some tightening of the upper thighs occurs.

Serson (1971, 1972) stressed geometric evaluation of the abdominal wall and described a low curved transverse incision that extended down onto the upper portion of the thighs.

Graser (1973) reported 44 abdominoplasties, two thirds of which were combined with other major surgical procedures (vaginal hysterectomy, rhytidectomy, rhinoplasty, etc.). Graser's incision differs from that of Pitanguy in that the lateral extension of the skin incision beyond a vertical line corresponding to the vertical projection of the anterior superior iliac spine extends straight laterally as opposed to downward as originally described by Pitanguy (see Figure 36–1). Graser notes that the resultant scar by his technique always lies within the bikini line rather than extending beyond the inguinal fold onto the thighs. Graser's scars are somewhat more concave than Pitanguy's and follow the natural skin lines of the lower abdominal wall and the inguinal region.

Regnault (1972, 1975, 1976) described abdominoplasty by the "W" technique, which is designed so that the length of the lower skin incision nearly equals the length of the superior incision in an attempt to prevent or reduce any folding of tissue that might result from inequality of incision lengths (see Figure 36–1). Approximation of flaps is facilitated by advancing and gathering toward the midline the remaining difference in incision lengths that occurs because the upper flap has been widely undermined and the lower incision is fixed in length.

Baker, Gordon, and Mosienko (1977) described a template method of abdominal lipectomy using a preestablished pattern to outline the area of the dermolipectomy prior to undermining the remaining portion of the abdominal wall. In their opinion, this method (1) allows a more symmetrical resection, wound closure, and scar, (2) reduces operating time, (3) does not pull the mons pubis superiorly, and (4) eliminates the need for a vertical scar.

Planas (1977) advocated the "vest over pants" abdominoplasty, with initial incision extending from the umbilicus bilaterally and diagonally downward to the lateral extensions of a planned low transverse incision. The upper abdomen is undermined and advanced downward over the lower abdominal skin. The line of resection is made at the lower edge of the "vest over the pants."

An extensive transverse incision extending circumferentially around the trunk was described by Somalo (1940), revised by González-Ulloa (1959, 1960) and modified by Vilain (1964). The "belt lipectomy" was designed to improve simultaneously deformities secondary to fatty deposits in the abdominal, gluteal, and dorsal regions. This

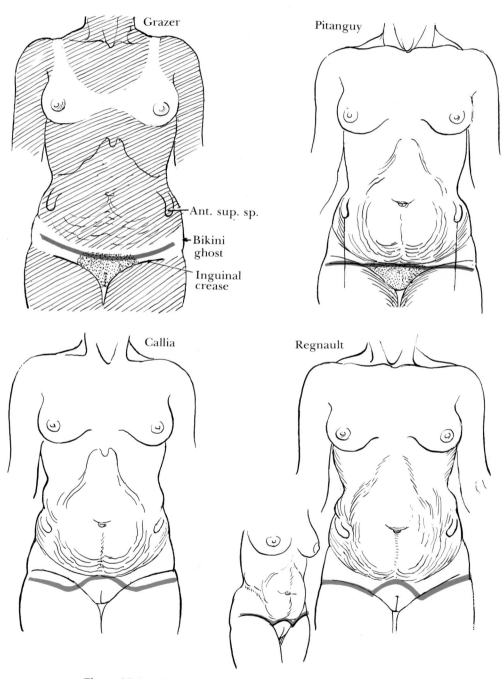

Figure 36–1.   The four most often used abdominoplasty incisions.

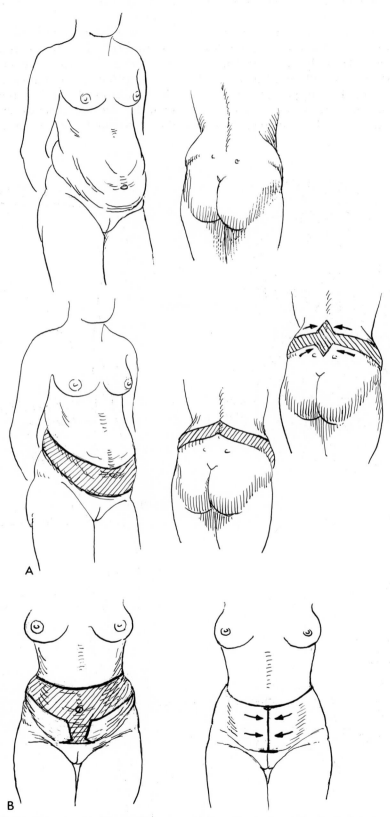

Figure 36–2. *A*, Belt lipectomy to simultaneously improve deformities in the abdominal, gluteal, and dorsal regions.

B, Modification of the "belt" permits vertical tissue excision when indicated.

technique is limited to special problem cases and priority for its use is low. Regnault (1975) described a modified belt lipectomy with vertical and horizontal excision of the abdominal wall (Figure 36–2). The umbilicus was maintained at the center of the excisions and the flaps were closed without undermining.

VERTICAL INCISIONS

Vertical incisions have been advocated when there is a large amount of horizontal excess abdominal skin and musculoaponeurotic laxity. Babcock (1916) described vertical ellipses of fat and skin with wide undermining and midline approximation in order to contour the waist and upper pelvis. Babcock wrote one of the few early articles that advocated wide undermining of the abdominal wall. His major emphasis in describing this procedure was on correction of the relaxed abdominal wall with the use of buried silver chain. Schepelman (1918) described a similar but wider vertical excision for dermolipectomy.

Rectangular vertical excision of the abdominal panniculus was described by Kuster (1926). Triangular wedges were then excised at the four corners of the rectangle.

Fischl (1971) recommended elliptical vertical xiphoid-to-pubis excision of "the crumpled tummy" that is deformed by stretched excess skin with numerous striae running in all directions. Fischl was of the opinion that the greatest amount of excess skin could be resected with a vertical incision and that the lateral-to-medial skin removal would produce a more desirable waistline.

COMBINATION PROCEDURES

At present, a combination of transverse and vertical incisions is mainly used when the abdominal skin flap cannot be pulled down far enough for the umbilical skin site to reach the suprapubic skin incision. Abdomens with a large amount of vertical and transverse skin redundancy or a massive panniculus adiposus are also best corrected with transverse and vertical incisions (Figure 36–3). The cloverleaf shaped excision technique described by Weinhold (1909) has been noted. Passot (1931) suggested circular periumbilical and lower midline resection of panniculous adiposus.

Galtier (1955) noted the importance of maintaining the umbilicus and described a technique of dividing the abdominal wall into quadrants, connecting symmetrical and equidistant points on the

quadrants, and resecting a star shaped section of the abdominal panniculus, leaving a cross-shaped scar. The umbilicus was preserved with a circular incision.

Dufourmentel and Mouly (1959) reported vertical and horizontal wedge excisions with slight to moderate undermining, umbilical transposition, and an inverted "T" shaped scar.

Castanares and Goethel (1967) described resection of severe cases of panniculus adiposus using a transverse incision two inches above the inguinal fold and two vertical midline triangles — the apex of the upper one directed toward the xiphoid and the apex of the lower one directed toward the pubis. Skin incisions are directed straight through the panniculus to the deep fascia, a block resection is performed, and no undermining is done. Wound closure as suggested by Castanares is performed with large Dazy buttons and retention sutures. The concept here is to remove the offending panniculus adiposus and keep operating time to a minimum. Regnault (1975) modified the Castanares technique and described a "fleur de lis" vertical and transverse excision.

Minilift Abdominoplasty. Limited abdominal resections, so-called "minilift abdominoplasty" as described by Elfaz (1971) and Glicenstein (1975), have very little use other than to correct very small amounts of abdominal wall excess skin.

PATIENT SELECTION AND PREOPERATIVE EVALUATION

Abdominoplasty, which is primarily an aesthetic repair of the anterior abdominal wall, is performed to correct deformities of the skin, adipose tissue, muscles, and fascia. Etiologies of these deformities are prior pregnancy, weight loss, adiposity, and previous surgical incisions. The vast majority of patients requesting abdominoplasty are females, although some males are candidates for this surgical procedure following weight loss. Patients with large abdominal wall aprons associated with obesity will not benefit from an "abdominoplasty." These patients require a direct surgical approach and resection without undermining (abdominal lipectomy).

Abdominoplasty has become a common operation. The reasons for this are (1) current society's emphasis on youth and vigor, (2) more liberal attitudes toward sex, (3) clothing fashions that reveal the body, (4) more time spent in leisure and recreational activities by all levels of society, and (5) the fact that in general, excellent surgical

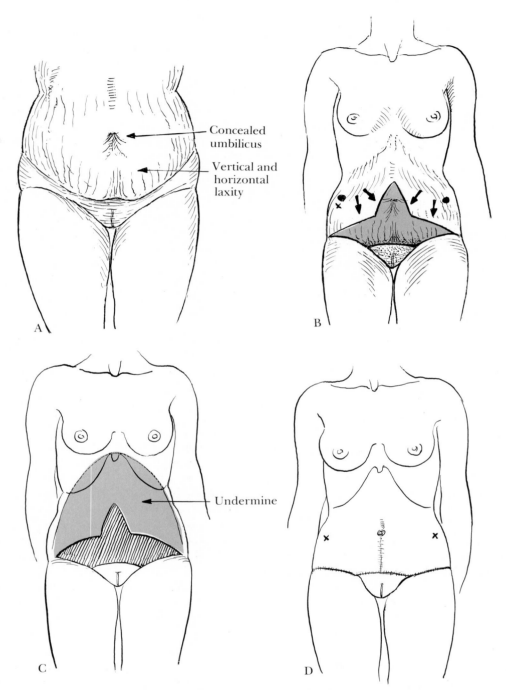

Figure 36–3. *A*, Large amounts of horizontal and vertical tissue redundancy require transverse and vertical resections.

B, Thick panniculus adiposus should be resected and closed without undermining.

C, When the adipose layer is thin or of moderate thickness, flaps can be elevated and advanced for closure.

D, The resultant scar is an inverted "T"

results can be obtained with an abdominoplasty operation.

Patient complaints are usually of two types: (1) when nude, or almost nude, as in current beachwear fashion, the striae-marred skin sags and wrinkles and the abdomen bulges and (2) in any clothing that fits the body contour, the abdomen protrudes. Social, leisure, and sexual activities are frequently limited in order to avoid the embarrassment of exposure of the abdomen. Most patients impose these limitations upon themselves, as they are rarely chastised by friends, husbands, or family members because of their abdomen. Occasionally, a patient reports diminution of sex life because her mate is "turned-off" by the appearance and "mushy feel" of the abdominal wall with these deformities.

The majority of patients requesting abdominoplasty have deformities that lie between the extremes of pure skin excess, "dermochalasis," and a fatty abdominal wall apron. Musculoaponeurotic laxity following one or more pregnancies increases the deformity. Vigorous exercise regimens will help increase muscle tone but will never improve the problem of skin excess, nor will it correct the postpartum "pot belly." Accompanying striae vary from a few on the low midabdomen to many extending above the umbilicus. Prior surgical scars may further increase the deformity.

The ideal candidate for abdominoplasty is normal in weight for her stature and height, does not plan further pregnancies, has the abdominal wall deformities noted, and will accept the inevitable surgical scars. As with all aesthetic procedures, motivation, psychologic state, and physiologic condition must be evaluated.

An abdominoplasty can be performed in conjunction with various other operative procedures, such as abdominal hysterectomy, vaginal hysterectomy, tubal ligation, cholecystectomy, ovarian cystectomy, herniorrhaphy, face lift, breast reduction, breast augmentation, and others in properly selected patients (Grazer, 1973; Hinderer, 1975; Baker, Gordon, Mosienko, 1977; DeCastro and Daher, 1978).

A carefully taken medical history is mandatory to point out any systemic disease that may contraindicate major abdominal wall surgery. Easy bruisability, prolonged bruising following relatively minor injuries, or other signs suggesting blood dyscrasia should be investigated. Prior transverse surgical scars in the upper quandrants of the abdominal wall or in the lower quandrants where they will not be excised during an abdominoplasty should be evaluated in regard to the potential for altering the vascularity to the distal abdominal wall flap. Old vertical incisions on the abdominal wall are not likely to cause flap survival problems but will limit inferior mobilization of the abdominal skin flap.

Abdominoplasty is contraindicated when (1) future pregnancies are planned, (2) the patient is psychologically unstable, (3) the patient is unrealistic in expectations of scars and postoperative results, and (4) there are previous abdominal incisions that will jeopardize blood supply to the abdominal wall flap.

Routine abdominal examination is performed with the patient in the supine position. The amount of excess skin may be roughly evaluated by placing the thumbs at the lateral borders of the symphysis pubis and grasping the abdominal wall skin between the thumbs and fingers of each hand. This assessment indicates the feasibility of bringing the periumbilical skin down to the suprapubic skin incision. Flexion of the hips further aids evaluation as it simulates the desired patient position for closure of the abdominal wall incision at the time of abdominoplasty.

When the skin of the periumbilical area can be approximated to the suprapubic incision, a vertical skin incision is not necessary. Striae above the umbilicus and in the flank areas will remain after maximal skin excision. However, the remaining striae will be improved in appearance as many are brought below the umbilicus, and stretching the skin makes them less obvious. The patient must be advised of striae that will remain after surgery.

The abdominal wall muscles are best evaluated as to mass and possible midline diastasis with the shoulders lifted off the examining table so as to tighten the abdominal wall muscles. The muscles and fascia are usually lax and diastatic in the midline. Occasionally, the muscle tone is quite good if the patient has been vigorously exercising in an attempt to flatten a "protruding tummy." However, aponeurotic laxity and muscular diastasis preclude the desired result being obtained by exercise.

The amount of abdominal protrusion, laxity, striae, wrinkling, and excess skin are also evaluated with the patient standing, as it is the deformities seen in this position that are often of most concern to the patient.

Informed Consent

The general details of the surgical procedure, risks, complications, and limitations should be explained to the patient in clear terms, in order to inform the patient sufficiently of the planned procedure. The patient can then decide if, in his or her opinion, the anticipated result justifies the surgery.

The exact location and contour of the planned surgical incision should be drawn on the patient's abdomen during consultation. Some patients may wish to have this drawn in indelible ink in order to show a concerned mate. Scar widths ranging from a thin line to wide hypertrophic scars should be discussed. The possibility of change in shape and character of the umbilicus should be pointed out. Preoperative and postoperative photographs of previous patients with similar deformities showing the range of results from poor to excellent may be shown. Photographs of patients used for demonstrative purposes should be used only with the patient's written consent.

Complications of abdominoplasty can be discussed in general terms, including infection, thrombophlebitis, pulmonary emboli, and death. The most frequent significant complications, hematoma and skin slough, should be noted as such.

Most realistic patients are aware that there are potential complications with any major surgical procedure before they are seen in consultation. A frank discussion of the factors above informs the patient of the risk involved with surgery and helps establish the kind of doctor-patient rapport needed should a complication occur.

CHOICE OF SURGICAL TECHNIQUE

The choice of incision and surgical technique for abdominoplasty depends upon the anatomic deformity and the surgeon's preference. Patients with excessive abdominal wall skin following childbirth or weight loss are usually ideal candidates for low transverse incisions, which can be hidden in bikini panties or bathing suits. The incisions described by Grazer, Regnault, Pitanguy, or Callia (see Figure 36–1) are excellent for this kind of patient. The gentle curve of Grazer's incision follows the natural skin lines of the lower abdominal wall and inguinal region and heals with a minimum of scarring. Lateral extensions to correct dogears are made straight laterally and are still hidden within the bikini pants line. The low horizontal incision described by Pitanguy follows the limit of the pubic hair growth and then crosses the inguinal crease across the vertical projection of the iliac spine. Curving the incision upward or downward laterally helps to compensate for the excessive length of the superior margin of the skin flap.

The low transverse incision described by Callia gently curves downward below the inguinal skin crease to help tighten the upper thighs. The open "W" design of the lower skin incision allows greater medial advancement of the longer superior skin flap. The "W" abdominoplasty technique described by Regnault produces near equal lengths of the upper and lower skin incisions in an attempt to prevent bunching and crowding of the abdominal wall flap that may result when there is inequality of the incision lengths.

Any of the four types of incisions can be modified according to the needs and preference of the surgeon. All the incisions will give excellent results when the surgical procedure is appropriately executed. In general, the author prefers an open "W" incision similar to that described by Callia, but with the lateral limbs of the incisions lying within the inguinal crease similar to that described by Regnault. This produces an incision that is quite similar to the Regnault incision except the "W" is more open than described by Regnault.

The degree of rectus muscle diastasis and musculoaponeurotic laxity varies among patients. However, all patients require musculoaponeurotic tightening. It is the musculoaponeurotic repair that (1) supports fascial weaknesses, (2) flattens abdominal bulges, and (3) slims the waistline. Inadequate musculoaponeurotic repair will lead to an unacceptable result.

Patients who have a thick layer of abdominal fat that is associated with a hernia or muscular diastasis require an incision that permits the maximal removal of abdominal wall tissue and musculofascial repair without creating and undermining abdominal wall flaps. The fleur de lis incision described by Regnault permits the largest dermolipectomy removal of the lower abdominal wall. The vertical portion of the fleur de lis incision can be extended up to the xiphoid process if necessary, and the width of the vertical portion of the fleur de lis incision can be widened and tailored as indicated. A "T" shaped incision can be used to resect large amounts of tissue from the upper abdominal wall. However, this will place a transverse incision on the upper abdomen in a location that will be difficult to conceal in some clothing. Patients with extensive lipodystrophy may require a belt lipectomy in order to permit appropriate resection in the abdominal, gluteal, and flank areas. This type of procedure is not within the category of abdominoplasty.

PREOPERATIVE PREPARATION

No aspirin-containing compounds should be taken for 10 days prior to surgery because aspirin decreases platelet cohesiveness, resulting in increased intraoperative bleeding. Patients taking birth control pills and other hormones such as estrogens seem to have greater intraoperative bleeding than others. When feasible, the medication should be discontinued 10 days preoperatively. A hematoma under the abdominal skin flap may be disastrous.

Careful bathing with pHisoHex for two days preceding surgery is advised. On the evening before surgery or on the morning of surgery prior to premedication, measurements and markings are outlined with indelible surgical marking ink. Markings should be made with the patient standing in order to (1) give better symmetry of the incision and (2) place the incision in the desired position regardless of incision design of choice.

The following markings and measurements are made to help in symmetrical undermining, flap division, dermofat resection, incision closure, and dogear correction (Figure 36–4): (1) vertical line from the xiphoid through the umbilicus to the midline of the pubis. It is noted if the xiphoid or umbilicus is out of line with the other structures. Asymmetrical abdominal walls are not uncommon. (2) The anterior superior iliac spines are marked. (3) Vertical projections of the iliac spines are drawn down across the inguinal crease on to the upper thighs. (4) A horizontal line is drawn passing through the umbilicus and extending laterally measured equal distance to each side. (5) A second horizontal line 3 cm above and parallel to (4) is drawn. (6) The planned surgical incision is marked and measured for symmetry on the two limbs from the midline. The length of the lateral extensions of the incision will depend on the amount of abdominal wall laxity and excess tissue. (7) Planned extensions of the skin incision to correct potential dogears are drawn and measured for symmetry of location and length.

The author's incision begins at the base of the midline vertical 1.5 cm inside the pubic hairline, extends transversely as a slightly curved line to the lateral margins of the pubic hair, turns inferiorly to the inguinal crease, and then extends laterally for several centimeters beyond the perpendicular line from the anterior superior iliac spine. The lateral lengths of the incision are measured for symmetry.

Following appropriate premedication and induction of suitable general anesthesia, the superior portion of the pubic hair is shaved to expose the previously drawn incision better. A Foley catheter is placed in the bladder to prevent intraoperative lower abdominal distension secondary to a full bladder and the need for the patient to move around in the immediate postoperative period to urinate. Antiembolic stockings or ace wraps are placed on the lower extremities from the toes to the midthigh to help prevent superficial venous pooling. Iodine surgical prep solution is used to wash the abdominal wall just before surgery.

The patient must be placed on the operating table in such a way that the patient can be flexed at the hips 100 to 120 degrees at the time of skin flap closure. With most standard operating tables, this is accomplished first by "flexion" of the table to its maximal extent, and second by elevation of the "back" to the necessary level. The lower legs should be 80 to 90 degrees to the thighs when the abdominal flap is sutured. It is helpful if the anesthesiologist is familiar with placing the patient in this position prior to covering the patient and table with surgical drapes. Care must be taken to prevent injury to the upper extremities when the operating table is flexed.

SURGICAL TECHNIQUE

The planned and marked surgical line is incised down to the muscle fascia along its entire length (Figure 36–5, A). Major vessels in the groins are avoided. The superficial epigastric and superficial circumflex iliac arteries should be cross clamped and suture ligated on the femoral side as they are encountered. The branches of the external pudendal arteries near the midline are small and can be electrocoagulated. Injured lymphatic channels should be electrocoagulated or suture ligated and injured lymph nodes should be removed in order to reduce the chance of a postoperative lymph collection. The abdominal wall flap is dissected with a scalpel or by electrocautery up to the level of the umbilicus (Fig. 36–5, B). The plane of dissection should be made so as to leave a filmy areolar layer on the surface of the muscle fascia rather than having the muscle fascia stripped bare. This reduces intraoperative bleeding, promotes postoperative fluid resorption, and cuts down on the chance of postoperative blood accumulation beneath the abdominal flap.

The umbilicus is outlined with ink and excised as an ellipse with the longest dimension placed transversely or vertically depending upon the shape of the original umbilicus (Fig. 36–5, C, D).

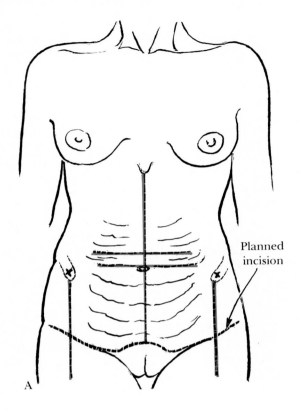

Planned
incision

Figure 36–4.   *A*, Preoperative markings include:
   (1) Xiphoid to symphysis.
   (2) Horizontal line through the umbilicus.
   (3) Horizontal line 3 to 4 centimeters above the umbilicus.
   (4) Anterior superior iliac spines.
   (5) Lower abdominal skin incision.

   B, The importance of these guidelines for flap dissection, draping, and resection is obvious.

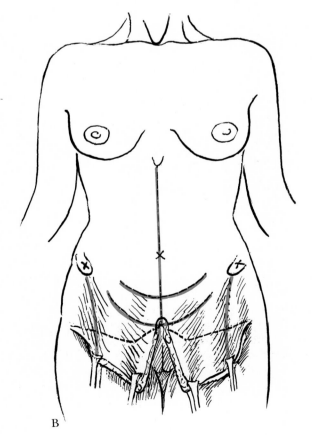

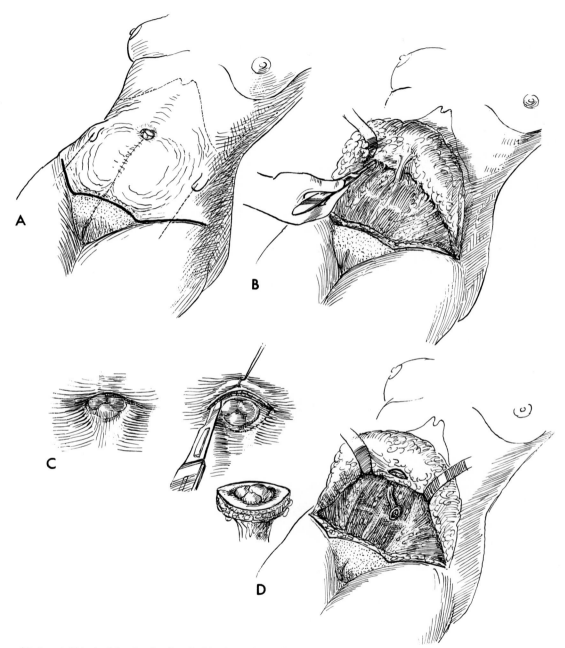

Figure 36–5. *A*, Skin incision begins just inside the pubic hairline and curves gently to the inguinal skin crease.

B, The plane of flap dissection leaves a filmy areolar layer on the surface of the rectus muscle fascia.

C and *D*, The umbilicus is excised in an elliptical fashion, either transverse or vertical, depending on the shape of the existing umbilicus. The umbilicus is freed from the abdominal flap.

The longest dimension of the umbilicus should not be more than 2 cm in length. Skin hook retraction makes it possible to excise the umbilicus with a smooth and symmetrical cut. A moderate layer of fat should be left on the umbilical stalk to insure appropriate vasculature for survival.

The abdominal flap is divided in the midline from the lower end of the skin flap to the umbilicus, thereby giving greater exposure for continued dissection of the upper portion of the abdominal flap (Figure 36–6, A).

Flap elevation is carried superiorly in the midline to the xiphoid process and laterally above the costal margins for 2 to 3 cm (Fig. 36–6, B, C).

An en bloc triangular resection of redundant tissues between the lower skin incision and the umbilicus is made when preoperative evaluation determines this can be done and permit satisfactory wound closure. The lengths of the superior limbs of the triangle should equal the length of the lower abdominal skin incision to permit wound closure without dogears (Figure 36–7).

Complete hemostasis is obtained with electrocautery and suture ligation of large vessels.

Diastasis of the rectus muscles is closed and musculoaponeurotic laxity is corrected by a series of buried horizontal mattress sutures (Figure 36–8, A, B). The midline of the muscle fascia is marked with ink from the xiphoid process down to the symphysis pubis in order to provide a guideline for symmetrical muscle approximation. The amount of plication indicated is estimated by grasping the muscle fascia with forceps in numerous locations along each side of the midline and judging the amount of tension that will be obtained by approximating the fascia from the two sides. When the rectus diastasis is extremely wide, the rectus fascia can be incised and closed in two layers down the midline. However, this is rarely indicated.

Midline muscle approximation should begin in the area of the abdomen where there is the greatest amount of laxity in the muscle fascia or the greatest amount of protrusion when the patient is standing. In some patients, the greatest amount of abdominal bulge is in the lower portion of the abdomen, whereas other patients have their greatest bulge above the umbilicus. Preoperative photographs available in the surgical theatre will be of benefit in confirming this decision. Regardless of where muscle plication is begun, plication must extend from the xiphoid to the pubis in all patients. Areas that are not plicated will bulge postoperatively.

Horizontal mattress sutures with the knots buried (Fig. 36–8, C) are placed approximately 1.5 cm apart from the xiphoid down to the suprapubic area. The suture material must have strong tensile strength but must be soft to reduce the chance of it being palpable in a thin walled abdomen. The author's choice of suture is 2–0 Neurolon.* All knots must be carefully buried; otherwise they will be palpable beneath the skin flap. The distance between each bite of the mattress stitch should be kept small to prevent bunching of the fascia within the suture knot, which will produce a lump that is palpable beneath the skin.

Approximation of the muscle fascia in the midline reduces mainly horizontal musculoaponeurotic laxity and to a lesser degree vertical laxity. When there is residual laxity of the muscular fascia following the vertical plication, a row of obliquely transverse plication sutures can be placed across the rectus fascia and into the external oblique fascia from the umbilicus to the iliac spines (Figure 36–9). This further reduces musculoaponeurotic laxity and helps slim and define the waistline (Jackson and Downie, 1978). Psillakis (1978) reported suturing the major oblique muscles to the rectus fascia in a vertical direction from the costal margin to near the iliac spine in an attempt to reduce musculoaponeurotic laxity further.

As the rectus muscle is sutured together in the midline and the fascia is plicated and rolled in, the stalk of the umbilicus is shortened as its base is rolled in with the muscle fascia (Figure 36–10, A). However, the umbilical stalk in many patients remains excessively long so that there would be a tendency for the umbilicus to protrude from the postoperative abdominal wall flap umbilical site. The necessary length of the umbilical stalk is judged according to the thickness of the abdominal wall flap, and the umbilicus is shortened appropriately. Permanent suture material is used to suture the stalk of the umbilicus to the muscle fascia with four quadrant stitches placed at 3, 6, 9, and 12 o'clock (Fig. 36–10, B). When the abdominal flap is appropriately thin, an identifying plastic button is temporarily sutured on top of the umbilicus with four quadrant stitches. Two of the stitches, in opposing quadrants, should anchor the umbilicus to the fascia to prevent it from moving about when the abdominal flap is advanced over it (Fig. 36–10, C). The button will be palpable through the abdominal flap after the lower abdominal incision has been closed and the patient temporarily is taken out of flexion. This permits exact determination of the new umbilical site after complete closure of the flap incision.

The surgical table is flexed, the back is elevat-

Text continued on page 1024.

*Ethicon Corp.

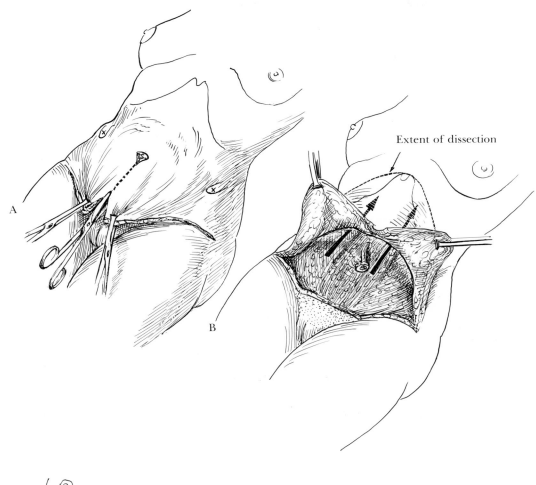

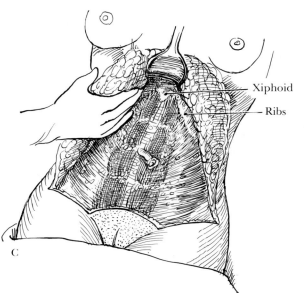

Figure 36–6. *A*, The abdominal flap is divided in the midline from the inferior margin of the skin flap up to the umbilicus. *B* and *C*, Dissection is continued superiorly above the costal margins and to the xiphoid process in the midline. Symmetrical dissection along the lateral margins of the abdominal skin flap is important.

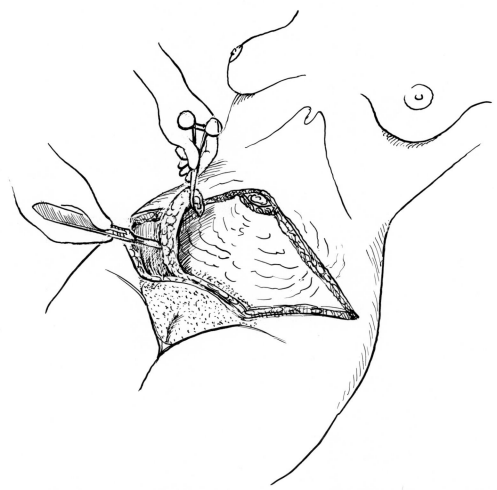

Figure 36–7.   When possible, en bloc triangular resection of redundant tissues expedites the operation.

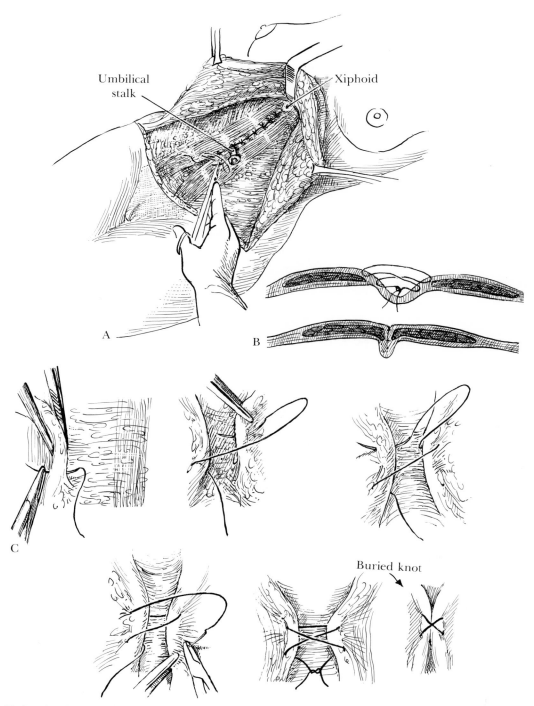

Figure 36–8. *A* and *B*, The midline of the abdominal fascia from the xiphoid process to symphysis pubis is marked with ink. Horizontal buried mattress sutures correct the fascial laxity.

C, Horizontal mattress sutures are placed with the knots buried beneath the approximated muscle fascia to prevent palpable knots postoperatively. The method of placing the buried knots is demonstrated.

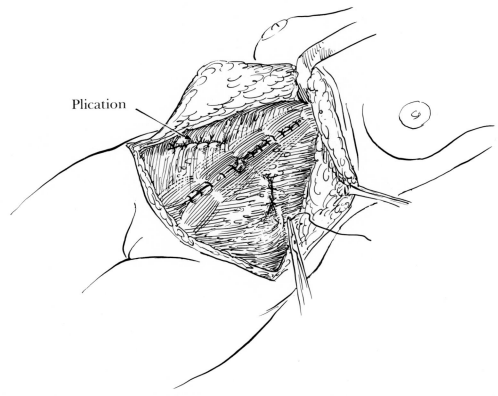

Plication

Figure 36–9.   Bilateral oblique transverse plication sutures can be placed across the rectus fascia and into the external oblique fascia from the umbilicus to the iliac spines when laxity of the abdominal wall musculature persists following vertical muscle approximation.

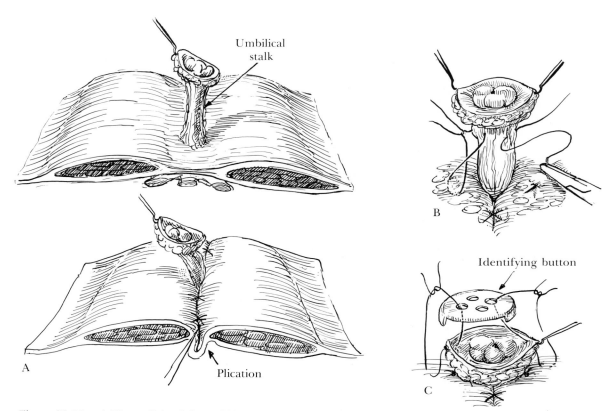

Figure 36–10. *A,* The pedicle of the umbilicus is shortened as its base is rolled in with plication of the muscle fascia.

B, When the umbilical pedicle continues to be longer than appropriate for the thickness of the abdominal flap, the umbilicus is shortened by suturing to the abdominal wall fascia with permanent sutures.

C, If the abdominal wall flap is thin, an identifying plastic button can be sutured to the umbilicus for ease in determining the umbilical site following closure of the abdominal wall skin flap. Temporary fixation sutures secure the button to the abdominal fascia adjacent to the umbilicus to prevent displacement when the abdominal flap is drawn inferiorly.

ed, and knees are raised to place the patient in flexion at the hips in order to approximate the old umbilical site to the suprapubic skin incision site without excess tension (Figure 36–11, *A*). The angle of the trunk to the thighs is usually 100 to 110 degrees but occasionally it must be 90 degrees. Equal traction is placed on the two halves of the divided abdominal wall flap as it is advanced downward (Figure 36–11, *B*). A temporary tacking suture is placed between the suprapubic skin, underlying abdominal wall fascia, and the skin flap in

order to secure the abdominal flap to its new position (Figure 36–11, *C*).

Symmetrical traction and resection of the two halves of the abdominal wall skin flap is facilitated by the preoperative horizontal markings placed on the abdominal skin. The direction of pull on the two halves of the split abdominal flap is downward and medial. Excess abdominal flap is measured and marked from the midline laterally by advancing the pubic and inguinal soft tissues upward while the flap is being pulled down (Figure 36–12,

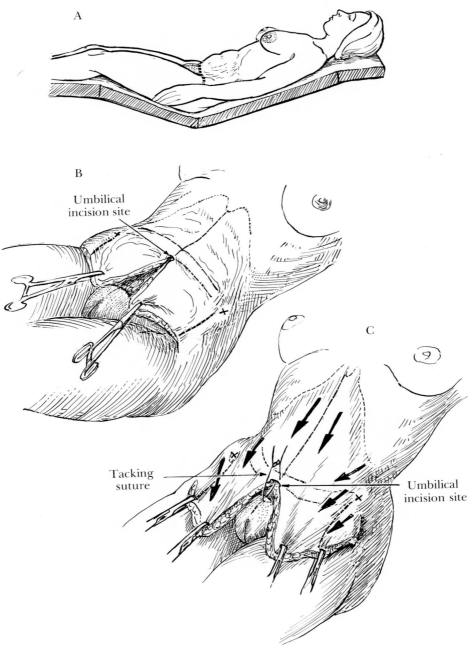

Figure 36–11.   The surgical table is flexed under the hips, back elevated, and knees raised. The angle of trunk to thighs is 100 to 110 degrees for flap closure. The old umbilical site is advanced to the midline symphysis marking and fixed with a temporary suture.

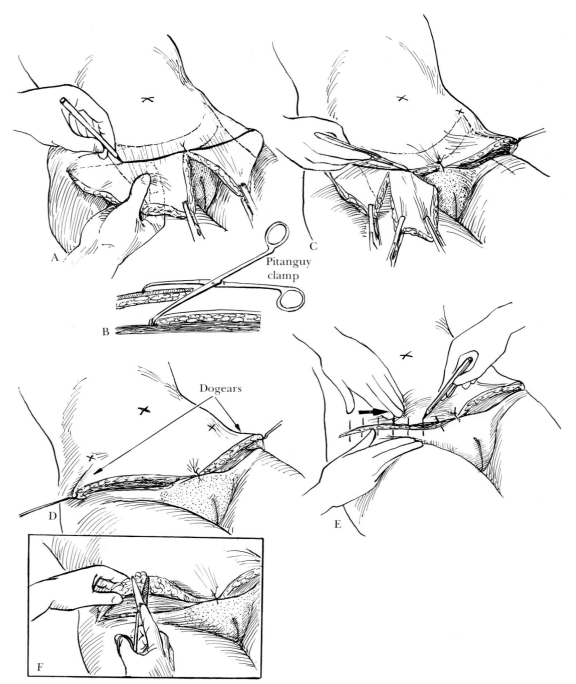

Figure 36–12. *A,* Preoperative markings assist symmetrical inferior and medial traction on the divided flap halves and symmetrical flap resection.

B, The Pitanguy clamp is useful in marking flap resections.

C, The halves of excess abdominal flap are further divided and resected.

D and *E,* Small dogears at the lateral limit of abdominal flap resection are removed by medial advancement of the abdominal flap and, if necessary, lateral extensions of the primary incision.

F, Fat is resected along the edge of the abdominal flap to correct discrepancy in thickness between the abdominal flap and suprapubic and inguinal skin edges.

A). The Pitanguy marking clamp (Fig. 36–12, *B*) is useful for making this determination, but it is also easily accomplished by manual flap manipulation. Excessive traction on the abdominal flap must be avoided.

When the two triangles of excess abdominal wall flap have been marked bilaterally, the triangles are further divided in half in order to facilitate symmetrical resection (Fig. 36–12, *C*). Small dogears at the lateral most extent of the resection of the abdominal wall flap are frequently removed by medial advancement of the lateral portion of the abdominal wall flap as it is sutured in position (Fig. 36–12, *D*). The open "W" lower skin incision permits this reduction in discrepancy between the lengths of the upper and lower skin incisions. When necessary, dogears are excised by appropriately directed lateral extensions of the primary incision.

The abdominal flap and the inguinal and suprapubic tissues are adjusted into position, where they should be approximated, and ink markings are made across the two skin edges (Fig. 36–12, *E*). Symmetrical markings on the two sides of the midline assure symmetrical flap suturing.

Fat along the lower edge of the abdominal wall skin flap is beveled so as to reduce the discrepancy between the thickness of the abdominal wall flap and the inguinal and suprapubic skin edges (Fig. 36–12, *F*). This is important in preventing a postoperative bulge along the incision line.

Some patients will not have enough excess skin between the umbilicus and the suprapubic skin incisions to permit moving the old umbilical site down to the suprapubic incision. In these patients, the old umbilical site must be changed to a small vertical ellipse and sutured in the subcutaneous and fat layer with an absorbable suture, with the skin approximated with an intracuticular Prolene suture (Figure 36–13). This will leave a small vertical incision on the lower abdomen, which is not desirable but is not usually objectionable. Patients should be advised of this possibility whenever there is any question as to the amount of excess skin. Occasionally, the preoperative evaluation may be misleading in terms of the amount of dermolipomatous excess.

Jackson-Pratt drains are placed beneath the abdominal wall skin flap through two small stab incisions made inside the pubic hair (Figure 36–14, *A*). A mosquito clamp is placed through the stab incisions and a Jackson-Pratt drain is pulled through the skin and placed in the desired position beneath the abdominal wall flap. This permits complete closure of the abdominal skin incision without drain sites. The pubic hair will hide the small scars left at the stab wounds. The drains permit removal of serosanguinous fluid or lymphatic fluid that may collect beneath the abdominal wall flap during the first 24 to 48 hours after surgery.

The abdominal wall skin flap is sutured into position in three layers. Five sutures of 2–0 Neurolon are placed between the lower edge of the abdominal flap and the lower abdominal wall fascia in order to anchor the abdominal flap securely in position and to prevent pulling up of the pubic hairline and groin skin in the postoperative course

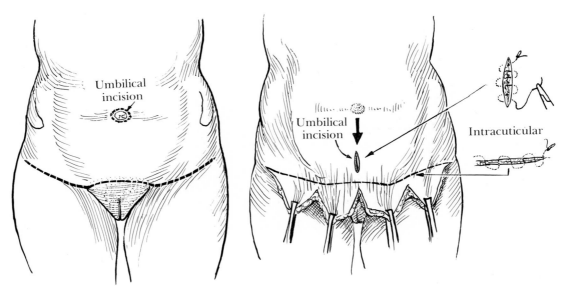

Figure 36–13. When the abdominal skin is not sufficiently redundant to permit transposition of the umbilical site to the suprapubic skin incision, the original umbilical site is converted to a vertical ellipse.

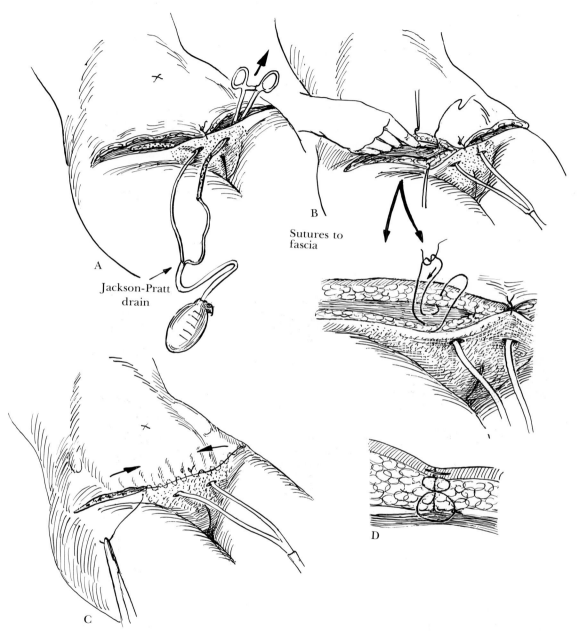

Figure 36–14. *A,* Drains are placed through small stab incisions within the pubic hair. The scars are hidden by hair when healed.

B, To prevent postoperative upward migration of the pubic hairline and inguinal skin, the lower edge of the abdominal flap is sutured to muscle fascia with several permanent sutures.

C and *D,* Subcutaneous tissue is sutured with absorbable suture material, and the skin is approximated with intracuticular Prolene.

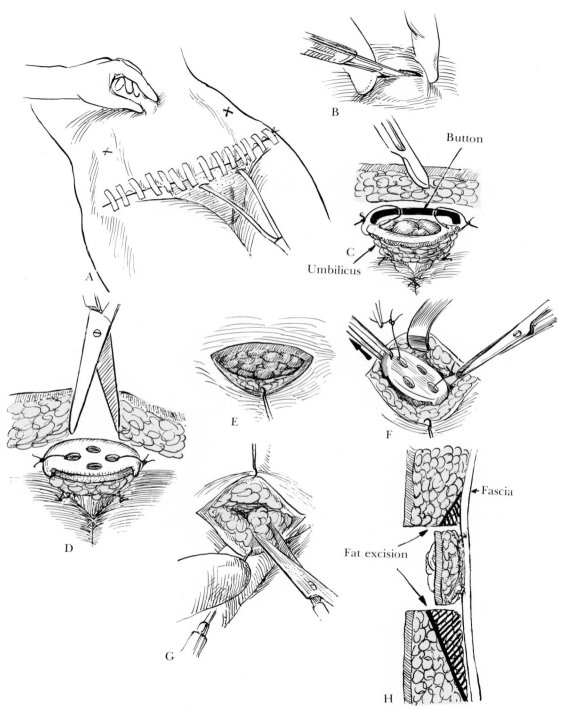

Figure 36–15. *A,* The surgical table is fully straightened until there is no flexion at the hips for accurate positioning of the abdominal flap over the underlying umbilicus. The plastic button is palpated.

B and *C,* A 1.5- to 1.75-cm incision is made through the skin and into subcutaneous tissue.

D and *E,* Skin hook retraction and scissor dissection expose the plastic button.

F, Temporary fixation sutures holding the button to the umbilicus and muscle fascia are removed.

G and *H,* An "inny" belly button with a small hood is fashioned by excising a greater amount of fat inferiorly and a lesser amount superior to the new umbilical site.

(Fig. 36–14, *B*). The subcutaneous tissue is sutured with absorbable sutures of 3–0 chromic catgut and the skin is approximated with an intracuticular 3–0 Prolene suture (Fig. 36–14, *C, D*). The skin incision is supported with steristrips and the patient is straightened out for accurate localization of the umbilicus.

Palpation of the abdominal wall locates the identifying button and determines the exact location of the new umbilical site (Figure 36–15, *A*). A 1.5 cm transverse incision, centered across the preoperative midline marking, is drawn directly over the identifying button. It is not necessary to curve this incision, as the traction on the abdominal wall will open the transverse incision to an ellipse. A single cut with the scalpel is made through skin and subcutaneous tissue over the button (Fig. 36–15, *B, C*). Skin hook retraction and spreading through the fat layer with small scissors easily locate the underlying button on the umbilicus (Fig. 36–15, *D, E*).

Sutures holding the button to the fascia and the umbilicus are cut, and the umbilicus is lifted by a skin hook into the incision (Fig. 36–15, *F*). The mobility of the umbilicus and its relationship to the thickness of the abdominal wall flap are determined. The umbilicus is released and the recipient site is prepared.

In patients with thick abdominal walls, the button may be difficult to palpate. In these patients, it is easier to find the new location of the umbilicus by straightening out the table and using bimanual determination prior to complete closure of the abdominal flap incision (Figure 36–16). Grazer (1973) suggested visualizing the umbilicus with the aid of a fiberoptic retractor placed under the anchored skin flap and passing a needle through the abdominal flap into the umbilicus, thus determining its position in the abdominal flap. Preoperative midline marking is helpful in centering the umbilicus.

With skin hook retraction for exposure, fat is excised from the underneath side of the abdominal wall flap superiorly and inferiorly to the new umbilical site (see Fig. 36–15, *G*). A greater amount of fat is excised below and a lesser amount is removed above the umbilical site in order to help create a small hood effect over the top of the umbilicus (see Fig. 36–15, *H*). The lateral sides of the umbilical site are likewise trimmed of fat in order to smooth out the contour between the superior and inferior fat resections.

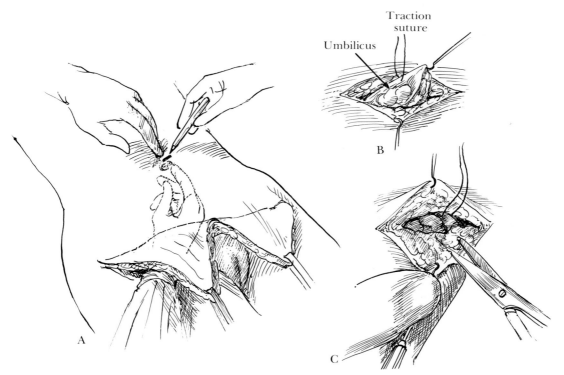

Figure 36–16. *A,* When the abdominal flap is too thick to permit palpation of an underlying button for umbilicus placement, the new site must be determined prior to flap suturing.

B and *C,* A temporary traction suture placed in the umbilicus permits return to abdominal flap closure. The new umbilical site is then prepared, and the umbilicus is sutured into position as described in Figures 36–15 and 36–17.

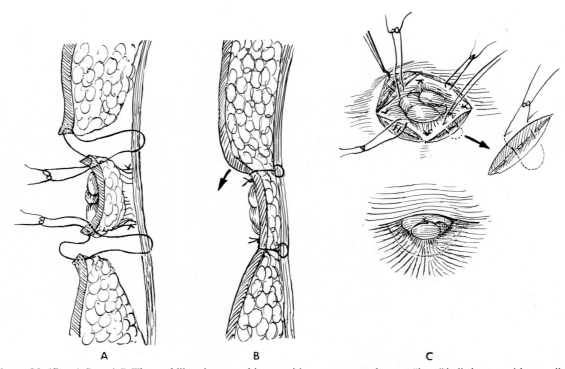

Figure 36–17. *A*, *B*, and *C*, The umbilicus is sutured into position so as to produce an "inny" belly button with a small superior hood and minimal scarring.

The goals of the umbilical reconstruction are (1) a nonprotruding umbilicus, (2) no suture marks surrounding the umbilicus, (3) a minimal periumbilical scar and (4) a small natural appearing hood over the upper half of an "inny belly button." The technique is as follows: Quadrant sutures are placed at 12, 3, 6, and 9 o'clock. The sutures go through the skin of the umbilicus and the superior portion of the umbilical stalk, then into the underlying muscle fascia, next intradermally in the abdominal skin but not piercing the epidermis, and then back into the dermis of the umbilicus and out through the epidermis (Figure 36–17, A). A suture placed in this manner produces a stitch that brings the umbilicus and the abdominal wall skin down to the muscle fascia, joins the abdominal wall skin to the umbilical skin, and places the knot, when tied, on the inside of the umbilical crater. Each of the quadrant sutures is placed and left

long. When all four sutures are in place, they are tied; an assistant provides pressure on the abdominal wall flap to reduce the tension and the chance of breaking a suture (Fig. 36–17, B). Small half buried mattress sutures of 5–0 nylon are placed from the umbilical skin into the dermis of the abdominal wall skin and tied (Fig. 36–17, C).

Placement of the sutures between the umbilicus and the abdominal wall as described provides good epithelial approximation, reducing the chance of a scar. No suture marks are placed on the periumbilical skin, and the suture marks inside the crater of the umbilicus heal readily and are not visible once healing is complete. Other techniques of umbilical plasty have been described by Baroudi (1975), Avelar (1978), and Freeman and Wiener (1978).

A small Telfa or folded gauze dressing is placed over the suture line. No plaster cast or wrap

A   B   C

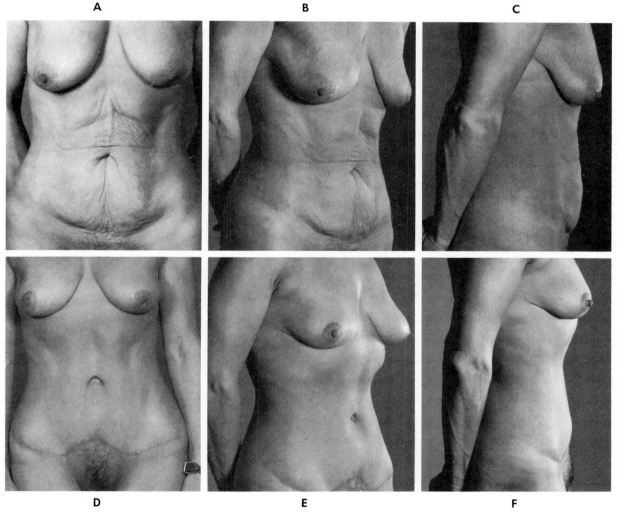

D   E   F

Figure 36–18. *A, B,* and *C,* A 45-year-old patient with dermolipomatous redundancy and slight midline rectus muscle separation following two full-term pregnancies and a recent 20-pound weight loss. Muscle tone was good due to vigorous exercise regimen. Also there is third-degree mammary ptosis.

D, E, and *F,* Twelve months following abdominoplasty by open "W" technique and mastopexy. The umbilical "hood" is similar to that present preoperatively.

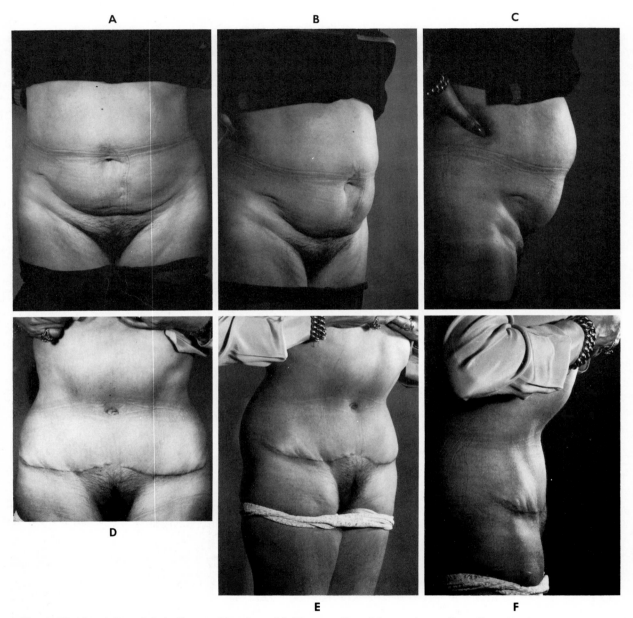

Figure 36–19.   *A, B,* and *C,* A 49-year-old patient with (1) protruding abdomen due to diastasis recti and musculoaponeurotic laxity, (2) minimal waistline contour, and, (3) right lower quadrant appendectomy scar.

D, E, and *F,* Photographs six months postoperatively. Musculoaponeurotic repair included vertical closure of diastasis recti and oblique plication of external oblique fascia to correct abdominal protrusion and create a curved waistline silhouette. The postoperative photographs suggest that the patient is voluntarily retracting her abdominal muscles. However, the photographs show the patient at rest.

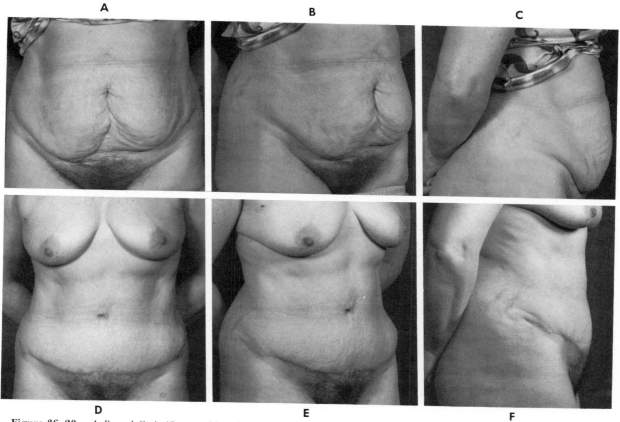

Figure 36–20. *A, B,* and *C,* A 42-year-old patient with a protruding abdomen following three pregnancies and two cesarean sections. A dermolipomatous apron is hanging anterior to the protruding abdominal wall.

D, E, and *F,* Eight months following musculoaponeurotic repair and resection of abdominal apron using a Grazer incision.

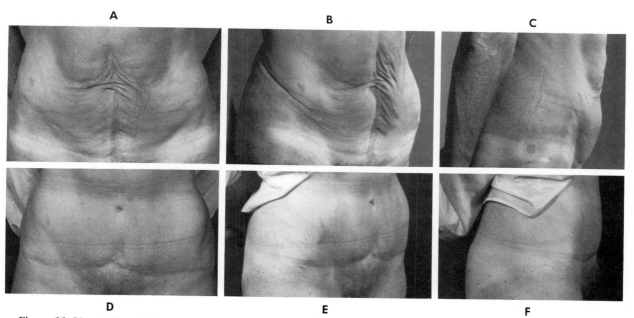

Figure 36–21. *A, B,* and *C,* A 39-year-old patient with abdominal skin redundancy and midline cesarean section scar.

D, E, and *F,* Fourteen months following musculoaponeurotic repair and excision of excess skin using a Pitanguy incision.

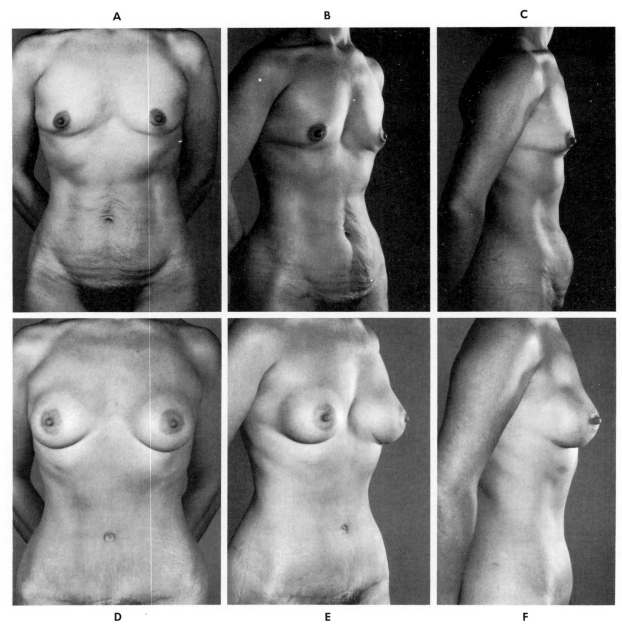

Figure 36–22. *A, B,* and *C,* A 35-year-old patient with breast tissue atrophy, abdominal skin excess, striae extending above the umbilicus and musculoaponeurotic laxity of the abdominal wall following two pregnancies.

D, E, and *F,* Sixteen months following augmentation mammaplasty and abdominoplasty. Note the significant resection of the striae and the improvement in appearance of the remaining striae.

around dressing is applied at this time because the skin flap is in its state of maximal "shock" from the undermining and tension produced by the wound closure. Figures 36–18 through 36–22 demonstrate results obtained by the technique described with various skin incisions.

POSTOPERATIVE CARE

When possible, the patient should be transferred from the operating table to a ward bed, bypassing a recovery room stretcher or bed. This reduces early postoperative pain and possibly lessens the chance of postoperative bleeding. The bed should remain flexed in the semi-Fowler position to take tension off the suture line for four to five days. Thereafter, a pillow under the knees will be comfortable and is usually adequate. Hospital beds with electric controls for changing bed position should not be plugged into an electric outlet, as the patient or a visitor may straighten out the patient and jeopardize the abdominal flap survival.

Lying on either side with the hips flexed is permitted as soon as the patient is comfortable enough to get into this position. Activity is limited during the first 48 hours postoperatively when chance of hematoma is greatest.

In order to promote venous return and reduce the chance of thrombophlebitis, ankle and knee flexion and extension exercise are encouraged for five minutes every hour while the patient is awake for the next few days. It also provides the patient a way to participate in postoperative care and helps divert attention from the abdominal wall discomfort.

Prior to having the patient stand at bedside on the first postoperative day, an elasticized expandable soft panty girdle is put on to support the abdomen; it is worn most of the time during the next two weeks. This provides support to the abdomen and security to the patient, and it helps keep the abdominal wall flap against the fascia. Many patients find the panty girdle comfortable when worn for the first month postoperatively.

The Foley catheter is removed when the patient can ambulate to the bathroom or to a bedside commode. Full trunk extension is unlikely for the first three to five postoperative days, depending upon how much tension there is on the skin flap. Ambulation is begun carefully, with assistance on the second morning after surgery. It progresses according to the individual patient's tolerance. Hemovac drains are removed on the second morning following surgery, or they may

be left in place another 24 hours if the amount of drainage warrants such. Suction is disconnected prior to removing the drain or bleeding may be started by pulling away a clot that has been adherent to a vessel and the tubing.

Intake of clear liquids is permitted on the first morning postoperatively if bowel sounds are present. Occasionally, adynamic ileus will prevent oral intake for two to three days postoperatively. When liquids are tolerated, a regular diet is begun cautiously.

Postoperative pain and discomfort is usually moderate but not severe. Severe pain requires examining the patient for possible hematoma. Pain tolerance is quite variable from patient to patient. Narcotic analgesics are usually necessary intermittently for the first two to three days following surgery. Anxious and apprehensive patients may require Valium or some other tranquilizer to help maintain a calm, peaceful, postoperative course. Antiemetics are necessary to reduce nausea and vomiting and may very well play a secondary role in preventing early postoperative hematoma formation.

Showering and bathing is permitted after five days. All sutures are removed by the 14th postoperative day. Normal activities are resumed slowly; vigorous activities such as golf, swimming, and tennis are restricted to the sixth postoperative week.

COMPLICATIONS

Abdominoplasty is a major surgical procedure and as such is associated with complications that vary from insignificant nuisances to death. In a retrospective questionnaire study with replies from 958 plastic surgeons, Grazer and Goldwyn (1977) obtained information on 10,490 abdominoplasties. Facts obtained from this study indicate that surgeons in practice eight or more years do not have fewer complications than those in practice for lesser periods of time, and surgeons performing a large number of abdominoplasties had the same type of complications to the same degree as those doing only a moderate number of abdominoplasties.

Hematoma and Seroma

Hematoma and/or serous fluid collection is the most frequent complication of abdominoplasty. Meticulous hemostasis during the surgical procedure is the best method of prevention. Electrocautery dissection for abdominal wall flap elevation allows rapid coagulation of vessels, produces a drier operating field, and reduces operating time. Large vessels, venous and arterial, should be ligated to prevent late postoperative bleeding. Transected vessels that retract beneath the abdominal wall fascia should be figure-of-eight suture ligated through the fascia as they are encountered. Otherwise, the vessel may contract and bleeding may cease but occur again in the postoperative period.

Large hematomas, usually the result of a single large vessel that has lost its tie or sloughed a cauterized end, requires immediate evacuation to prevent vascular compromise and sloughing of the abdominal wall skin. This type of hematoma usually occurs within the first 24 hours after the operation and is associated with increased discomfort, swelling, and ecchymosis. When present, the diagnosis is obvious. If the skin flap appears pale and avascular, sutures should be clipped while waiting for the patient to return to the operating room. Most often, a large bleeding vessel is found in either the superior or inferior flap edge. Removal of all sutures may be necessary to explore the wound adequately. A fiberoptic light source retractor may be of great value. General anesthesia is necessary for hematoma evacuation for several reasons: (1) the patient is usually extremely apprehensive, (2) local anesthesia is inadequate, and (3) positioning for resuturing flap margins is too uncomfortable for the nonanesthetized patient.

The incidence of serous fluid collection is reduced by (1) flap dissection so as to leave a thin areolar layer over the abdominal wall muscular aponeurosis and (2) avoidance of injury to the lymph nodes and lymph channels in the inguinal area. Jackson-Pratt drains are routinely placed under the abdominal wall flap and brought out through stab incisions in the pubic hair, where a very small resultant scar will be hidden. Although drains are of questionable value in preventing hematoma, the removal of serosanguinous fluid during the first 36 to 48 hours reduces the amount the abdominal tissues must reabsorb, allows the flap to adhere, and reduces the risk of infection.

Serous fluid collections appear after three to five days and may be of a large volume (100 to 150 cc). Transected lymph channels in the inguinal region and exudate from the flap surface are better reabsorbed when the areolar tissue remains on the muscle aponeurosis. Serous collections are usually ballotable and easily detected beneath the skin flap. Aspiration with a large bore needle using strict aseptic technique is necessary for the flap to stick down in its normal position. A firm elastic panty girdle helps slow reaccumulation. A second or third aspiration may occasionally be necessary.

Skin Slough

Skin slough is one of the worst complications of abdominoplasty. Fortunately, it is rare. Previous transverse surgical incisions above the level of skin that will be resected may be a contraindication to abdominoplasty. The cause of skin slough is inadequate blood supply to maintain the distal portion of the abdominal flap. The arterial supply to an abdominal flap that has been elevated to the xiphoid process and costal margins and resected from the level of the umbilicus to the suprapubic incision is from (1) branches from the lateral thoracic vessels, (2) perforating branches from the intercostal vessels, and (3) perforating branches from the internal mammary vessels. Skin slough is most likely to occur when (1) excess tension is placed on the skin flap by transverse skin resection, (2) excess tension is placed on the skin flap by vertical skin resection, (3) an unrecognized hematoma produces vascular compromise of the skin flap, and (4) the flap is not handled gently during the surgical procedure.

In the absence of a hematoma or some unusual but obvious injury to the skin flap, a skin slough may be expected if during the first 12 to 36 hours postoperatively the distal flap appears dusky to purplish, ecchymosis is present, and capillary filling is slow or absent. Over a period of three to five days, the devitalized area will demarcate. The final devitalized area is likely to be larger than it was initially, as poorly vascularized fat necroses, taking with it skin that was surviving on the subdermal plexus.

When a potential skin slough is noted during the first few to 48 hours postoperatively, consideration should be given to cutting the sutures holding the skin flap to the lower abdominal fascia and skin incision. Careful explanation to calm the patient will probably obtain their cooperation.

The author has had experience with two patients whose abdominal flaps became dusky and the blood from the cut flap end became dark even before the excess flap was excised. No mechanical problems could be determined. Both patients subsequently sloughed a large area below the umbilicus. The only other similarity in these two patients was that they smoked three and one half to four packs of cigarettes per day.

Small skin sloughs near the incision lines should be debrided conservatively, trimming the edges of the eschar as separation occurs. The wound is permitted to granulate and epithelize. Scar excision and revision is possible for the less extensive sloughs after an appropriate time has passed for the skin in the area in question to loosen up.

Large areas of skin slough should be debrided, kept clean with good principles of wound care, and permitted to contract. If the patient's cooperation and confidence in the surgeon can be maintained, a very large area of slough of the abdominal wall flap will contract down to a relatively small area over several weeks. The final repair may be a rather simple skin approximation.

If for some reason, immediate wound closure is necessary, a split thickness skin graft is applied as soon as healthy granulation tissue is present. In the author's opinion, this is the lesser of the two alternatives for managing a large slough in terms of the final scar appearance.

Dehiscence

Dehiscence not related to other complications is most often due to excess tension on the skin flap following overly generous dermolipectomy.

Dehiscence can occur following abdominoplasty if there is sudden movement of the patient to a fully extended torso putting stress on the nonhealed flap margins, or if the patient accidentally falls while resuming ambulation in the early postoperative period. Dehiscence may occur owing to hematoma or wound infection.

Dehiscence caused by excess tension should be repaired immediately. Permanent sutures placed between the lower edge of the skin flap and the abdominal wall muscle fascia as described for primary wound closure will do much to take tension off the skin edge. Dehiscence associated with infection or hematoma requires the usual principles of wound management.

Infection

Infection is rare in the author's experience. However, the retrospective study of 10,490 abdominoplasties performed by 958 surgeons as reviewed by Grazer and Goldwyn (1977) noted an infection rate incidence of 7.3 percent. Staphylococcus, Streptococcus, *E. coli*, and pseudomonas were the most common pathogens. Undrained hematomas can act as a nidus for infection, or contamination and infection can follow an attempt

to remove collected blood or serum. Aseptic technique is mandatory in evacuating a hematoma or seroma.

Scars

Scar hypertrophy and keloid formation may occur following abdominoplasty. Because of the wound tension usually present, it is not surprising that a widened hypertrophic abdominal scar sometimes develops. Keloids, which are more common in deeply pigmented individuals, are rare. Keloids are notoriously difficult to treat whenever or wherever they occur; the abdomen is no exception. Fortunately, except for the periumbilical scar, incisions are usually designed so as to be hidden in a bikini or other small articles of clothing. Hypertrophic scars are often improved with the passage of time and intralesional steroid injections. Patience and good rapport with the patient are important during this trying time.

Umbilical Necrosis

Umbilical necrosis may occur if (1) the umbilical stalk is excessively "defatted" so that its blood supply is compromised or (2) the blood supply to the umbilical stalk is strangulated by musculoaponeurotic plication sutures. Loss of a normal appearing umbilicus produces a severe aesthetic deformity of the abdominal wall. The umbilicus is important as a reference point for establishing the upper and lower half of the abdominal wall and the midline between the right and left halves. An absent or distorted umbilicus is readily noticeable and gives a strange appearance to the abdomen. Neoumbilicaneoplasty by defatting around a new umbilical site and suturing the abdominal skin to the underlying muscle fascia has been described by Baroudi (1975). This gives an improvement over a nonexistent umbilicus but the results are less than desirable.

Umbilical Scars

Periumbilical scars can be unsightly. Umbilical scars result from inherent healing characteristics or partial umbilical necrosis and slough. The umbilicus should be removed as an ellipse rather than excised in a circular fashion and reimplanted in a like fashion. A circular scar contracture may occur following circumferential excision. The umbilical stump must be shortened and the thickness of the abdominal adipose tissue must be resected in such a fashion as to give an umbilicus of the desired shape, which is usually most aesthetically pleasing if it is not protruding from the abdominal wall. Sutures should be placed so that the main pressure of the knots lie on the inside of the depressed portion of the umbilicus — therefore reducing to a minimum the likelihood of a periumbilical scar secondary to sutures.

An excessively wide umbilicus is most often due to an umbilicus recipient site in the abdominal flap that is made too large. For most patients, an umbilical diameter greater than 1.75 cm appears large. Umbilical stenosis is due to (1) initially cutting out the umbilicus too small, (2) failure to make an adequate recipient site, or (3) a rim of scar tissue contracting around the junction of the umbilicus and the abdominal flap. Treatment requires releasing the contracted scar and is difficult.

Umbilical Malposition

Placement of the umbilicus too high, too low, or too laterally is an error in surgical judgment. Appropriate preoperative marking of the abdomen with indelible ink provides vertical and horizontal reference points for symmetrical undermining, flap traction, dermolipectomy, and umbilical placement. Correction of a malpositioned umbilicus may require flap elevation, fat and skin resection, and possibly complete umbilical transposition to the indicated location.

Abdominal Asymmetry

Asymmetry of the abdominal wall in shape and scar location may occur if flap undermining, flap traction, flap resection, fat resection, or musculoaponeurotic tightening is not performed symmetrically. The preoperative markings and measurements must be followed throughout the operation.

Thrombophlebitis and Pulmonary Embolus

This is the most severe complication of abdominoplasty. Patients who undergo surgical procedures that position the body so as to impede venous return, or by the nature of the surgical procedure decrease venous return in the lower extremities or produce an increased pressure or inflammatory response in the lower abdomen or pelvis are at a greater risk of postoperative thrombophlebitis and pulmonary embolus. In the retrospective study of Grazer and Goldwyn (1977), 115 patients were reported to have deep phlebitis (an incidence of 1.1 percent of reported patients). Pulmonary emboli were reported in 0.8 percent of the patients, and six deaths were reported to be caused by pulmonary embolus following abdominoplasty. According to this study, there was no relationship between the time of ambulation and the incidence of phlebitis, pulmonary embolus, or death. Surgical stockings or ace wraps from the toes to the midthighs to help prevent superficial venous stasis and early flexion and extension exercises at the ankles and/or knees to help promote venous return are possibly of some benefit in reducing thrombophlebitis and pulmonary embolus. No single position in bed should be maintained in a rigid fashion for more than a couple of hours. Intermittent variation in the degree of flexion at the hips may be of some benefit in promoting venous blood flow.

Nerve Injury

This is one of the least common complications of abdominoplasty, and few references to it are found in the literature. The lateral femoral cutaneous nerve, a branch of the second and third lumbar nerves, passes from the lateral border of the psoas muscle, crosses the ilium obliquely toward the anterior superior iliac spine, and passes behind the inguinal ligament into the thigh. Sutures placed between the advanced abdominal wall flap and the fascia in the area of the inguinal ligament may injure the lateral femoral cutaneous nerve, producing paresthesia and disturbance in sensation on the anterolateral surface of the thigh (by definition, *Meralgia paresthetica* or Bernhardt's syndrome). In the author's experience, symptoms are initial numbness followed by a burning sensation or tingling but with complete abatement by three to four weeks following surgery. It is conceivable that symptoms could persist, making nerve exploration a real consideration.

Sensory Changes

Most patients have some loss of sensitivity of the abdominal wall for several weeks from the level of the umbilicus down to the end of the abdominal flap. Normal sensitivity returns with time. The area of usual dermolipectomy removes a portion of the dermatones supplied by posterior spinal roots T10, T11, T12. T9, which is initially at the upper level of the umbilicus, is moved down to the suprapubic skin incision (Guilherme de Silveira Carvalho, Baroudi, Keppke, 1977). The only practical importance of the dermatone change would be if the patient were later to have abdominal surgery under spinal anesthesia.

(For list of references, see pages 1071 and 1072.)

Chapter 37

Buttocks and Thighs

SHERRELL J. ASTON, M.D., F.A.C.S.

BUTTOCK REDUCTION

History

The history of dermolipectomy of the thighs and buttocks is limited. In 1952, Correa Iturrospe reported reduction of fat thighs as part of the surgical treatment of obesity. Lewis (1957) described resection of redundant thigh skin and fat using a long vertical incision extending down the medial thigh from the groin to near the knee. In his book *Atlas of Aesthetic Plastic Surgery* (1973), Lewis states he first performed procedures for reduction of trochanteric lipodystrophy and correction of ptotic buttocks in 1954. Farina (1961) discussed in detail trochanteric lipodystrophy and described correction by a long vertical incision down the lateral side of the thigh, flap elevation and rotation, and excision of a triangle of tissue posterior to the iliac crest.

In 1964, Pitanguy described extensive trochanteric dermolipectomy using an incision that followed the gluteal crease posteriorly and extended laterally toward the anterior superior iliac spine in such a way that the entire incision could be hidden in a bikini bathing suit. It was this procedure that stimulated the interest of plastic surgeons and the public press. Procedures later described by Delerm and Girotteaue (1973), Guerrero-Santos (1976), Planas (1975), Vilain (1975), Grazer (1976), and others have contributed variations in technique and extensions of applicability of the Pitanguy type incision.

Guerrero-Santos (1976) described a "rotated, shaved and buried flap" technique for advancing the lateral trochanteric prominence beneath a "sandwich-type" gluteal flap to reduce trochanteric prominence and add tissue to lateral gluteal depressions. Grazer (1976) described the "tuck-and-roll thigh plasty," which also suspends the thigh on a buried de-epithelized flap and creates a new infragluteal fold. Better contour of the buttocks is made the tighter the roll flaps are packed. The techniques of Guerrero-Santos and Grazer are designed to correct the depression between the greater trochanter and ilium that frequently accompanies trochanteric lipodystrophy or, as modified procedures without tissue resection, to correct postoperative or posttraumatic depressions.

Vilain, Dardour, and Bzowski (1977) described burying a de-epithelized triangular flap of dermis and fat created from the excess skin of the lateral trochanteric bulge area to correct trochanteric lipodystrophy and create a rounded buttock contour. The lateral length of the incision with this technique is shorter than the usual Pitanguy technique incision for correction of trochanteric lipodystrophy. The disadvantage of this technique is that it is only applicable in cases of pure subtrochanteric fat bulge.

Agris (1977) reported a dermal-fat suspension flap sutured anteriorly to the inguinal fascia and posteriorly to the fascia lata in an attempt to support the weight of the thigh skin and subcutaneous tissue and ideally to prevent recurrent lateral thigh depressions and inferior scar migration. This technique is similar to that previously described by Guerrero-Santos.

Grazer (1979) presented a classification of frequently seen buttock and thigh deformities and a classification of hip and thigh plasty in an attempt to aid verbal and written communication among plastic surgeons throughout the world. Grazer's Classification of Deformities is Type I—crural excess, Type II—trochanteric deformity or riding breeches, Type III—gluteal recess or medial half deformity. Type IV—composite of II and III, Type V—obesity. Type VI—asymmetry and traumatic deformity, and Type VII—aging or atrophy.

INDICATION FOR SURGERY

The demand for aesthetic surgery of the buttocks and thighs is increasing. The complaints of patients seeking buttock and thigh surgery are of two types: unaesthetic appearance and difficulty with fitting clothes. The chief indication for most buttock and thigh "lifts" is for the aesthetic improvement anticipated.

Current society's emphasis on youth-oriented concepts, physical fitness, revealing clothing fashions, and more liberal attitudes toward sex increases the psychologic stress on patients with buttock and thigh deformities. Some patients with trochanteric lipodystrophy or large hanging buttocks limit their social and leisure activities in order to avoid the embarrassment of exposure of the buttocks and thighs. However, many patients who request correction of medial thigh ptosis frequently engage in social and leisure activities such as swimming and tennis that expose their deformity when dressed appropriately for the sport.

Patients with grotesque lipodystrophies (either localized or generalized), massively obese patients, and patients with large hanging folds of skin and fat following extensive weight loss have more extensive deformities than do the majority of patients requesting aesthetic buttock and thigh surgery. The primary goal of surgery in patients with massive amounts of excess tissue is to remove bulk for a functional improvement. The main emphasis in this chapter is on aesthetic buttock and thigh surgery.

Patient Evaluation

A carefully taken medical history and complete physical examination are necessary to detect any systemic disease that may contraindicate buttock and thigh surgery. The general body habitus is noted. Examination from the waist to the ankles is important to evaluate the full extent of the patient's deformity. Thighs, hips, and buttocks are evaluated for redundancy, laxity, and lipomatous deposits. Any asymmetry of the two sides is noted and pointed out to the patient. The lower extremities are examined for evidence of venous, arterial, or lymphatic disease. The pretibial areas and ankles are inspected for possible edema. Attention is given to the anatomic deformity of the patient's chief complaint. The potential for improvement with a surgical procedure is determined. Specific deformities will be discussed in the appropriate sections of this chapter.

Planned surgical incisions are drawn on the patient's skin with indelible ink in order for the patient to inspect the location of the scars later when at home. Often the location of the scars are of interest to a patient's mate.

Easy bruisibility, problem bleeding, or other signs suggesting blood dyscrasia should be investigated. Patients should be specifically questioned about frequent aspirin ingestion. No aspirin containing compounds should be taken for at least ten days prior to surgery because aspirin decreases platelet cohesiveness resulting in an increase in bleeding during surgery.

Informed Consent

The general details of the planned operative procedure are explained in clear terms to the patient. The most common complication, wide hypertrophic scars, is noted. Thigh and buttock surgery causes some of the least desirable scars produced by aesthetic surgery. This is due in part to the location of the scars and the constant tension exerted on them.

The possibility of a severe complication such as thrombophlebitis, pulmonary embolus, and death is pointed out.

Preoperative and postoperative photographs of patients showing the range of surgical results can be shown to the prospective patient. A textbook or journal article may be useful for this purpose.

Preoperative Preparation

Two days prior to surgery, the patient begins twice daily pHisoHex showers to reduce the surface bacteria and decrease the potential for wound infection. On the evening prior to surgery, the patient takes a pHisoHex shower, which is repeated the next morning. Planned surgical incisions and markings are made with indelible ink on the prior evening or the morning of surgery before the patient receives premedication. Patient cooperation is thus better, and it avoids embarrassment of markings made in a busy operating room just prior to induction of anesthesia. Measurements and markings are made with the patient in the standing position.

Patients having buttock and/or trochanteric reduction will not be permitted to flex the hips or sit for two weeks after surgery. On the evening prior to surgery, these patients are taught to "log roll" out of bed. Having practiced getting out of bed in this manner makes it easier to do so following surgery when the surgical wounds are painful. The patient rolls over in bed without flexing the hips to the prone position, uses hands and arms to turn approximately 45 degrees to the vertical of the bed, and then pushes off the bed feet first, knees and hips straight, and stands. Returning to bed is just the reverse.

After induction of suitable endotracheal anesthesia, a Foley catheter is placed in the bladder and ace bandages are placed on the lower extremities from the feet to above the knees. The patient is placed on the operating table in either a supine or prone position according to the procedure planned. Routine presurgical preparation is carried out. When surgery is planned on both the anterior thighs and the buttock area, the surgical field must be draped so that the patient can be turned from the supine position to the prone or vice versa, without contaminating the sterile area.

TROCHANTERIC LIPODYSTROPHY

Lipomatosis refers to a circumscribed or encapsulated deposit of fat rather than to the more diffuse accumulation of fat that is associated with excessive caloric intake. Two topographic varieties of lipomatoses occur in the trochanteric, pelvic, gluteal, and crural areas: (1) that localized to a specific area and (2) that which is regional and diffuse, extending from the waist to the knees.

Trochanteric lipodystrophy, a bilateral lipomatous collection in the trochanteric region, produces the so-called "riding breeches" deformity, which is the most common deformity seen in patients requesting posterior thigh and buttock reduction. The trochanteric bulges are often accompanied by overlying depressions on the lateral sides of the buttocks, producing an aesthetically unattractive silhouette.

In normal anatomy, there is a small depression between the ilium and the lateral upper thigh and buttock. The depressions associated with trochanteric lipodystrophy are accentuated by trochanteric and pelvic lipomatoses (Figure 37–1, *A*). Pelvic and crural lipodystrophy to some degree accompanies the trochanteric lipodystrophy in many patients. This specific localized lipodystrophy is often found in patients who are otherwise thin or normal in body habitus. The waist and lower thighs are frequently of normal size.

Patients with trochanteric lipodystrophy are often limited in the kind of clothing they can wear. Sports clothing, beachwear, and the like are never worn by some of these patients. Rigorous dieting, weight loss, and exercise programs do little, if anything to change the size of the involved areas.

Evaluation and Treatment of Trochanteric Lipodystrophy

With the patient standing, the buttocks and thighs are evaluated for symmetry, the amount and location of the lipomatous deposits, lateral thigh depressions above the fat deposits, skin laxity, medial thigh redundancy, and buttock ptosis (Fig. 37–1, *A*).

Bikini panties or bathing suits of the style the patient wishes to wear postoperatively are outlined and removed (Fig. 37–1, *B*). It is not always possible to have the scars confined to the bikini area, especially with current mini-bikini fashions. The patient should be so advised.

The superior margin of a fusiform area of dermolipectomy is determined and marked along

Text continued on page 1047.

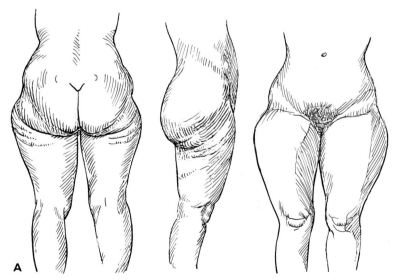

Figure 37–1.   *A*, "Riding breeches" deformity associated with lateral buttock depressions causing an aesthetically unpleasing silhouette anteriorly, posteriorly, and laterally.

Illustration continued on the following page.

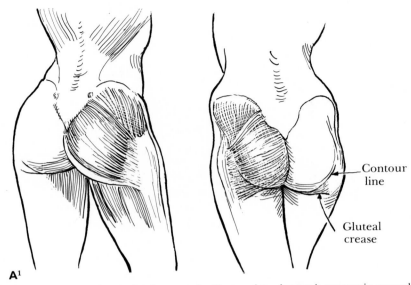

A¹

Contour
line

Gluteal
crease

Figure 37–1 *Continued.*   *A¹*, A slight depression between the ilium and trochanter is present in normal anatomy. Pelvic and trochanteric lipomatosis often accentuates the depression.

Figure 37–1 *Continued.*   *B* and *C*, Bikini panties provide a guideline for incision placement. The superior limit of fusiform resection lies at the superior limit of the lateral buttock depression.

D and *E*, The amount of tissue to be resected is determined.

F, Measurements for symmetry.

See illustration on the opposite page.

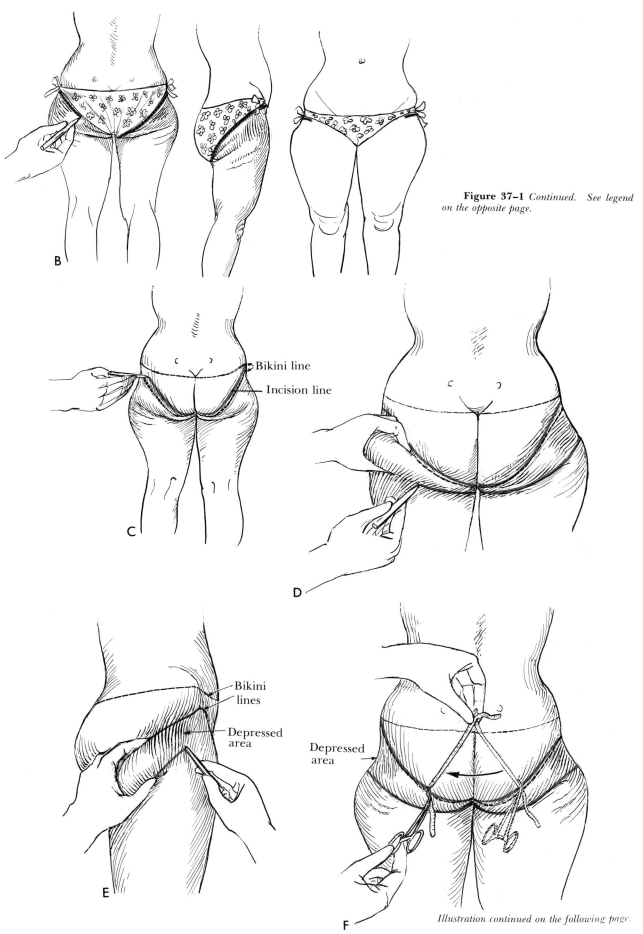

Figure 37–1 *Continued. See legend on the opposite page.*

Bikini line

Incision line

B

C

D

Bikini lines

Depressed area

E

Depressed area

F

Illustration continued on the following page.

1043

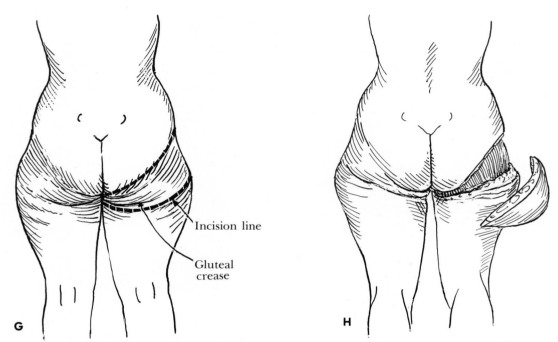

Incision line

Gluteal crease

G

H

Figure 37–1 *Continued.*   G, The inferior medial incision remains near the gluteal crease.

H, Fusiform resection is made as discussed in the text.

Illustration continued on the opposite page.

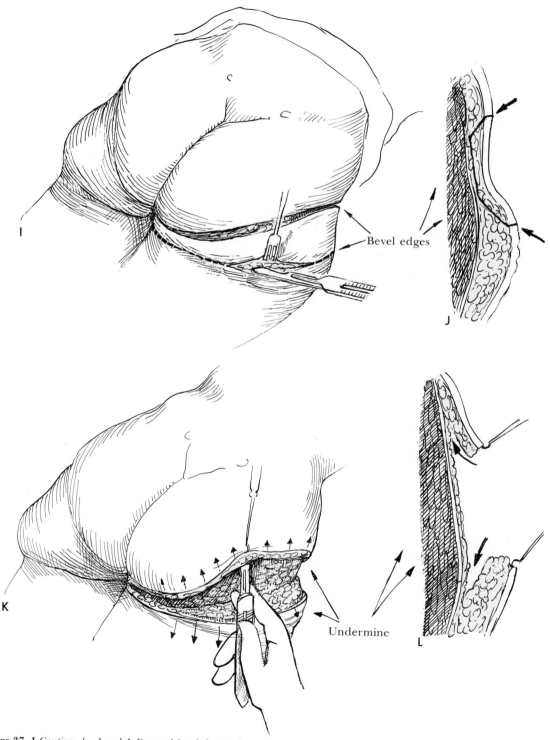

Figure 37–1 *Continued.*   *I* and *J,* Fat excision is beveled toward the center of the skin excision to preserve the fat to help fill the depression.

K and *L,* Flaps are undermined for a short distance for mobilization and wound closure.

Illustration continued on the following page.

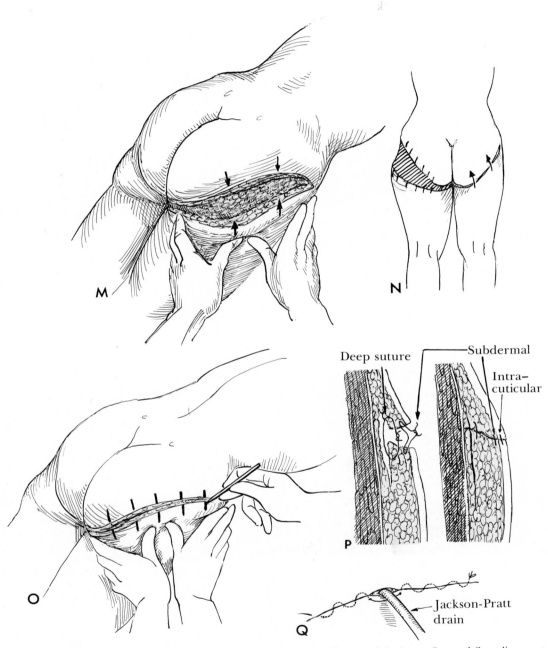

Figure 37–1 *Continued.*   *M, N,* and *O,* Superior and medial advancement of the lower flap and flap alignment.

P and *Q,* The wound is closed in three layers with a vacuum suction drain placed in the base.

the superior limit of the posterior lateral buttock depression. It extends anteriorly toward the anterior superior iliac spine (Fig. 37–1, C). The medial margin of the superior and inferior skin incisions at the gluteal cleavage are determined by grasping the tissues of the buttock and upper posterior thigh between the thumb and the fingers and determining the amount of tissue to be resected without producing excess tension (Fig. 37–1, D). The entire area of dermolipectomy is determined in a similar manner (Fig. 37–1, E). The inferior incision must be near the gluteal crease medially to prevent downward migration of the scar onto the thigh a few weeks postoperatively (Fig. 37–1, G).

Judgment of the amount of skin and fat to be excised will improve with experience as one learns to take into account the thickness of the fat and the mobility of the skin flaps on each side of the area to be resected. Tense fat thighs require less skin resection than do buttocks of similar size with skin laxity. If there is associated medial thigh laxity, the incisions are extended medially in the inguinal crease and resection is performed as described in the section on the correction of medial thigh laxity.

Symmetry of measurements and markings are assured by a tape fixed at the coccyx and swung alternately from side to side (Fig. 37–1, F).

Any depression of the posterior lateral buttock should be marked on the skin so that its extent can be determined after the patient is in the prone position in the operating theater.

Following preoperative preparation (discussed earlier in this chapter), the planned area of dermolipectomy is excised (Fig. 37–1, H). The upper and lower fat excisions are beveled away from the skin incisions so as to preserve fat to be advanced into the posteriolateral depressed area. When the depression is deep, only skin is removed from the depressed area (Fig. 37–1, I, J). The superior and inferior skin flaps are undermined along the depressed area in order that the flaps can be approximated and the fat can be redistributed into the depression (Fig. 37–1, K, L).

The inferior flap is rotated in a superior medial direction and aligned for proper fit to the superior flap edge (Fig. 37–1, M, N). An assistant marks with ink the indicated points of flap approximation (Fig. 37–1, O). A Jackson-Pratt drain is placed in the base of the resected area and brought out through the skin incision (Fig. 37–1, Q).

Flaps are sutured in three layers: 2–0 chromic

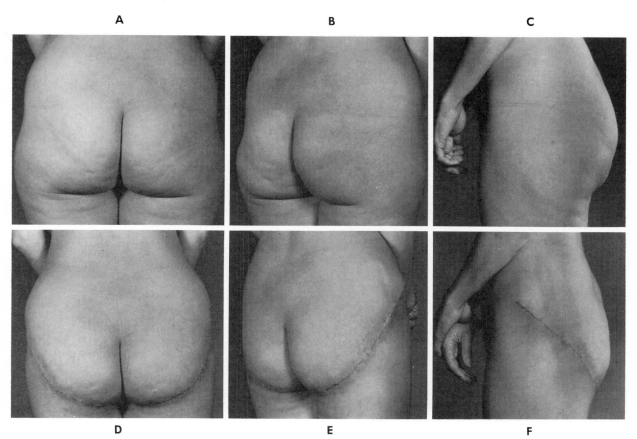

Figure 37–2.   *A, B,* and *C,* Trochanteric lipodystrophy and medial gluteal excess.

D, E, and *F,* One month postoperatively.

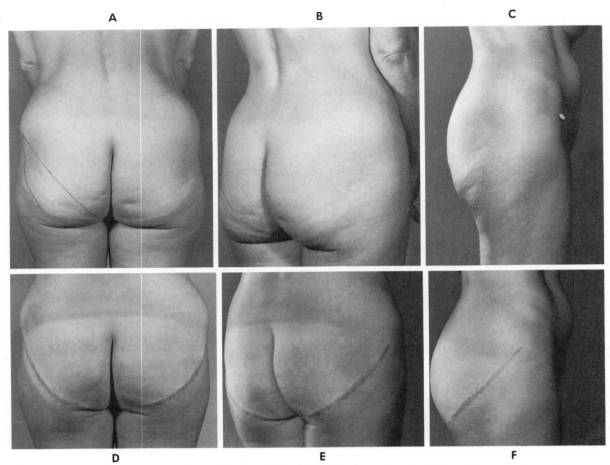

Figure 37–3. *A, B,* and *C,* Trochanteric lipodystrophy, medial gluteal excess, and mild lateral buttock depression.

D, E, and *F,* One year following resection by the technique described. Scars that were initially hypertrophic have flattened but widened.

in the deep tissues to secure the flaps in position, 3–0 chromic with buried knots in the subcutaneous tissues, and 3–0 intracuticular Prolene for skin approximation (Fig. 37–1, *P*), supported by steri-trips for epithelial approximation. (See Figures 37–2 and 37–3.)

Correction of Postoperative Lateral Thigh Depression

The most common unfavorable result following surgery for correction of trochanteric lipodystrophy with posterior lateral gluteal depressions is an accentuation of the depression. This is caused by (1) too low a placement of the superior margin of the fusiform skin excision, (2) failure to redistribute fat from the lateral bulge in the trochanteric area into the depression, and/or (3) resection of too much fat in the already depressed area (Figure 37–4, *A*). The increased depression is often accompanied by a persistent large lipomatous collection over the trochanteric area and a surgical scar passing through the depression (Figs. 37–4, *B*

and 37–5). The author has had some success in improving this kind of deformity using the following technique.

The superior limit of the depression and the area of depression is marked with the patient standing, and the amount of skin redundancy, if any, is determined and marked in a fusiform fashion as described in the technique for resection of trochanteric lipodystrophy (Fig. 37–4, *C*). The amount of skin redundancy in the lateral thigh is usually maximal along the area of depression. The inferior limit of the trochanteric bulge is marked.

The patient is prepared in the operating room and a full-thickness skin incision is made along the margins of the fusiform outline (Fig. 37–4, *D*). The clearly demarcated area of the depression is de-epithelialized and the remainder of the excess skin is removed full thickness (Fig. 37–4, *E*). Fat resection and contouring is made along the posterior portion of the buttocks if indicated (Fig. 37–4, *F*).

The superior incision is deepened approximately halfway to the fascia (Fig. 37–4, *G*) to establish a sewing edge. The inferior incision is deepened to the fascia lata and the lower flap is

Text continued on page 1054.

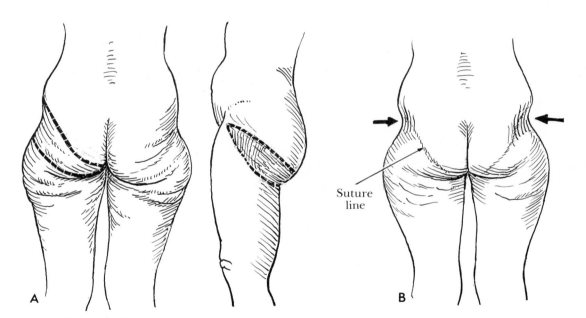

Figure 37–4.   *A*, Preoperative "riding breeches" deformity and lateral gluteal depressions.

B, Postoperative result with deeper lateral depressions.

Illustration continued on the following page.

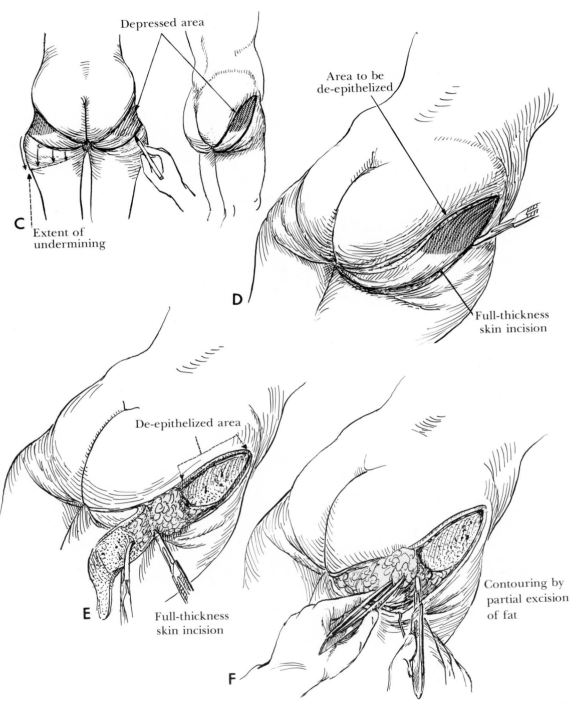

Figure 37–4 *Continued.   C,* Preoperative markings establish (1) superior limit of depression; (2) area of depression; (3) lower limit of trochanteric bulge; and (4) any skin redundancy.

D, Full-thickness skin incisions.

E and *F,* The area of depression is de-epithelized to maintain tissue bulk. Skin and fat are resected as indicated.

Illustration continued on the opposite page.

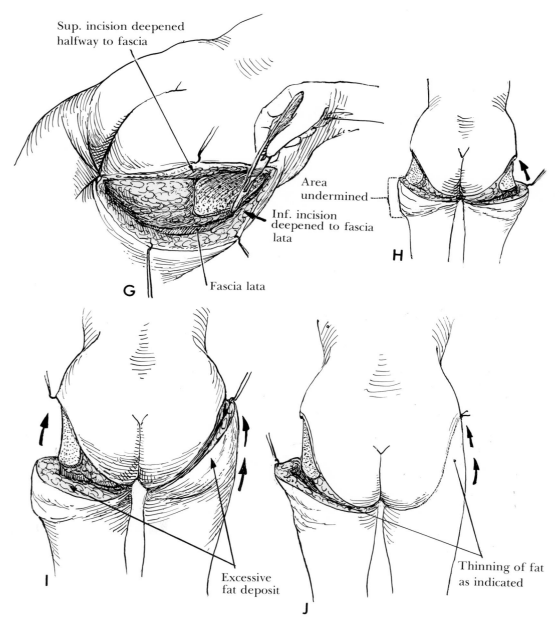

Sup. incision deepened
halfway to fascia

Area
undermined

Inf. incision
deepened to fascia
lata

Fascia lata

G

H

I

Excessive
fat deposit

J

Thinning of fat
as indicated

Figure 37–4 *Continued.*   G, The superior incision deepened.

H, The trochanteric bulge undermined at the level of the fascia lata.

I and *J*, The flap is advanced superomedially and fat is resected as indicated.

Illustration continued on the following page.

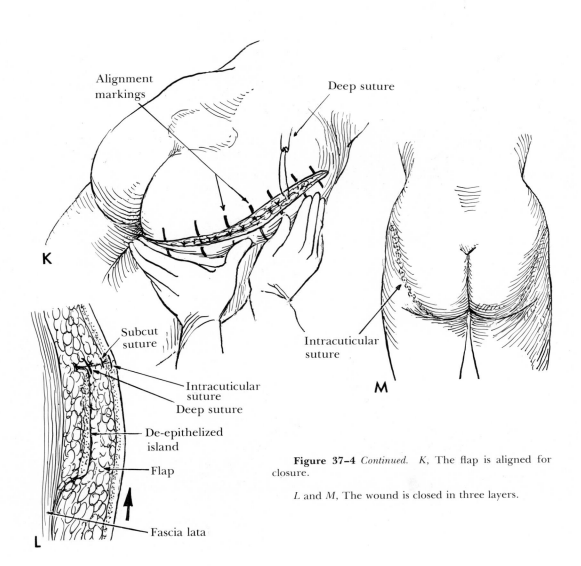

Alignment markings

Deep suture

K

Subcut suture

Intracuticular suture

Deep suture

De-epithelized island

Flap

Fascia lata

L

Intracuticular suture

M

Figure 37–4 *Continued.* *K*, The flap is aligned for closure.

L and *M*, The wound is closed in three layers.

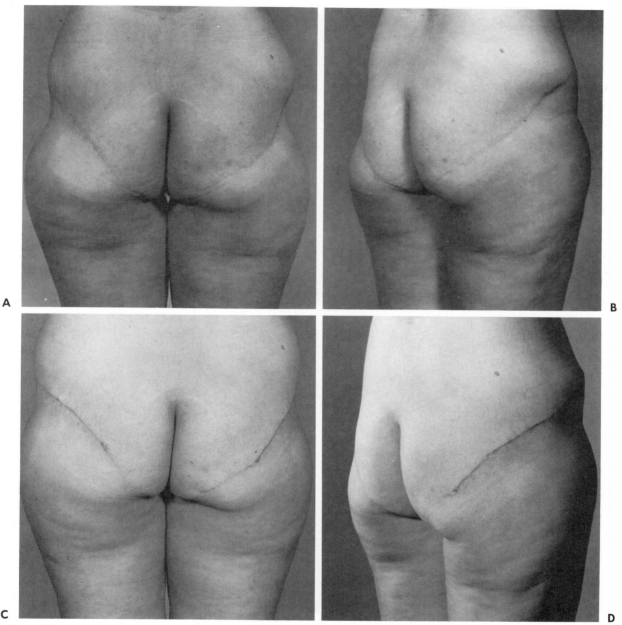

Figure 37–5.   *A* and *B*, Large trochanteric lipodystrophy bulges and deep lateral buttock depressions two years postoperatively.

C and *D*, Improvement of deformity 10 months following the technique described in Figure 37–4.

then undermined at the level of the fascia to the lower limit of the trochanteric bulge as marked with the patient standing (Fig. 37–4, *G, H*). The flap is advanced over the dermis-fat island and checked for thickness (Fig. 37–4, *I*). If the fat flap is too thick, it can be beveled with the scalpel to the desired thickness (Fig. 37–4, *J*). The borders of the two flaps are aligned and cross marked with ink as an aid in placing sutures between the flaps (Fig. 37–4, *K*). If necessary, the upper flap can be undermined to obtain a sewing edge. Flaps are sutured in three layers: 2–0 chromic deep, 3–0 chromic with buried knots in the subcutaneous tissue, and 3–0 Prolene intracuticular suture to approximate the skin (Fig. 37–4, *L, M*). (See Figure 37–5.)

PTOSIS AND REDUNDANCY OF BUTTOCKS

Ptosis and redundancy of the buttocks may be due to aging and musculocutaneous laxity, weight loss or small flat gluteal muscles such that the skin and subcutaneous tissue hang loosely in the area where the gluteal crease should be. Patients with this deformity are concerned with their appearance when nude or in tight fitting or revealing clothing such as bathing suits and slacks.

Frequently, ptosis and redundancy of the but-tocks is associated with trochanteric lipodystrophy. Dermolipectomy of the trochanteric lipodystrophy is performed at the same time as correction of the drooping buttocks.

Technique

With the patient standing, the amount of skin redundancy responsible for the drooping buttocks is carefully evaluated by pinching together and rolling in the excess skin on the upper and lower sides of the gluteal crease (Figure 37–6, *A*). The exact amount of excess tissue is determined and outlined in a fusiform fashion. The medial and lateral lengths of the excision will depend on the amount of skin excess. Markings of medial thigh laxity and redundancy and/or trochanteric lipodys-trophy, when present, are outlined for simultane-ous correction.

With the patient prepared for surgery in the prone position on the operating table, the pre-viously outlined fusiform skin excess is excised. Judicious resection and contouring removes a small amount of subcutaneous tissue and any ex-cess fat (Fig. 37–6, *B*). Initial removal of skin without simultaneous removal of fat prevents the possibility of overresection, which will produce a flat buttock.

After excision of an appropriate amount of fat, the thigh flap is elevated in an upward and

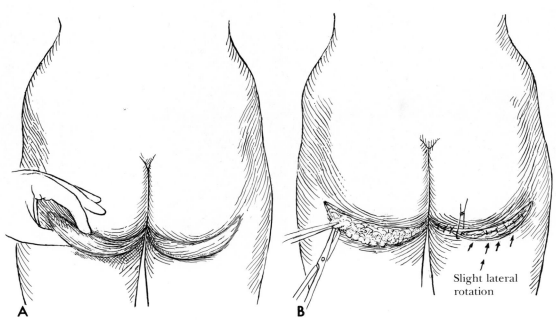

Slight lateral rotation

Figure 37–6. *A*, The amount of excess skin and subcutaneous tissue evaluated for correction of drooping buttocks.

B, After excision of excess skin, the subcutaneous tissue and fat are judiciously resected.

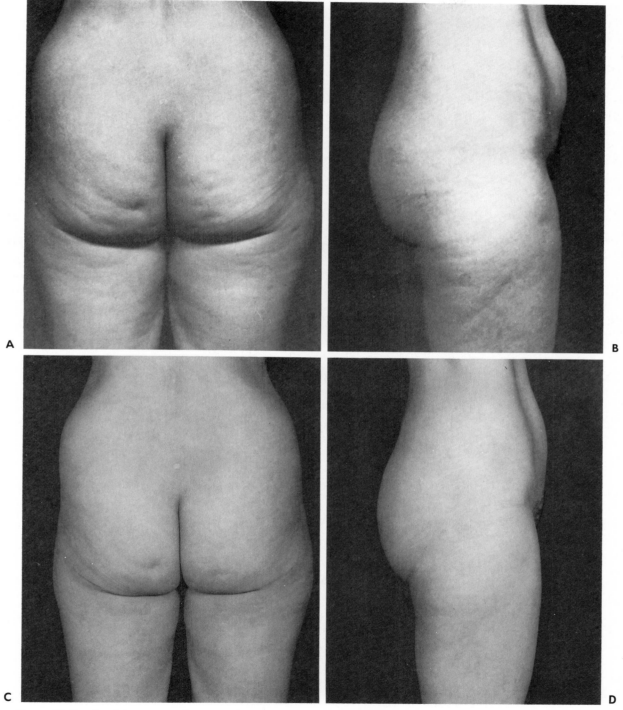

Figure 37-7. *A* and *B*, Preoperative status showing heavy, hanging buttocks.

C and *D*, Eighteen months after correction by the technique described in Figure 37–6. Note that the scars are camouflaged in the gluteal crease.

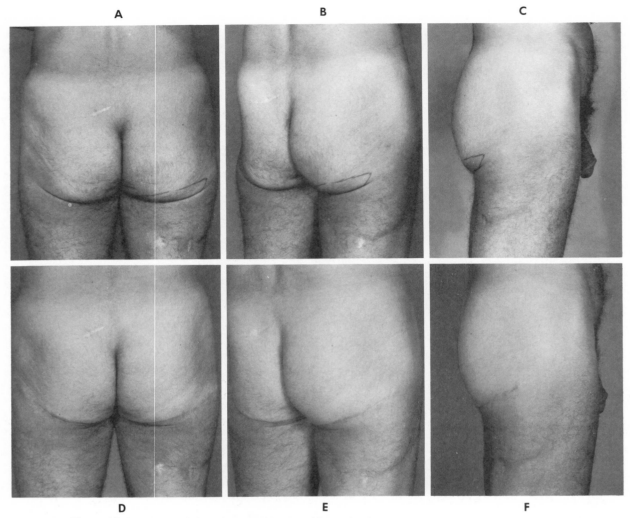

A   **B**   **C**

D   **E**   **F**

Figure 37–8.   *A, B,* and *C,* A 40-year-old male with sagging buttocks.

D, E, and *F,* One year after resection of the excess skin and a small amount of subcutaneous tissue.

slightly lateral direction. The flaps are aligned and sutured into position in three layers (Fig. 37–6, *B*): (1) 3–0 chromic catgut sutures with buried knots are used to approximate the deepest level of resection, (2) a layer of subdermal 4–0 chromic catgut sutures is created and (3) the skin is approximated with intracuticular 3–0 Prolene sutures and supported with steristrips. (See Figures 37–7 and 37–8.)

MEDIAL THIGH PTOSIS AND REDUNDANCY

Ptosis and laxity of the skin of the upper medial thighs occurs with aging as in other areas of the body. Redundancy of medial thigh skin is often associated with weight loss. Medial thigh deformities often accompany posterior and lateral buttock and thigh deformities. The skin of the upper inner thigh near the groin is relatively thin, as is the underlying fat layer. The force of gravity is constantly pulling this area when the patient is standing, folding it when sitting, and allowing it to fall posteriorly when supine. Therefore, it is not surprising that with time there is some ptosis and redundancy of the skin in this area (See Fig. 37–9, *A*).

Many patients requesting correction of medial thigh ptosis are active in leisure activities such as tennis or water sports in which the laxity and redundancy show below the usual clothing.

Often, it is difficult to obtain as much correction of the medial thigh laxity and redundancy as desired and still have an acceptable surgical scar. Incisions placed in the inguinal crease tend to spread and pull down onto the upper thigh below the level covered by underwear or a normal bathing suit. Extensive resection may produce tension in the inguinal area and spread the labia majoria, causing great discomfort to the patient. Vertical incisions placed on the thighs permit maximal thigh reduction and modeling, but the scars are unsightly and unacceptable for an aesthetic operation.

Lewis (1957, 1966, 1973) described the "thigh lift" using an elliptical excision in the inguinal crease anteriorly, an elliptical excision along the inferior crease of the buttock posteriorly, and a boomerang shaped excision extending down the posteromedial aspect of the thigh to a point proximal to the knee. A minimum of skin undermining was advised.

Delerm and Girotteau (1973) used horizontal gluteal crease incisions and created dermal flaps on the upper thigh flap in order to suspend the thigh to the ischial tuberosity medially and the fascia lata laterally. While this technique is designed to correct posterior buttock laxity, inguinal fold and upper medial thigh laxity is also improved.

Planas (1975) described incisions extending from the gluteal crease to the crural area and then going vertically upward from the ischion for approximately 15 cm onto the lower abdominal wall before curving laterally. The direction of traction is made vertically and the medial thigh flap is suspended on the abdominal wall anteriorly and to the gluteal region posteriorly. Wide undermining and flap elevation was advised. The scars on the anterior abdominal wall make this procedure less than ideal.

Technique

The amount of redundancy and laxity of the upper medial thighs is estimated and marked with the patient standing (Figure 37–9, A, B). The thickness of the tissue to be resected is determined by the thickness of the subcutaneous fat in the upper medial thigh. When the thigh is thin or when the mantle of subcutaneous fat has descended, the indicated resection may be skin alone. Excess removal of fat from the upper medial thigh will produce an unsightly depressed inguinocrural scar. The superior border of excision lies in the inguinal crease. Lateral extension of the incision will be determined by the amount of excess tissue. Rarely does this go beyond a vertical line dropped from the anterior superior iliac spine. The medial limit of excision is tailored toward the buttock crease (Fig. 37–9, C). If buttock laxity and/or trochanteric lipodystrophy is present, as is frequently associated with medial thigh laxity, the resection is planned posteriorly and all incisions are outlined (Fig. 37–9, D).

After the patient is prepared in the operating room, the tissue to be excised from the upper medial thigh can be removed in either of two ways: (1) the planned fusiform resection is excised directly (Fig. 37–9, E), and the defect is closed by superior, medial advancement and posterior rotation of the thigh flap or (2) the superior incision along the inguinal crease is made (Fig. 37–9, F), the flap of excess tissue is undermined to the level of the estimated resection, the flap is advanced superiorly and medially producing a posterior rotation to the anterior medial thigh, and exact markings and resection are made (Fig. 37–9, G). The skin edges are approximated and marked for aligning wound closure (Fig. 37–9, H). The flaps are sutured in three layers (Fig. 37–9, I, J, K): (1) permanent sutures with buried knots are anchored between the fascia of the mobile lower flap and the fixed fascia in the inguinal crease. This helps anchor the thigh flap superiorly and prevent inferior flap displacement. Sutures of 3–0 chromic catgut complete this deep layer of fascia to fascia. (2) The subcutaneous tissue is sutured with 4–0 interrupted chromic catgut sutures (3) Skin is sutured with 3–0 intracuticular Prolene. Steristrips are applied for epithelial approximation. If correction of buttock laxity or dermolipectomy of trochanteric lipodystrophy is indicated, the patient is turned to the supine position and the planned surgical procedure is performed. (See Figures 37–10 and 37–11.)

OBESITY AND HEAVY FAT THIGHS

Patients with heavy, fat, thick thighs from the groin to the knees have a variant of localized lipodystrophy. Some of these patients are normal in size throughout the remainder of the body, although most have pelvic and crural lipomatous accumulation. Patients with this type of deformity are not good candidates for buttock and thigh reduction surgery.

Patients who are generally obese are poor candidates for buttock and thigh surgery prior to a significant weight loss. In addition to the usual problems associated with operating through thick layers of fat (such as fat necrosis and wound infection), patients with fat thighs owing to obesity or lipodystrophy obtain a limited improvement with surgery.

CELLULITE

"Cellulite" is a term used by the public press and some practitioners when referring to the pebbly or cobblestone appearance of the thighs and

Text continued on page 1065.

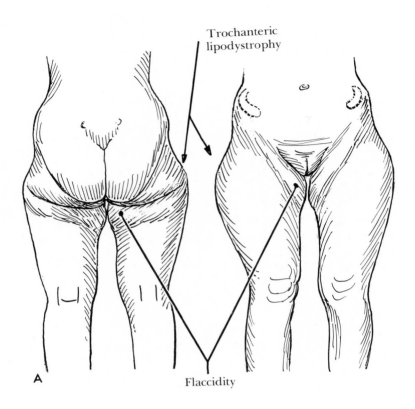

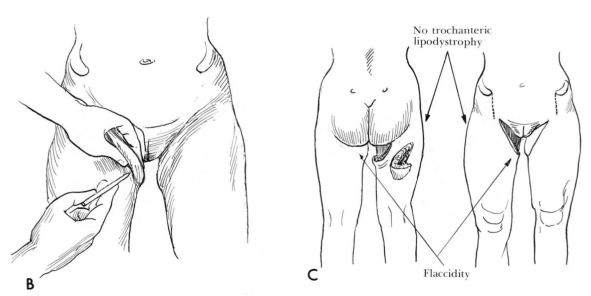

Figure 37–9.   *A,* Medial thigh flaccidity and redundancy associated with lateral gluteal deformities.

B, The excess medial thigh tissue is marked with the patient standing.

C, The incision lies in the inguinal crease anteriorly and extends medially and posteriorly toward the gluteal crease.

Illustration continued on the opposite page.

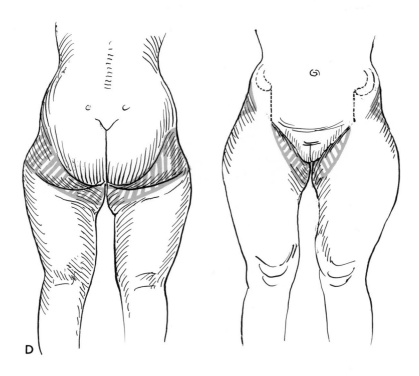

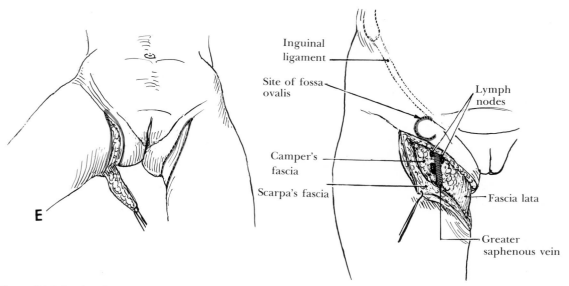

Figure 37–9 *Continued.*   *D,* The anterior, posterior, and lateral deformities are outlined and corrected simultaneously.

E, The elliptical full-thickness excision of the medial thigh excess as outlined.

Illustration continued on the following page.

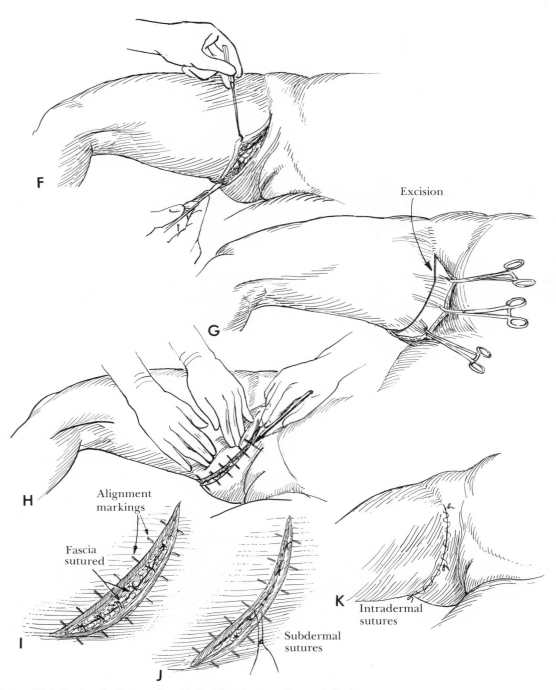

Figure 37–9 *Continued.   F,* Superior skin incision down to Camper's fascia.

G, The medial thigh excess is undermined and excised.

H, The medial thigh flap is advanced cephalad and medially. The flap is aligned for closure.

I, J, and *K,* The fascia-to-fascia permanent buried sutures help prevent inferior flap displacement. The subcutaneous tissue is closed with chromic catgut sutures, and the skin is approximated with intracuticular 3–0 Prolene.

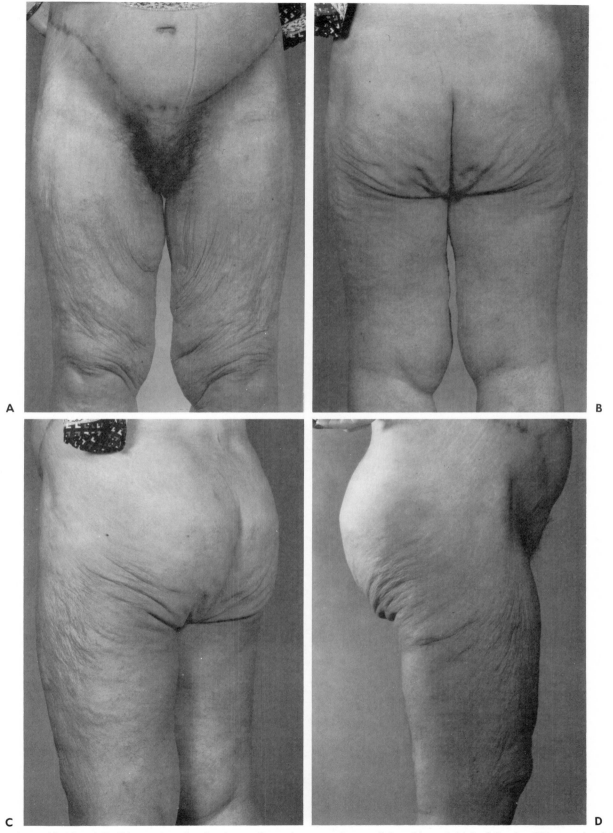

Figure 37–10. *A–D*, Skin ptosis and redundancy of anterior, posterior, medial, and lateral thighs following 200-pound weight loss. Previous abdominoplasty was performed elsewhere.

Illustration continued on the following page.

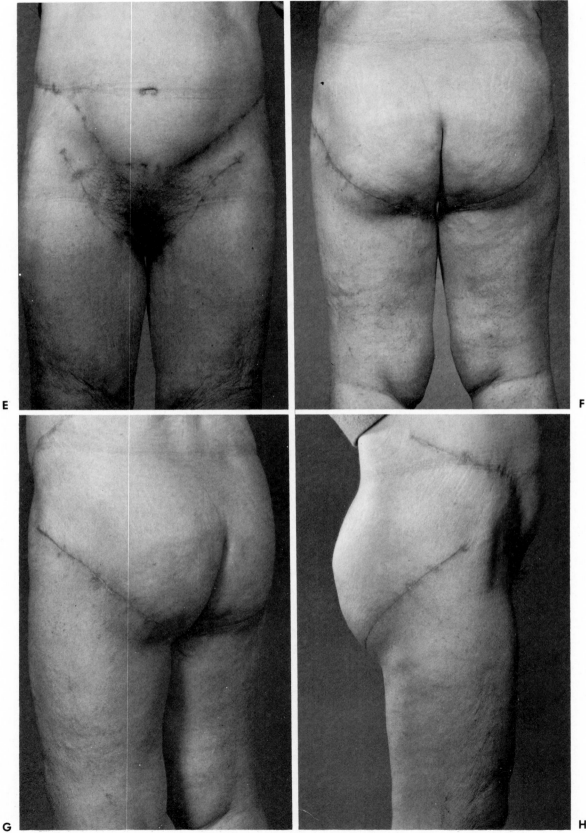

Figure 37–10 *Continued.   E–H,* The medial thigh correction by flap undermining, as described in Figure 37–9 *F–K.* The medial portion of the incision has migrated below the inguinal crease. The buttock and lateral thigh corrections are as described in previous sections.

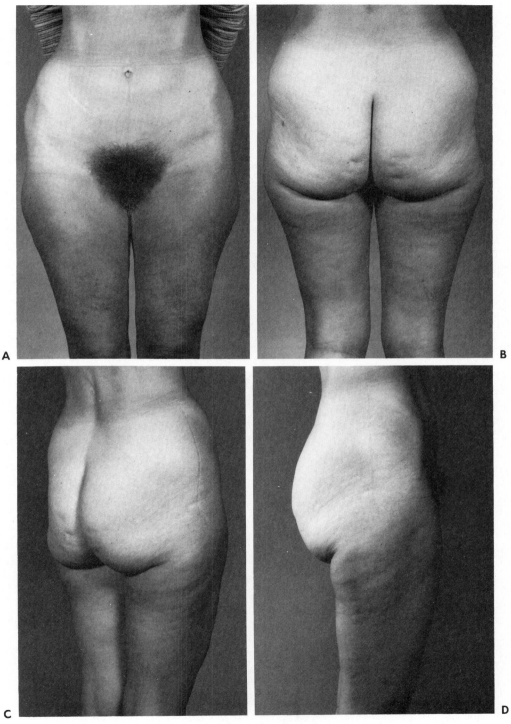

Figure 37–11. *A–D*, Preoperative status showing trochanteric lipodystrophy, lateral buttock depressions, gluteal excess, and upper medial thigh fullness.

Illustration continued on the following page.

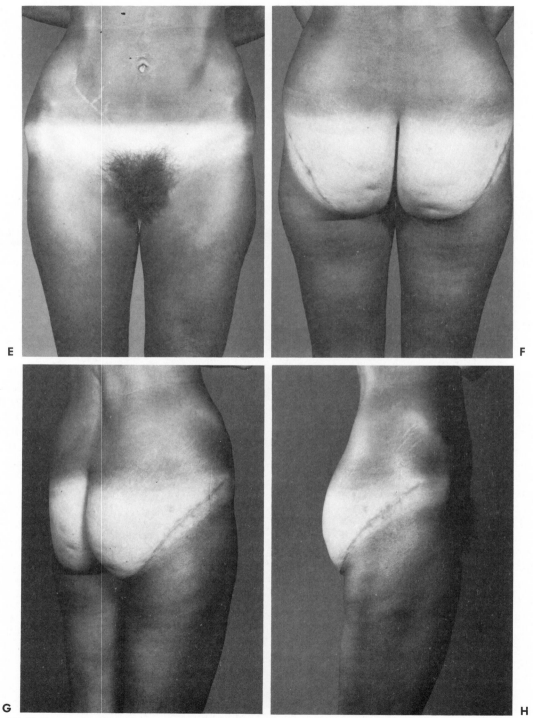

Figure 37–11 *Continued.* *E–H*, Postoperative status 10 months following correction. Note that all scars are hidden within bikini coverage area.

buttocks caused by the small fat accumulations lying between the fibrous connections of the subcutaneous tissue to the dermis of the skin

Frequent massage and manipulation of the area involved may break down some of the fat, thereby slightly improving the appearance. In many cases, the improved appearance is probably due to a small amount of edema in the area that has been frequently massaged.

There is no specific surgical treatment for cellulite alone. When cellulite accompanies medial thigh laxity and redundancy, trochanteric lipodystrophy, or ptosis of the buttocks, it will persist following surgery except for those areas directly removed by the surgical procedure.

POSTOPERATIVE CARE

The incisions are dressed with thin Telfa bandages and paper tape. Bulky dressings are not necessary.

When possible, the patient is transferred directly from the operating table to the bed that will be used for the next few days. This eliminates the discomfort associated with temporarily moving the patient to a recovery room stretcher or bed.

Postoperative pain is usually moderate. Analgesics should be given as necessary to keep the patient comfortable. Severe pain suggests a possible hematoma and requires immediate examination. Tranquilizers may help overly anxious patients during the initial postoperative period.

After correction of trochanteric lipodystrophy or sagging buttocks, a low residue diet is begun on the morning following surgery and maintained for approximately four days in order to reduce the need for a bowel movement. The Foley catheter is removed on the second morning following surgery.

On the first morning after correction of buttock laxity or trochanteric lipodystrophy, the patient is "log rolled" out of bed without flexion at the hips and stands at bedside. Ambulation is begun on the second morning after surgery and progresses as tolerated. Flexion and extension exercises at the ankles are advised for five minutes every hour while the patient is awake for the first three days after surgery to promote venous return in the lower extremities. Antiembolic stockings or ace wraps from the toes to midthighs also may help prevent venous stasis.

Drains are removed from the incisions and the intracuticular stitch is pulled and tightened to close the drain site two days following surgery. Intracu-

ticular sutures are removed 14 days postoperatively.

The patient is not permitted to sit for the first 14 days following buttock and trochanteric reduction. Standing and walking is permissible. Most normal activities are resumed slowly after four weeks, and vigorous activities such as golf, running, and tennis are permitted by the sixth postoperative week.

COMPLICATIONS

Scars

The most common complications following surgical correction of laxity of the medial thighs, buttocks, and trochanteric lipodystrophy involve the surgical scars. The position of the scars is such that they are under constant stress and tension and, therefore, have a tendency to widen and become hypertrophic. This is especially true of scars on the posterior lateral buttocks. Scars in the inguinocrural area have less tendency to become hypertrophic but they often spread in width.

Scars in the inguinocrural area following medial thigh lifting may migrate inferiorly below the level covered by normal swimwear even when there is not a great deal of tension on the incision. Permanent anchoring sutures in the deep fascia as described help retard the inferior migration but will not prevent it. A low inguinocrural incision can be improved in some patients by deepithelialization and repositioning. However, further full-thickness skin excision should not be made or the problem may become worse. Posterior scars will migrate down out of the gluteal crease if there is excess resection from the upper portion of the posterior thigh. Scars that become displaced too low posteriorly are difficult to correct because of the distortion in shape of the buttock associated with a scar that has pulled down, and the constant downward pull of the thigh exacerbates the problem.

Interlesional injection of steroids frequently helps improve hypertrophic scars. Some will benefit from excision and revision after two or three years, but fresh scars may likewise become hypertrophic.

Hematoma

The incidence of hematoma in buttock reduction surgery is low, as the small amount of flap undermining and approximation keeps dead space beneath the flaps to a minimum. Jackson-Pratt drains placed in the base of the resected area remove serosanginous drainage but will not prevent a hematoma. Excessive pain in the early postoperative period suggests a hematoma and requires immediate examination. Hematomas should be evacuated under sterile surgical conditions as soon as possible.

Wound Infection

Wound infection following buttock reduction surgery is rare. An undiagnosed hematoma may serve as a nidus for bacterial growth. Meticulous hemostasis reduces the chance of hematoma formation and likewise reduces the chance of a wound infection. An appropriate intraoperative blood level of a broad spectrum antibiotic may further reduce the likelihood of a wound infection.

Wound Dehiscence

Wound dehiscence following buttock reduction surgery may result from one of several causes: (1) improper approximation of the flaps at the time of the surgical procedure, (2) excessive activity or sitting by the patient prior to adequate healing, (3) wound infection or hematoma, and (4) too early removal of sutures.

Asymmetry of the Buttocks

Asymmetry of the buttocks and thighs may result because of the difficulty of evaluation when the patient is in the supine or prone position. Careful preoperative markings and measurements taking into account any asymmetry of the buttocks and thighs combined with an appropriately measured resection during the operative procedure will help prevent significant asymmetry.

Lateral Thigh Depressions

In normal anatomy, there is a depression between the greater trochanter and the ilium on the lateral upper thigh and buttock. Frequently, the depression associated with trochanteric lipodystrophy appears greater than normal because of the lipomatous collection in the buttocks, upper thighs, over the area of the greater trochanter, and in the pelvis. Planned resection of fat in the area of depression should be carefully noted during preoperative evaluation and marking. This is discussed in the section on correction of trochanteric lipodystrophy. Correction of postoperative depressions is discussed in a separate section.

(For list of references, see page 1072.)

REFERENCES

Breast Reduction and Mastoplexy/Mammary Augmentation

Abu al Qasim al-Zahrawi or Albucasis: Albucasis de C Chirurgia. Channing, J. (tr.). Oxford, Clarendon Press, 1778.

Adams, W. M.: Free composite grafts of the nipples in mammaryplasty. South. Surg. 13:715, 1947.

Adams, W. M.: Labial transplant for correction of loss of the nipple. Plast. Reconstr. Surg. 4:295, 1949.

Aegineta, P.: On male breasts resembling the female. In Adams, F. (tr.): The Seven Books of Paulus Aegineta. London, Sydenham Society, 1946, Vol 2, Book t, Sect. 46, p. 334.

Arion, H. G.: Retromammary prosthesis. C.R. Soc. Fr. Gynecol. No. 5, May 1965.

Arons, M. S.: Reduction of very large breasts: The inferior flap technique of Robertson. Br. J. Plast. Surg. 29:137, 1976.

Arufe, H. N., Erenfryd, A., and Saubidet, M.: Mammaplasty with single vertical superiorly-based pedicle to support the nipple-areola. Plast. Reconstr. Surg. 60:221, 1977.

Ashley, F. L.: A new type of breast prosthesis. Plast. Reconstr. Surg. 45:421, 1970.

Ashley, F. L.: Further studies on the natural-Y breast prosthesis. Plast. Reconstr. Surg. 49:414, 1972.

Aston, S. J.: Personal experience, 1978.

Auber, V.: Hypertrophie mammaire de la puberté, resection partielle restauratrice. Arch. Franco-Belges Chir. 3:287, 1923.

Aufricht, G.: Mammaplasty for pendulous breasts: Empiric and geometric planning. Plast. Reconstr. Surg. 4:13, 1949.

August, G. P., Chandra, R., and Hung, W.: Prepubertal male gynecomastia. J. Pediatr. 80:259, 1972.

Axhausen, G.: Ueber Mammaplastik, Med. Klin. 22:976, 1926.

Bader, K., Pellettiere, E., and Curtin, J. W.: Definitive surgical therapy for the "pre-malignant" or equivocal breast lesion. Plast. Reconst. Surg. 46:120, 1970.

Baker, J. L., Jr., Bartels, R. J., and Douglas, W. M.: Closed compression technique for rupturing a contracted capsule around breast implants. Plast. Reconstr. Surg. 58:137, 1976.

Bames, H. O.: Breast malformations and a new approach to the problem of small breasts. Plast. Reconstr. Surg. 5:499, 1950.

Bames, H. O.: Augmentation mammaplasty by lipotransplant. Plast. Reconstr. Surg. 11:404, 1953.

Barsky, A. J., Kahn, S., and Simon, B. E.: The development of a technique for the surgical correction of gynecomastia. Transactions of the International Society of Plastic Surgeons, 2nd Congress, London, 1959. Edinburgh, E. and S. Livingstone Ltds., 1960, pp. 527–531.

Barsky, A. J., Kahn, S., and Simon, B. E.: Principles and Practice of Plastic Surgery. II. New York, McGraw-Hill Book Co., 1964, pp. 564–569.

Becker, K. L.: Clinical and therapeutic experiences with Klinefelter's syndrome. Fertil. Steril. 23:568, 1972.

Benjamin, J. L., and Guy, C.: Calcification of implant capsules following augmentation mammaplasty. Plast. Reconstr. Surg. 59:432, 1977.

Berson, M.: Dermal-fat transplants used in building up the breasts. Surgery 15:451, 1945.

Biesenberger, H.: Eine neue Method der Mammaplastik. Zentralbl. Chir. 55:2382, 1928.

Biggs, T. M., Brauer, R. C., and Wolf, L. E.: Mastopexy in conjunction with subcutaneous mastectomy. Plast. Reconstr. Surg. 60:1, 1978.

Boo-Chai, K.: The complications of augmentation mammaplasty by silicone injection. Br. J. Plast. Surg. 22:281, 1969.

Brightmore, T. G. J.: Cystic lesion of a dorsal supernumerary breast in a male. Proc. R. Soc. Med. *64*:662, 1971.

Campos, F.: Sobre um caso de ginecomastia, bilateral e seu tratamento cirurgico. Arg. Cir. Clin. Exp. *6*:703, 1942.

Capozzi, A., DuBou, R., and Pennisi, V. R.: Distant migration of silicone gel from a ruptured breast implant (case report). Plast. Reconstr. Surg. *62*:302, 1978.

Carlsen, L., and Tershakowec, M. G.: Variation of Biesenberger technique of reduction mammaplasty. Plast. Reconstr. Surg. *55*:653, 1975.

Chaplin, C. H.: Loss of both breasts from injection of silicone (with additive). Plast. Reconstr. Surg. *44*:447, 1969.

Cocke, W. M., Leathers, H. K., and Lynch, J. B.: Foreign body reaction to polyurethane covers of some breast prostheses. Plast. Reconstr. Surg. *56*:527, 1973.

Cogswell, H. D., and Czerny, E. W.: Carcinoma of an aberrant breast in the axilla. Am. J. Surg. *27*:388, 1961.

Cohen, I. K.: On the use of soluble steroid within inflatable breast prostheses (Letter to the Editor). Plast. Reconstr. Surg. *62*:105, 1978.

Cohen, I. K., Goodman, H., and Theogaraj, S. D.: Xeromammography — A reason for using saline-filled breast prostheses. Plast. Reconstr. Surg. *60*:886, 1977.

Conway, H.: Mammaplasty: Analysis of 110 consecutive cases with end results. Plast. Reconstr. Surg. *10*:303, 1952.

Conway, H.: and Dietz, G. H.: Augmentation mammaplasty. Surg. Gynecol. Obstet. *114*:573, 1962.

Conway, H., and Smith, J.: Breast plastic surgery: Reduction mammaplasty, mastopexy, augmentation mammaplasty and mammary construction. Plast. Reconstr. Surg. *21*:8, 1958.

Copeland, M. M., and Geschickter, C. F.: Diagnosis and treatment of premalignant lesions of the breast. Surg. Clin. North Am. *30*:1717, 1950.

Cordoso de Castro, C.: Mammaplasty with curved incisions. Plast. Reconstr. Surg. *57*:596, 1976.

Corso, P. F.: Plastic surgery for the unilateral hypoplastic breast. A report of eight cases. Plast. Reconstr. Surg. *50*:134, 1972.

Courtiss, E. H., and Goldwyn, R. M.: Breast sensation before and after plastic surgery. Plast. Reconstr. Surg. *58*:1, 1976.

Courtiss, E. H., and Goldwyn, R. M.: Reduction mammaplasty by the inferior pedicle technique. Plast. Reconstr. Surg. *59*:500, 1977.

Cronin, T. D., and Gerow, F.: Augmentation mammaplasty: a new "natural feel" prosthesis. *In* Transactions of the Third International Congress of Plastic Surgery. Amsterdam, Excerpta Medica, 1964, pp. 41–49.

Cuenca, C. R., and Becker, K. L.: Klinefelter's syndrome and cancer of the breast. Arch. Intern. Med. *121*:159, 1968.

Cutler, M.: Tumors of the Breast. London, Pitman Publishing Ltd., 1961.

Czerny, V.: Plastischer Ersatz der Brustdruse durch ein lipoma. Chir, Kong. Verhandl. *2*:126, 1895.

Dartigues, L.: Procédé de suspension et mastopéxie par voie axillotomique. Bull. Soc. Méd. Paris *16*:145, 1924.

Dartigues, L.: Traitement chirurgical du prolapsus mammaire. Arch. Franco-Belg. Chir. *28*:313, 1925.

Dartigues, L.: État actuel de la chirurgie esthétique mammaire. Les différentes procédés, de mastoplastie en général et de la greffe aréolomammélonnair en particulier. Monde Méd. *38*:75, 1928.

De Cholnoky, T.: Augmentation mammaplasty. Survey of complications of 10,941 patients by 265 surgeons. Plast. Reconstr. Surg. *45*:573, 1970.

De Cholnoky, T.: Supernumerary breast. Arch. Surg. *39*:926, 1939.

De Cholnoky, T.: Accessory breast tissue in the axilla. N.Y. State J. Med. *51*:2245, 1951.

Dehner, J.: Mastopexie zur Beseitgung der Hängebrust. Munch. Med. Wochenschr. *55*:1878, 1908.

Dempsey, W. C., and Latham, W. D.: Subpectoral implants in agumentation mammaplasty. Plast. Reconstr. Surg. *42*:515, 1968.

Domanskis, E. J., and Owsley, J. Q. Jr.: Histological investigation of the etiology of capsule contracture following augmentation mammaplasty. Plast. Reconstr. Surg. *58*:689, 1976.

Dufourmentel, L.: La mastopéxie par déplacement souscutané avec transposition du mamelon. Bull. Mem. Soc. Chir. Paris, *20*, 1925.

Dufourmentel, C., and Mouly, R.: Plastie mammaire par la méthode oblique. Ann. Chir. Plast. *6*:45, 1961.

Dufourmentel, C., and Mouly, R.: Dévelopments récents de la plastie mammaire par la méthode oblique latérale. Ann. Chir. Plast. *10*:227, 1965.

Dufourmentel, C., and Mouly, R.: Modification of "periwinkle shell operation" for small ptotic breast. Plast. Reconstr. Surg. *41*:523, 1968.

Dukes, C. E., and Mitchley, M. I.: Polyvinyl sponge implants: Experimental and clinical observations. Br. J. Plast. Surg. *15*:225, 1962.

Durston, W.: Concerning the death of the big-breasted woman. Phil. Trans. Vol. IV, for Anno 1669, pp. 1068–1069. London, Royal Society, 1670.

Durston, W.: Concerning a very sudden and excessive swelling of a woman's breasts. Phil. Trans., Vol. IV, for Anno 1669, pp. 1047–1049. London, Royal Society, 1670.

Durston, W.: Observations about the unusual swelling of the breasts. Phil. Trans. Vol. IV, for Anno 1669, pp. 1049–1050. London, Royal Society, 1670.

Edgerton, M. T., McClary, A. R.: Augmentation mammaplasty. Plast. Reconstr. Surg. *21*:279, 1958.

Edgerton, M.T., Meyer, E., and Jacobson, W. E.: Augmentation mammaplasty. II. Further surgical and psychiatric evaluation. Plast. Reconstr. Surg. *27*:279, 1961.

Eisenberg, H. V., and Bartels, R. J.: Rupture of silicone baggel breast implant by closed compression capsulotomy. Plast. Reconstr. Surg. *59*:849, 1977.

Elbaz, J. S., and Verheecke, J.: La cicatrice en L dans les plasties mammaires. Ann. Chir. Plast. *17*:283, 1972.

Ellenberg, A. H.: Marked thinning of the breast skin flaps after the insertion of implants containing triamcinolone. Plast. Reconstr. Surg. *60*:755, 1977.

Feliberti, M. C., Arrillaga, A., and Colon, G. A.: Rupture of inflated breast implants in closed compression capsulotomy. Plast. Reconstr. Surg. *59*:848, 1977.

Felix, E. R., Sethi, S. M., Ransdell, A. M., and Lissner, A. B.: Strombeck mammaplasty with free nipple grafts. Plast. Reconstr. Surg. *45*:47, 1970.

Frantz, P., and Herbst, C. A.: Augmentation mammaplasty, irradiation and breast cancer. Cancer *36*:1147, 1975.

Fredricks, S.: Management of mammary hypoplasia. *In* Goldwyn, R. M. (ed.): Plastic and Reconstructive Surgery of the Breast. Boston, Little, Brown and Co., 1976, p. 387.

Freeman B. S.: Subcutaneous mastectomy for benign breast lesions with immediate or delayed prosthetic replacement. Plast. Reconstr. Surg. *30*:676, 1962.

Freeman, B. S.: Complications of subcutaneous mastectomy with prosthetic replacement, immediate or delayed. South Med. J. *60*:1277, 1967.

Freeman, B. S.: Technique of subcutaneous mastectomy with replacement: Immediate and delayed. Br. J. Plast. Surg. *22*:161, 1969.

Georgiade, N. G.: Reconstructive Breast Surgery. St. Louis, C. V. Mosby Co., 1976.

Gersuny, R.: Cited by Thorek, M.: Plastic Surgery of the Breast and Abdominal Wall. Springfield, Ill., Charles C Thomas, Publisher, 1942.

Gifford, S.: Emotional attitudes toward cosmetic breast surgery: loss and restitution of the "ideal self." *In* Goldwyn, R. M. (ed.): Plastic and Reconstructive Surgery of the Breast. Boston, Little, Brown and Co., 1976.

Gillies, H., and McIndoe, A. H.: The technique of mammaplasty in conditions of hypertrophy of the breast. Surg. Gynecol. Obstet. *68*:658, 1939.

Girard, C.: Über Mastoptose und Mastopexie. Verh. Dsch. Ges. Chir. *39*:200, 1910.

Gobell, R.: Mamma pendula und heftiger Mastodynie. Munch. Med. Wochenschr. 61:1760, 1914.

Goin, J. M.: High pressure injection of silicone gel into an axilla – A complication of closed compression capsulotomy of the breast (case report). Plast. Reconstr. Surg. 62:891, 1978.

Goin, M. K., Goin, J. M., and Gianini, M. H.: The psychic consequences of a reduction mammaplasty. Plast. Reconstr. Surg. 59:530, 1977.

Goldman, L. D., and Goldwyn, R. M.: Some anatomical considerations of subcutaneous mastectomy. Plast. Reconstr. Surg. 51:501, 1973.

Goldwyn, R. M. (ed.): Plastic and Reconstructive Surgery of the Breast. Boston, Little, Brown and Co., 1976.

Goulian, D.: Dermal mastopexy. Clin. Plast. Surg. 3:171, 1976.

Goulian, D.: Dermal mastopexy. Plast. Reconstr. Surg. 47:105, 1971.

Goulian, D., and Conway, H.: Correction of the moderately ptotic breast, a warning. Plast. Reconstr. Surg. 43:478, 1969.

Goulian, D., Jr., and McDivitt, R. W.: Subcutaneous mastectomy with immediate reconstruction of the breasts using the dermal mastopexy technique. Plast. Reconstr. Surg. 50:211, 1972.

Griffiths, C., Jr.: The submuscular implant in augmentation mammaplasty. In Transactions of the 4th International Congress of Plastic Surgeons, pp. 1009–1015. Amsterdam, Excerpta Medica, 1968.

Grindlay, J. H., and Clagett, O. T.: Plastic sponge prosthesis for use after pneumonectomy. Proc. Staff Meet. Mayo Clin. 24:538, 1949.

Grindlay, J. H., and Waugh, J. M.: Plastic sponge which acts as framework for living tissues. Arch. Surg. 63:288, 1951.

Grossman, A. R.: The current status of augmentation mammaplasty. Plast. Reconstr. Surg. 52:1, 1973.

Gsell, F.: Reduction mammaplasty for extremely large breasts. Plast. Reconstr. Surg. 53:643, 1974.

Haagensen, C. D.: Diseases of the Breast, ed. 2. Philadelphia, W. B. Saunders Company, 1971.

Hamblen, E. C.: Endocrinology of Women. Springfield, Ill., Charles C Thomas, Publisher, 1945.

Hamilton, W. J., Boyd, J. D., and Mossman, H. W.: Human Embryology. Baltimore, Williams and Wilkins Co., 1945.

Hanson, E., and Segovia, J.: Dorsal supernumerary breast (case report). Plast. Reconstr. Surg. 61:441, 1978.

Harmon, J., and Aliapoulios, M. A.: Gynecomastia in marihuana users. N. Engl. J. Med. 287:936, 1972.

Hausner, R. J., Schoen, F. J., and Pierson, K. K.: Foreign-body reaction to silicone gel in axillary lymph nodes after an augmentation mammaplasty. Plast. Reconstr. Surg. 62:381, 1978.

Hayes, H.: Breast implants and possible late hematogenous infection (Letter to the Editor). Plast. Reconstr. Surg. 60:104, 1977.

Hiraide, K., and Akai, S.: A case of carcinoma arising in accessory mammary tissue. Jap. J. Cancer Clin 14:964, 1968.

Hollenberg, C.: An investigation of polyurethane foam in experimental animals. Can. J. Surg. 6:371, 1963.

Hoopes, J. E., Edgerton, M. T., and Shelley, W.: Organic synthetics for augmentation mammaplasty: Their relation to breast cancer. Plast. Reconstr. Surg. 39:263, 1967.

Horton, C. E., Adamson, J. E., Mladick, R. A., and Carraway, J. H.: Simple mastectomy with immediate reconstruction. Plast. Reconstr. Surg. 53:42, 1974.

Huang, T. T., Blackwell, S. J., and Lewis, S. R.: Migration of silicone gel after the "squeeze technique" to rupture a contracted breast capsule (case report). Plast. Reconstr. Surg. 61:277, 1978.

Hueston, J.: Unilateral agenesis and hypoplasia: difficulties and suggestions. In Goldwyn, R. M. (ed.): Plastic and Reconstructive Surgery of the Breast. Boston, Little, Brown and Co., 1975, pp. 361–374.

Hughes, E. S. R.: The development of the mammary gland. Ann. R. Coll. Surg. Engl. 6:99, 1950.

Imber, G., Schwager, R. G., Guthrie, R. H., and Gray, G. F.: Fibrous capsule formation after subcutaneous implantation of synthetic materials in experimental animals. Plast. Reconstr. Surg. 54:183, 1974.

Jarrett, J. R., Cutler, R. G., and Teal, D. F.: Subcutaneous mastectomy in small, large, or ptotic breasts with immediate submuscular placement of implants. Plast. Reconstr. Surg. 62:381, 1978.

Jenny, H.: Personal communication, 1969.

Johnson, M., and Lloyd, H. E. D.: Bilateral breast cancer 10 years after an augmentation mammaplasty (case report). Plast. Reconstr. Surg. 53:88, 1974.

Johnstone, G.: Prepubertal gynecomastia in association with an interstitial-cell tumor of the testis. Br. J. Urol. 39:211, 1967.

Joseph, J.: Zur Operation der hypertrophischen Hängebrust. Dtsch. Med. Wochenschr. 51:1103, 1925.

Kahn, S., Hoffman, S., and Simon, B. E.: Correction of non-hypertrophic ptosis of the breasts. Plast. Reconstr. Surg. 41:244, 1968.

Kaplan, I.: Reduction mammaplasty. Nipple-areola survival on a single breast quadrant. Plast. Reconstr. Surg. 61:27, 1978.

Kausch, W.: Die Operation der mammahypertrophie. Zentralbl. Chir. 43:713, 1916.

Kaye, B. L.: Axillary breasts: an aesthetic deformity of the trunk. Clin Plast. Surg. 2:397, 1975.

Kelley, A. P., Jacobson, H. S., Fox, J. I., and Jenny, H.: Complications of the Cronin Silastic mamary prosthesis. Plast. Reconstr. Surg. 37:438, 1966.

Kopf, E. H., Vinnik, C. A., Bongiovi, J. J., and Dombrowski, D. J.: Complications of silicone injections. Rocky Med. J. 73:77, 1976.

Kraske, H.: Operative treatment of hypertrophied mamma. München. Med. Wochenschr. 70:672, 1923.

Ksander, G. A., Vistnes, L. M., and Fogarty, D. C.: Experimental effects on surrounding fibrous capsule formation from placing steroids in a silicone bag-gel prosthesis before implantation. Plast. Reconstr. Surg. 62:873, 1978.

Letterman, G., and Schurter, M.: Gynecomastia. In Georgiade, N. G. (ed.): Reconstructive Breast Surgery. St. Louis, C. V. Mosby Co., 1976, pp. 229–250.

Letterman, G., Schurter, M.: Surgical correction of gynecomastia. Plast. Reconstr. Surg. 49:259, 1972.

Lewis, J. R., Jr.: The augmentation mammaplasty with special reference to alloplastic materials. Plast. Reconstr. Surg. 35:51, 1965.

Lexer, E.: Hypertrophie bie der mammae. München. Med. Wochenschr. 59:2702, 1912.

Lilla, J. A., and Vistnes, L. M.: Long-term study of reactions to various silicone breast implants in rabbits. Plast. Reconstr. Surg. 57:637, 1976.

Longacre, J. J.: The use of the local pedicle flaps for reconstruction of the breast after sub-total extirpation of the mammary gland and for the correction of distortion and atrophy of the breast due to excessive scar. Plast. Reconstr. Surg. 11:380, 1953.

Longacre, J. J.: Surgical reconstruction of the flat discoid breast. Plast. Reconstr. Surg. 17:358, 1956.

Longacre, J. J.: Breast reconstruction with local dermal and fat pedicle flaps. Plast. Reconstr. Surg. 24:563, 1959.

Lotsch, F.: Über Hängebrustplastik. Zentralbl. Chir. 50:1241, 1923.

Lotsch, F.: Über Hängebrustplastik. Klin. Wochenschr. 7:603, 1928.

Malbec, E. F.: Gynecomastia; surgical technics. Rev. Fac. Med. Bogota 14:380, 1945.

Maliniac, J. W.: Plastic repair of pendulous breasts. M.J. Rec. 136:312, 1932.

Maliniac, J. W.: Two-stage mammaplasty in relation to blood supply. Am. J. Surg. 68:55, 1945.

Maliniac, J. W.: Breasts and Their Repair. New York, Grune and Stratton, 1950.

Maliniac, J.: Harmful fallacies in mammaplasty. Personal communication. Abstract, International Congress of Plastic Surgery, London, 1959.

Marino, H.: Glandular mastectomy: Immediate reconstruction. Plast. Reconstr. Surg. *10*:204, 1952.

May, H.: Breast plasty in the female. Plast. Reconstr. Surg. *17*:351, 1956.

McIndoe, A. H., and Rees, T. D.: Mammaplasty: Indications, technique and complications. Br. J. Plast. Surg. *10*:307, 1958.

McKissock, P. K.: Reduction mammaplasty with a vertical dermal flap. Plast. Reconstr. Surg. *49*:245, 1972.

Mendes Filho, A., and Ludovici, C. O.: Importancia da mamografia nas plasticas mamarias. Rev. Lat. Am. Cir. Plast. *12*:131, 1968.

Meyer, R., and Kesselring, U.: Reduction mammaplasty with an L-shaped suture line. Plast. Reconstr. Surg. *55*:139, 1975.

Millard, R. D., Jr., Mullin, W. R., and Lesavoy, M. A.: Secondary correction of the too-high areola and nipple after a mammaplasty. Plast. Reconstr. Surg. *58*:568, 1976.

Mladick, R. A.: Possible dangers of placing implant subpectorally immediately after subcutaneous mastectomy. (Letter to the Editor). Plast. Reconstr. Surg. *62*:289, 1978.

Moore, A. M., and Brown, J. B.: Investigations of polyvinyl compounds for use as subcutaneous prostheses (polyvinyl sponge, Ivalon). Plast. Reconstr. Surg. *10*:453, 1952.

Morestin, H.: De l'ablation esthétique des tumeurs du sein. Bull. Mém. Soc. Chir. Paris *29*:561, 1903.

Morestin, H.: Hypertrophie mammaire. Bull. Mém. Soc. Anat. Paris *80*:682, 1905.

Morestin, H.: Hypertrophie mammaire traitée par la rèsection discöide. Bull. Mém. Soc. Chir. Paris *33*:649, 1907, 1909.

Mornard, P.: Mastopéxie esthétique par transplantation du mamelon, pratique chirurgicale illustrée (Pauchet). Paris, G. Doin et Cie, 1926.

Nedkoff, N.: New corrective method for breast hypertrophy. Zentralbl. Chir. *65*:1503, 1938.

Nöel, A.: Aesthetische Chirurgie der weiblichen Brust. Ein neues Verfahren zur Korektur der Hängebrust. Med. Welt *2*:51, 1928.

Nosnachuk, J. S.: Injected dimethylpolysiloxane fluid: a study of the antibody and histologic response. Plast. Reconstr. Surg. *42*:562, 1968.

Nydick, M., Bustos, J., Dale, J. H., and Rawson, R. W.: Gynecomastia in adolescent boys. J.A.M.A. *178*:106, 1961.

O'Conor, C. M.: Glandular excision with immediate mammary reconstruction. Plast. Reconstr. Surg. *33*:57, 1964.

Oppenheimer, B. S., Oppenheimer, E. T., and Stout, A. P.: Sarcomas induced in rodents by embedding various plastic films. Proc. Soc. Exp. Biol. Med. *79*:366, 1952.

Ortiz-Monasterio, F., and Trigos, I.: Management of patients with complications from injections of foreign material into the breasts. Plast. Reconstr. Surg. *50*:42, 1972.

Pangman, W. J., II: Comments on breast plasty. South. Gen. Pract. Med. Surg. *115*:256, 1953.

Pangman, W. J., and Wallace, R. M.: The use of plastic prostheses in breast plastic and other soft tissue surgery. Read before the 6th Congress of the Pan-Pacific Surgical Association, October 7, 1954.

Papillon, J.: Pros and cons of subpectoral implantation. Clin. Plast. Surg. *3*(2):321, 1976.

Parsons, R. W., and Thering, H. R.: Management of the silicone-injected breast. Plast. Reconstr. Surg. *60*:534, 1977.

Passot, R.: La correction esthétique du prolapsus mammaire par le procédé de la transposition du mamelon. Presse Méd. *33*:317, 1925.

Peacock, E. E., Jr.: Biological basis for management of benign disease of the breast. Plast. Reconstr. Surg. *55*:14, 1975.

Penn, J.: Breast reduction. II. Transactions of the International Society of Plastic Surgeons, 2nd Congress, London, 1959. Edinburgh, E. and S. Livingstone, Ltd., 1960.

Pennisi, V. R.: Xeromammography — A reason for using saline-filled breast prostheses (voice of polite dissent). Plast. Reconstr. Surg. *61*:107, 1978.

Pennisi, V. R., Capozzi, A., and Terez, F. M.: Subcutaneous mastectomy data: A preliminary report. Plast. Reconstr. Surg. *59*:53, 1977.

Pennisi, V. R., Capozzi, A., Walsh, J., and Christensen, N.: Obscure breast carcinoma encountered in subcutaneous mastectomies. Plast. Reconstr. Surg. *47*:17, 1971.

Perras, C., and Papillon, J.: The value of mammography in cosmetic surgery of the breast. Plast. Reconstr. Surg. *52*:132, 1973.

Perrin, E. R.: The use of soluble steroids within inflatable breast prostheses. Plast. Reconstr. Surg. *57*:163, 1976.

Persoff, M. M.: Problems with the use of soluble steroids within inflatable breast prostheses (Letter to the Editor). Plast. Reconstr. Surg. *62*:106, 1978.

Peterson, H. D., and Burt, G. B.: Role of steroids in prevention of circumferential capsular scarring in augmentation mammaplasty. Plast. Reconstr. Surg. *54*:28, 1974.

Pickrell, K.: An evaluation of Etheron as an augmentation material in plastic and reconstructive surgery. A long-term clinical and experimental study. Presented at the annual meeting of the American Society of Plastic and Reconstructive Surgery, Hawaii, October, 1962.

Pickrell, K. L., Puckett, C. L., and Given, K. S.: Subpectoral augmentation mammaplasty. Plast. Reconstr. Surg. *60*:325, 1977.

Pitanguy, I.: Breast hypertrophy. Transactions of the International Society of Plastic Surgeons, 2nd Congress, London, 1959. Edinburgh, E. and S. Livingstone, Ltd., 1960.

Pitanguy, I.: Transareolar incision for gynecomastia. Plast. Reconstr. Surg. *38*:414, 1966.

Pitanguy, I.: Amastia and mammary asymmetries. The International Microform Journal of Aesthetic Plastic Surgery. Transactions of the 2nd Congress of the International Society of Aesthetic Plastic Surgery, 1974-D.

Pousson, M., and Michel, L.: Sur un cas de mastopéxie. J. Méd. Bordeux *27*:495, 1897.

Ragnell, A.: Operative correction of hypertrophy and ptosis of the female breast. Acta Chir. Scand. *94*:113, 1946.

Ragnell, A.: Operative correction of hypertrophy and ptosis of the female breast. IVAR Haeggstroms Boktryckeri A. B., Stockholm, 1946.

Ragnell, A.: Further experience of preservation of lactation capacity and nipple sensitivity in breast reduction. Transactions of International Society of Plastic Surgeons, 1st Congress, Sweden, 1955. Baltimore, Williams and Wilkins Co., 1957.

Redfern, A. B., Ryan, J. J., and Su, C. T.: Calcification of the fibrous capsule about mammary implants. Plast. Reconstr. Surg. *59*:249, 1977.

Rees, T. D.: Plastic surgery of the breast. *In* Converse, J. M. (ed.): Reconstructive Plastic Surgery, Vol. 5. Philadelphia, W. B. Saunders Company, 1964, p. 1903.

Rees, T. D.: Plastic surgery of the breast. *In* Converse, J. M. (ed.): Reconstructive Plastic Surgery, Vol. 7. Philadelphia, W. B. Saunders Company, 1977, p. 3661.

Rees, T. D., and Aston, S. J.: The tuberous breast. Clin. Plast. Surg. *3*:339, 1976.

Rees, T. D., Ballantyne, D. L. J., Seidman, I., and Hawthorne, G. A.: Visceral response to subcutaneous and intraperitoneal injections of silicone in mice. Plast. Reconstr. Surg. *39*:402, 1967.

Rees, T. D., and Dupuis, C. C.: Unilateral mammary hypoplasia. Plast. Reconstr. Surg. *41*:307, 1968.

Rees, T. D., and Flagg, S.: Untoward results and complications following breast reduction mammaplasty. *In* Goldwyn, R. M. (ed.): The Unfavorable Results in Plastic Surgery: Avoidance and Treatment. Boston, Little, Brown and Co., 1972.

Rees, T. D., Guy, C. L., and Coburn, R. J.: The use of inflatable breast implants. Plast. Reconstr. Surg. *52*:609, 1973.

Regnault, P.: Partially submuscular breast augmentation. Plast. Reconstr. Surg. *59*:72, 1977.

Regnault, P.: Reduction mammaplasty by the "B" technique. Plast. Reconstr. Surg. *53*:19, 1974.

Regnault, P.: Breast ptosis. Definition and treatment. Clin. Plast. Surg. *3*:193, 1976.

Reiffel, R. L., Rees, T. D., Guy, C. L., and Aston, S. J.: Comparison of fibrous capsule contracture between breast augmented with silicone gel or saline-filled implants. (In press)

Ribeiro, L.: A new technique for reduction mammaplasty. Plast. Reconstr. Surg. 55:330, 1975.

Rigdon, R. H.: Local reaction to polyurethane — a comparative study in the mouse, rat, and rabbit. J. Biomed. Mater. Res. 7:79, 1973.

Rintala, A. E., and Svinhufvud, U.M.: Effect of augmentation mammaplasty on mammography and thermography. Plast. Reconstr. Surg. 54:390, 1974.

Robbins, T. H.: A reduction mammaplasty with the areola-nipple based on an inferior dermal pedicle. Plast. Reconstr. Surg. 59:64, 1977.

Robertson, D. C.: The technique of inferior flap mammaplasty. Plast. Reconstr. Surg. 40:372, 1967.

Robertson, J. L. A.: Changed appearance of mammograms following breast reduction. Plast. Reconstr. Surg. 59:347, 1977.

Robles, J. M., Zimman, O. A., and Lee, J. C.: A larger subpectoral pocket for breast implants. Plast. Reconstr. Surg. 61:78, 1978.

Rubin, L. R.: The cushioned augmentation repair after a subcutaneous mastectomy. Plast. Reconstr. Surg. 57:23, 1976.

Rudolph, R., Abraham, J., Vecchione, T., Guber, S., and Woodward, M.: Myofibroblasts and free silicon around breast implants. Plast. Reconstr. Surg. 62:185, 1978.

Schatten, W. E., Hartley, J. H., Crow, R. W., and Griffin, J. M.: Further experience with lateral wedge resection mammaplasties. Br. J. Plast. Surg. 28:37, 1975.

Schatten, W. E., Hartley, J. H., Jr., and Hamm, W. G.: Reduction mammaplasty by the Dufourmentel-Mouly method. Plast. Reconstr. Surg. 48:306, 1971.

Schonfeld, W. A.: Body-image disturbances in adolescents with inappropriate sexual development. Am. J. Orthopsychiatry 34:493, 1964.

Schwarzmann, E.: Die Technik der mammaplastik. Der Chirurg. 2:932, 1930.

Shipley, R. H., O'Donnell, J. M., and Bader, K. F.: Personality characteristics of women seeking breast augmentation. Comparison to small-busted and average-busted controls. Plast. Reconstr. Surg. 60:369, 1977.

Shipley, R. H., O'Donnell, J. M., and Bader, K. F.: Psychological effects of cosmetic augmentation mammaplasty. Aesth. Plast. Surg. 2:429, 1978.

Silver, H. L.: Treating the complications of augmentation mammaplasty. Plast. Reconstr. Surg. 49:637, 1972.

Simon, B. E., and Hoffman, S.: Correction of gynecomastia. In, Goldwyn, R. M. (ed.): Plastic and Reconstructive Surgery of the Breast. Boston, Little, Brown and Co., 1976, pp. 305–322.

Simon, B. E., Hoffman, S., and Kahn, S.: Classification and surgical correction of gynecomastia. Plast. Reconstr. Surg. 51:48, 1973.

Simon, B. E., Hoffman, S., and Kahn, S.: Treatment of asymmetry of the breasts. A report of 30 cases of development origin. Clin. Plast. Surg. 2:375, 1975.

Skoog, T.: Inverted nipples. In Skoog, T.: Plastic Surgery. Philadelphia, W. B. Saunders Company, 1974, pp. 384–390.

Skoog, T.: Inverted nipples. In: Skoog, T.: Plastic Surgery. New Methods and Refinements. Stockholm, Almqvist and Wiksell, 1974, p. 382.

Skoog, T.: A technique of breast reduction, transposition of the nipple on a cutaneous vascular pedicle. Acta Chir. Scand. 126:453, 1963.

Smahel, J.: Tissue reactions to breast implants coated with polyurethane. Plast. Reconstr. Surg. 61:80, 1978.

Smith, G. M. R., and Greening, W. P.: Carcinoma of aberrant breast tissue. Br. J. Surg. 59:89, 1972.

Snyder, R. E.: Commentary on xeromammography — A reason for using saline-filled breast prostheses (voice of polite dissent). Plast. Reconstr. Surg. 61:107, 1978.

Snyderman, R. K., and Lizardo, J. G.: Statistical study of malignancies found before, during or after routine breast plastic operations. Plast. Reconstr. Surg. 25:253, 1960.

Strömbeck, J. O.: Mammaplasty: Report of a new technique based on the two pedicle procedure. Br. J. Plast. Surg. 13:79, 1960.

Strömbeck, J. O.: Reduction mammaplasty. In Gibson T. (ed.): Modern Trends in Plastic Surgery. London, Butterworth and Co., 1964, p. 237.

Strömbeck, J. O.: Reduction mammaplasty. In Grabb, W. C., and Smith, J. W. (eds.): Plastic Surgery. A Concise Guide to Clinical Practice. Boston, Little, Brown and Co., 1968, pp. 821–835.

Strömbeck, J. O.: Reduction mammaplasty. Surg. Clin. North Am. 51:453, 1971.

Strömbeck, J. O.: Reduction mammaplasty. In Grabb, W. C., and Smith, J. W. (eds.): Plastic Surgery. Boston, Little, Brown and Co., 1973.

Tabari, K.: Augmentation mammaplasty with simaplast implant. Plast. Reconstr. Surg. 44:468, 1969.

Thomas, T. G.: On the removal of benign tumours of the mamma without mutilation of the organ. N. Y. Med. J. Obstet. Rev. 35:337, 1882.

Thomson, H. G.: The fate of the pseudosheath pocket around silicone implants. Plast. Reconstr. Surg. 51:667, 1973.

Thorek, M.: Possibilities in the reconstruction of the human form. N. Y. Med. J. Rec. 116:572, 1922.

Thorek, M.: Plastic Surgery of the Breast and Abdominal Wall. Springfield, Ill. Charles C Thomas, Publisher, 1942.

Thorek, M.: Plastic reconstruction of the breast and free transplantation of the nipple. J. Int. Coll. Surg. 9:194, 1946.

Tolhurst, D. E.: "Nutcracker" technique for compression rupture of capsules around breast implants. Plast. Reconstr. Surg. 61:795, 1978.

Trier, W. C.: Complete breast absence. Plast. Reconstr. Surg. 36:430, 1965.

Uchida, J.: Clinical application of cross-linked dimethylpolysiloxane; restoration of breast, cheeks, atrophy of infantile paralysis, funnel-shaped chest, etc. Jap. F. Plast. Reconstr. Surg. 4:303, 1961.

Verchère, F.: Mastopéxie latérale contre la mastoptose hypertrophique. Méd. Mod. 9:340, 1898.

Vilain, R.: Modification of the Biesenberger procedure. In Goldwyn, R. M. (ed.): Plastic and Reconstructive Surgery of the Breast. Boston, Little Brown and Co., 1976, pp. 155–163.

Villandre, C.: Cited by Dartigues, L.: Arch. Franco-Belg. Chir. 28:325, 1925.

Vinnik, C. A.: The hazards of silicone injections. J.A.M.A. 236:959, 1976.

Vinnik, C. A.: Spherical contracture of fibrous capsules around breast implants. Prevention and treatment. Plast. Reconstr. Surg. 58:555, 1976.

Vistnes, L. M., Bentley, J. W., and Fogarty, D. C.: Experimental study of tissue response to ruptured gel-filled mammary prostheses. Plast. Reconstr. Surg. 59:31, 1977.

Vistnes, L. M., Ksander, G. A., and Kosek, J.: Effects of local instillation of triamcinolone on the capsules around silicone bag-gel prostheses in animals. Plast. Reconstr. Surg. 62:739, 1978.

Watson, J.: Some observations on free fat grafts, with reference to their use in mammaplasty. Br. J. Plast. Surg. 12:263, 1959.

Webster, J. P.: Mastectomy for gynecomastia through a semicircular intra-areola incision. Ann. Surg. 124:557, 1946.

Weiner, D. L., Aiache, A. E., Silver, L., and Tittiranonda, T.: A single dermal pedicle for nipple transposition in subcutaneous mastectomy, reduction mammaplasty, or mastopexy. Plast. Reconstr. Surg. 51:115, 1973.

Wilflingseder, P., Propst, A., and Mikuz, G.: Constrictive fibrosis following silicone implants in mammary augmentation. Chir. Plast. 2:215, 1974.

Williams, C., Aston, S., and Rees, T. D.: The effect of hematoma on the thickness of pseudosheaths around silicone implants. Plast. Reconstr. Surg. 56:194, 1975.

Williams, J. E.: Experience with a large series of silastic breast implants. Plast. Reconstr. Surg. 49:253, 1972.

Williams, J. E.: Augmentation mammaplasty inframammary approach. *In* Georgiade, N.: Reconstructive Breast Surgery. St. Louis, C. V. Mosby Co., 1976, pp. 50–67.

Wise, R. J.: A preliminary report of a method of planning the mammaplasty. Plast. Reconstr. Surg. *17*:367, 1956.

Wise, R. J., Gannon, J. P., and Hill, J. R.: Further experience with reduction mammaplasty. Plast. Reconstr. Surg. *32*:12, 1963.

Wise, R. J.: Surgical management of the hypertrophic breast. *In* Masters, F. W., and Lewis, J. R. (eds.): Symposium of Aesthetic Surgery of the Face, Eyelid and Breast. St. Louis, C. V. Mosby Co., 1972.

Wise, R. J.: Treatment of breast hypertrophy. Clin. Plas. Surg. *3*:289, 1976.

Wolfe, J. N.: On mammography in the presence of breast implants (Letter to the Editor). Plast. Reconstr. Surg. *62*:286, 1978.

Breast Reconstruction After Mastectomy

Bostwick, J., Vasconez, L. O., and Jurkiewicz, M. J.: Breast reconstruction after a radical mastectomy. Plast. Reconstr. Surg. *61*:682, 1978.

Bostwick, J., et al.: Sixty latissimus dorsi flaps. Plast. Reconstr. Surg. *63*:31, 1979.

Brent, B., and Bostwick, J.: Nipple-areola reconstruction with auricular tissues. Plast. Reconstr. Surg. *60*:353, 1977.

Broadbent, T. R., Metz, P. S., and Woolf, R. M.: Restoring the mammary areola by a skin graft from the upper inner thigh. Br. J. Plast. Surg. *30*:220, 1977.

Cronin, T. D., and Gerow, F.: Augmentation mammaplasty—A new "natural feel" prosthesis. *In* Transactions of the Third International Congress of Plastic Surgeons, pp. 41–49. Amsterdam, Excerpta Medica, 1964.

Freeman, B. S.: Subcutaneous mastectomy for benign breast lesions with immediate or delayed prosthetic replacement. Plast. Reconstr. Surg. *30*:676, 1962.

Gillies, H. O., and Millard, D. R.: The Principles and Art of Plastic Surgery, Vol. 2. Boston, Little, Brown and Co., 1957, p. 429.

Haagensen, C. D.: Diseases of the Breast, 2nd Ed. Philadelphia, W. B. Saunders Company, 1971, p. 449.

Halsted, W. D.: The results of radical operations for the cure of cancer of the breast. Ann. Surg. *46*:1, 1907.

Horton, C. E., et al.: Simple mastectomy with immediate reconstruction. Plast. Reconstr. Surg., *53*:42, 1974.

Identification of breast cancer patients with risk of early recurrence after radical mastectomy. A report of primary therapy breast cancer study group. Cancer *42*:2809, 1978.

Jarrett, J. R., Cutler, R. G., and Teal, D. F.: Subcutaneous mastectomy in small, large or ptotic breasts with immediate submuscular placement of implants. Plast. Reconstr. Surg. *62*:702, 1978.

Reinhard, W.: Total mastoneoplasty following amputation of the breast. Dtsch. Zeitschr. Chir. *236*:309, 1932.

Abdominoplasty

Aston, S. J., and Pickrell, K. L.: Reconstructive surgery of the abdominal wall. *In* Converse, J. M. (ed.): Reconstructive Plastic Surgery, 2nd Ed. Philadelphia, W. B. Saunders Company, 1977, Vol. 7, pp. 3727–3762.

Avelar, J.: Abdominoplasty—Systematization of a technique without external umbilical scar. Aesth. Plast. Surg. *2*:141, 1978.

Babcock, W.: The correction of the obese and relaxed abdominal wall with especial reference to the use of buried silver chain. Phila. Obstet. Society, May 4, 1916.

Babcock, W.: On diseases of women and children. Am. J. Obstet. Gynecol. *74*:596, 1916.

Baker, T. J., Gordon, H. L., and Mosienko, P.: A template (pattern) method of abdominal lipectomy. Aesth. Plast. Surg. *1*:167, 1977.

Baroudi, R., Keppke, E. M., and Netto, F. T.: Abdominoplasty. Annual Meeting of American Society Aesthetic Plastic Surgery, March 11, 1973, California.

Baroudi, R.: Umbilicalplasty. Clin. Plast. Surg. *2*:431, 1975.

Cardoso De Gastro, C., and Daher, M.: Simultaneous reduction mammaplasty and abdominoplasty. Plast. Reconstr. Surg. *61*:36, 1978.

Castanares, S., and Goethel, J. A.: Abdominal lipectomy: a modification in technique. Plast. Reconstr. Surg. *40*:378, 1967.

Desjardin, A.: Lipectomy for extreme obesity. Paris Chir. *3*:466, 1911.

Dufourmentel, C., and Mouly, R.: Chirurgie Plastique. Paris, Flammarion, 1959, pp. 381–389.

Edgerton, M. T., and Knorr, N. J.: Motivational patterns of patients seeking cosmetic (esthetic) surgery. Plast. Reconstr. Surg. *48*:551, 1971.

Elbaz, J. S., and Flageul, G.: Chirurgie plastique de l'abdomen. Paris, Masson, 1971.

Fischl, R. A.: Vertical abdominoplasty. Annual Meeting of the American Society of Plastic and Reconstructive Surgery, October 4, 1971, Canada.

Flesch-Thbesius, J., and Weisheimer, K.: Die operation des Hangebauches. Chirurt. *3*:841, 1931.

Freeman, B. S., and Wiemer, D. R.: Abdominoplasty with special attention to the construction of the umbilicus: technique and complications. Aesth. Plast. Surg. *2*:65, 1978.

Galtier, M.: Obésité de la paroi abdominale. Presse Méd. *70*: 135, 1962.

Galtier, M.: Surgical therapy of obesity of the abdominal wall with ptosis. Mem. Acad. Chir. *81*:341, 1955.

Glicenstein, J.: Difficulties of surgical treatment of abdominal dermodystrophies. Ann. Chir. Plast. *20*:147, 1975.

González-Ulloa, M.: Belt lipectomy. Br. J. Plast. Surg *13*:179, 1960.

González-Ulloa, M.: Circular lipectomy with transposition of the umbilicus and aponeurolytic technique. Circugia, *27*:394, 1959.

Grazer, F. M.: Abdominoplasty. Plast. Reconstr. Surg. *51*:617, 1973.

Grazer, F. M., and Goldwyn, R. M.: Abdominoplasty assessed by survey, with emphasis on complications. Plast. Reconstr. Surg. *59*:513, 1977.

Guilherme da Silveira Carvalho, C., Baroudi, R., and Keppke, E. M.: Anatomical and technical refinements for abdominoplasty. Aesth. Plast. Surg. *1*:217, 1977.

Hinder, U. T.: The dermolipectomy approach for augmentation mammaplasty. Clin. Plast. Surg. *2*:359, 1975.

Jackson, I. T., and Downie, P. A.: Abdominoplasty—the waistline stitch and other refinements. Plast. Reconstr. Surg. *61*:180, 1978.

Jolly, R.: Abdominoplasty. Berl. Klin. Wochenschr. *48*:1317, 1911.

Kamper, M. J., Galloway, D. V., and Ashley, F.: Abdominal panniculectomy after massive weight loss. Plast. Reconstr. Surg. *50*:441, 1972.

Kelly, H. A.: Excision of the fat of the abdominal wall lipectomy. Surg. Gynecol. Obstet. *10*:299, 1910.

Kelly, H. A.: Report of gynecological cases. John Hopkins Med. J. *10*:197, 1899.

Lagache, G., and Vandenbussche, F.: Indications, contre indications et résultats de la technique de Callia dans le traitement des ptoses cutanées abdominales, avec où sans surcharge graisseuse. Ann. Chir. Plast. *16*:37, 1971.

Masson, J. K.: Lipectomy: the surgical removal of excess fat. Postgrad. Med. *32*:481, 1962.

McGraw, L. H.: Surgical rehabilitation after massive weight reduction: case report. Annual Meeting of the American Society of Aesthetic Plastic Surgery, March 12, 1973, California.

Pitanguy, I.: Abdominoplastias. Hospital (Rio de Janeiro) 71(6):1541, 1967.

Pitanguy, I.: Abdominal lipectomy: an approach to it through an analysis of 300 consecutive cases. Plast. Reconstr. Surg. 40:384, 1967.

Pitanguy, I.: Technique for trunk and thigh reductions. In: Transactions of the 5th International Congress of Plastic and Reconstructive Surgery. Melbourne, Butterworths, 1971, pp. 1204–1210.

Pitanguy, I.: Surgical reduction of the abdomen, thighs, and buttocks. Surg. Clin. North Am. 51:479, 1971.

Planas, J.: The "vest over pants abdominoplasty." Plast. Reconstr. Surg. 61:694, 1978.

Psillakis, J. M.: Abdominoplasty: some ideas to improve results. Aesth. Plast. Surg. 2:205, 1978.

Regnault, P.: Abdominal dermolipectomies. Clin. Plast. Surg. 2:411, 1975.

Regnault, P.: Abdominal lipectomy, a low "W" incision. Internal microfilm. Aesth. Plast. Surg. 1972.

Regnault, P.: Abdominoplasty by the "W" technique. Plast. Reconstr. Surg. 55:265, 1975.

Sanders, R. J., DiClementi, D., and Ireland, K.: Principles of abdominal wound closure. Arch. Surg. 112:1188, 1977.

Schepelman, E.: Bauchdeckenplastik mit besonderer Berucksichtigung des Hangebauches. Reitr. Klin. Chir. 3:372, 1918.

Schwartz, A. W.: A technique for excision of abdominal fat. Br. J. Plast. Surg. 27:44, 1974.

Serson, D.: Planeamento geometrico la dero lipectomia abdominal. Rev. Esp. Cir. Plast 4:37, 1971.

Serson, D., and Martins, L. C.: Cermolipectomia abdominal; abordage geometrico. Rev. Lat. Am. Cir. Plast. 16:13, 1972.

Somalo, M.: Circular dermolipectomy of trunk. Sem. Med. 1:1435, 1940.

Somalo, M.: Cruciform ventral dermolipectomy, swallow-shaped incision. Prensa Med. Argent. 33:75, 1946.

Thorek, M.: Plastic Surgery of the Breast and Abdominal Wall. Springfield, Ill., Charles C Thomas, Publisher, 1924.

Thorek, M.: Plastic reconstruction of the female breast and abdomen. Am. J. Surg. 43:268, 1939.

Thorek, P.: Anatomy in Surgery. Philadelphia, J. B. Lippincott Co., 1951, pp. 363–397.

Vernon, S.: Umbilical transplantation upward and abdominal contouring in lipectomy. Am. J. Surg. 94, 1957.

Vilain, R.: Some considerations in surgical alteration of the feminine silhouette. In: Clinics in Plastic Surgery, W. B. Saunders, Philadelphia, 2(3):449, 1975.

Vilain, R., and Dubousset, J.: Technique et indications de la lipectomie circulaire. 150 observations. Ann. Chir. 18:289, 1964.

Weinhold, S.: Bauchdeckenplastik. Zentralbl. F. Gynak. 38:1332, 1909.

Zook, E. G.: Massive weight loss patient. Clin. in Plastic Surgery, W. B. Saunders, Philadelphia, 2(3):457, 1975.

Buttocks and Thighs

Agris, J.: The use of dermal-fat suspension flaps for thigh and buttock lifts. Plast. Reconstr. Surg. 59:817, 1977.

Correa, I. M.: Tratamiento quirurgico de la obesidad. Rev. Med. Argent. 66:340, 1952.

Delerm, A., and Girotteau, Y.: Plastie, Cruro'femoro'fessiere Ou Crcum Fessiere. Ann. Chir. Plast. 18:31, 1973.

Farina, R., Baroudi, R., Golcman, B., and DeCastro, O.: Riding trousers–like type of pelvicrural lipodystrophy (trochanteric lipomatosis). Br. J. Plast: Surg. 13:174, 1961.

Farina, R., Baroudi, R., Golcman, B., and DeCastro, O.: Lipodistrofia pelvo-crurol tipo calcos de montaria (lipomatose trocanterica). Hospital (Rio de Janeiro), 57:717, 1960.

Grazer, F.: The tuck and roll thigh plasty. Presented for Education Courses at the Annual Meeting of the American Society of Plastic and Reconstructive Surgery. Boston, 1976.

Grazer, F.: Classification of thigh, hip and gluteal contour, deformity, classification of hip and thigh plasty. Personal communication, 1979.

Guerrero-Santos, J.: Lipectomies and body sculpture. Presented for Education Courses at the Annual Meeting of the American Society of Plastic and Reconstructive Surgery. Boston, 1976.

Hoffman, S., and Simon, B. E.: Experiences with the Pitanguy method of correction of trochanteric lipodystrophy. Plast. Reconstr. Surg. 55:551, 1975.

Lewis, J. R.: The thigh lift. J. Int. Coll. Surg. 27:330, 1957.

Lewis, J. R.: Correction of ptosis of the thighs: the thigh lift. Plast. Reconstr. Surg. 37:494, 1966.

Lewis, J. R.: Atlas of Aesthetic Plastic Surgery. Boston, Little, Brown and Co., 1973.

Pitanguy, I.: Dermolipectomy of the abdominal wall, thighs, buttocks and upper extremity. In Converse, J. M. (ed.): Reconstructive Plastic Surgery. Philadelphia, W. B. Saunders Company, 1977.

Pitanguy, I.: Technique for trunk and thigh reduction. In Transactions of the Fifth International Congress of Plastic and Reconstructive Surgery. Melbourne, Butterworths, 1971, p. 1204.

Pitanguy, I.: Lipodistrofia trocanterica. Rev. Bras. Cir. 47:69, 1964.

Pitanguy, I.: Surgical reduction of the abdomen, thighs, and buttocks, Surg. Clin. North Am. 51:479, 1971.

Pitanguy, I.: Trochanteric lipodystrophy, Plast. Reconstr. Surg., 34:280, 1964.

Planas, J.: The "Crural meloplasty," for lifting of the thighs, Clinics in Plast. Surg. 2:495, 1975.

Vilain, R.: Surgical correction of steatomeries, Clinics in Plastic Surgery, 2:467, 1975.

Vilain, R.: Some considerations in surgical alteration of the fibrocinial silhouette, Clinics in Plast. Surg. 2:449, 1975.

Vilain, R. C., Dardour, J. C., and Bzowski, A.: Use of Dermal-fat flaps in treating abdominal scars, in abdominoplasty, and in subtrochanteric lipectomy. Plast. Reconstr. Surg. 60:876, 1977.

INDEX